Integrative Dermatology

Integrative Medicine Library

Published and Forthcoming Volumes

SERIES EDITOR

Andrew Weil, MD

Donald I. Abrams and Andrew Weil: *Integrative Oncology*

Timothy Culbert and Karen Olness: *Integrative Pediatrics*

Daniel A. Monti and Bernard D. Beitman: *Integrative Psychiatry*

Victoria Maizes and Tieraona Low Dog: *Integrative Women's Health*

Gerard Mullin: *Integrative Gastroenterology*

Randy Horwitz and Daniel Muller: *Integrative Rheumatology, Allergy, and Immunology*

Stephen DeVries and James Dalen: *Integrative Cardiology*

Robert Norman, Philip Shenefelt, and Reena Rupani: *Integrative Dermatology*

Myles Spar and George Munoz: *Integrative Men's Health*

Robert A. Bonakdar and Andrew W. Sukiennik: *Integrative Pain Management*

Integrative Dermatology

EDITED BY

Robert A. Norman, DO, MPH
Associate Professor
Nova Southeastern University College of Osteopathic Medicine
Associate Professor
University of Central Florida School of Medicine
Integrative Dermatology Lecturer for the AZCIM Fellowship
Tampa, Florida

Philip D. Shenefelt, MD
Professor of Dermatology and Cutaneous Surgery
College of Medicine
University of South Florida
Tampa, Florida

Reena N. Rupani, MD, FAAD
Associate Program Director
Assistant Professor of Dermatology
SUNY Downstate Medical Center
Brooklyn, New York

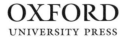
OXFORD
UNIVERSITY PRESS

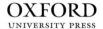

Oxford University Press is a department of the University of Oxford.
It furthers the University's objective of excellence in research, scholarship,
and education by publishing worldwide.

Oxford   New York

Auckland   Cape Town   Dar es Salaam   Hong Kong   Karachi
Kuala Lumpur   Madrid   Melbourne   Mexico City   Nairobi
New Delhi   Shanghai   Taipei   Toronto

With offices in

Argentina   Austria   Brazil   Chile   Czech Republic   France   Greece
Guatemala   Hungary   Italy   Japan   Poland   Portugal   Singapore
South Korea   Switzerland   Thailand   Turkey   Ukraine   Vietnam

Oxford is a registered trademark of Oxford University Press
in the UK and certain other countries.

Published in the United States of America by
Oxford University Press
198 Madison Avenue, New York, NY 10016

Library of Congress Cataloging-in-Publication Data

Integrative dermatology / edited by Robert A. Norman, Philip D. Shenefelt, Reena N. Rupani.
p. ; cm.—(Integrative medicine library)
Includes bibliographical references and index.
ISBN 978-0-19-990792-2 (alk. paper)
I. Norman, Robert A., 1955– editor of compilation.   II. Shenefelt, Philip D., editor of compilation.
III. Rupani, Reena N., editor of compilation.   IV. Series: Weil integrative medicine library.
[DNLM: 1. Skin Diseases—therapy.   2. Complementary Therapies—methods.   3. Integrative Medicine—
methods.   4. Nutrition Therapy—methods. WR 650]
RL71
616.5—dc23   2013033235

This material is not intended to be, and should not be considered, a substitute for medical or other
professional advice. Treatment for the conditions described in this material is highly dependent on the
individual circumstances. And, while this material is designed to offer accurate information with respect
to the subject matter covered and to be current as of the time it was written, research and knowledge about
medical and health issues is constantly evolving and dose schedules for medications are being revised
continually, with new side effects recognized and accounted for regularly. Readers must therefore always
check the product information and clinical procedures with the most up-to-date published product
information and data sheets provided by the manufacturers and the most recent codes of conduct and safety
regulation. The publisher and the authors make no representations or warranties to readers, express or
implied, as to the accuracy or completeness of this material. Without limiting the foregoing, the publisher
and the authors make no representations or warranties as to the accuracy or efficacy of the drug dosages
mentioned in the material. The authors and the publisher do not accept, and expressly disclaim, any
responsibility for any liability, loss or risk that may be claimed or incurred as a consequence of the use and/
or application of any of the contents of this material.

1 3 5 7 9 8 6 4 2
Printed in the United States of America
on acid-free paper

DISCLOSURES

Whitney P. Bowe is a consultant for Johnson & Johnson Consumer Products (Skillman, NJ) and Tria Beauty (Pleasanton, CA). She also holds a provisional patent for the use of bacteriocin-like inhibitory substance (BLIS) for the treatment of acne.

FOREWORD

ANDREW WEIL, MD

Series Editor

Integrative dermatology is such an obvious concept that the paucity of practitioners offering it to patients is disappointing. Nutritional status strongly influences skin health; dietary change and dietary supplements should be first-line interventions in managing skin conditions. The folk medical traditions of the world include many herbal remedies for skin problems; botanical medicine has much to offer dermatology. The skin (along with the gastrointestinal tract) is the most common site of expression of stress-related ailments. I would like to see more dermatologists use or refer patients for mind/body interventions like hypnosis and visualization. (Strong evidence supports the success of mindfulness training and journaling in the treatment of psoriasis.) Whole system approaches such as Ayurvedic and Traditional Chinese Medicine have good track records with atopic dermatitis and other chronic skin disorders.

Presumably, the reason that more dermatologists are not offering patients integrative treatment plans is that conventional medical and specialty training still do not include sufficient information on nutrition and health, botanical medicine, mind/body therapies, whole systems, and other subjects that make up the curriculum of the integrative medicine fellowship offered by the University of Arizona Center for Integrative Medicine. Our Center has now graduated more than 1,000 physicians from this intensive training—men and women from all specialties—but to date, few dermatologists have enrolled.

The editors of this volume have done a great service in assembling a solid roster of experts from a wide range of disciplines to help physicians access evidence-based information essential to the field of integrative dermatology. I hope it will inspire more practitioners to broaden and improve their practice by incorporating the philosophical principles and safe and effective methods of integrative medicine.

Tucson, Arizona
January 2014

PREFACE

Integrative techniques have been employed in dermatology since the earliest recorded healers and patients. As mentioned in our chapter on the history of integrative dermatology, the term is relatively new, but its origins in medicine reach back before the advent of "miracle drugs" and to the earliest use of plants and incantations for healing the skin. Over the last 50 years, integrative approaches to healing employing both conventional and alternative options have gained popularity for patients and physicians alike. As the reader will discover in our history chapter, "Integrative dermatology is as much a philosophy as it is a method; it looks to reverse causal factors rather than just stop symptoms. The truest nature of integrative dermatology is to approach the patient with a more all-encompassing holistic and more diverse worldview than is available or offered in modern Western practice."

As integrative practitioners, we pay great attention to storytelling and approach the patient's medical history with care: What is the essence of the individual, and why does he or she come for treatment at this time? What is the central generative principle behind his or her skin disorder? Correct diagnosis in the individualized context is key to providing a comprehensive treatment and healing strategy. As Dr. Andrew Weil often states, alternative therapies are not meant to replace traditional therapies, but instead should be used in conjunction with them in integrated fashion to achieve the most favorable result. Therefore, we always must ask: Which combination of our many modalities will yield the best results in this given individual (not just in this diagnostic condition)?

One of the key factors in integrative medicine is prevention; from a healthcare perspective, prevention is preferable to cure. An individual who takes steps to prevent a disease avoids both the symptoms and the recovery process. As you discover how to avert or allay early skin conditions for your patients, your family, and yourself, your enthusiasm for integrative methods will grow. As a practitioner of integrative dermatology, you will have the skills to incorporate prevention into each patient encounter.

By incorporating integrative techniques into your dermatology practice, you may also increase your relationships with nontraditional practitioners and broaden the reach and influence of your work. Greater attention to history-taking (via previsit questionnaires, staff support, and motivational interviewing) will elucidate details such as environmental or dietary factors likely to be affecting skin health. A practitioner of functional medicine, then, can help you modify the stream of allergens contributing to an inflammatory response rather than just cooling down the inflammation medically. A nutritionist, similarly, can be a tremendous asset in the team approach to care. As you read through the chapters included here, you can begin to incorporate the healing modalities that make sense to your patients and practice, as well as begin to develop your local referral network for adjunctive care providers.

You can choose the extent of involvement you wish to have in integrative dermatology, and this book aims to provide an extensive introduction to the field. If you wish to be conversationally literate with the subject, there are plenty of facts and wonderful narrative here, written by many of the most knowledgeable providers and researchers in the world of integrative dermatology. You can also use each chapter as a springboard for further research and more extensive practical training, which is available now through many centers for integrative medicine (the flagship program being at the University of Arizona in Tucson).

Enjoy, and thank you for joining us on this path toward holistic healing. We hope our words and pictures greatly benefit you and your patients, and that this text helps expand the philosophical and practical approaches to dermatologic care.

Robert D. Norman, Philip A. Shenefelt, and Reena N. Rupani

ACKNOWLEDGMENTS

Many thanks to Rebecca Suzan, Andrea Seils, and all the editors and assistants at Oxford University Press who have worked and who have guided us to bring this book to fruition. Special thanks to all the contributing writers who took their valuable time to create these fine chapters and help craft each part of this collection into a truly wonderful book. Appreciation goes out to Dr. Andrew Weil for his invitation to edit this book and great respect and admiration for all the work he has done to help grow the field of Integrative Medicine. Much love to our families, teachers, fellow healers, friends, and patients and to all those who love learning and helping others.

Robert A. Norman, DO
Philip D. Shenefelt, MD
Reena N. Rupani, MD, FAAD

CONTENTS

CONTRIBUTORS

Adekemi Akingboye, MD
Department of Dermatology
   State University of New York
   Downstate Medical Center
   Brooklyn, New York

Saba Alaqili, OMSIV
Lake Erie College of Osteopathic
   Medicine
   Bradenton, Florida

Falguni Asrani, MD
Department of Dermatology
   State University of New York
   Downstate Medical Center
   Brooklyn, New York

Hilary Baldwin, MD
Associate Professor of Dermatology
   State University of New York
   Downstate Medical Center
   Brooklyn, New York

Paul Blackcloud, MS, BA
Department of Dermatology
   Columbia University College
   of Physicians & Surgeons
   New York, New York

Whitney P. Bowe, MD
Department of Dermatology
   State University of New York
   Downstate Medical Center
   Brooklyn, New York

Patrick Brennan, OMS IV
Lake Erie College of Osteopathic
   Medicine
   Bradenton, Florida

Katy Burris, MD
Department of Dermatology
   State University of New York
   Downstate Medical Center
   Brooklyn, New York

Daniel C. Butler, BS
Department of Dermatology
   University of Arizona
   College of Medicine
   Tucson, Arizona

Alan M. Dattner, MD
Holistic Dermatology
   New York, New York

Kristopher Denby, MD
Department of Dermatology
University of Rochester
  Medical Center
Rochester, New York

Nana Duffy, MD, MSCE
Genesee Valley Laser Centre
  Rochester, New York

Jaimie B. Glick, MD
Department of Dermatology
  State University of New York
  Downstate Medical Center
  Brooklyn, New York

Andrea M. Hui, MD
Department of Dermatology
  State University of New York
  Downstate Medical Center
  Brooklyn, New York

Jeanette Jacknin, MD
Private Practice
  Scottsdale, Arizona

Rebecca F. Jacobson, MST
Department of Dermatology
  Brown University
  Providence, Rhode Island

Vasant Lad, BAMS, MASc
The Ayurvedic Institute
  Albuquerque, New Mexico

Shoshana Landow, MD
Clinical Assistant Professor of
  Dermatology Brown University
  Providence, Rhode Island

Kachiu C. Lee, MD, MPH
Department of Dermatology
  Brown University
  Providence, Rhode Island

Peter A. Lio, MD
Assistant Professor of Clinical
  Dermatology & Pediatrics
  Northwestern University Feinberg
  School of Medicine
  Chicago, Illinois

Raman Madan, MD
Drexel University College of Medicine
  Philadelphia, Pennsylvania

Niandra Reid, MD, MBA
Department of Dermatology
  Brown University
  Providence, Rhode Island

Leslie Robinson-Bostom, MD
Professor of Dermatology
  Brown University
  Providence, Rhode Island

Nicole E. Rogers, MD, FAAD
Assistant Clinical Professor of
  Dermatology Tulane University
  School of Medicine
  New Orleans, Louisiana

Joseph Salhab, OMSIV
Lake Erie College of Osteopathic
  Medicine
  Bradenton, Florida

Daniel M. Siegel, MD, MS
Clinical Professor of Dermatology
State University of New York
Downstate Medical Center
Brooklyn, New York

Francisco Tausk, MD
Professor of Dermatology and
Psychiatry University of
Rochester School of Medicine
Rochester, New York

Mary Teeple, MD
Department of Dermatology
Brown University
Providence, Rhode Island

Erin N. Wilmer, BS
Department of Community Health
and Family Medicine University
of Florida College of Medicine
Gainesville, Florida

Integrative Dermatology

1

Diet for Healthy, Youthful Skin

JEANETTE JACKNIN, MD

Key Concepts

♣ The healthy skin diet incorporates a low-glycemic, anti-inflammatory, Mediterranean-style diet rich in fruits, vegetables, low-glycemic whole grains, legumes, monounsaturated fats such as olive oil, and a fatty acid ratio higher in omega-3 than in omega-6 fatty acids.

♣ The healthy skin diet also must be rich in antioxidants, which help reduce the chronic inflammation that is associated with aging of the skin and the development of wrinkles, sagging, and discoloration.

♣ Dietary choices are an important part of the patient's environment and influence which genes are turned on and which genes are turned off. A high-glycemic diet can lead in susceptible individuals to insulin resistance and pro-inflammatory changes, while a low-glycemic diet can help to reduce or avoid insulin resistance and be generally anti-inflammatory.

♣ The healthy skin diet includes whole unprocessed foods rich in low-glycemic whole grains, legumes, fruits, vegetables, and lean protein along with adequate hydration. Organic and, where possible, locally grown products are preferred. Avoid sugar, excess alcohol, and excess caffeine, and consider instead in moderation red wine, tea, and high-cocoa-content dark chocolate.

♣ Herbs and spices such as oregano, parsley, turmeric, ginger, garlic, chili peppers, cinnamon, rosemary, thyme, and others contain antioxidants and anti-inflammatory agents and are recommended for the healthy skin diet.

Introduction

As an integrative health practitioner, one of the first things to emphasize with patients is that a nourishing diet is one of the crucial building blocks of the skin's good health and appearance. A diet that is healthy for the whole body will reflect quickly in youthful, less-aged skin. In this chapter, we will look at what a healthy diet really consists of in terms of the overall proportion of carbohydrates, fats, and proteins, and the nourishing foods and spices that help protect and preserve your patients' skin. The importance of drinking enough pure water every day cannot be stressed enough. We also will look at certain foods and spices that can be very helpful for specific diseases that affect the skin. Supplements to recommend to your patients will be discussed in the next chapter.

Diet

The healthy skin diet recommended below incorporates the tenets of the Mediterranean, anti-inflammatory, and low-glycemic diets. The Mediterranean diet is based upon fruits, vegetables, whole grains, legumes, monounsaturated fats like those found in olive oil, and a healthy ratio of omega-3 to omega-6 polyunsaturated fatty acids. It has been linked with improved longevity and better cardiovascular, cognitive, and metabolic health (Galland, 2010; Kastorini et al., 2011), as well as a decreased incidence of cancer (Caperle et al., 996).

The Mediterranean diet is also beneficial for the skin, as its anti-inflammatory effect is due in part to its emphasis on extra-virgin olive oil, which is high in compounds that modulate oxidative stress and quell inflammatory reactions. Oleocanthal, one of the components of olive oil, has been recently been shown to possess anti-inflammatory actions similar to ibuprofen (Galland, 2010; Lucas et al., 2011). In one hospital-based study in Italy, researchers compared medical history, sun exposure habits, and dietary patterns from over 300 controls to over 300 patients with cutaneous melanoma. Carefully controlling for sun exposure and pigmentary characteristics, shellfish, fish rich in omega-3 fatty acids, regular tea drinking, and greater consumption of fruits and vegetables (in particular carrots, cruciferous and leafy vegetables, and citrus fruits) were associated with protection from cutaneous melanoma (Fortes et al., 2008). Thus, it has been suggested that a nutritional approach to sun protection using the Mediterranean diet would be a useful complement to externally applied sun protection strategies (Shapira, 2010).

To maintain healthy skin, one's diet must be rich in antioxidants, which are also anti-inflammatory. Free radical damage has been shown to be an important factor in the aging process and in the development of cancer. Chronic inflammation has been discovered to be the root cause of many diseases, including heart disease, cancer, and Alzheimer's disease. It is also thought to be the root cause of wrinkles and aging skin with sagging, discoloration, enlarged pores, and lack of radiance. When applied topically, antioxidants have also been shown to provide powerful anti-inflammatory, photoprotective, and anti-aging skin benefits (Camouse et al., 2009; Graf et al., 2010; Haftek et al., 2008; Kerscher et al., 2011; Kohen et al., 2009; Oresajo et al., 2008, 2010; Puizina-Ivic et al., 2010; Yuan et al., 2011). Dietary choices significantly influence the extent of inflammation, so it needs to be emphasized to patients that they do have a lot of control over their skin's health and appearance. The diet recommended below for healthy, youthful skin incorporates the principles of the anti-inflammatory diet, which has become popular in the past 10 years.

The suggested diet also incorporates the principles of a low-glycemic approach as well as the ideas of nutrigenomics and gene expression. This is a new science that studies the effects of foods and food constituents on gene expression. It is about how our environment, including our food choices, affects activation or deactivation of specific portions of our DNA, which is transcribed into mRNA and then to proteins. It provides a basis for understanding the biological activity and effects of foods and food components.

Following a low-glycemic diet is also an important key to good health as well as clear skin. This is a diet that is low in refined carbohydrates and processed foods and high in vegetable produce and lean protein, helping to keep blood sugar levels stable. A high-glycemic diet can lead to insulin resistance, where the body needs to produce ever-increasing amounts of the hormone insulin to clear glucose from the blood. Based on the accelerated rate of aging seen in diabetics, chronic glucose exposure has long been known to affect how the body ages by a process called glycation (van Boekel et al., 1991). Insulin resistance has been linked to high blood pressure, diabetes, and heart disease, and there is evidence that it also leads to acne and more skin inflammation and aging. It has been shown that insulin resistance and inflammation disrupt sebum production, cause collagen malformation, and excite epidermal growth factor receptors, which are involved in skin tissue renewal. Insulin resistance can also stimulate inflammatory reactions in skin cells (Cosgrove et al., 2007; Epstein et al., 2010; Nagata et al., 2010; Piccardi & Manissier, 2009). In the human body, once sugars enter the circulation they attach themselves to the amino groups of tissue proteins such as collagen to slowly rearrange their youthful structure into the main culprits of damage, called advanced glycation end products (AGEs). AGE molecules are particularly destructive since they can undergo extensive cross-linking with other proteins, causing once-healthy collagen fibers to lose their elasticity, becoming rigid, more brittle, and prone to breakage (Danby, 2010; Pageon & Asselineau, 2005; Pageon et al., 2008).

Glycation occurs naturally in all tissues of the body but is accelerated by a high-sugar diet and, within the skin, by excessive sun exposure (Avery, 2006; Danby, 2010; Pageon, 2010).

Not surprisingly, collagen abnormalities in aging and diabetes share similar roots, and both cause thinning, discoloration, and loss of elasticity of the skin, with a tendency to rashes and infections. Laboratory research shows that once formed, AGEs can then be self-perpetuating, directly inducing the cross-linking of collagen even in the absence of glucose (Sajithlal et al., 1998). Glycation also induces fibroblast apoptosis (cell death), which in turn switches fibroblasts from a matrix-producing to a matrix-degrading state (Alikhani et al., 2005). In this state, the secretion of collagen-degrading enzymes, called matrix metalloproteinases (MMPs), increases and levels of their inhibitors decline. In fact, glycation directly increases the release of MMP-1, which preferentially breaks down collagen (Pageon et al., 2007). The North American diet contains excessive amounts of simple carbohydrates and saturated fats, which has been shown numerous times to correlate with an increased appearance of skin wrinkles (Cosgrove et al., 2007; Epstein et al., 2010; Nagata et al., 2010; Piccardi & Manissier, 2009). Epidemiologic data also suggest that a high-glycemic diet may contribute to inflammatory skin conditions such as acne, rosacea, psoriasis, and eczema (Cosgrove et al., 2007; Smith et al., 2008; Veith & Silverberg, 2011).

The glycemic index (GI) was introduced in 1981 by nutritionist Dr. David Jenkins to determine which carbohydrate foods were best suited to a diabetic diet. The GI ranking is a measure of how a food affects blood sugar levels. The faster a food breaks down into simple sugars during digestion, the higher the GI. Navigating the GI is not difficult. It is simply a scale based on glucose, which is rated at 100. The lower the GI of the food, the less it will trigger the release of insulin. Other factors, such as when one last ate and what else one is eating at the time, can alter the insulin impact. As a general guide, though, Boxes 1.1, 1.2, and 1.3 give some examples of high-, medium-, and low-glycemic foods (Saran, 2008).

Poor dietary habits and dietary nutrient deficiencies increase a person's susceptibility to skin disorders. This is largely due to the fact that skin-cell turnover time is so short. Skin cells are produced, die, and are replaced by new cells every few weeks. The condition of the skin is therefore a good mirror of a person's overall nutritional status. Also, many vitamins and minerals in a healthy diet help to maintain good circulation to the skin, increase the skin-cell levels of nutrients and oxygen, and remove the waste materials. A poor diet and crash diets can lead to brittle nails and hair loss as well.

Also important is the concept of multiple marginal nutrient deficiencies. This means there are minor deficiencies in several nutrients, which together

Box 1.1 High-Glycemic Foods (71–100+ on the scale)

- Tofu frozen dessert 115
- Dates 103
- French bread 95
- Crisped rice cereal 88
- Baked potato 85
- Cornflakes cereal 84
- Pretzels 81
- Jellybeans 80
- Donut 76
- French fries 76
- Frozen waffle 76
- Graham crackers 74
- Corn chips 73
- Mashed potatoes 73
- Bagel 72
- Watermelon 72
- Carrots 71

render the body less effective at fighting off disease and cancer. In this country, with the typical American diet, multiple marginal nutrient deficiencies are very common—much more so than deficiencies of single nutrients. These marginal nutrient deficiencies are very important, as they can lead to or cause flare-ups in infectious disease, carcinogenesis, and reduced immunity. They also make the skin look aged and unhealthy. Nutritional deficiencies are even more common in older adults, whose recommended daily intake of vitamins is actually higher than that of younger people, but whose diets tend to be poorer.

Box 1.2 Medium-Glycemic Foods (55–70 on the scale)

- White bread 70
- Instant oatmeal 66
- Table sugar 65
- Raisins 64
- Ice cream 61
- Granola bar 61
- Blueberry muffin 59
- White rice 56
- Brown rice 55

Box 1.3 Low-Glycemic Foods (less than 55 on the scale)

- Sweet potato 54
- Long-grain rice 47
- Heavy, mixed-grain bread 30–45
- Fettuccini 32
- Fat-free milk 32
- Peach 28
- Lentils 28
- Plum 24
- Cherries 22
- Soybeans 18
- Tomatoes 15
- Broccoli 15
- Asparagus 15
- Cucumber 15

Thus, the healthy skin diet incorporates the features of the Mediterranean, anti-inflammatory, and low-glycemic diets, all of which have been studied by numerous researchers and found to significantly improve the appearance and health of the skin.

A Healthy Preventive Diet

In general, a balanced diet of whole, unprocessed foods that is rich in whole grains, legumes, fruits, vegetables, and lean protein will provide the necessary nutrients for healthy skin, hair, and nails. Forty percent to 50% of calories should be from carbohydrates, 30% from fat, and 20% to 30% from protein (Weil, 2012). Figure 1.1 shows Dr. Andrew Weil's recommended anti-inflammatory diet in easy-to-understand pyramid form (Weil, 2012). This is in keeping with the antiglycemic, Mediterranean diet that is recommended here for optimal skin health.

- Include carbohydrates, fat, and protein at each meal as much as possible.
- Eat smaller, more frequent meals: four to six a day.
- Choose fruits and vegetables from all parts of the color spectrum, especially berries, tomatoes, orange and yellow fruits, soy, cabbage, and dark leafy greens. To get maximum natural protection against

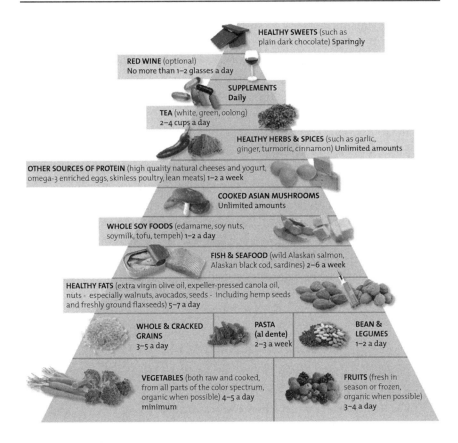

FIGURE 1.1 The Anti-Inflammatory Diet Pyramid

age-related diseases, including the appearance of wrinkles and aging, as well as to reduce repeated exposure to food toxins, your patients should eat a wide variety of fruits, vegetables, and mushrooms.

- Choose organic produce whenever possible and avoid or soak off pesticide residues.
- Choose locally grown products whenever possible.
- Avoid foods containing additives, preservatives, aspartame (NutraSweet), caffeine, and refined sugar as much as possible. Avoid highly processed foods, which have high levels of additives but relatively little nutritive value and may contain concentrated toxins. Alcohol, caffeine, sugar, and fried foods, which are sources of harmful free radicals, should be avoided as much as possible. I know this is a big change from the typical American diet and can be a difficult change for your patients to completely effect, but it is definitely worth the effort.

- Have your patients try to switch to tea instead of coffee, or at least limit their intake of coffee to one cup a day. Good-quality white, black, green, and oolong teas are good sources of antioxidants, in contrast to coffee, which has a lot of acid that can increase insulin production and inflammation, and ultimately cause wrinkling.
- If your patients drink alcohol, suggest red wine with its anti-inflammatory resveratrol.
- Suggest plain dark chocolate in moderation, preferably with a minimum cocoa content of 70%. Of course your patients should limit their intake of candy and carbonated soft drinks as much as possible.
- Have your patients avoid eating burned foods, especially meats; burning leads to increased formation of carcinogenic compounds.
- Nondairy sources of calcium include sardines, greens, broccoli, and various sea vegetables, such as nori, dulse, and kombu. In addition, tofu, sesame seeds, calcium-fortified orange juice, and fortified soy milk can be good calcium sources (Weil, 2012).

PROPER HYDRATION WITH PURE WATER

- Drink six to eight cups of pure or sparkling water with or without lemon throughout the day.
- Use bottled water or get a home water purifier.

It takes at least six to eight cups of pure water each day to keep the skin and body well hydrated. Good hydration is necessary for the skin to feel and look smooth. Hair looks and feels brittle and dry if one is not drinking enough water. Also, dehydration is often mistaken for hunger, and people may be tempted to overeat if they don't realize that it is really water that their body craves. The source of the water should be pure and filtered. Patients need to be educated to the fact that drinks containing caffeine are actually diuretics. As a substitute for soft drinks that are filled with sugar, artificial sweeteners, preservatives, and artificial flavorings and colorings, they can enjoy naturally carbonated water such as Perrier™ water or club soda flavored with lemon.

CARBOHYDRATES

Carbohydrates in the form of starchy vegetables and grains have a high GI, whereas unrefined grains and vegetables with a low GI release glucose into the bloodstream more slowly and therefore will not as readily cause rapid spikes in the body's glucose and insulin levels after meals. Ceramides make up the lipid-rich protective layer in the epidermis, but their concentration decreases with age. One can get more ceramides through foods such as rice bran, wheat flour, and wheat germ oil. Because they play an important role in preventing dehydration in the skin, oral plant-based ceramides may help to combat skin dryness and breakdown associated with aging (Bak et al., 2011; Cho et al., 2011; Jennemann et al., 2011). In a randomized trial, 51 women with dry skin were given either 350 mg of a wheat extract containing ceramides or placebo for three months. A significant increase in skin hydration and an improvement in the clinical signs of dryness were observed at the end of three months in those eating the wheat extract containing ceramides (Guillou et al., 2011).

- **Fruits:** Recommend three or four servings per day (one serving is equal to one medium-sized piece of fruit, a half-cup of chopped fruit, or a quarter-cup of dried fruit). Fruits are rich in flavonoids and carotenoids, which have both antioxidant and anti-inflammatory activity. Resveratrol derived from the skin of grapes and other fruits is especially important. Although data on this substance are mixed, resveratrol has been shown to have cancer chemopreventive activity in assays representing the three major stages of carcinogenesis, and it inhibits tumorigenesis in the mouse skin cancer model (Athar et al., 2007; Jang et al., 1997). Berries, peaches, nectarines, oranges, pink grapefruit, red grapes, plums, pomegranates, cherries, apples, and pears are all lower in glycemic load than most tropical fruits.
- **Vegetables:** Recommend four or five servings per day (one serving equals two cups of salad greens or a half-cup of vegetables). Lightly cooked dark leafy greens (spinach, collard greens, kale, Swiss chard), cruciferous vegetables (broccoli, cabbage, Brussels sprouts, kale, bok choy, cauliflower), carrots, beets, onions, peas, squashes, sea vegetables, and washed raw salad greens are all good. Vegetables are also rich in flavonoids and carotenoids with both antioxidant and anti-inflammatory activity. Tomatoes and tomato paste are a great dietary source of lycopene. It was shown that it was possible to protect against UV light-induced erythema by 40% after eating 40 grams of tomato paste a day for 10 weeks (Stahl et al., 2007). Ellagic acid is another polyphenol found abundantly in various fruits, nuts, and vegetables. It has also been shown to inhibit chemically induced cancer in the skin of rodents.
- **Cooked Asian mushrooms:** Encourage your patients to enjoy unlimited amounts of shiitake, enokidake, maitake, and oyster mushrooms. They contain compounds that enhance immune function. One should never eat raw mushrooms, and avoid the non-nutritious button and Portobello varieties.

- **Beans and legumes:** Recommend one or two servings per day (one serving is equal to a half-cup of cooked beans or legumes). Anasazi, adzuki, and black beans as well as chickpeas, black-eyed peas, and lentils are all very healthy. Beans are a great low-glycemic-load food.
- **Whole and cracked grains:** Recommend three to five servings a day (one serving is equal to a half-cup of cooked grains). Brown rice, basmati rice, wild rice, buckwheat, groats, barley, quinoa, and steel-cut oats are great. "Whole grains" means grains that are intact or in a few large pieces, not whole-wheat bread or other products made from whole-wheat flour. Whole grains digest slowly, lowering the frequency of spikes in blood sugar that promote inflammation.
- **Pasta (al dente):** Recommend two or three servings per week (one serving is equal to a half-cup of cooked pasta). Organic pasta, rice noodles, bean thread noodles, and part whole-wheat and buckwheat noodles like Japanese udon and soba are all considered "good" pasta. Note that pasta cooked al dente has a lower GI than fully cooked pasta.
- Eat unrefined grains and vegetables that are high in complex carbohydrates.
- "Good" carbs include apples, beans, winter squashes, sweet potatoes, and oatmeal.
- Eat whole grains such as basmati and brown rice and bulgur wheat, in which the grain is intact or in a few large pieces; they release glucose at a slow rate, especially when eaten with other foods. These are more desirable than whole-wheat flour products, which have about the same GI as white flour products.
- Avoid foods made with wheat flour and sugar, especially bread and packaged snack foods, including chips and pretzels.
- Avoid products made with high-fructose corn syrup, which is most of our "junk" food.
- Healthy sweets—suggest unsweetened dried fruit, dark chocolate, and fruit sorbet. Dark chocolate with at least 70% pure cocoa provides antioxidant activity together with a satisfying taste.
- Alcohol: If your patients want to drink alcohol, organic red wine, one or two glasses a day, with its high antioxidant activity is the healthiest of the choices.

FATS

Fats and oils are more concentrated sources of energy than carbohydrates, but these need to be converted into glucose to be used by the body. Some fat is essential, but one needs the right balance and type of fat. Within the skin, fatty acids are an integral component of cell membranes. Not enough fat actually causes skin inflammation, susceptibility to skin infection, and hair loss. The cutaneous effects of a diet deficient in essential fatty acids are hyperdesquamation, causing a characteristic scaly skin disorder; increased transepidermal water loss; and altered lipid profiles; these are all also characteristics of inflammatory dermatoses (Bibel et al., 1989; Ziboh et al., 2000). Because fatty acids are antimicrobial, the stratum corneum in mice that were fed diets deficient in essential fatty acids supported 100-fold more bacteria than mice fed a healthy diet, and the mice with the deficient diet were the only group from which *Staphylococcus aureus* was routinely isolated (Bibel et al., 1989). Clinical studies show that the healthy balance of fatty acids in skin dramatically decreases with aging and increased oxidative stress, such as that caused by chronic sun exposure. Therefore, getting the correct amount and type of fats through diet or supplementation is critical to maintaining healthy skin as one ages. Omega-3 fatty acids help to keep normal skin healthy by maintaining its natural oil barrier and making it look younger, less wrinkled, and clearer. Traditional and non-Westernized diets offer a healthier balance of omega-6 to omega-3 fatty acids, typically at a ratio of about 4:1 (Simopoulos et al., 2011; Taylor et al., 2011). The current North American diet unfortunately provides a ratio of about 15:1 of omega-6 fatty acids to omega-3 fatty acids (Simopoulos, 2011; Wertz et al., 2010). Omega-6 fat is found in relatively high amounts in egg yolks, poultry skin, and organ meats from animals fed corn-based diets. It contains arachidonic acid, which has an inflammatory effect on the body and skin. Alternatively, fish oil rich in the omega-3 oils eicosapentaenoic and docosahexaenoic acids (EPA and DHA) inhibits the formation of inflammatory molecules and generates anti-inflammatory and antiproliferative metabolites (Ziboh et al., 2000). It has also been shown that extra-virgin olive oils, a key feature of the Mediterranean diet, are very rich in phenolic antioxidants, squalene, and oleic acid, which help to protect against skin cancer and aging by inhibiting oxidative stress (Owen et al., 2000). With this ability to modulate inflammation, omega-3 fatty acids are also effective in the management of inflammatory skin conditions, such as acne, psoriasis, eczema, and rosacea (Koku et al., 2011; Taylor et al., 2011).

Up to 30% of calories a day can come from fats, as long as most of that amount is from monounsaturated oils such as olive oil and foods high in omega-3 fatty acids: oily fishes (salmon, sardines, mackerel), flax seeds, and some nuts (Weil, 2005).

- Recommend five to seven servings per day of omega-3 fatty acids (one serving is equal to one teaspoon of oil, two walnuts, one tablespoon of flaxseed, or one ounce of avocado).

- Use extra-virgin olive oil or expeller-pressed organic canola oil for cooking oil.
- Organic, expeller-pressed, high-oleic sunflower or safflower, walnut, and hazelnut oils can all be used in salads.
- Eat salmon (preferably fresh or frozen wild or canned sockeye), sardines packed in water or olive oil, herring, black cod, sablefish, or butterfish; omega-3–fortified eggs; hemp seeds and flaxseeds; and whole soy products, all high in omega-3 fatty acids.
- Eat avocados and nuts, especially walnuts, cashews, almonds, and nut butters made from these nuts. They are all high in omega-3 fatty acids.
- Avoid margarine, vegetable shortening, and all products made with partially hydrogenated oils of any kind.
- Avoid eating plain safflower, sunflower, corn, cottonseed, and mixed vegetable oils.
- Avoid butter, cream, high-fat cheese, unskinned chicken, fatty meats, and products made with palm kernel oil, which are all high in saturated fat.

PROTEIN

We need proteins to build, maintain, and repair the body, but they can also be converted to glucose and serve as an energy source when needed. Proteins are built from 20 different amino acids, 10 of which must be regularly supplied by foods in our diet because our body cannot produce them itself.

- Protein should constitute about 20% to 30% of one's diet, and vegetable proteins from beans and soybeans should be substituted for animal ones as often as possible. Grilled salmon, tuna, and other fish, low-fat natural cheese and yogurt, omega-3–enriched egg whites, skinless poultry, and grass-fed lean meats are also good choices.
- On a 2,000-calorie-a-day diet, daily intake of protein should be between 80 and 120 grams.
- Whole soy foods: Recommend at least one or two servings per day (one serving is equal to a half-cup of tofu or tempeh, one cup of soymilk, a half-cup cooked edamame, or one ounce of soynuts). Recent research has confirmed the antioxidant and DNA-protective effects of soy isoflavones on the skin. It is the protective effect of genistein in soy that is believed to block UV-induced cellular damage (Accorsi-Neto et al., 2009). In addition to the photoprotective benefits, soy protein peptides stimulate collagen and hyaluronic acid production within the dermis in vitro (Sudel et al., 2005). Since they exert weak estrogenic activity, soy isoflavones may also help to delay accelerated skin aging

due to hormonal decline in postmenopausal women (Accorsi-Neto et al., 2007; Izumi et al., 2007). To assess the effect of soy isoflavones on skin aging, 30 postmenopausal women were given 100 mg/day of an isoflavone-rich soy extract for 6 months. At the end of this time, researchers observed that over 86% of the women experienced significant increases in skin thickness, collagen and elastin fibers, and microcapillary density (Accorsi-Neto et al., 2009). In another trial, skin benefits were observed when 40 mg soy isoflavones were taken daily for 12 weeks (Izumi et al., 2007).

- Fish and seafood: At least two to six servings, four ounces each, are recommended per week. Wild Alaskan salmon, especially sockeye, herring, sardines, black cod, and sablefish are best, as they are rich in omega-3 fats, which are strongly anti-inflammatory.
- If your patients eat chicken, suggest they choose organic, cage-free skinned chicken.
- If they eat eggs, choose omega-3–enriched eggs or organic eggs from free-range chickens.
- If they are lactose tolerant and eat dairy, have them use organic, reduced-fat products, especially low-fat yogurt or low-fat Swiss, Jarlsberg, or Parmesan cheese.
- If they have lactose intolerance or are allergic to milk protein (as do many of Asian and African-American descent), have them avoid cow milk, cheese, and other dairy products as much as possible.

FIBER

- Recommend to your patients that they eat at least 40 grams of fiber a day. They can do this by increasing the amount of fruit (especially berries), beans, vegetables, and whole grains they consume.
- Eating some form of fiber with every meal is ideal, as this speeds the passage of toxins through the intestinal tract.
- Ready-made cereals that provide 4 to 5 grams of bran per one-ounce serving should be chosen.

TEA

- Drinking two to four cups per day of white, green, or oolong teas is healthy and is thought to be much better for one's skin than coffee. Tea is rich in catechins, inflammation-reducing antioxidant compounds. Green tea also exhibits antimutagenic activity in vitro and inhibits carcinogen-induced skin tumors in rodents.

The most active anticarcinogenic component of green tea is (-)-epigallocatechin-3-gallate (EGCG), the major constituent in the green tea polyphenols fraction (Stoner & Mukhtar, 1995). In vitro and in vivo animal and human studies suggest that green tea polyphenols are photoprotective in nature and can be used as pharmacological agents for the prevention of solar UVB light-induced skin disorders, including photoaging, melanoma, and nonmelanoma skin cancers (Baliga & Katiyar, 2006; Katiyar, 2003; Nichols & Katiyar, 2010).

HEALTHY HERBS AND SPICES

Herbs and spices are an overlooked but very important part of most people's diets. Some of them are extremely powerful antioxidants and anti-aging powerhouses. In 2001 the USDA/Tufts team published their research on the free radical quenching activity or oxygen radical absorbance capacity (ORAC) score of 27 culinary herbs. They found oregano to be the most potent, followed by bay leaf, dill, winter savory, coriander, orange mint, thyme, rosemary, basil, sage, and parsley. Unlimited amounts of turmeric, curry powder containing turmeric, ginger, garlic, chili peppers, basil, cinnamon, rosemary, and thyme are recommended. Turmeric, ginger, and garlic are especially powerful anti-inflammatory agents that improve the look and clarity of the skin. Topical application of curcumin, the yellow pigment in turmeric and curry, strongly inhibits tumor production in mouse skin (Huang et al., 1988) and markedly inhibits arachidonic acid-induced epidermal inflammation (ear edema) in mice (Huang et al., 1991; Stoner & Mukhtar, 1995). It has also been observed that there is an inverse relationship between consumption of Mediterranean herbs such as rosemary, sage, parsley, and oregano and certain types of cancer. One component extracted from the leaves of rosemary, carnosol, has been evaluated for anticancer properties in skin cancer and other cancers with promising results. Studies have provided evidence that carnosol targets multiple deregulated pathways associated with inflammation and cancer, and more preclinical studies with carnosol as a cancer chemoprevention and anticancer agent are being done (Johnson, 2011).

Dr. Nicholas Perricone (2004) introduced what he considers to be the most important groups of "superfoods" to help reduce inflammation and rejuvenate the body and skin. They are (1) acai; (2) allium vegetables such as onions and garlic; (3) barley; (4) buckwheat; (5) green food such as wheat grass and algae; (6) beans and lentils; (7) hot chili peppers; (8) nuts and seeds; (9) yogurt and kefir; (10) sprouts; and (11) maitake mushrooms. He also talks in depth about his other favorites: salmon, blueberries, chia seeds, watercress, and organic coconut oil. In addition he talks about the exciting new field of nutrigenomics, a combination of nutrition and genomics. By eating many of the foods included in an anti-inflammatory diet, our protective genes can be switched on and genes that can have a negative effect on our health are switched off (Perricone, 2010). Molecular tags attach directly to the DNA or to the proteins surrounding the DNA, the histones. These molecular tags can be semipermanent and even passed on to the next generation. This means that we can change the way our genes and our children's genes are expressed by eating healthy foods and nutrients. Foods that have significant effects on gene expression include tea, cocoa, blueberries, and watercress (Perricone, 2010).

Conclusion

What we eat helps to determine the health and appearance of our body and our skin. This chapter details the anti-inflammatory, antiglycemic, whole-food diet that has been shown in numerous studies to positively affect the well-being and youthfulness of our skin.

REFERENCES

Accorsi-Neto, A., Haidar, M., Simões, R., et al. (2009). Effects of isoflavones on the skin of postmenopausal women: a pilot study. *Clinics (Sao Paulo), 64*(6), 505–510.

Alikhani, Z., Alikhani, M., Boyd, C.M., et al. (2005). Advanced glycation end products enhance expression of pro-apoptotic genes and stimulate fibroblast apoptosis through cytoplasmic and mitochondrial pathways. *Journal of Biological Chemistry, 280*(13), 12087–12095.

Athar, M., Back, J. H., Tang, X., et al. (2007). Resveratrol: a review of preclinical studies for human cancer prevention. *Toxicology & Applied Pharmacology, 224*(3), 274–283.

Avery, A. (2006). Organic diets and children's health. *Environmental Health Perspectives, 114*(4), A210–A211.

Bak, J. F., Møller, N., Schmitz, O., et al. (1992). In vivo insulin action and muscle glycogen synthase activity in type 2 (non-insulin-dependent) diabetes mellitus: effects of diet treatment. *Diabetologia, 35*(8), 777–784.

Baliga, M. S., & Katiyar, S. K. (2006). Chemoprevention of photocarcinogenesis by selected dietary botanicals. *Photochemical & Photobiological Sciences, 5*(2), 243–253.

Bhattacharyya, T. K., Jackson, P., Patel, M. K., et al. (2012). Epidermal cell proliferation in calorie-restricted aging rats. *Current Aging Science, 5*(2), 96–104.

Bibel, D. J., Miller, S. J., Brown, B. E., et al. (1989). Antimicrobial activity of stratum corneum lipids from normal and essential fatty acid-deficient mice. *Journal of Investigative Dermatology, 92*(4), 632–638.

Caperle, M., Maiani, G., Azzini, E., et al. (1996). Dietary profiles and anti-oxidants in a rural population of central Italy with a low frequency of cancer. *European Journal of Cancer Prevention, 5*(3), 197–206.

Cho, H. J., Chung, B. Y., Lee, H. B., et al. (2011). Quantitative study of stratum corneum ceramides contents in patients with sensitive skin. *Journal of Dermatology.* doi: 10.1111/j.1346-8138.2011.01406.x.

Cosgrove, M. C., Franco, O. H., Granger, S. P., et al. (2007). Dietary nutrient intakes and skin-aging appearance among middle-aged American women. *American Journal of Clinical Nutrition, 86*(4), 1225–1231. Erratum in *American Journal of Clinical Nutrition* 2008;88(2):480.

Danby, F. W. (2010). Nutrition and aging skin: sugar and glycation. *Clinical Dermatology, 28*(4), 409–411.

Epstein, H. A. (2010). Food for thought and skin. *Skinmed, 8*(1), 50–51.

Fortes, C., Mastroeni, S., Melchi, F., et al. (2008). A protective effect of the Mediterranean diet for cutaneous melanoma. *International Journal of Epidemiology, 37*(5), 1018–1029.

Galland, L. (2010). Diet and inflammation. *Nutrition in Clinical Practice, 25*(6), 634–640.

Guillou, S., Ghabri, S., Jannot, C., et al. (2011). The moisturizing effect of a wheat extract food supplement on women's skin: a randomized, double-blind placebo-controlled trial. *International Journal of Cosmetic Science, 33*(2), 138–143. doi: 10.1111/j.1468-2494.2010.00600.x.

Huang, M. T., Lysz, T., Ferraro, T., Abidi, T. F., et al. (1991). Inhibitory effects of curcumin on in vitro lipoxygenase and cyclooxygenase activities in mouse epidermis. *Cancer Research, 51*(3), 813–819.

Izumi, T., Saito, M., Obata, A., Arii, M., et al. (2007). Oral intake of soy isoflavone aglycone improves the aged skin of adult women. *Journal of Nutrition Science & Vitaminology, 53*(1), 57–62.

Jacknin, J. (2001). *Smart medicine for your skin.* New York, NY: Penguin Putnam.

Jang, M., Cai, L., Udeani, G. O., et al. (1997). Cancer chemopreventive activity of resveratrol, a natural product derived from grapes. *Science, 275*(5297), 218–220.

Jennemann, R., Rabionet, M., Gorgas, K., et al. (2012). Loss of ceramide synthase 3 causes lethal skin barrier disruption. *Human Molecular Genetics, 21*(3), 586–608.

Johnson, J. J. (2011). Carnosol: a promising anti-cancer and anti-inflammatory agent. *Cancer Letters, 305*(1), 1–7.

Kastorini, C. M., Milionis, H. J., Ioannidi, A., et al. (2011). Adherence to the Mediterranean diet in relation to acute coronary syndrome or stroke nonfatal events: a comparative analysis of a case/case-control study. *American Heart Journal, 162*(4), 717–724.

Katiyar, S. K. (2003). Skin photoprotection by green tea: antioxidant and immunomodulatory effects. *Current Drug Targets: Immune, Endocrine & Metabolic Disorders, 3*(3), 234–242.

Lucas, L., Russell, A., & Keast, R. (2011). Molecular mechanisms of inflammation. Anti-inflammatory benefits of virgin olive oil and the phenolic compound oleocanthal. *Current Pharmaceutical Design, 17*(8), 754–768.

Nagata, C., Nakamura, K., Wada, K., et al. (2010). Association of dietary fat, vegetables and antioxidant micronutrients with skin ageing in Japanese women. *British Journal of Nutrition, 103*(10), 1493–1498.

Nichols, J. A., & Katiyar, S. K. (2010). Skin photoprotection by natural polyphenols: anti-inflammatory, antioxidant and DNA repair mechanisms. *Archives of Dermatological Research*, *302*(2), 71–83.

Owen, R. W., Giacosa, A., Hull, W. E., et al. (2000). Olive-oil consumption and health: the possible role of antioxidants. *Lancet Oncology*, *1*, 107–112.

Pageon, H. (2010). Reaction of glycation and human skin: the effects on the skin and its components, reconstructed skin as a model. *Pathologie Biologie*, *58*(3), 226–231.

Pageon, H., & Asselineau, D. (2005). An in vitro approach to the chronological aging of skin by glycation of the collagen: the biological effect of glycation on the reconstructed skin model. *Annals of the New York Academy of Science*, *1043*, 529–532.

Pageon, H., Bakala, H., Monnier, V. M, et al. (2007). Collagen glycation triggers the formation of aged skin in vitro. *European Journal of Dermatology*, *17*(1), 12–20.

Pageon, H., Técher, M. P., & Asselineau, D. (2008). Reconstructed skin modified by glycation of the dermal equivalent as a model for skin aging and its potential use to evaluate anti-glycation molecules. *Experimental Gerontology*, *43*(6), 584–588.

Perricone, N. (2000). *The wrinkle cure*. New York, NY:Rodale Books.

Perricone, N. (2003). *The acne prescription*. New York, NY:HarperCollins.

Perricone, N. (2004). *The Perricone promise*. New York, NY:Warner Books.

Perricone, N. (2010). *Forever young*. New York, NY:Atria Books.

Piccardi, N., & Manissier, P. (2009). Nutrition and nutritional supplementation: Impact on skin health and beauty. *Dermatoendocrinology*, *1*(5), 271–274.

Razny, U., Polus, A., & Kiec-Wilk, B. (2010). Angiogenesis in Balb/c mice under beta-carotene supplementation in diet. *Genes & Nutrition*, *5*(1), 9–16.

Sajithlal, G. B., Chithra, P., & Chandrakasan, G. (1998). Advanced glycation end products induce crosslinking of collagen in vitro. *Biochimica et Biophysica Acta*, *1407*(3), 215–224.

Sampson, H. A., & McCaskill, C. C. (1985). Food hypersensitivity and atopic dermatitis: evaluation of 113 patients. *Journal of Pediatrics*, *107*(5), 669–675.

Saran, K. B. (2008). Acne and carbs. Retrieved from *Dermadoctor.com* on March 3, 2012. http://www.dermadoctor.com/article_Acne-And-Carbs_249.html

Shapira, N. (2010). Nutritional approach to sun protection: a suggested complement to external strategies. *Nutrition Review*, *68*(2), 75–86.

Simopoulos, A. P. (2011). Importance of the omega-6/omega-3 balance in health and disease: evolutionary aspects of diet. *World Review of Nutrition & Dietetics*, *102*, 10–21.

Smith, R. N., Mann, N., Mäkeläinen, H., et al. (2008). A pilot study to determine the short-term effects of a low glycemic load diet on hormonal markers of acne: a non-randomized, parallel, controlled feeding trial. *Molecular Nutrition & Food Research*, *52*(6), 718–726.

Stahl, W., Heinrich, U., Wiseman, S., et al. (2001). Dietary tomato paste protects against ultraviolet light-induced erythema in humans. *Journal of Nutrition*, *131*(5), 1449–1451.

Stoner, G. D., & Mukhtar, H. (1995). Polyphenols as cancer chemopreventive agents. *Journal of Cell Biochemistry Supplement*, *22*, 169–180.

Südel, K. M., Venzke, K., Mielke, H., et al. (2005). Novel aspects of intrinsic and extrinsic aging of human skin: beneficial effects of soy extract. *Photochemistry & Photobiology, 81*(3), 581–587.

Teng, N. I., Shahar, S., Manaf, Z. A., et al. (2011). Efficacy of fasting calorie restriction on quality of life among aging men. *Physiology & Behavior, 104*(5), 1059–1056

van Boekel, M. A. (1991). The role of glycation in aging and diabetes mellitus. *Molecular Biology Reports, 15*(2), 57–64.

Veith, W. B., & Silverberg, N. B. (2011). The association of acne vulgaris with diet. *Cutis, 88*(2), 84–91.

Weil, A. Anti-inflammatory diet & pyramid. *Dr.Weil.com.* Retrieved March 3, 2012, from http://www.drweil.com/drw/u/PAG00361/anti-inflammatory-food-pyramid.html

Ziboh, V. A., Miller, C. C., & Cho, Y. (2000). Metabolism of polyunsaturated fatty acids by skin epidermal enzymes: generation of antiinflammatory and antiproliferative metabolites. *American Journal of Clinical Nutrition, 71*(1 Suppl), 361S–366S.

2

Nutrition and Supplements for Healthy Skin

JEANETTE JACKNIN, MD

Key Concepts

♣ Adequate nutrition is key to healthy skin. The Western diet may be deficient in important micronutrients such as B vitamins, vitamin C, vitamin E, folic acid, iron, or zinc, with deleterious effects on the skin. Nutritional supplements may be important for skin health in patients who are not motivated to, or for some other reason cannot, change to a healthier diet.

♣ Supplemental antioxidants such as vitamins A, C, and E as well as beta-carotene, other carotenoids, selenium, zinc, chromate, B vitamins, coenzyme Q10, and vitamin D can promote normally functioning, healthy skin.

♣ Essential fatty acids that cannot be made by the body may require dietary supplementation. Omega-3 fatty acids found in fish oils and flaxseed oil tend to be anti-inflammatory, countering the proinflammatory effects of omega-6 fatty acids, including arachidonic acid found in animal proteins.

Introduction

The skin is the largest and most visible organ in the body, so it is a great indicator of general health as well as organ health. "Your skin is the fingerprint of what is going on inside your body, and all skin conditions, from psoriasis to acne to aging, are the manifestations of your body's internal needs, including its nutritional needs," says Georgiana Donadio, PhD, DC, MSc, founder and director of the National Institute of Whole Health in Boston (Bouchez & Grayson, 2012). Vitamins, minerals, and other nutrients give the skin a more radiant, healthy, and youthful glow. Studies have shown that a deficiency of vitamins B12, B6, C, and E, folic acid, iron, or zinc appears to mimic radiation in damaging DNA, causing single- and double-strand breaks, oxidative lesions, or both. Many common micronutrient deficiencies, such as those of iron or biotin, also cause mitochondrial decay with oxidant leakage, leading to accelerated aging (Ames, 2004).

It is best to get essential nutrients for one's skin through dietary intake, but usually this is not entirely possible. Oral supplements and topical creams help. Dietary supplements include vitamins, minerals, herbs or other botanicals, amino acids, and substances such as enzymes. We will leave the discussion of herbs to another chapter.

Have your patients begin by taking supplemental antioxidants—such as vitamins A, C, and E. Antioxidants fight against free radicals that damage collagen and elastin, the fibers that support skin structure, causing wrinkles and other signs of aging. Free radicals and reactive oxygen species are synthesized endogenously (e.g., in energy metabolism and the antimicrobial defense system of the body) and produced as reactions to exogenous exposure (e.g., cigarette smoke, poor diet, over-exercise, environmental pollutants, and food contaminants). Human dietary intervention studies based on the use of antioxidant compounds show how they can protect from endogenous and exogenous environmental assaults and neutralize sun-induced effects on the skin. The future challenge will be to combine the strategic use of "cosmeceuticals" and "nutraceuticals" in preventing the damaging effects of ultraviolet radiation and environmental pollutants on the many biological processes involving skin aging and cancer (Morganti, 2009).

Beta-carotene, selenium, and zinc as well as the fatty acids found in fish oil, the B vitamins, and vitamin D—are also very important for the normal functioning of healthy skin. Studies have shown that groups of oral antioxidants taken together help to create and restore youthful skin. Thirty-nine volunteers with healthy skin were divided into three groups and supplemented for a period of 12 weeks (Heinrich et al., 2006). Group 1 received a mixture of lycopene (3 mg/day), lutein (3 mg/day), beta-carotene (4.8 mg/day), alpha-tocopherol (10 mg/day), and selenium (75 mcg/day). Group 2 received a mixture of lycopene (6 mg/day) and no lutein but the other supplements remained the same. Skin density and thickness were significantly increased and roughness and scaling were improved in groups 1 and 2 compared to the placebo control group. Other studies have confirmed and expanded on these results. A clinical, randomized, double-blind, parallel-group, placebo-controlled study was conducted in healthy young female volunteers investigating the preventive, photoprotective effect of oral supplementation with Seresis™, an antioxidative combination containing beta-carotene, lycopene, vitamins C and E, selenium and proanthocyanidins. Seresis™ was able to slow the time of the development and grade of UVB-induced erythema by decreasing the UV-induced expression of collagen-degrading enzymes, called matrix metalloproteinases (MMPs) MMP-1 and 9, which Greul and colleagues (2002) hypothesized was important in photoprotective processes. Miquel and colleagues studied menopausal women and emphasized the important role of the B vitamins, the key antioxidant vitamins C and E, as well as beta-carotene, lipoic acid, and the soy isoflavones (Miquel et al., 2006). These nutrients may help to prevent antioxidant deficiency and thus protect the mitochondria against premature oxidative damage with loss of adenosine triphosphate (ATP) synthesis and specialized cellular functions, including that of the skin. Therefore, Miquel concluded that the administration of synergistic combinations of some of the above-mentioned antioxidants in the diet as well as topically may have favorable effects on the health and quality of life of women, especially of menopausal age and older.

These and other supplements can be taken in capsule, pill, or liquid form. In the 1980s, patented spray and liquid forms of vitamins, minerals, and other nutrients were introduced. They are absorbed directly into the body though the tissues lining the mouth. Manufacturers claim that they provide an over 90% absorption rate within 30 seconds, nine times as fast as pills or capsules (Jacknin, 2001).

Today, more than 50% of all Americans take dietary supplements. Patients should inform their doctors which supplements and herbs they are taking, as some can interact with certain pharmaceutical drugs. Rarely, a nutritional supplement may cause an unwanted side effect. The Office of Dietary Supplements was established in 1994 at the National Institutes of Health (NIH). Around 2000, the NIH launched an online database devoted entirely to dietary supplements that cited studies from more than 3,000 scientific journals at that time. With the increasing popularity of alternative medicine and the emphasis on individuals assuming greater responsibility for their own healthcare, the over-the-counter supplement business has expanded rapidly in the last 15 years. It promises to grow even larger in the years to come.

Necessary Nutrients for Healthy, Youthful Skin

At the current time, the vitamins and nutrients below are those that are recommended as being the most important for patients to take daily to ensure healthy, youthful skin and to fight the appearance of aging (Jacknin, 2001; Perricone, 2000, 2004). The antioxidants can be most conveniently taken as part of a daily multivitamin/multimineral supplement that also provides at least 400 micrograms of folic acid. The vitamins all have anti-aging, antioxidant, and anti-inflammatory benefits. Patients should take these supplements with their largest meal. Of course, these recommendations will expand as our knowledge of the biochemistry of the skin increases.

1. Mixed carotenoids, 10,000 to 25,000 international units (IU) daily, with meals. This should include astaxanthin, 2 to 4 mg daily, and beta-carotene, 8,000 to 25,000 IU daily.
2. B100 complex daily
3. Vitamin C, 500 mg twice a day, and asorbyl palmitate–vitamin C ester, 500 mg daily
4. Bioflavonoids and quercetin, 300 mg three times a day, before meals
5. Vitamin D, at least 2,000 IU daily
6. Vitamin E, 400 IU of natural mixed tocopherols
7. Calcium citrate, 600 mg, plus magnesium, 200 mg once or twice daily, for women, depending on whether or not they have osteopenia. Men should avoid supplemental calcium.
8. Selenium, 200 mcg daily
9. Zinc, 20 mg daily
10. Alpha-lipoic acid (ALA), 250 mg twice a day
11. Acetyl-L-carnitine, 250 to 750 mg twice a day
12. CoQ10, 60 to 120 mg a day in divided doses with food
13. DMAE, 75 mg twice a day
14. Omega-3/6 in a 2:1 ratio in molecularly distilled products certified to be free of heavy metals and other contaminants. Omega-3, 1,000 mg fish oil twice a day, and omega-6, 750 mg twice a day.
15. Copper, 3 mg a day; can be taken in a trace mineral pill or liquid
16. Chromium, 150 mg a day
17. If patients are not regularly eating ginger and turmeric, advise them to add these spices to their foods.

Let us look at these nutrients and supplements in more depth.

Vitamins

VITAMIN A

Vitamin A is very important for the maintenance and repair of skin tissue. If vitamin A levels in the body drop even a little below normal, this can be reflected in the skin, including a dry, flaky complexion (Bouchez & Grayson, 2012). Vitamin A augments immunity to infection, protects against damage from pollution, helps to block cancer formation, slows the aging process, and is essential for the maintenance and repair of normal skin tissue and mucous membranes (Jacknin, 2001). It is one of the very helpful antioxidants that neutralize damaging free radicals. Forms of vitamin A include beta-carotene, astaxanthin, and other carotenoids, and one takes these supplements instead of the vitamin itself. It is thought that, on average, people need 5,000 IU vitamin A daily. Vitamin A should not be taken in large amounts by pregnant women, children, or people with liver disease. Overdosage can cause headaches, nausea, itchy skin, brittle nails, liver toxicity, bone pain, and birth defects. Potent oral vitamin A derivatives have been very useful in the treatment of severe acne, psoriasis, and other, less common skin disorders. Acitretin (Soriatane), a powerful oral vitamin A derivative, has been very important in the treatment of difficult psoriasis cases.

It is topical vitamin A that makes a real difference in one's skin. Medical studies show a reduction in lines and wrinkles, good acne control, and some psoriasis relief, all from using creams containing derivatives of vitamin A (Jacknin, 2001). A study involving 72 individuals of varying ages was done to see if the topical application of natural vitamin A could improve function in both naturally aged, sun-protected, and photoaged skin. In one of the study groups of people 80-plus years of age, topical application of vitamin A for seven days increased fibroblast growth and collagen synthesis while reducing levels of the collagen-degrading skin enzyme, MMP. The overall findings indicated that naturally aged, sun-protected, and photoaged skin all show connective tissue damage, elevated MMP levels, and reduced collagen production. Topical vitamin A treatment reduced MMP expression and stimulated collagen synthesis in naturally aged and sun-protected skin, as it did in photoaged skin. Synthetic vitamin A drugs such as topical tretinoin have shown even more profound effects in reversing both photodamaged and naturally aged skin (Varani et al., 1998).

Other skin diseases that respond to exfoliating agents and keratolytics, products that remove a keratin plug from a hair follicle or sweat gland, also are improved with topical vitamin A derivatives. These conditions include actinic keratoses, flat warts, keratosis piliaris, ichthyoses, pityriasis rubra pilaris, and mycosis fungoides. Some vitamin A derivatives are available by prescription only, such as tretinoin, while others, like retinol, are available over the counter. Retinol is a nonprescription form of vitamin A useful for diminishing the dark spots and changes in the tone, texture, and moisture level of the skin that accompany aging. Prescription retinoids decrease the production of the melanin in the skin, increase the rate of skin-cell turnover, and affect the growth and differentiation of skin cells. These are best used for the reduction of fine wrinkles, mottled increased skin pigmentation, and roughness of facial skin.

A newer formulation, tretinoin gel microsphere, is as effective as the original tretinoin, but with less skin irritation. Adapalene, another topical prescription retinoid used for acne, claims to be less irritating and expensive than the original tretinoin. Another retinoid, tazarotene, is indicated for the treatment of stable plaque psoriasis that covers up to 20% of the body, and for mild to moderate facial acne. Thus, vitamin A and its derivatives are very important in maintaining healthy skin and treating skin disease (Jacknin, 2001).

ASTAXANTHIN AND OTHER MIXED CAROTENOIDS

Carotenoids are yellow-orange pigments that come from plants and give nature its wide variety of colors—from carrots to flamingos. They are converted to vitamin A in the liver. Astaxanthin is thought to be one of the most important carotenoids. It comes from the microalgae *Haematococcus pluvialis*, plentiful in Arctic marine environments. It is the most potent of all of the carotenoids and is a powerful anti-inflammatory, 10 times stronger than beta-carotene and 100 times stronger than vitamin E. Wild Alaskan salmon, lobster, rainbow trout, shrimp, crawfish, crab, and red caviar all owe their rich colors to their astaxanthin-rich algae diets (Bouchez & Grayson, 2012).

In Lyons and O'Brien (2002) early study, the ability of an algal extract to protect against UVA-induced DNA alterations was examined in human skin fibroblasts and human melanocytes. The protective effects of the proprietary algal extract, which contained a high level of astaxanthin, were compared with synthetic astaxanthin. The synthetic astaxanthin prevented UVA-induced DNA damage at all concentrations (10 nM, 100 nM, 10 microM) tested. The algal extract displayed protection against UVA-induced DNA damage when the equivalent of 10 microM astaxanthin was added. In skin fibroblasts pre-incubation (18 hours) with 10 microM of either the synthetic astaxanthin or the algal extract prevented UVA-induced induction of cellular superoxide dismutase activity, coupled with a marked decrease in cellular glutathione content. This work suggested a role for the algal extract as a potentially beneficial antioxidant (Lyons and O'Brien, 2002). Astaxanthin's linear, polar-nonpolar-polar molecular layout equips it to precisely insert into the membrane and span its entire width. In this position, it can intercept reactive molecular species within the membrane's hydrophobic interior and along its hydrophilic boundaries. In double-blind, randomized controlled trials, astaxanthin blocked oxidative DNA damage, lowered C-reactive protein and other inflammation biomarkers, and boosted immunity. It improved blood flow in an experimental microcirculation model and protected the mitochondria against endogenous oxygen radicals, conserved their redox (antioxidant) capacity, and enhanced their energy production efficiency in cultured cells (Kidd, 2011). In his review article Kidd summarized that astaxanthin's clinical success extends beyond protection against oxidative stress and inflammation, to demonstrable promise for slowing age-related functional decline. Repetitive exposure of the skin to UVA radiation elicits sagging more frequently than wrinkling, which is mainly attributed to its biochemical mechanism to upregulate the expression of MMP-1 and skin fibroblast elastase/neutral endopeptidase (SFE/NEP) respectively (Suganuma et al., 2010). The addition of astaxanthin at concentrations of 4 to 8 microM immediately after UVA exposure significantly attenuated the induction of MMP-1 and SFE/NEP expression elicited by UVA at the gene, protein, and activity levels. Thus, he hypothesized that astaxanthin would have a significant benefit in terms of protecting against UVA-induced skin photoaging seen as sagging and wrinkles.

Other mixed carotenoids such as beta-carotene, alphacarotenes, lycopenes, lutein, and zeaxanthin are also good antioxidants. Beta-carotene has been used to treat various photosensitivity disorders for more than 30 years. The main indication for its use is in the treatment of the photosensitivity associated with erythropoietic protoporphyria (Anstey, 2002). When beta-carotene was applied as such or in combination with alpha-tocopherol for 12 weeks, erythema formation induced with a solar light simulator was diminished from week 8 on. Similar effects were also achieved with a diet rich in lycopene. Ingestion of tomato paste corresponding to a dose of 16 mg lycopene per day was studied over 10 weeks. At week 10, erythema formation was significantly lower in the group that ingested the tomato paste as compared to the control group. No significant difference was found at week 4 of treatment. Such protective effects of carotenoids were also demonstrated in cell culture. The in vitro data indicate that there is an optimal level of protection for each carotenoid (Stahl & Sies, 2002). In a study published in the *British Journal of Dermatology in 1996*, Naldi and colleagues found that foods high in beta-carotene also reduced the risk of psoriasis. Significant inverse relations with psoriasis were observed for the intake of carrots, tomatoes, and fresh fruit, and the index of beta-carotene intake (Naldi et al., 1996).

Although the skin can turn yellow-orange if you eat very large amounts of carotenoids, no overdose can occur, so it is relatively safe. However, people who have diabetes or underactive thyroid glands should not take carotenoid supplements, as people with these conditions often have difficulty converting carotenoids into vitamin A (Jacknin, 2001).

B VITAMINS

The B vitamins are coenzymes that should always be taken together. The single most important B vitamin for the epidermis is biotin, as it is important for cell growth and for the formation and maintenance of strong nails and healthy hair and skin. Biotin is needed to process fats, carbohydrates, and proteins, and in the utilization of the other B vitamins. The body needs 300 micrograms of biotin a day, but deficiencies are rare. Most people normally get enough biotin in the foods they eat, and biotin can also be produced by the body from ingested foods. If there is even a mild biotin deficiency, however, itchy, scaly skin and hair loss can result (Bouchez & Grayson, 2012). Nicotinamide (the amide form of vitamin B3) has been used in dermatology for more than 40 years for a diverse range of conditions including acne, rosacea, autoimmune bullous dermatoses, and recently the treatment and prevention of photoaging and photoimmunosuppression. Nicotinamide's effects are due to its role as a cellular energy precursor, a modulator of inflammatory cytokines, and an inhibitor of the nuclear enzyme poly-adenosine diphosphate-ribose polymerase-1, which plays a significant role in DNA repair (Surjana & Damian, 2011). Vitamin B12 (cobalamin) and folic acid are critical to the formation of red blood cells and the production of DNA, and these two vitamins often work together synergistically to magnify each other's effects. Niacin is the B vitamin with the greatest potential to cause unwanted side effects, such as flushing and liver toxicity, especially if it is taken in high doses and over long periods of time. Its ongoing use should therefore be closely monitored (Jacknin, 2001).

Importantly, topical preparations containing B vitamins, especially niacin, can help give your patients' skin an almost instant healthy glow, hydrating cells and increasing overall skin tone. Topical niacin helps the skin retain moisture, making one's complexion appear younger. Its anti-inflammatory properties also help to soothe dry, irritated skin. In higher concentrations, niacin in creams can also work as a lightening agent, evening out blotchy skin tone (Bouchez & Grayson, 2012).

VITAMIN C

Vitamin C, or ascorbic acid, protects against the harmful effects of pollution, increases immunity, aids in interferon and anti-stress-hormone production, and thereby helps to prevent cancer. By increasing immunity, it also helps to guard against infection. Vitamin C is an antioxidant essential for the manufacture of collagen and is important in reducing bruising and blood-clotting problems, strengthening blood-vessel walls, and healing wounds. There is also evidence suggesting that vitamins C and E work together synergistically. The February 2005 *Journal of Investigative Dermatology* reported that people who supplemented their diet with vitamins C and E reduced their sunburns due to UVB. A reduction of factors linked to DNA damage within skin cells was also found, indicating that vitamins C and E protect against

DNA damage (Bouchez & Grayson, 2012). Using data from the first National Health and Nutrition Examination Survey, Cosgrove and colleagues examined associations between nutrient intakes and skin aging in 4,025 women (40 to 74 years of age). Nutrients were estimated from a 24-hour recall. Higher intakes of oral vitamin C and linoleic acid and lower intakes of fats and carbohydrates were associated with better skin-aging appearance, with a less wrinkled appearance, dryness, and atrophy. These associations were independent of age, race, education, sunlight exposure, income, menopausal status, body mass index, supplement use, physical activity, and energy intake (Cosgrove et al., 2007).

The antioxidant vitamin C increases the production of the proteins collagen and elastin, which are necessary to maintain firm skin that does not sag or wrinkle. Vitamin C also neutralizes free radicals caused by ultraviolet light and promotes skin-cell renewal, thereby inhibiting skin aging. Thus, it is very important in reducing the appearance of fine lines and wrinkles, returning and maintaining youthful skin resilience, and lightening and evening skin tones. Vitamin C is available in many over-the-counter cosmetics, lotions, creams, eye-lift gels, and transdermal patches that are applied to the wrinkled areas and left on between one and eight hours, depending on the strength (Jacknin, 2001).

In a 2002 double-blind study, a topical vitamin C complex was applied to half of the face and a placebo gel to the opposite side. Clinical evaluation of wrinkling, pigmentation, inflammation. and hydration was done before the study and at weeks 4, 8, and 12. There was a statistically significant improvement of the vitamin C-treated side at 12 weeks, with overall facial improvement and decreased photoaging scores of the cheeks and the perioral area. Biopsies showed increased collagen formation in the vitamin C side only (Fitzpatrick et al., 2002).

Considerable interest has been generated about combining antioxidants with sunscreens to provide enhanced protection. Vitamins C and E have both been shown to be effective in different models of photodamage. In a study done on swine skin, vitamin C provided additive protection against acute sunburn cell formation when combined with a sunscreen. When vitamins E and C were combined, very good protection from a UVB insult occurred. Vitamin C, however, was significantly better than vitamin E at protecting against a UVA-mediated phototoxic insult in Darr and colleagues' animal model (Darr et al., 1996).

Cantaloupe, collards, currants, grapefruit, green peas, kale, lemons, mangos, mustard greens, onions, oranges, papayas, parsley, persimmons, pineapple, radishes, spinach, strawberries, sweet peppers, tomatoes, turnip greens, and watercress all contain an abundance of vitamin C. Supplementation to increase vitamin C levels is thought to help both preventively and therapeutically. The oral esterified polyascorbate form of vitamin C (such as Ester-C) is best to supplement the diet with, as it enters the bloodstream, tissues, and white blood cells four times as quickly as does the usual vitamin C product. In this form, ascorbic acid is bound to calcium, magnesium, potassium, zinc, and/or sodium, with any one of these minerals allowing for more rapid absorption. High doses of vitamin C can cause diarrhea. Additionally, if you take large doses of vitamin C, your body gets used to these doses. Therefore, if you choose to reduce your patient's intake, taper off gradually to avoid a rebound vitamin C deficiency (Jacknin, 2001).

VITAMIN D

In its active form as calcitriol, vitamin D contributes to skin-cell metabolism, growth, and repair. It optimizes the skin's immune system and helps to destroy free radicals, which can cause premature aging. In fact, vitamin D *has been found to be more effective in reducing lipid peroxidation and increasing enzymes that protect against oxidation than vitamin E (Sardar et al., 1996).* Age, skin color, latitude, seasonal variations in availability of sunlight, and sunscreen use make it difficult for one to produce all the vitamin D one needs from sun exposure. Unfortunately, between the ages of 20 and 70, *one's skin loses about 75% of its ability to produce vitamin D3*—the metabolic precursor of calcitriol (Holick, 2004). There is now overwhelming scientific data suggesting that the human body requires a blood level of 25(OH) D above 30 ng/mL for maximum health. To increase the blood level to the minimum 30 ng/mL requires at least 1,000 IU vitamin D orally per day for adults (Holick, 2010).

The skin is the last organ of the body to receive antioxidants from the food and supplements one eats (Tavakkol et al., 2004). Much of the active vitamin D that the body produces is used to help build and maintain strong bones. *Rates of cell division and differentiation are triggered by growth factors and other molecules that are controlled by the presence of vitamin D (Matsumoto et al., 1991).* If adequate amounts of vitamin D are not available, the epidermis will not differentiate optimally. As a result, the outer layer of the skin becomes thinner and more fragile. It begins to sag from lack of adequate support, and dryness and wrinkles set in as moisture is gradually lost to the outside (Oda et al., 2009). This is why vitamin D is essential to the maintenance of healthy-looking skin. However, if supplemental oral vitamin D is taken, or topical vitamin D is applied *topically*, protection for the skin can be enhanced.

A vitamin D derivative, calcipotriene (Dovonex™), can be used topically to treat psoriasis.

VITAMIN E

Vitamin E, or tocopherol, is an antioxidant that also helps to improve blood circulation to the skin, promote normal clotting, repair tissue, improve healing, and reduce scarring. It helps to maintain the integrity of cell membranes, and it is needed to synthesize DNA. Like vitamin C, it inhibits free radicals, thereby preventing cell damage, helping to prevent cancer, and retarding the signs of aging (Jacknin, 2001). Cold-pressed vegetable oils, whole grains, dark-green leafy vegetables, nuts, seeds, and legumes are great sources of vitamin E. Additional sources include dry beans, sweet potatoes, brown rice, oatmeal, cornmeal, wheat germ, eggs, milk, and organ meats.

Duke University researcher Sheldon Pinnell and colleagues demonstrated in 2002 that "appreciable photoprotection can be obtained from topical vitamins C and E." They found that supplementation with vitamin E 400 mg per day reduced photodamage and wrinkles and improved skin texture. It was reported in *The Journal of Investigative Dermatology* in February 2005 that people who take vitamins C and E reduced the amount of their sunburns over time. Further, researchers saw a reduction of factors linked to DNA damage within skin cells, leading them to conclude that these antioxidant vitamins help protect against DNA damage (Bouchez & Grayson, 2012). Vitamin E scavenges for harmful oxygen radicals in the cell membranes, while vitamin C works in biologic fluids to attack free radicals. Vitamin E also works better when taken with selenium and zinc. Iron supplements should not be taken at the same time as vitamin E. Vitamin E applied topically is very soothing and moisturizing, and therefore has been very popular in skin care. It is available in stick, oil, and cream form for use on the face, lips, and body, as a moisturizer and anti-aging cream, and to reduce the prominence of healing scars.

Minerals

SELENIUM

Selenium, zinc, and copper are involved in cellular respiration and utilization of oxygen, DNA and RNA reproduction, maintenance of cell membrane integrity, and destruction of free radicals. Superoxide radicals are reduced to hydrogen peroxide by superoxide dismutases in the presence of copper and zinc cofactors. Hydrogen peroxide is then reduced to water by the selenium–glutathione peroxidase couple. Efficient removal of these superoxide free radicals maintains the integrity of skin cell membranes, reduces the risk of cancer, and slows the aging process (Chan et al., 1998). Selenium also has anti-aging and anti-inflammatory effects (Puizina-Ivić et al., 2010), aids in the production of antibodies, protects the immune system, and helps prevent cancers, including skin cancer. In *Photodermatology, Photoimmunology, and Photomedicine* in 1991, scientists reported that oral selenium as well as copper helped reduce the formation of sunburn cells in human skin. In *The Journal of the American Medical Association* in 1996, researchers showed that skin cancer patients who took 200 micrograms of selenium per day had 37% fewer skin cancer malignancies and a 50% reduced risk of death from skin cancer. Later, Césarini and colleagues investigated the capacity of an oral antioxidant complex consisting of selenium, lycopene, beta-carotene, and alpha-tocopherol to reduce UV-induced damage in 25 individuals. After 7 weeks, many parameters of the epidermal defense against UV-induced damage were significantly improved, including an elevation of the actinic erythema threshold, a general reduction of the UV-induced erythema, and a parallel reduction of the lipoperoxide levels (Césarini et al., 2003). A 12-week course of oral selenium together with other antioxidants was given to 26 of 39 patients in a later study. Their skin density and thickness was significantly increased and roughness, scaling, smoothness, and wrinkling of the skin were improved (Heinrich et al., 2006). Topically, selenium also helps protect the skin from sun damage and sunburn (Bouchez & Grayson, 2012). Our bodies need 70 micrograms of selenium a day, but over 200 micrograms a day can be toxic. Early evidence of overdosage includes a metallic taste in the mouth; later signs include fragile or black nails and hair loss (Jacknin, 2001).

ZINC

Zinc is also involved in cellular respiration and utilization of oxygen, DNA and RNA reproduction, maintenance of cell membrane integrity, and sequestration of free radicals. It helps to maintain the integrity of skin cell membranes, reduces the risk of skin cancer, and slows the aging process (Chan et al., 1998). Zinc is an essential mineral required for protein synthesis and collagen formation, promoting the healing of wounds. It is also important to help keep the immune system healthy and to maintain the proper concentration of vitamin E in the blood. Mahoney and colleagues' six-week study of 21 women demonstrated that cream containing 0.1%

copper-zinc malonate cream had the propensity to increase elastin synthesis in human skin in vivo, and that regeneration of elastic fibers may contribute to decreased wrinkles in female patients with photoaged facial skin (Mahoney et al., 2009). A daily intake of approximately 15 milligrams of zinc is desirable. Interestingly, while consuming up to 100 milligrams of zinc daily enhances the body's immune response, taking in more than 100 milligrams a day actually depresses immunity. In too-large quantities, zinc can cause nausea, vomiting, diarrhea, and abdominal pain and can deplete copper stores in the body (Jacknin, 2001).

CHROMIUM

Chromium is involved in the metabolism of glucose or sugar and is needed for energy and the synthesis of cholesterol, fats, and protein. It helps to maintain lower blood sugar and insulin levels, helping to prevent glycation and inflammation, which ages cells and the organism as a whole. Many people do not get enough chromium through diet alone, as there is a lack of chromium in our water and soil, and because the typical American diet high in refined white sugar, flour, and junk foods is deficient in chromium. It often needs to be supplemented at a dose of 150 micrograms per day (Jacknin, 2001).

COPPER

Copper is also involved in the cellular utilization of oxygen, DNA and RNA reproduction, maintenance of cell membrane integrity, and elimination of free radicals. Superoxide radicals are reduced to hydrogen peroxide by superoxide dismutases in the presence of copper and zinc cofactors. Removal of these superoxide free radicals helps to maintain skin cell membranes, reduces the risk of skin cancer, and slows the aging process (Chan et al., 1998). Copper aids in the formation of hemoglobin and red blood cells and therefore is important for healthy circulation of blood to the skin. This mineral also works in balance with zinc and vitamin C to form elastin and collagen (Jacknin, 2001). A study on 20 volunteers showed that after 30 days the formation of pro-collagen, a precursor of collagen, increased by 70% compared with 50% formation with vitamin C and 40% due to tretinoin (www.dermadoctor.com). In the skin, copper also helps to stimulate the formation of the extracellular cement between skin cells, thus improving skin strength and reducing fragility. Copper also stimulates the formation of glycosaminoglycans, helping to thicken the dermis and firm the skin. Topical applications of copper-rich creams have been found to firm the skin and help restore some elasticity. Studies conducted at the University of Pennsylvania and presented in 2002 found that when compared with a popular skin-care treatment and a placebo, a cream containing copper peptides demonstrated rapid, visual overall improvements in skin roughness, clarity, fine lines, wrinkling, and overall photodamage. In similar studies, this same team of researchers found that copper peptides noticeably improved skin elasticity and thickness (Bouchez & Grayson, 2012). Copper is naturally found in most vegetables, nuts, and seafood. Most people are able to get the 3 milligrams of copper they need from their diet every day and do not need to supplement (Jacknin, 2001).

Other Nutrients

BIOFLAVONOIDS AND QUERCETIN

Bioflavonoids, while not true vitamins, enhance the absorption of vitamin C and should be taken with it. Quercetin is one well-known bioflavonoid that is particularly effective in allergenic skin reactions. Bioflavonoids act together with vitamin C to preserve the structure of capillaries and to reduce symptoms of oral herpes. Bioflavonoids also promote good blood circulation and have an antibacterial effect. In 2005 a study from Uruguay took plant extracts containing potent antioxidants such as quercetin, mixed them with a cosmetic base, and applied this combination to the skin of the back of rabbits. Afterwards, the rabbits' skin was exposed to 1 hour of UV radiation. The production of hydroxyl radicals was measured in the irradiated areas. Dr. Morquio concluded that the cosmetic preparation reduced hydroxyl radicals secondary to its high concentration of quercetin and other flavonoids (Morquio et al., 2005). Casagrande and colleagues' Brazilian study (2006) also investigated the ability of quercetin-containing topicals to inhibit UVB radiation-induced oxidative damage in mice. Two different quercetin formulations were shown to inhibit this oxidative damage. In their 2010 study, Chondrogianni and colleagues (2010) identified both quercetin and its derivative, quercetin caprylate, as antioxidants that increase cellular lifespan, survival, and viability of human fibroblasts. When these compounds are added to already senescent fibroblasts, a rejuvenating effect was observed. Finally, Chondrogianni and colleagues showed that quercetin and quercetin caprylate have a whitening effect when applied to skin cells. These data again demonstrate that topical quercetin and quercetin caprylate can be very effective natural anti-aging ingredients in humans.

COENZYME Q10

Coenzyme Q10 (CoQ10), or ubiquinone, is a vitamin-like substance similar to vitamin E but even more powerful as an antioxidant. It is an essential part of the mitochondria, the energy-producing part of almost all the cells in the body. It acts similarly to acetyl-L-carnitine, assisting in energy production within the mitochondria. Energy production declines as a cell ages and the cell's ability to repair itself also declines. Therefore, CoQ10 plays a key role in the effectiveness of the immune system and in delaying the aging process.

A standardized multistep method to assess the anti-inflammatory properties and photoprotective properties and to compare the oxidative stress-protection capacity of topical antioxidants was devised in 2005 (McDaniel et al., 2005b). Correlation and trends between in vitro and in vivo results were established. The overall oxidative protection capacity scores of 95, 80, 68, 55, 52, and 41 were obtained for idebenone, dl-alpha tocopherol, kinetin, ubiquinone, L-ascorbic acid, and dl-alpha lipoic acid, respectively. The higher the score, the more effective the overall oxidative stress-protection capacity of the antioxidant. Idebenone is an antioxidant lower-molecular-weight analogue of CoQ10 and ubiquinone is another form of CoQ10. Thus, idebenone had the highest oxidative stress protection compared to the other topical antioxidants in this study (McDaniel et al., 2005b). Idebenone is a key ingredient in the much-advertised Prevage FACE Advanced Anti-Aging Serum.

McDaniel and colleagues also did a clinical study to establish the efficacy of idebenone in a topical skincare formulation for the treatment of photodamaged skin (McDaniel et al., 2005a). In this double-blind non-vehicle control study, 0.5% and 1.0% idebenone commercial formulations were evaluated in a clinical trial for topical safety and efficacy in photodamaged skin. Forty-one female subjects, aged 30 to 65, with moderately photodamaged skin were randomized to use a blind-labeled skincare preparation twice daily. After six weeks' use of the 1.0% idebenone formula, a 26% reduction in skin roughness/dryness, a 37% increase in skin hydration, a 29% reduction in fine lines/wrinkles, and a 33% improvement in overall global assessment of photodamaged skin were observed. For the 0.5% idebenone formulation, a 23% reduction in skin roughness/dryness, a 37% increase in skin hydration, a 27% reduction in fine lines/wrinkles, and a 30% improvement in overall global assessment of photodamaged skin were observed. The immunofluorescence staining revealed an increase in collagen I for both concentrations (McDaniel et al., 2005a). Prahl and colleagues found that topical application of CoQ10 rapidly improves mitochondrial function in skin in vivo (Prahl et al., 2008). As the functional loss of mitochondria represents an inherent part in the cutaneous aging process, CoQ10 has an anti-aging effect in skin. The effect of CoQ10 on human dermal and epidermal cells was further examined (Muta-Takada et al., 2009). CoQ10 promoted proliferation of fibroblasts but not keratinocytes. It also accelerated production of basement membrane components and showed protective effects against cell death in keratinocytes. These results suggested that protection of the epidermis against oxidative stress and enhancement of production of epidermal basement membrane components may be involved in the anti-aging properties of CoQ10 in skin.

CoQ10 also reduces the effects of histamine, so it is valuable in dealing with allergic skin problems and hives. It is thought that this nutrient can also enhance the skin's natural immunologic ability (Jacknin, 2001). Importantly, in an eight-year prospective study of 117 patients with melanoma, CoQ10 plasma levels predicted the risk of metastasis: CoQ10 levels were significantly lower in patients than in control subjects and in patients who developed recurring melanoma than those who did not (Rusciani, 2006). The amount of CoQ10 stored in a person's cells declines with age, so supplements are recommended. At least 60 to 120 mg CoQ10 a day should be added to the average American diet to maintain mitochondria that function effectively. CoQ10 is also available in topical form, added to various moisturizers, anti-aging creams, and sunscreens.

ESSENTIAL FATTY ACIDS

Essential fatty acids (EFAs) are polyunsaturated fatty acids that cannot be made by the body and therefore must be supplied by the diet. There are several different families of EFAs, the most important being the omega-3 essential fatty acids. EFAs have anti-inflammatory and antiglycation effects, enhancing the immune system and stabilizing blood sugar levels, thereby reducing the aging of cells.

Not ingesting enough fat actually causes skin inflammation, susceptibility to skin infection, and hair loss. The cutaneous effects of a diet deficient in EFAs are hyperdesquamation, resulting in a characteristic scaly skin disorder; increased transepidermal water loss; and altered lipid profiles, all of which are also characteristics of inflammatory dermatoses (Bibel, 1989; Ziboh, 2000). Because fatty acids are antimicrobial, the stratum corneum in mice fed diets deficient in EFAs supported 100-fold more bacteria than mice fed a healthy diet, and the deficient mice were the only group from which *Staphylococcus aureus* were routinely isolated (Bibel, 1989). Clinical studies show that the healthy balance of fatty acids in the skin dramatically decreases with aging and increased oxidative stress, such as that caused by chronic sun exposure. Therefore, getting the correct amount and type of fats through diet or supplementation is critical to maintaining healthy skin as one ages. Omega-3 fatty acids help to keep normal skin healthy by maintaining its natural oil barrier and making it look younger, less wrinkled, and clearer. Traditional and non-Westernized diets offer a healthier balance of omega-6 to omega-3 fatty acids, typically at a ratio of about 4:1 (Simopoulos, 2011). The current North American diet unfortunately provides a ratio of about 15:1 of omega-6s to omega-3s (Simopoulos, 2011). Omega-6 fat is found in relatively high amounts in egg yolks, poultry skin, and organ meats from animals fed corn-based diets. It contains arachidonic acid, which has an inflammatory effect on the body and skin. Alternatively, fish oil rich in the omega-3 oils eicosapentaenoic and docosahexaenoic acids (EPA and DHA) inhibits the formation of inflammatory molecules and generates anti-inflammatory and antiproliferative metabolites (Ziboh, 2000). It has also been shown that extra-virgin olive oils are very rich in phenolic antioxidants, squalene, and oleic acid, which help to protect against skin cancer and aging by inhibiting oxidative stress (Owen, 2000). With this ability to modulate inflammation, omega-3 fatty acids are also effective in the management of inflammatory skin conditions such as acne, psoriasis, eczema, and rosacea.

The daily requirement for EFAs is satisfied if they make up about 15% of total daily caloric intake, but there aren't any known adverse effects to consuming larger amounts. Pure, cold-pressed, nonhydrogenated fortified flaxseed oil, primrose oil, black-currant seed oil, and other vegetable oils contain high amounts of linoleic acid, an important EFA. Evening primrose oil contains the highest amount of gamma-linolenic acid, another EFA, of any food substance and is often used in the treatment of atopic dermatitis. Flaxseed from the herb flax contains those omega-3 essential fatty acids necessary for the proper synthesis of immune and anti-inflammatory compounds. One to two tablespoons of cold-pressed flaxseed oil should be taken daily, preferably with other foods, in those with healthy skin (Jacknin, 2001).

ALPHA-LIPOIC ACID

Alpha-lipoic acid (ALA) is a superior anti-inflammatory, penetrating all portions of the cell, as it is both fat and water soluble. ALA helps turn off an inflammatory messenger known as nuclear factor kappa B (NFkB). Factors that suppress NFkB inhibit skin-damaging inflammatory processes (Saliou et al., 2001). ALA also increases the body's ability to take glucose into the cells. This increased sensitivity to insulin results in decreased blood sugar levels, further reducing glycation and aging of the cells (Bouchez & Graystone, 2012). Another benefit to having abundant quantities of ALA in the skin is its ability to regulate a collagen-regulating factor known as AP-1. When ALA activates AP-1, it turns on enzymes that digest only glycation-damaged collagen. As we age, proteins become glycated, resulting in the formation of nonfunctioning cross-linked tissues or advanced glycated end products (AGEs). The accumulation of these cross-links is a hallmark molecular characteristic of visible skin aging. ALA is the only antioxidant that can boost cellular levels of glutathione, a very important antioxidant for overall health and longevity. Glutathione also rapidly depletes with age, stress, the environment, and less-than-optimal health, and its replenishment is critical to help skin's defense against accelerated skin aging. Glutathione deficit shows up on the skin as dullness, severe loss of elasticity, deep wrinkles, dryness, and visible changes in the skin's texture. Studies have shown that a major contributor to aging can be ameliorated by feeding old rats the normal mitochondrial metabolites acetyl carnitine and lipoic acid at high levels (Ames, 2004).

Topical ALA is also very effective in reducing the appearance of wrinkles and increasing firmness, tone, moisture, texture, and radiance of the skin. Thirty-three women, mean age 54 years, were included in a controlled study where half the face was treated twice daily for 12 weeks with the ALA cream and the other half with the control cream. Twelve weeks of treatment with a cream containing 5% ALA improved clinical characteristics related to photoaging of facial skin using four different parameters (Beitner, 2003).

DIMETHLAMINOETHANOL (DMAE)

DMAE is an analogue of the B vitamin choline and is a precursor of acetylcholine. Growing evidence points to acetylcholine as a ubiquitous cytokine-like molecule that regulates basic cellular processes such as proliferation, differentiation, locomotion, and secretion. Indeed, this modulatory role may contribute to the cutaneous activity of DMAE (Grossman, 2005). DMAE is a naturally occurring powerful anti-inflammatory, helping to increase skin firmness and tone and reduce wrinkling and brown spots (Jacknin, 2001). It has a very strong affinity for free radicals, stabilizing the membrane around the outside of each skin cell so that assaults from sun damage and cigarette smoke are reduced. DMAE also prevents the formation of lipofuscin, the brown pigment that becomes the basis for age spots. As with ALA, DMAE is available in supplements and in topical creams. Three percent DMAE facial gel applied daily for 16 weeks in a randomized placebo-controlled trial was shown to be efficacious in reducing forehead lines and periorbital fine wrinkles, and in the overall appearance of aging skin. Acute skin-firming effects of DMAE were confirmed by quantitative measures of cutaneous tensile strength. In vitro studies in peripheral blood lymphocytes indicated that DMAE is a moderately active anti-inflammatory agent, and that the skin is an active site of acetylcholine synthesis, storage, secretion, metabolism, and receptivity (Grossman, 2005).

The recommended oral dose is 50 to 100 milligrams per day, taken with meals. It is thought that DMAE can make epilepsy and bipolar depression worse; thus, it is advised that those with these health problems avoid DMAE. DMAE can also be overstimulating for some people, causing muscle tension or insomnia, in which case it should be discontinued (Bouchez & Graystone, 2012). For optimal health and beauty, advise your patients to take DMAE supplements and apply a topical lotion containing DMAE to the face, neck, and body.

Conclusion

Whether patients have skin problems or not, their health professional should suggest that they eat a balanced, healthy diet to meet as many of their vitamin and mineral needs as possible. Doctors should also suggest that their patients take supplements to keep their skin healthy, including vitamins B, C, D, E, and carotenoids; bioflavonoids and quercetin; the minerals copper, selenium, zinc, chromium, calcium, and magnesium; omega-3 and omega-6 fatty acids in a 2:1 dosage; and the nutrients CoQ10, ALA, acetyl-L-carnitine, and DMAE. Because it is difficult to take so many different individual supplements a day, it is recommended that multivitamins and multiminerals be taken that combine as many of the nutrients in the appropriate doses as possible.

REFERENCES

Ames, B. N. (2004). A role for supplements in optimizing health: the metabolic tune-up. *Archives of Biochemistry & Biophysics, 423*(1), 227–234.

Anstey, A. V. (2002). Systemic photoprotection with alpha-tocopherol (vitamin E) and beta-carotene. *Clinical & Experimental Dermatology, 27*(3), 170–176.

Beitner, H. (2003). Randomized, placebo-controlled, double blind study on the clinical efficacy of a cream containing 5% alpha-lipoic acid related to photoageing of facial skin. *British Journal of Dermatology, 149*(4), 841–849.

Bibel, D. J., Miller, S. J., Brown, B. E., Pandey, B. B., Elias, P. M., Shinefield, H. R., & Aly, R. (1989). Antimicrobial activity of stratum corneum lipids from normal and essential fatty acid-deficient mice. *Journal of Investigative Dermatology, 92*(4), 632–638.

Bouchez, C., & Grayson C. (2012). *Nutrients for healthy skin: inside and out.* Retrieved March 3, 2012, from *WebMD.com.* http://www.webmd.com/skin-problems-and-treatments/features/skin-nutrition

Casagrande, R., Georgetti, S. R., Verri, W. A. Jr, et al. (2006). Protective effect of topical formulations containing quercetin against UVB-induced oxidative stress in hairless mice. *Journal of Photochemistry & Photobiology B, 84*(1), 21–27.

Césarini, J. P., Michel, L., Maurette, J. M., et al. (2003). Immediate effects of UV radiation on the skin: modification by an antioxidant complex containing carotenoids. *Photodermatology, Photoimmunology & Photomedicine, 19*(4), 182–189.

Chan, S., Gerson, B., & Subramaniam, S. (1998). The role of copper, molybdenum, selenium, and zinc in nutrition and health. *Clinical Laboratory Medicine, 18*(4), 673–685.

Chondrogianni, N., Kapeta, S., Chinou, I., et al. Anti-ageing and rejuvenating effects of quercetin. *Experimental Gerontology, 45*(10), 763–771.

Clark, L. C., Combs, G. F., Turnbull, B. W., Slate, E. H., Chalker, D. K., Chow, J.,...& Taylor, J. R. (1996). Effects of selenium supplementation for cancer prevention in patients with carcinoma of the skina randomized controlled trial. *JAMA: the Journal of the American Medical Association, 276*(24), 1957–1963.

Cosgrove, M. C., Franco, O. H., Granger, S. P., et al. (2007). Dietary nutrient intakes and skin-aging appearance among middle-aged American women. *American Journal of Clinical Nutrition, 86*(4), 1225–1231.

Darr, D., et al. (1996). Effectiveness of antioxidants (vitamin C and E) with and without sunscreens as topical photoprotectants. *Acta Dermato-Venereologica, 76*(4), 264–268.

Fitzpatrick, R. E., et al. (2002). Double-blind, half-face study comparing topical vitamin C and vehicle for rejuvenation of photodamage. *Dermatologic Surgery, 28*(3), 231–236.

Greul, A. K., Grundmann, J. U., Heinrich, F., et al. (2002). Photoprotection of UV-irradiated human skin: an antioxidative combination of vitamins E and C, carotenoids, selenium and proanthocyanidins. *Skin Pharmacology & Applied Skin Physiology, 15*(5), 307–315.

Grossman, R. (2005). The role of dimethylaminoethanol in cosmetic dermatology. *American Journal of Clinical Dermatology, 6*(1), 39–47.

Heinrich, U., Tronnier, H., & Stahl, W. (2006). Antioxidant supplements improve parameters related to skin structure in humans. *Skin Pharmacology & Physiology, 19*(4), 224–231.

Holick, M. F. (2004). Sunlight and vitamin D for bone health and prevention of autoimmune diseases, cancers, and cardiovascular disease. *American Journal of Clinical Nutrition, 80*(6 Suppl), 1678S–1688S.

Holick, M. F. (2010). Vitamin D: extraskeletal health. *Endocrinology & Metabolism Clinics of North America, 39*(2), 381–400.

Jacknin, J. (2001). *Smart medicine for your skin.* New York, NY:Penguin Putnam.

Kidd, P. (2011). Astaxanthin, cell membrane nutrient with diverse clinical benefits and anti-aging potential. *Alternative Medicine Review, 16*(4), 355–364.

La Ruche, G., & Cesarini, J. P. (1991). Protective effect of oral selenium plus copper associated with vitamin complex on sunburn cell formation in human skin. *Photodermatology, Photoimmunology & Photomedicine, 8*(6), 232.

Lyons, N. M., & O'Brien, N. M. (2002). Modulatory effects of an algal extract containing astaxanthin on UVA-irradiated cells in culture. *Journal of Dermatological Science, 30*(1), 73–84.

Mahoney, M. G., Brennan, D., Starcher, B., et al. (2009). Extracellular matrix in cutaneous ageing: the effects of 0.1% copper-zinc malonate-containing cream on elastin biosynthesis. *Experimental Dermatology*, *18*(3), 205–211.

Matsumoto, K. Y., Azuma, M., Kiyok, M., et al. (1991). Involvement of endogenously produced 1,25-dihydroxyvitamin D-3 in the growth and differentiation of human keratinocytes. *Biochimica et Biophysica Acta*, *1092*(3), 311–318.

McDaniel, D. H., Neudecker, B. A., DiNardo, J. C., et al. (2005a). Clinical efficacy assessment in photodamaged skin of 0.5% and 1.0% idebenone. *Journal of Cosmetic Dermatology*, *4*(3), 167–173.

McDaniel, D. H., Neudecker, B. A., DiNardo, J. C., et al. (2005b). Idebenone: a new antioxidant—Part I. Relative assessment of oxidative stress protection capacity compared to commonly known antioxidants. *Journal of Cosmetic Dermatology*, *4*(1), 10–17.

Miquel, J., Ramírez-Boscá, A., Ramírez-Bosca, J. V., et al. (2006). Menopause: a review on the role of oxygen stress and favorable effects of dietary antioxidants. *Archives of Gerontology & Geriatrics*, *42*(3), 289–306.

Morganti, P. (2009). The photoprotective activity of nutraceuticals. *Clinical Dermatology*, *27*(2), 166–174.

Morquio, A., Rivera-Megret, F., & Dajas, F. (2005). Photoprotection by topical application of *Achyrocline satureioides* ('Marcela'). *Phytotherapy Research*, *19*(6), 486–490.

Muta-Takada, K., Terada, T., Yamanishi, H., et al. (2009). Coenzyme Q10 protects against oxidative stress-induced cell death and enhances the synthesis of basement membrane components in dermal and epidermal cells. *Biofactors*, *35*(5), 435–441.

Naldi, L., Parazzini, F., Peli, L., et al. (1996). Dietary factors and the risk of psoriasis. Results of an Italian case-control study. *British Journal of Dermatology*, *134*(1), 101–106.

Oda, Y., Uchida, Y., Moradian, S., et al. (2009). Vitamin D receptor and coactivators SRC2 and 3 regulate epidermis-specific sphingolipid production and permeability barrier formation. *Journal of Investigative Dermatology*, *129*(6), 1367–1378.

Owen R. W., Giacosa A., Hull W. E., et al. (2000). Olive-oil consumption and health: the possible role of antioxidants. *Lancet Oncol*. 1:107–12.

Perricone, N. (2000). *The wrinkle cure*. New York, NY:Rodale Books.

Perricone, N. (2004). *The Perricone promise*. New York, NY:Warner Books.

Prahl, S., Kueper, T., Biernoth, T., et al. (2008). Aging skin is functionally anaerobic: importance of coenzyme Q10 for anti aging skin care. *Biofactors*, *32*(1–4), 245–255.

Puizina-Ivić, N., Mirić, L., Carija, A., et al. (2010). Modern approach to topical treatment of aging skin. *Collegium Anthropologicum*, *34*(3), 1145–1153.

Rusciani L., Proietti I., Rusciani A. (2006). Low plasma coenzyme Q10 levels as an independent prognostic factor for melanoma progression. *J Am Acad Dermatol*. 54(2):234–41.

Saliou, C., et al. (2001). Solar ultraviolet-induced erythema in human skin and nuclear factor-kappa-B-dependent gene expression in keratinocytes are modulated by a French maritime pine bark extract. *Free Radicals in Biology & Medicine*, *30*(2), 154–160.

Sardar, S., Chakraborty, A., & Chatterjee, M. (1996). Comparative effectiveness of vitamin D3 and dietary vitamin E on peroxidation of lipids and enzymes of the hepatic antioxidant system in Sprague-Dawley rats. *International Journal of Vitamin & Nutrient Research, 66*(1), 39–45.

Simopoulos A. P. (2011). Evolutionary aspects of diet: the omega-6/omega-3 ratio and the brain. *Mol Neurobiol.* 44(2):203–15.

Stahl, W., & Sies, H. (2002). Carotenoids and protection against solar UV radiation. *Skin Pharmacology & Applied Skin Physiology, 15*(5), 291–296.

Suganuma, K., Nakajima, H., Ohtsuki, M., et al. (2010). Astaxanthin attenuates the UVA-induced up-regulation of matrix-metalloproteinase-1 and skin fibroblast elastase in human dermal fibroblasts. *Journal of Dermatological Science, 58*(2), 136–142.

Surjana, D., & Damian, D. L. (2011). Nicotinamide in dermatology and photoprotection. *Skinmed, 9*(6), 360–365.

Tavakkol, A., Nabi, Z., Soliman, N., & Polefka, T. G. (2004). Delivery of vitamin E to the skin by a novel liquid skin cleanser: comparison of topical versus oral supplementation. *Journal of Cosmetic Science, 55*(2), 177–187.

Varani, J., et al. (1998). Molecular mechanisms of intrinsic skin aging and retinoid-induced repair and reversal. *Journal of Investigative Dermatology Symposium Proceedings, 3*(1), 57–60.

Ziboh, V. A., Miller, C. C., & Cho, Y. (2000). Metabolism of polyunsaturated fatty acids by skin epidermal enzymes: generation of antiinflammatory and antiproliferative metabolites. *The American Journal of Clinical Nutrition, 71*(1), 361s–366s.

3

Therapeutic Diets For Skin Disorders

JEANETTE JACKNIN, MD

Key Concepts

♣ Diet can affect some inflammatory skin diseases such as acne. The Western diet, for example, promotes acne, while a therapeutic low-glycemic diet and a diet low in milk fat and moderate in iodine helps to reduce acne.

♣ Food allergies may play a role in atopic dermatitis, especially in children. A therapeutic diet avoiding eggs, peanuts, milk products, and any food allergens known for a given individual may help to lessen atopic dermatitis in some patients. Juices derived from anti-inflammatory fruits and vegetables may also lessen atopic dermatitis.

♣ For psoriasis, red meat and dairy may induce flares. Fasting and low-calorie diets, diets rich in omega-3 fatty acids such as certain fish and flaxseed oil, and whole-food vegetarian diets may improve psoriasis.

♣ Rosacea may flare with hot beverages, spicy foods, and alcohol consumption. Therapeutic diets minimizing animal fats and any known food allergens for the individual, avoiding refined sugars, and including ample dark-green vegetables may help to lessen rosacea.

Because certain foods are richer in one nutrient or another, specific foods are naturally helpful for certain disorders. For example, garlic is one of the strongest natural broad-spectrum antibacterial agents, and eating raw garlic cloves is a great boost to antibacterial activity. Onion is also a strong natural antibiotic, as are honey and wine. Still other foods have antiviral activity. Apples, blueberries, cranberries, grapes, grapefruit juice, mushrooms, peaches, plums, sage, tea, and red wine all have antiviral activity. Other foods help to reduce inflammation. These include apples, black currants, fatty fish such as sardines and salmon, garlic, ginger, onion, pineapple, sage, and hot chili peppers. Garlic, shiitake mushrooms, and yogurt greatly stimulate the immune system. So do fruits, vegetables, nuts, grains, and shellfish. Natural compounds found in many fruits and vegetables can interfere with some stages in the development of cancerous cells. Citrus fruits, tomatoes, broccoli, carrots, brown rice, oats, and soybeans are among the many foods that have natural anticancer activity. Food can also change your mood by affecting the body's level of serotonin, a key brain neurotransmitter. Caffeine, ginger, honey, and sugar are all known to elevate mood. Carbohydrates, folic acid (found in green leafy vegetables), and selenium (in seafood, grains, and nuts) also work to heighten your mood. Caffeine, chili peppers, cloves, garlic, ginger, licorice, onion, peppermint, and sugar all have analgesic, or painkilling, activity (Jacknin, 2001).

For various skin disorders a specific diet is very important as part of a treatment plan.

For Acne

A study by Loren Cordain, PhD, looked at the skin of more than 1,300 Islanders of Papua New Guinea and the hunter-gatherers of Paraguay who ate traditional diets (Cordain et al., 2002). None had an active case of acne. In contrast, of those eating a typical Western diet between 79% and 95% of adolescents were battling acne and between 40% and 54% of adults 25 and older were still breaking out. The typical Western diet is heavy in refined-grain breads, sugar-laden soft drinks, French fries, and processed treats like cookies and cakes. The Islanders ate mainly fruit, fish, and tubers. Likewise, the hunter-gatherers of Paraguay ate mostly whole foods found locally: peanuts, wild game, and the sweet native root manioc. Cordain and colleagues' study theorizes that our high-glycemic diet spikes insulin levels, which then indirectly bumps up sebum and skin-cell production in pores, flaring acne. Cordain later reviewed the literature (Cordain, 2005) and concluded that a large body of evidence existed showing how diet may directly or indirectly influence five causes of acne: (1) increased proliferation of basal keratinocytes within the pilosebaceous duct, (2) incomplete separation of ductal corneocytes from one another and subsequent obstruction of the pilosebaceous duct, (3) androgen-mediated increases in sebum production, (4) colonization of the comedo by *Propionibacterium acnes*, and (5) inflammation both within and adjacent to the comedo. Cordain's findings were confirmed when 43 male acne patients aged 15 to 25 years old were studied (Smith et al., 2005, 2007) during a 12-week, experimental treatment with a low-glycemic-load diet composed of 25% energy from protein and 45% from low-glycemic-index carbohydrates. The control acne patients ate carbohydrate-dense foods, ignoring the glycemic index. At 12 weeks, mean acne lesion counts had decreased more in the low-glycemic-load group than in the control group. The experimental diet also resulted in greater improvement in insulin sensitivity than did the control.

- Dr. Perricone (Perricone, 2003) recommends a three-day skin-clearing diet to get a quick visible reduction in acne lesions. It is a strict anti-inflammatory, low-glycemic diet and consists of lots of spring water, egg whites, salmon, oatmeal, ground flaxseed, cantaloupe, blueberries, green or black tea, sardines, olive oil, romaine lettuce, apples, yogurt, pumpkin seeds, fresh-squeezed lemon juice, steamed vegetables, turkey breast, pecans, and almonds.
- Food sensitivities can also cause flare-ups of acne and need to be evaluated. Blood tests for food allergens that cause delayed reactions can be done. Immediate food sensitivities can be discovered through the careful use of a food diary in which the patients record everything they eat and their skin's and body's apparent reactions. Suspect foods can then be avoided (Jacknin, 2001).
- It is important to limit milk and milk products to one or two servings a day, as data suggest that dairy products can be problematic for people with acne and other inflammatory skin conditions. Dairy products may cause the body to produce more androgens, which cause more oil and sebum to clog pores. Also, dairy produced in nonorganic farms may contain external hormones and pesticides, which can flare existing skin conditions. Acne patients can eat calcium-rich vegetables such as spinach and collard greens in lieu of more dairy.
- Too much iodine can irritate pores and cause flare-ups. Have your patients limit foods that have high levels of iodine: iodized salt, fast foods, sea vegetables, kelp tablets, milk, and shellfish (Jacknin, 2001).

For Dry Skin

Suggest to your patients that they:
- Keep well hydrated with a minimum of eight glasses of pure or sparkling water a day. Limit dehydrating coffee, alcohol, and colas.
- Eat fish, rolled oats, and ground flaxseeds frequently, as they are high in omega-3 essential fatty acids, which help the skin to retain moisture.

- Eat plenty of carrots, tomatoes, green leafy vegetables, cantaloupes, and apricots. These foods supply carotenoids from which the body manufactures vitamin A, which is essential for skin cell growth and repair.
- Eat plenty of whole grains, legumes, wheat germ, and nutritional yeast. These are good sources of pantothenic acid, important in the synthesis of much-needed fats and oils.
- Sorbitol helps the skin retain moisture and is found in grapes, berries, plums, pears, and seaweeds and algae.

Eczema and Atopic Dermatitis

Food allergens can be a big flare factor in eczema. One hundred thirteen patients with severe atopic dermatitis were evaluated (Sampson, 1985) for food hypersensitivity with double-blind placebo-controlled oral food challenges. Fifty-six percent of children experienced 101 positive food challenges; skin symptoms developed in 84% of the challenges. Eggs, peanut, and milk accounted for 72% of the hypersensitivity reactions induced. When patients were given appropriate restrictive diets based on oral food challenge results, most showed significant improvement in their clinical course compared with patients in whom no food allergy was documented. The role of foods in the exacerbation of atopic eczema was also studied (Sloper et al., 1991) by offering a food elimination diet and subsequent random-order, double-blind food challenges to 91 eczematous children. Eczema improved in 74% of patients after stopping cows' milk, eggs, and various other foods, with significant decreases in erythema, excoriation, lichenification, and extent of the eczema. Sloper and colleagues suggested that a standard elimination diet avoiding cows' milk, egg, tomato, colors, and preservatives should help up to three quarters of children with moderate or severe eczema.

- Eczema can clear within a few days to several weeks after the offending food allergens are removed from the diet. Use an elimination or exclusion diet to pinpoint foods that cause flare-ups. There is also blood testing for delayed-sensitivity allergens, foods that cause symptoms one to three days after the food is eaten. Many allergists suggest a rotation diet after the initial evaluation of the food allergens. Different foods are rotated into the diet over a period of four to seven days, so that the same food is not eaten twice during this period. This can increase patients' ability to tolerate foods to which they previously reacted and decreases the risk of developing new food sensitivities that will cause a flare-up of eczema. Clinical ecologists think that between 10% and 30% of people in industrialized countries have food and chemical sensitivities that sometimes manifest as eczema. Abnormal intestinal bacteria or enzyme deficiencies may magnify the food sensitivities and secondarily the eczema.

- Juice made from anti-inflammatory fruits and vegetables such as black-currants, red grapes, carrots, beets, spinach, celery, cucumber, parsley, green juices, and wheatgrass can help reduce flares of eczema (Jacknin, 2001). A glass of 16 to 24 ounces of vegetable juice at night can be very helpful in controlling eczema. This vegetable juice should consist mostly of dark-green vegetables such as parsley, kale, cucumber, zucchini, green pepper, and celery, with an apple added for sweetness.

Hair Loss and Scalp Problems

- Hair is made up mostly of protein. Therefore, it is necessary to eat enough protein as part of a healthy diet to maintain normal hair production.
- Vitamins B6, B12, biotin, and folic acid are also important for proper hair development and health. Good sources of vitamin B6 include bananas, potatoes (both white and sweet), and spinach. Citrus fruits, tomatoes, whole-grain and fortified grain products, beans, and lentils contain lots of folic acid. Major sources of B12 include meat, poultry, fish, and dairy products. Suggest your patients include plenty of whole soy foods in their diet, as soybeans are a rich source of biotin, or vitamin B7 which is also important for healthy skin and hair (Jacknin, 2001).
- Essential fatty acids—especially omega-3 fatty acids—play a key role in hair development and maintenance. One should eat some of these foods every day if possible: salmon, tuna, mackerel, and other fatty fish, flaxseed oil, walnuts, and almonds.
- Because magnesium and zinc also affect the health of hair, make sure your patients' diets are rich in these trace minerals.

Nail Problems

- Fresh carrot juice containing calcium and phosphorus is great for strengthening the nails.
- Suggest that your patients' diets include foods high in biotin, a B vitamin essential for strong and healthy nails. Good sources of biotin

include egg yolks, whole soy products, cereals, yeast, cauliflower, lentils, milk, and peanut butter.
- Lots of protein, vitamin C, and zinc are essential for strong nails.

Psoriasis

Diet is thought to be key in controlling psoriasis, both in terms of the many suspected sensitivities that may keep the skin reacting and as a major factor in determining the alkalinity of the blood. In two recent reviews (Araujo et al., 2009; Wolters, 2005) it was noted that omega-3, fasting, low-calorie, and vegetarian diets improved psoriatic symptoms in some studies. Each of these diets modifies the polyunsaturated fatty acid metabolism and influences the eicosanoid profile so that inflammatory processes are suppressed. Some patients with psoriasis also show an elevated sensitivity to gluten and improve after a gluten-free diet. In general, the whole-foods diet with lots of fresh yellow and green vegetables, soybeans, chickpeas, lentils, black beans, sesame seeds, lean proteins, and low-fat fish that I have recommended is great for psoriatic patients.

- Food sensitivities need to be assessed and treated, either by professional testing or by elimination and then careful reintroduction of one food at a time, noting any flare-ups of symptoms along the way. Usually, if your patients itch, it is something they ate the previous day or earlier in the day that their skin cannot tolerate and is reacting to. Suspects to test for possible allergy or sensitivity to include wheat, milk, eggs, meat, dairy products, shellfish, aromatic spices, citrus fruits and juices, and nuts. In a study published in the *California Medicine Journal* in 1980, an elimination diet was shown to significantly help patients' psoriasis.
- Have your patients limit their intake of protein. As far back as the early 1900s, Dr. L. Duncan Bulkley reported in a speech to the Dermatology Section of the AMA that a low-protein, mainly vegetarian diet is best for people with psoriasis. In 1932, Dr. Jay Schamberg, a highly respected professor of dermatology at the University of Pennsylvania, wrote in the *Journal of the American Medical Association* that in his patients with psoriasis, "a low-protein diet, without any other internal or external treatment, causes a disappearance of the greater part of the eruptions." The growth of skin cells can also be curbed by fasting, and many people with psoriasis have noted improvement on a fasting and vegetarian regimen.
- Many natural-medicine experts recommend that the blood of psoriasis patients be kept slightly alkaline, with a pH of 7.3 to 7.5, in order

to maintain the optimal internal chemical milieu for strong immunity, efficient removal of toxins, and clearing of the skin lesions. The daily diet should consist of 80% alkaline-forming foods and 20% acid-forming foods. Fruits, vegetables, and fiber form the core of the diet. Exceptions to this are the citrus fruits and vegetables of the nightshade family. Citrus fruits and juices, strawberries, tomatoes, tobacco, eggplant, white potatoes, peppers, paprika, and hot, spicy foods should be eliminated from the diet of people with psoriasis.

- Recommend that your patients eat a high-fiber diet to speed removal of toxins via the bowel.
- Red meat and dairy products contain arachidonic acid, which increases inflammation, flaring lesions.
- Fish like salmon, sardines, mackerel, herring, and tuna are high in omega-3 essential fatty acids, which can help reduce itchiness and inflammation. Free fatty acid levels are abnormal in psoriatic skin. At least one tablespoon of olive oil, cod liver oil, flaxseed oil, or canola oil should be added to food each day to increase the intake of oils with beneficial omega-3 fatty acids.
- Have your patients choose whole-grain products over white bread and foods made with white flour. In studies, people intermittently following a strict rice diet found that their psoriasis cleared significantly. Sugar, tea, animal fats, food additives, vinegar, and carbonated beverages increase the body's acidity and should also be limited as much as possible.
- Juicing is very helpful for psoriatics. Fresh vegetable juices, particularly beet, carrot, cucumber, lettuce, parsley, and spinach, are healthy. Suggested combinations include apple and carrot, cucumber and grape, or beet, carrot, and garlic juice mixed together. Have your patients avoid citrus juices.
- Coffee, caffeine, and alcohol impair liver function and should be avoided, if possible.
- Drinking six to eight glasses of pure, filtered water every day in addition to any other liquids is particularly important in aiding the elimination of toxins and acidity problems.

Rosacea

- Investigate the possibility of food allergies and sensitivities that may cause flare-ups.
- Hot coffee, tea, and hot chocolate can all flare rosacea. Suggest your patients decrease the temperature of hot drinks in order to reduce

flares. Also, they should try decreasing the number of cups they drink down to one or two a day.

- Avoid alcohol and spicy foods, which usually aggravate rosacea.
- Patients should identify and avoid other foods that aggravate their unique case of rosacea. People with rosacea have reported a wide variety of foods that trigger flare-ups in their individual cases. Examples include cheese, sour cream, yogurt, citrus fruit, liver, chocolate, vanilla, soy sauce, yeast extract, vinegar, eggplant, avocados, spinach, broad-leafed beans and pods, and foods high in histamine or niacin. Taking an antihistamine about two hours before a meal may offset the effects of histamine, while aspirin may reduce the effects of niacin-containing foods in rosacea patients affected by them.
- Have your patients eat plenty of dark-green vegetables, which are rich in vitamin B12, important in healing rosacea.
- Patients should avoid animal and hydrogenated fats, which promote inflammation in rosacea. That means eliminating dairy products, red meat, fried foods, and margarine as much as possible.
- Have your patients avoid junk food, refined sugars, and artificial flavorings and preservatives, all of which are toxic for their skin and can flare rosacea.

Conclusion

Specific dietary modulation can help the signs and symptoms of some of your patients' skin disorders. In particular, anecdotal reports of successful dietary manipulation have been confirmed in studies on acne, dry skin, eczema, hair and nail disorders, psoriasis, and rosacea.

REFERENCES

Araujo, M. L., Burgos, M. G., & Moura, I. S. (2009). [Nutritional influences in psoriasis]. *Anais Brasileiros de Dermatologia, 84*(1), 90–92.

Cordain, L. (2005). Implications for the role of diet in acne. *Seminars in Cutaneous Medicine & Surgery, 24*(2). 84–91.

Cordain, L., Lindeberg, S., Hurtado, M., et al. (2002). Acne vulgaris: a disease of Western civilization. *Archives of Dermatology, 138*(12), 1584–1590.

Jacknin, J. (2001). *Smart medicine for your skin.* New York, NY:Penguin Putnam.

Perricone, N. (2003). *The acne prescription.* New York, NY:HarperCollins.

Sampson, H. A., & McCaskill, C. C. (1985). Food hypersensitivity and atopic dermatitis: evaluation of 113 patients. *The Journal of Pediatrics, 107*(5), 669–675.

Sloper, K. S., Wadsworth, J., & Brostoff, J. (1991). Children with atopic eczema. I: Clinical response to food elimination and subsequent double-blind food challenge. *Quarterly Journal of Medicine, 80*(292), 677–693.

Smith, R. N., Mann, N. J., Braue, A., et al. (2005). A low-glycemic-load diet improves symptoms in acne vulgaris patients: a randomized controlled trial. *Dermatological Surgery, 31*(7 Pt 2), 855–860.

Smith, R. N., Mann, N. J., Braue, A., et al. (2007). The effect of a high-protein, low glycemic-load diet versus a conventional, high glycemic-load diet on biochemical parameters associated with acne vulgaris: a randomized, investigator-masked, controlled trial. *Journal of the American Academy of Dermatology, 57*(2), 247–256.

Wolters, M. (2005). Diet and psoriasis: experimental data and clinical evidence. *British Journal of Dermatology, 153*(4), 706–714.

4

Skin-Influencing Factors in Daily Life

KATY BURRIS, MD, ANDREA M. HUI, MD,
AND ADEKEMI AKINGBOYE, MD

Key Concepts

♣ UVA and UVB light cause the majority of effects on the skin, which can be short term and/or long term.

♣ A large body of evidence supports the role of several vitamins in photoaging.

♣ Emollients are the foundation of dermatologic treatment and help maintain normal skin function.

♣ Ceramides represent 40% of the lipid content in the human stratum corneum and play a vital role in maintaining the epidermal barrier.

♣ Our body works to maintain homeostasis despite potential external influences such as UV light, heat, humidity, and chemicals.

Introduction

There is no question that the external environment plays a significant role in the maintenance of skin health. Numerous factors may influence the overall health and appearance, many of which will be reviewed in this chapter.

Ultraviolet Exposure

It is well known and accepted that ultraviolet radiation (UVR) exposure can have numerous effects on the skin. UVR is a part of the electromagnetic spectrum and is usually subdivided into UVA (400 to 315 nm), UVB (315 to

290 nm), and UVC (290 to 200 nm); UVA is then further subdivided into UVA1 (400 to 340 nm) and UVA2 (340 to 315 nm) (Bolognia et al., 2008). Fortunately, the most energetic form of UVR, UVC, is largely absorbed by the atmospheric ozone layer and normally does not reach the surface of the earth (Polefka et al., 2012). UVB is blocked by window glass while UVA is not. UVA and UVB therefore cause the majority of effects on the skin, which can be short term and/or long term.

SHORT-TERM EFFECTS OF UVR

Visible, short-term effects of UVR on the skin include sunburn and tanning. The most immediate response of human skin to UVR exposure is sunburn erythema, caused principally by UVB and short-wavelength UVA (Clydesdale et al., 2001). The ability to induce sunburn rapidly declines with increasing wavelength. UV light with a wavelength of 360 nm is significantly less erythemogenic than light with a wavelength of 300 nm (Bolognia et al., 2008).

UVB-induced sunburns reach their peak between 6 and 24 hours after exposure. An immediate erythematous reaction is rarely observed after UVB exposure, whereas an immediate erythema is regularly observed after exposure to a high dose of UVA (Bolognia et al., 2008). UVA induces immediate tanning and persistent pigment darkening through oxidation of preexisting melanin or melanogenic precursors, as opposed to UVB-induced delayed tanning, which requires the activation of melanocytes (Wolber et al., 2008) via the development of pigment from de novo synthesis of melanin. Delayed tanning peaks approximately 3 days after sun exposure (Clydesdale et al., 2001).

UV light also exerts numerous effects on the immune system. UVR suppresses T-cell–mediated immune reactions, which are the critical cellular mediators of the vast majority of inflammatory dermatoses (Schwarz, 2010), thus allowing for phototherapy as treatment of conditions such as psoriasis or atopic dermatitis. However, chronic exposure to UVR is also responsible for suppressing key elements of the human immune system, such as in immune surveillance. In addition to being a risk factor for skin cancer, UVR-induced immunosuppression has been linked to altered responses to infectious agents, interference with vaccinations, and the expression of latent viruses such as herpes virus and human papilloma virus (Norval, 2006).

LONG-TERM EFFECTS OF UVR

One of the most important long-term associations is that between UV damage and the risk of skin cancer. There are three major types of skin cancer: basal cell carcinoma, squamous cell carcinoma, and melanoma. Chronic exposure to UVR is the predominant cause of non-melanoma skin cancers. Over 80% of these cancers develop on parts of the body exposed to the sun, including the face, neck, and arms (Alberts & Hess, 2008). Carcinogenesis is viewed as a multistep process involving initiation, promotion, and progression. Unlike any other carcinogen, UVR is considered to be a complete carcinogen; it not only initiates the mutagenic event (similar to most carcinogens) but also promotes and advances the progression of cancerous cells (Bickers & Athar, 2006). Epidemiological data indicate that excessive or cumulative sunlight exposure takes place years before the resulting skin cancers develop. The most important defense mechanisms that protect human skin against UVR involve melanin synthesis and active repair mechanisms. DNA is the major target of direct or indirect UV-induced cellular damage, leading to the development of skin cancers years later (Rass & Reichrath, 2008).

Another important long-term side effect of UV exposure is its contribution to the skin's natural aging process, known as photoaging. Photoaged skin is characterized by dryness, mottled pigmentation, sallowness, deep furrows and wrinkles, telangiectasia, significant laxity, precancerous lesions, rough texture, and a leathery appearance (Rabe et al., 2006). Histologically, the classic finding is solar elastosis; thinning of the stratum corneum and flattening of the dermoepidermal junction are also seen. The UVA and UVB in sunlight both promote photoaging proportionally to the intensity, duration, and frequency of exposure.

Other than sun avoidance, sunscreens are the first line of defense against UVR. Many UV filters have been developed in recent years that enhance product efficacy, safety, and cosmesis. Topically applied sunscreens protect by absorbing or reflecting UVR at the skin surface. UV filters can be grouped into two broad categories: chemical and physical. Polyphenols are naturally occurring compounds found in foods that may potentially have sunscreen capabilities. Most of the natural polyphenols are pigments, typically yellow, red, or purple, and can absorb UVR. It is believed that when applied topically, they may be able to prevent penetration of the UVR into the skin. The UVR that polyphenols can absorb includes the entire UVB spectrum of wavelengths and part of the UVC and UVA spectra (Nichols & Katiyar, 2010). This is exciting as they may have the potential to serve more specifically as recognized UV filters in the future.

Recent attention has developed in regards to the theory of chemoprevention, which is defined as a means of cancer control that is based on the use of specific natural or synthetic chemical substances that can suppress, retard, or reverse the process of carcinogenesis (Nichols & Katiyar, 2010). UVR is known to generate hydrogen peroxide and other reactive oxygen species free radicals, which frequently damage DNA, RNA, lipids, and proteins in human skin (Jagdeo & Brody, 2011). Some studies have demonstrated that alternative therapies such as caffeine and green tea polyphenols may serve as potential antioxidants. Alpha-hydroxy acids (AHAs) are compounds derived from dairy products (lactic acid), fruit (malic acid and citric acid), or sugar cane (glycolic acid). Topical treatment of photodamaged skin with AHA has been reported to improve wrinkling, roughness, and dyspigmentation within months of daily application (Stiller et al., 1996).

There is a large body of evidence supporting the role of several vitamins in photoaging. In particular, there is strong evidence to suggest the benefit of topical retinols, vitamin C, vitamin B3, and vitamin E in the treatment and prevention of photoaging (Zussman et al., 2010). Retinols and carotenoids are the two most common forms of vitamin A studied for their role in protecting the skin from UV-induced damage. Although the data are lacking for carotenoids, vast funds of unequivocal scientific data support the use of retinol and its derivatives for the treatment of the clinical manifestations of photoaging via increasing epidermal thickness and collagen production. Additionally, there are studies that raise the possibility that topical retinoids may have a place in the chemoprevention of skin cancers as well (Cho et al., 2005).

Vitamin C plays an important role as it is critical in the synthesis of collagen and elastin as well as an important antioxidant in the skin, modulating the effects of UV-induced reactive oxygen species (ROS) damage (Zussman et al., 2010). However, there is controversy regarding exogenous ascorbic acid. It is innately unstable in formulation and it is unclear how much, if any, intact molecule remains on the skin with topical application (Gaspar & Campos, 2007). Vitamin E is thought to play an important role in skin aging because of its antioxidant properties and its contribution to the regulation of collagen breakdown. Vitamin E functions within biological membranes to halt lipid peroxidation from the formation of free radicals (Zussman et al., 2010).

Vitamin B3, also known as niacinamide, has been shown to increase collagen production in both mouse studies and in human fibroblast cell culture. Both topical niacinamide and oral niacin are effective in preventing UV-induced immunosuppression and carcinogenesis. Niacin is a precursor to nicotinamide-adenine dinucleotide (NAD), which is largely involved in DNA surveillance and repair proteins, namely p53 and poly (adenosine 5'-diphosphoribose-ribose) polymerase activity (Zussman et al., 2010). Although nicotinamide has photoprotective effects against carcinogenesis and immune suppression in mice (Damian, 2010), it remains to be seen in clinical trials if it is photoimmunoprotective in humans as well.

Humidity and Dryness

The principal role of the skin is to provide protection against physical injury, regulate temperature, and prevent loss of body water. Variations in humidity in the environment with the changing of seasons and environment are correlated with worsening of skin conditions such as atopic dermatitis and psoriasis (Wilkinson & Rycroft, 1992). Accordingly, these conditions are exacerbated during the winter and in arid climates, where low humidity can further impair normal epidermal barrier function and cause skin dryness.

Skin dryness is described by visible, textural, and sensory changes to the skin (Linde, 1992). It is a disturbance in the normal physiological processes of healthy skin, which may result in a change in a patient's perception of his or her skin's health. Redness, flakiness, scaliness, and fissures are all visible symptoms of skin dryness. The skin may feel rough and bumpy (Linde, 1992). The patient may complain of sensations such as tightness, itching, burning, and pain, due to the activation of unmyelinated C nerve fibers (Kakigi & Mochizuki, 2011). The prolongation of skin dryness may inevitably lead to breakdown of the skin barrier and worsening of inflammatory dermatoses.

Water is vital to the function of the stratum corneum. Enzymes within the stratum corneum require water in order to degrade the corneodesmosomes and allow normal desquamation (Menon et al., 1992). As keratinocytes terminally differentiate from the basal layer of the epidermis, the cells flatten out and extrude lipids. The keratinocytes then cornify to become corneocytes, developing a thick, protein-rich cornified envelope.

The cornified envelope contains keratin bundles, which are highly cross-linked and provide an insoluble barrier (Downing, 1992). The corneocytes are held together intercellularly by lipids. The lipid layer comprises mostly cholesterol, free fatty acids, and ceramides (Popa et al., 2012). The stratum corneum is constantly renewing itself and is highly efficient at repairing itself after normal wear.

Another important component of the stratum corneum is natural moisturizing factor (NMF), which accounts for 20% to 30% of its total dry weight and comprises amino acids and its metabolic byproducts. It is formed from the breakdown of filaggrin and released by lamellar granules and is ultimately deposited in the stratum corneum (Rawlings & Harding, 2004). The extremely hydrophilic NMF acts as a humectant and allows the stratum corneum to absorb water in a low-humidity environment (Rawlings et al., 1994). When NMF is removed from the skin in vitro, the stratum corneum is significantly less able to absorb water (Laden & Spitzer, 1967). NMF is also important for the maintenance of stratum corneum elasticity (Imokawa et al., 1991). Clinically, NMF deficiency manifests as severe scaliness and dryness of skin, which may be seen in a genetic skin disorder called ichthyosis vulgaris (Kawasaki et al., 2011). NMF levels decline as people age, which correlates with the drier skin commonly observed in the elderly population (White-Chu & Reddy, 2011).

When skin is dry, the desmosomes persist, hindering desquamation and allowing the abnormal aggregation of corneocytes on the uppermost surface of the skin. This results in scaling and flakiness, which compromises the skin barrier (Rawlings et al., 1994). The stratum corneum requires water to maintain its suppleness and softness. The loss of water in the stratum corneum can cause corneocytes to become brittle and eventually crack. The glass transition temperature, or the temperature below which a substance becomes brittle, is highly influenced by humidity levels. Normally, the glass transition temperature of keratins within the stratum corneum is slightly below body temperature. When the ambient humidity decreases, the glass transition temperature increases above body temperature, thus resulting in brittle corneocytes at normal body temperature. Skin cracks then become apparent (Ananthapadmanabhan et al., 2004). When the stratum corneum is dry and brittle, it is necessary to hydrate the skin with water before applying lipid-based substances such as petrolatum or oils. The hydrophilic portions of the stratum corneum are dependent upon water to maintain the normal function of its intercellular lipids and keratin fibers (Elias, 1981).

Dysregulation of the normal epidermal barrier results in inflammation (Denda et al., 1998). In environments with low humidity, inflammatory conditions such as pruritus, atopic dermatitis, and psoriasis are often exacerbated. The pro-inflammatory cytokine interleukin-1α (IL-1α), preformed within keratinocytes, is immediately released when the skin barrier is disrupted. IL-1α then upregulates the release of other pro-inflammatory cytokines, such as intercellular adhesion molecule-1 (ICAM-1), IL-6, IL-8, and granulocyte colony-stimulating factor, further increasing inflammation of the skin (Barker et al, 1991; Wood et al., 1992).

Humidity levels of less than 10% can cause the stratum corneum to actively lose moisture. Studies have shown that humidity levels of 70% or higher are able to restore moisture to the skin but are not required to maintain skin health and comfort. Patients should be instructed to adjust their humidifiers to a setting of 45% to 60%, which can maintain humidity such that levels in the home environment do not drop below 10% (Cohen-Mansfield & Jensen, 2005).

Winter months and cold climates pose a challenge due to low ambient humidity caused by evaporation from cold winds and use of home heating systems. Summer months and tropical climates can also cause low humidity by the use of air conditioners and dehumidifiers. Patients should be instructed to adjust their thermostats cooler (for winter months) or warmer (for summer months) while maintaining safety and comfort. Humidifiers should be used during winter months.

Patients should be advised to take short, tepid showers. Harsh soaps, combined with frequent long hot showers, remove the naturally occurring lipids on the skin surface. In those with already dry skin and/or inflammatory dermatoses, this further damages the skin and compromises skin barrier. In addition to changing bathing habits, patients should be instructed to regularly apply emollients as often as needed to maintain healthy skin (discussed later). Emollients should be applied while skin is still damp after bathing (within 5 minutes), and throughout the day (Hon et al., 2005).

Heat

Temperature regulation is a vital function of skin. The core body temperature for humans is maintained at approximately 36°C to 37.5°C (96.8°F to 99.5°F) (Bolognia et al., 2008). The daily environment can affect the body's temperature, requiring the skin to undergo many processes that maintain the ideal temperature by giving off excess heat or insulating against cold.

Several million eccrine sweat glands are present on the surface of human skin (Sato et al., 1989). When the ambient temperature is excessively hot or energy is internally generated through physical exertion, the skin allows the body to release excess heat through evaporative cooling by sweating. This mechanism protects the body against high temperatures at which proteins begin to denature, at approximately 45°F to 50°C (Sato et al., 1989). The eccrine sweat glands are under neurological control, secreting a plasma-like fluid while resorbing sodium in the ducts. The sweat is therefore hypotonic (Sato et al., 1989).

Excess heat is eliminated by release of sweat from the eccrine sweat glands, resulting in an evaporative cooling from the skin's surface. The importance of sweating is best demonstrated by conditions in which the sweat glands are absent, such as in the genetic disease hypohidrotic ectodermal dysplasia (Sato et al., 1989). Normal activities such as exercise place these patients at high risk of sudden death from high body temperature, due to the inability of the body to regulate excessively high core temperature through sweating. If a patient with hypohidrotic ectodermal dysplasia wishes to exercise, water may be sprayed on the patient to create an evaporative cooling effect (Jammersen et al., 2011).

Emollients

Emollients are the foundation of dermatologic treatment and help maintain normal skin function. The terms "emollients" and "moisturizers" are often used interchangeably. Emollients often contain humectants, which provide hydration to the stratum corneum, and occlusive agents, which effectively "seal in" moisture.

As soon as a patient applies an emollient, a smoothening effect is noted. This is because the emollient fills in the gaps between desquamated corneocytes, flattening out curled edges and improving cohesion between individual corneocytes (Leveque et al., 1987). Humectants then provide moisture to the skin to maintain a healthy, protective barrier against the harsh environment. Normal skin also functions to regulate transepidermal water loss, which then regulates body temperature and homeostasis. The main goal of all emollients is to improve the hydration of the stratum corneum and normalize epidermal barrier function. To best recommend an emollient, the practitioner must understand the different types of ingredients present in most commercially available emollients.

Occlusive Ingredients

Occlusive ingredients function to delay transepidermal water loss by coating the stratum corneum (Loden & Lindberg, 1991) and are generally oily substances (Table 4.1). This allows the epidermis to gradually replace any areas deficient in moisture through movement of water from the dermis and basal layer of the epidermis (Wu et al., 1983). However, transepidermal water loss is still a necessary aspect of skin barrier function, as it initiates barrier repair and synthesis of intercellular lipids (Jass & Elias, 1991).

Petrolatum is considered one of the most superior emollients and can significantly decrease transepidermal water loss by up to 99% while allowing the necessary cellular signals to initiate barrier repair (Friberg & Ma, 1993). It is often the gold standard occlusive to which other occlusive ingredients are clinically compared (Morrison, 2000). Petrolatum comprises purified hydrocarbons derived from petroleum. Its hydrocarbon molecules prevent oxidation, which result in a long shelf life. However, petrolatum application results in a

Table 4.1. Occlusive Ingredients

Class	Examples
Silicones	Dimethicone, cyclomethicone
Hydrocarbon oils and waxes	Petrolatum, mineral oil, paraffin, squalene
Wax esters	Lanolin, beeswax
Sterols	Ceramides, cholesterol
Polyhydric alcohols	Propylene glycol
Fatty alcohols	Lanolin alcohol, cetyl alcohol
Fatty acids	Lanolin acid, stearic acid
Vegetable wax	Carnauba wax
Vegetable oils	Soybean oil, castor oil, corn oil

greasy sensation, which may be cosmetically disagreeable. It may be combined with other less oily ingredients to improve its texture.

Direct replenishment of stratum corneum lipids may be accomplished by adding lipids and fats to topical emollients. Commonly used ingredients lanolin, triglycerides, ceramides, cholesterol, oil, waxes, and silicone, are also effective in coating the skin and preventing evaporative water loss. Lanolin is a popular occlusive ingredient. It is produced from sheep sebum and contains cholesterol, a vital component of the lipid bilayer within the stratum corneum (Lee & Warshaw, 2008). However, contact sensitization to lanolin may occur, leading manufacturers to regularly omit lanolin from their products (Stalder, 2005). Cholesterol itself may be used as an emulsifier in topical emollients to stabilize water-and-oil preparations (Barany et al., 2000).

Triglycerides may be oil (liquid) or fat (solid). Vegetable and fish oils contain essential fatty acids (EFAs) such as omega-3 and omega-6 fatty acids (McCusker & Grant-Kels, 2010). These fatty acids are derived from linoleic and alpha-linoleic acid. The most abundant EFA in the skin is linoleic acid (McCusker & Grant-Kels, 2010). EFAs play a major role in epidermal physiology, eicosanoid production, and cell signaling, and are also incorporated in ceramides, which maintain normal barrier function (Hansen & Jensen, 1985; Rodrigues et al., 2012).

Ceramides represent 40% of the lipid content in the human stratum corneum (Downing et al., 1987) and play a vital role in maintaining the epidermal barrier. Ceramides are not present below the layer of the stratum granulosum and are therefore a product of terminal keratinocyte differentiation. The direct application of ceramide-containing topical emollients has been shown to significantly improve inflammatory dermatoses such as atopic dermatitis by replenishing missing ceramides (Kircik & Del Rosso, 2011).

Humectants

When ambient humidity decreases below 80%, water is drawn into the stratum corneum from the underlying epidermis and dermis, and then water is lost into the environment, resulting in a continuous cycle of dryness. The addition of humectants to emollients improves the stratum corneum's ability to absorb water from the environment and also from the underlying epidermis (Idson, 1992). The corneocytes within the stratum corneum become hydrated and swell, creating a sensation of smoothness and suppleness. Commonly used humectants include propylene glycol, AHAs, beta-hydroxy acids (BHAs), glycerin, hyaluronic acid, and urea (Table 4.2).

Hydroxy acids function as both a humectant and exfoliant. These organic acids are naturally occurring; for example, glycolic acid is derived from sugar

Table 4.2. Humectant Ingredients

Class	Examples
Hydroxy acids	Glycolic acid, lactic acid, malic acid, citric acid, salicylic acid
NMF	Urea, lactic acid
Others	Glycerin, propylene glycol

cane, malic acid from apples, and lactic acid from sour milk. Lactic acid is also a component of NMFs and was the first AHA used for the treatment of ichthyosis (Stern, 1946). Lactic acid has been show in vitro and in vivo to stimulate production of ceramides by keratinocytes (Thueson et al., 1998), thus decreasing transepidermal water loss. Salicylic acid, a BHA derived from willow bark, also works well as a humectant and exfoliant. Additionally, salicylic acid acts as an effective comedolytic and is often added to over-the-counter acne treatments to improve comedonal acne (Green et al., 2009).

AHAs and BHAs have been clinically shown to normalize epidermal keratinization and exfoliation by degrading intercellular desmosomes (Van Scott & Yu, 1974). The disadhesion occurs at the level of the stratum granulosum (Van Scott & Yu, 1984). At the low concentrations present in commercially available emollients, AHAs and BHAs help to thin the stratum corneum, which in turn creates a more flexible, smooth surface and improved skin barrier (Van Scott & Yu, 1974). Hydroxy acids can be used regularly to help slough corneocytes for the improvement of thick calluses, seborrheic keratosis, and warts (Van Scott & Yu, 1984). Additionally, AHAs confer an anti-inflammatory benefit by decreasing erythema after UV exposure (Perricone & DiNardo, 1996).

Glycerin (glycerol) is a powerful humectant that allows the stratum corneum to effectively retain water in a dry environment (Choi et al., 2005). Urea is a component of NMF and functions similarly to glycerin (Rawlings & Harding, 2004). Hyaluronic acid is a naturally occurring glycosaminoglycan that is widely distributed in epithelial tissues. It is highly hygroscopic and effectively absorbs water from the atmosphere (Monheit & Coleman, 2006). It is probably best known as a dermal filler to correct facial wrinkles and has thus been marketed for its "anti-wrinkle" effects, although it does not penetrate the epidermis when applied topically (Denda et al., 1998). Propylene glycol functions as a humectant and occlusive and increases penetration of other topically applied products (Barany et al., 2000).

Other Ingredients

Preservatives are necessary to prevent bacterial growth in topical emollients. An optimal preservative should be safe and stable, should exhibit broad antimicrobial activity, and should not affect the consistency and efficacy of the emollient. Most emollients contain a combination of preservatives (Wade et al., 2000). Parabens are a common preservative. Antioxidants such as tocopherol, ascorbic acid (vitamin C), and butylated hydroxytoluene (BHT) react with free radicals to inhibit rancidity of the emollient. Chelating agents such as citric acid, tartaric acid, and EDTA react with heavy-metal ions and thus increase antioxidant activity (Wade et al., 2000).

Topical Formulations

There are several types of emollients depending on their oil and water composition. Ointments are highly viscous, greasy emollients made up of mostly oil with some water and are the best at occluding the skin surface and preventing transepidermal water loss. Ointments typically contain paraffins, animal fats, vegetable oils, and waxes (White-Chu & Reddy, 2011). Creams are an emulsion consisting of equal parts of oil and water. They are less greasy than ointments and are therefore more cosmetically elegant. Lotions have a higher water content than creams, which decreases their viscosity and allows easier application (Elson, 2011). Gels are mostly water, with some oil and a carbomer gelling agent. When applied topically, the gelling agent quickly dissipates and then allows the oil and water to spread evenly (Elson, 2011). Liquids are mostly made of water and can be formulated as emulsions or solutions.

Conclusion

Our skin is under regulation from internal as well as external factors. Our body works to maintain homeostasis despite potential external influences such as UV light, heat, humidity, and chemicals. To maintain this balance requires a thorough understanding of these factors and their effect on the skin, as well as knowledge of the treatments available.

REFERENCES

Alberts, D., & Hess, L. M. (2008). *Fundamentals of cancer prevention*. Verlag Berlin Heidelberg: Springer.

Ananthapadmanabhan, K. P., Moore, D. J., Subramanyan, K., Misra, M., & Meyer, F. (2004). Cleansing without compromise: the impact of cleansers on the skin barrier and the technology of mild cleansing. *Dermatologic Therapy, 17,* 16–25.

Barany, E., Lindberg, M., & Loden, M. (2000). Unexpected skin barrier influence from nonionic emulsifiers. *International Journal of Pharmacy, 195*(1–2), 189–195.

Barker, J. N., Mitra, R. S., Griffiths, C. E., Dixit, V. M., & Nickoloff, B. J. (1991). Keratinocytes as initiators of inflammation. *Lancet, 337*(8735), 211–214.

Bickers, D. R., & Athar, M. (2006). Oxidative stress in the pathogenesis of skin disease. *Journal of Investigative Dermatology, 126*(12), 2565–2575.

Bolognia, J. L., Jorizzo, J. L., & Rapini, R. P. (2008). *Dermatology* (Vol. 2, 2nd ed.). London: Elsevier.

Cho, S., Lowe, L., Hamilton, T. A., Fisher, G. J., Voorhees, J. J., & Kang, S. (2005). Long-term treatment of photoaged human skin with topical retinoic acid improves epidermal cell atypia and thickens the collagen band in papillary dermis. *Journal of the American Academy of Dermatology, 53*(5), 769–774.

Choi, E. H., Man, M-Q., Wang, F., et al. (2005). Is endogenous glycerol a determinant of stratum corneum hydration in humans? *Journal of General Internal Medicine, 20*(5), 288–293.

Cohen-Mansfield, J., & Jensen, B. (2005). The preference and importance of bathing, toileting and mouth care habits in older persons. *Gerontology, 51*(6), 375–385.

Clydesdale, G. J., Dandie, G. W., & Muller, H. K. (2001). Ultraviolet light induced injury: immunological and inflammatory effects. *Immunology & Cell Biology, 79*(6), 547–568.

Damian, D. L. (2010). Photoprotective effects of nicotinamide. *Photochemistry & Photobiology Science, 9*(4), 578–585.

Denda, M., Sato, J., Tsuchiya, T., Elias, P. M., & Feingold, K. R. (1998). Low humidity stimulates epidermal DNA synthesis and amplifies the hyperproliferative response to barrier disruption: Implication for seasonal exacerbations of inflammatory dermatoses. *Journal of Investigative Dermatology, 111*(5), 873–878.

Downing, D. T. (1992). Lipid and protein structures in the permeability barrier of mammalian epidermis. *Journal of Lipid Research, 33*(3), 301–313.

Downing, D. T., Stewart, M. E., Wertz, P. W., Colton, S. W., Abraham, W., & Strauss, J. S. (1987). Skin lipids: an update. *Journal of Investigative Dermatology, 88*(3 Suppl), 2s–6s.

Elias, P. M. (1981). Lipids and the epidermal permeability barrier. *Archives of Dermatological Research, 270*(1), 95–117.

Elson, D. (2011). Use of emollients in dry skin conditions. *Nursing Times, 107*(47), 20–21.

Friberg, S. E., & Ma, Z. (1993). Stratum corneum lipids, petrolatum and white oils. *Cosmetics & Toiletries, 107*, 55–59.

Gaspar, L. R., & Campos, P. M. (2007). Photostability and efficacy studies of topical formulations containing UV-filters combination and vitamins A, C and E. *International Journal of Pharmacy, 343*(1–2), 181–189.

Green, B. A., Yu, R. J., & Van Scott, E. J. (2009). Clinical and cosmeceutical uses of hydroxyacids. *Clinical Dermatology, 27*(5), 495–501.

Hammersen, J. E., Neukam, V., Nusken, K. D., & Schneider, H. (2011). Systematic evaluation of exertional hyperthermia in children and adolescents with hypohidrotic ectodermal dysplasia: an observational study. *Pediatrics Research, 70*(3), 297–301.

Hansen, H. S., & Jensen, B. (1985). Essential function of linoleic acid esterified in acyl-glucosylceramide and acylceramide in maintaining the epidermal water permeability barrier. Evidence from feeding studies with oleate, linoleate, arachidonate, columbinate and alpha-linolenate. *Biochimica et Biophysica Acta, 834*(3), 357–363.

Hon, K. L. E., Leung, T. F., Wong, Y., So, H. K., Li, A. M., & Fok, T. F. (2005). A survey of bathing and showering practices in children with atopic eczema. *Clinical and Experimental Dermatology, 30*(4), 351–354.

Idson, B. (1992). Dry skin: moisturizing and emolliency. *Cosmetics & Toiletries, 107,* 69.

Imokawa, G., Kuno, H., & Kawai, M. (1991). Stratum corneum lipids serve as a bound-water modulator. *Journal of Investigative Dermatology, 96*(6), 845–851.

Jagdeo, J., & Brody, N. (2011). Complementary antioxidant function of caffeine and green tea polyphenols in normal human skin fibroblasts. *Journal of Drugs in Dermatology, 10*(7), 753–761.

Jass, H. E., & Elias, P. M. (1991). The living stratum corneum: implications for cosmetic formulation. *Cosmetics & Toiletries, 106,* 47–53.

Kakigi, R., & Mochizuki, H. (2011). [Mechanisms of intracerebral pain and itch perception in humans]. *Brain Nerve, 63*(9), 987–994.

Kawasaki, H., Kubo, A., Sasaki, T., & Amagai, M. (2011). Loss-of-function mutations within the filaggrin gene and atopic dermatitis. *Current Problems in Dermatology, 41,* 35–46.

Kircik, L. H., & Del Rosso, J. Q. (2011). Nonsteroidal treatment of atopic dermatitis in pediatric patients with a ceramide-dominant topical emulsion formulated with an optimized ratio of physiological lipids. *Journal of Clinical & Aesthetic Dermatology, 4*(12), 25–31.

Klaus, M. V., Wehr, R. F., Rogers, R. S., 3rd, Russell, T. J., & Krochmal, L. (1990). Evaluation of ammonium lactate in the treatment of seborrheic keratoses. *Journal of the American Academy of Dermatology, 22*(2 Pt 1), 199–203.

Laden, K., & Spitzer, R. (1967). Identification of a natural moisturizing agent in skin. *Journal of the Society of Cosmetic Chemists, 18,* 351–360.

Lee, B., & Warshaw, E. (2008). Lanolin allergy: history, epidemiology, responsible allergens, and management. *Dermatitis, 19*(2), 63–72.

Leveque, J. L., Grove, G. L., de Rigal, J., Corcuff, P., Kligman, A. M., & Saint Leger, D. (1987). Biophysical characterization of dry facial skin. *Journal of the Society of Cosmetic Chemists, 38*(3), 171–178.

Loden, M., & Lindberg, M. (1991). The influence of a single application of different moisturizers on the skin capacitance. *Acta Dermato-Venereologica, 71*(1), 79–82.

Linde, Y. W. (1992). Dry skin in atopic dermatitis. *Acta Dermato-Venereologica Supplement, 177,* 9–13.

McCusker, M. M., & Grant-Kels, J. M. (2010). Healing fats of the skin: the structural and immunologic roles of the omega-6 and omega-3 fatty acids. *Clinical Dermatology, 28*(4), 440–451.

Menon, G. K, Ghadially, R., Williams, M. L., & Elias, P. M. (1992). Lamellar bodies as delivery systems of hydrolytic enzymes: implications for normal and abnormal desquamation. *British Journal of Dermatology, 126*(4), 337–345.

Monheit, G. D., & Coleman, K. M. (2006). Hyaluronic acid fillers. *Dermatologic Therapy*, *19*(3), 141–150.

Morrison, D. S. (2000). Petrolatum. In: M. Loden & H. I. Maibach (Eds.), *Dry skin and moisturizers* (p. 251). Boca Raton, FL: CRC Press.

Nichols, J. A., & Katiyar, S. K. (2010). Skin photoprotection by natural polyphenols: anti-inflammatory, antioxidant and DNA repair mechanisms. *Archives of Dermatological Research*, *302*(2), 71–83.

Norval, M. (2006). The mechanisms and consequences of ultraviolet-induced immunosuppression. *Progress in Biophysics & Molecular Biology*, *92*(1), 108–118.

Perricone, N. V., & DiNardo, J. C. (1996). Photoprotective and antiinflammatory effects of topical glycolic acid. *Dermatological Surgery*, *22*(5), 435–437.

Polefka, T. G., Meyer, T. A., Agin, P. P., & Bianchini, R. J. (2012). Effects of solar radiation on the skin. *Journal of Cosmetic Dermatology*, *11*(2), 134–143.

Popa, I., Remoue, N., Osta, B., et al. (2012). The lipid alterations in the stratum corneum of dogs with atopic dermatitis are alleviated by topical application of a sphingolipid-containing emulsion. *Clinical & Experimental Dermatology*, *23*(10), 1365–2230.

Rabe, J. H., Mamelak, A. J., McElgunn, P. J., Morison, W. L., & Sauder, D. N. (2006). Photoaging: mechanisms and repair. *Journal of the American Academy of Dermatology*, *55*(1), 1–19.

Rass, K., & Reichrath, J. (2008). UV damage and DNA repair in malignant melanoma and nonmelanoma skin cancer. *Advances in Experimental Medicine & Biology*, *624*, 162–178.

Rawlings, A. V., & Harding, C. R. (2004). Moisturization and skin barrier function. *Dermatologic Therapy*, *17*, 43–48.

Rawlings, A. V., Scott, I. R., Harding, C. R., & Bowser, P. A. (1994). Stratum corneum moisturization at the molecular level. *Journal of Investigative Dermatology*, *103*(5), 731–740.

Rawlings, A. V., Watkinson, A., Rogers, J., Mayo, A. M., Hope, J., & Scott, I. R. (1994). Abnormalities in stratum corneum structure, lipid composition and desmosome degradation in soap-induced winter xerosis. *Journal of the Society of Cosmetic Chemists*, *45*, 203–230.

Rodrigues, H. G., Vinolo, M. A., Magdalon, J., et al. (2012). Oral administration of oleic or linoleic acid accelerates the inflammatory phase of wound healing. *Journal of Investigative Dermatology*, *132*(1), 208–215.

Sato, K., Kang, W. H., Saga, K., & Sato, K. T. (1989). Biology of sweat glands and their disorders. I. Normal sweat gland function. *Journal of the American Academy of Dermatology*, *20*(4), 537–563.

Schwarz, T. (2010). The dark and the sunny sides of UVR-induced immunosuppression: photoimmunology revisited. *Journal of Investigative Dermatology*, *130*(1), 49–54.

Stalder, J. F. (2005). [Allergy to lanolin: myth or reality?] *Annales de Dermatologie et de Venereologie*, *132*(5), 506–509.

Stern, E. C. (1946). Topical application of lactic acid in the treatment and prevention of certain disorders of the skin. *Urologic & Cutaneous Review*, *50*, 106.

Stiller, M. J., Bartolone, J., Stern, R., et al. (1996). Topical 8% glycolic acid and 8% L-lactic acid creams for the treatment of photodamaged skin. A double-blind vehicle-controlled clinical trial. *Archives ofr Dermatology, 132*(6), 631–636.

Thueson, D. O., Chan, E. K., Oechsli, L. M., & Hahn, G. S. (1998). The roles of pH and concentration in lactic acid-induced stimulation of epidermal turnover. *Dermatological Surgery, 24*(6), 641–645.

Van Scott, E. J., & Yu, R. J. (1974). Control of keratinization with alpha-hydroxy acids and related compounds. I. Topical treatment of ichthyotic disorders. *Archives of Dermatology, 110*(4), 586–590.

Van Scott, E. J., & Yu, R. J. (1984). Hyperkeratinization, corneocyte cohesion, and alpha hydroxy acids. *Journal of the American Academy of Dermatology, 11*(5 Pt 1), 867–879.

Wade, A., Weller, P. J., & Kibbe, A. H. (2000). *Handbook of pharmaceutical excipients* (3rd ed.). Washington, DC: American Pharmaceutical Association, Pharmaceutical Press.

White-Chu, E. F., & Reddy, M. (2011). Dry skin in the elderly: Complexities of a common problem. *Clinics in Dermatology, 29*(1), 37–42.

Wilkinson, J. D., & Rycroft, R. J. G. (1992). Contact dermatitis. In: R. H. Champion, J. L. Burton, & F. J. G. Ebling (Eds.), *Textbook of dermatology* (5th ed.). Oxford: Blackwell Scientific Publications.

Wolber, R., Schlenz, K., Wakamatsu, K., et al. (2008). Pigmentation effects of solar-simulated radiation as compared with UVA and UVB radiation. *Pigment Cell & Melanoma Research, 21*(4), 487–491.

Wood, L. C., Jackson, S. M., Elias, P. M., Grunfeld, C., & Feingold, K. R. (1992). Cutaneous barrier perturbation stimulates cytokine production in the epidermis of mice. *Journal of Clinical Investigation, 90*(2), 482–487.

Wu, M. S., Yee, D. J., & Sullivan, M. E. (1983). Effect of a skin moisturizer on the water distribution in human stratum corneum. *Journal of Investigative Dermatology, 81*(5), 446–448.

Zussman, J., Ahdout, J., & Kim, J. (2010). Vitamins and photoaging: do scientific data support their use? *Journal of the American Academy of Dermatology, 63*(3), 507–525.

5

Topical Botanicals and the Skin

ANDREA M. HUI, MD AND DANIEL M. SIEGEL, MD

Key Concepts

- ♣ A significant focus has more recently been placed upon naturally occurring botanical compounds in complementary dermatologic therapy as compared with synthetic molecules.
- ♣ Patients often request botanically-based products, as they view them as safer and more "natural" alternatives to standard medical therapy; this has been reflected in a substantial increase in the use of botanical extracts in over-the-counter medications and skin care preparations as manufacturers respond to patient demands.
- ♣ Botanical compounds may consist of extracts from whole plants, seeds, roots, rhizomes, leaves, and flowers, or any part of the plant that is considered biologically active.
- ♣ Many botanical extracts demonstrate anti-inflammatory, antimicrobial, and antioxidant properties, which are quite useful in a wide range of dermatologic diseases, from atopic dermatitis and psoriasis to wound healing.

Introduction

Modern medicine derives much from traditional botanical medicine. Plants and other natural compounds have always played a role in medicines and treatments across the world, and even in modern times, traditional botanical methods continue to find use. Not surprisingly, a significant focus has more recently been placed upon naturally occurring botanical compounds in complementary dermatologic therapy as compared with synthetic molecules. Botanical compounds may consist of extracts from whole plants, seeds, roots, rhizomes, leaves, and flowers, or any part of the plant that is considered biologically active.

Patients often request botanically-based products, as they view them as safer and more "natural" alternatives to standard medical therapy. This has been reflected in a substantial increase in the use of botanical extracts in over-the-counter medications and skin care preparations as manufacturers respond to patient demands. Cosmetic skin preparations with active botanical compounds fall within the category of "cosmeceuticals," or items that have a measurable effect but are unregulated in contrast to "drugs."

Topical products based on botanicals are generally unregulated by the U.S. Food and Drug Administration (FDA) because they are considered additives or supplements (Thornfeldt, 2005) and instead fall under the Dietary Supplement Health and Education Act of 1994 (DSHEA). Therefore, botanical compounds have not yet been vigorously tested in clinical studies for safety and efficacy. Currently, no standards on potency, concentration, safety, or efficacy exist for most topical botanicals in the United States. In comparison, a regulatory committee in Germany known as Commission E has thoroughly reviewed clinical evidence for over 300 topical and systemic botanicals, which has helped establish their clinical safety and efficacy. Additionally, an herbal compendium known as *Physicians Desk Reference for Herbal Medicines,* based on work by Commission E, provides extensive reference regarding use and safety for over 400 herbs.

Many botanical extracts demonstrate anti-inflammatory, antimicrobial, and antioxidant properties, which are quite useful in a wide range of dermatologic diseases, from atopic dermatitis and psoriasis to wound healing. This chapter presents both laboratory and clinical evidence of several of the most popular botanicals used in dermatology.

Aloe Vera (*Aloe barbadensis*)

Aloe vera (*Aloe barbadensis*) (Fig. 5.1) is a perennial succulent originating from northern Africa with a wide range of therapeutic uses. For centuries, the clear gel of aloe vera, extracted from its leaf, has been used in a myriad of cosmetics, pharmaceuticals, and foods. It is composed of 99.5% water mixed with mucopolysaccharides, amino acids, hydroxyquinone glycosides, and minerals. Aloe vera has demonstrated a myriad of effects such as increased blood flow, enhanced wound healing, reduced inflammation, and decreased bacterial colonization (Draelos, 2001).

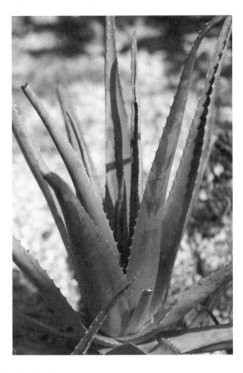

FIGURE 5.1 *Aloe barbadensis*

Wound healing is the major indication for aloe vera gel use. Various animal models have shown that aloe vera greatly promotes wound healing, via increased collagen synthesis and enhanced collagen turnover in the wounded tissue (Chithra et al., 1998; Gallagher & Gray, 2003; Rodriguez-Bigas et al., 1988). Several human studies have demonstrated aloe vera to be effective in accelerating the burn wound healing process in humans by increasing the rate of re-epithelialization compared with conventional treatments (Maenthaisong et al., 2007; Visuthikosol et al., 1995). Aloe has been widely accepted in treating radiation and stasis ulcers, especially given its antimicrobial and antifungal properties (Klein & Penneys, 1988).

Aloe vera demonstrates significant anti-inflammatory effects. In a randomized double-blinded placebo-controlled study of aloe vera extract 0.5% in a hydrophilic cream for the treatment of psoriasis, 25 of 30 patients in the aloe group showed complete clearing compared with 2 of 30 patients in the placebo group (Syed et al., 1996). Aloe vera is known to work via inhibition of the arachidonic pathway by cyclooxygenase.

Recently, aloe vera has been studied for its anticarcinogenic effects. Emodin, a naturally occurring hydroxyanthraquinone in aloe vera leaves, has shown strong inhibition of Merkel cell carcinoma proliferation while remaining nontoxic to normal cells (Fenig et al., 2004; Wasserman et al., 2002). Aloe vera has also demonstrated immunomodulating effects. In UVB-exposed skin, aloe vera prevented UVB-induced immunosuppression by repairing UVB-damaged epidermal Langerhans cells, which are vital to skin's cancer surveillance (Lee et al., 1997, 1999).

Evening Primrose Oil (*Oenothera biennis*)

Evening primrose oil (EPO) is an extract derived from the mature seeds of *Oenothera biennis*. EPO has demonstrated various effects on the skin, including alteration and improvement of lipid content and modulation of immunological and antitumor effects.

Given the concern for adverse effects regarding use of topical corticosteroids (Charman et al., 2000), EPO has been studied as a possible alternative for treatment in atopic dermatitis, both topically and orally. Topical EPO has been shown to penetrate the skin and increase cell proliferation in a pig model (Morris et al., 1997). In humans, topical EPO demonstrated the ability to stabilize the stratum corneum barrier function in patients with atopic dermatitis after a four-week treatment period. In this study by Gehring and colleagues, the vehicle was important factor, as topical EPO was effective only as a water-in-oil emulsion compared with an amphiphilic emulsion (Gehring et al., 1999).

EPO is rich in linoleic acid and gamma-linoleic acid (GLA), containing 72% and 10%, respectively (Schafer & Kragballe, 1991). Defective delta-6-desaturase, resulting in decreased GLA, has been demonstrated as a factor causing dry skin in atopic dermatitis (Manku et al., 1982). A study by Yoon and colleagues (2002) showed that oral administration of EPO to patients with atopic dermatitis significantly decreased the severity of skin lesions and pruritus in all patients, with concomitant normalization of serum interferon-gamma levels. In several randomized prospective studies, oral GLA has been shown to favorably increase the lipid content of the epidermis in patients with atopic dermatitis, with improvement of itching, dryness, and redness (Schafer & Kragballe, 1991; Wright, 1985; Yates et al., 2009).

Another mechanism whereby EPO may exert its effects is through conversion of GLA to dihomo-GLA, an essential component of cell signaling and enzyme regulation. Dihomo-GLA is also a precursor of arachidonic acid, itself a precursor of many anti-inflammatory molecules such as prostaglandins, leukotrienes, and platelet-activating factor (Puri, 2004).

EPO has also shown antitumorigenic effects both orally and topically. Oral EPO was shown to significantly inhibit the growth of melanoma in an athymic mouse model (Pritchard, 1990). In another mouse model, topically applied EPO significantly inhibited the formation of papillomas during the promotion stage of a skin carcinogenesis model. Additionally, an increase in lipid peroxidation was noted, which is a marker of tumor inhibition. EPO inhibited the binding of benzo(α)-pyrene to skin cell DNA, suggesting that this could be a mechanism by which EPO prevented papilloma development (Ramesh & Das, 1998).

Overall, EPO has shown promise as a topical and oral modulator of inflammatory and carcinogenic skin conditions.

Green Tea (*Camellia sinesis*)

Human skin possesses an innate antioxidant system, which effectively handles UV-induced oxidative stress but at times may be overcome by excessive UV exposure. This, in turn, results in oxidative stress, immunosuppression, premature photoaging, and subsequently development of skin cancers. Green tea polyphenols (GTPs) have been studied extensively in vitro and in vivo for their antioxidant effects and health benefits such as reduction of heart disease and cancer.

Green tea is produced from the young leaf buds of *Camellia sinensis*. Its production results in the least amount of oxidation and polymerization of the plant's polyphenols, compared with other teas (Graham, 1992). In dermatology, GTP has been investigated for its role in prevention of UV-induced photodamage and photocarcinogenesis, as well as its role in modulation of UV-induced immunosuppression and its antioxidant effects. Green tea contains four major polyphenols, of which epigallocatechin-3-gallate (EGCG) is considered to be the most effective suppressor of UV-induced carcinogenesis (Gensler et al., 1996; Vayalil et al., 2003). The efficacy of GTPs is dependent upon their vehicle; they are most effective when administered in a hydrophilic ointment (Vayalil et al., 2003).

The first animal model by Wang and colleagues (1991) showed that GTPs administered in drinking water and applied topically to SKH-1 hairless mice resulted in a dose-dependent delay of the mean time to tumorigenesis when mice were subjected to a photocarcinogenesis protocol. Several other studies demonstrated similar findings when GTPs was applied topically (Gensler et al., 1996; Mittal et al., 2003; Vayalil et al., 2003).

GTPs have demonstrated anti-photoaging effects through various mechanisms. In a pivotal study by Vayalil and colleagues, EGCG applied topically for 10 weeks to UVA-irradiated hairless mice demonstrated a significant reduction in skin wrinkling and sagging compared to vehicle. EGCG inhibited UVA-induced collagenase gene expression and subsequently prevented UVA-induced reduction in collagen synthesis (Kim et al., 2001). Additionally, topical EGCG application inhibited UV-induced production of matrix metalloproteinases (MMP)-2, -3, -7, and -9, which degrade collagen and result in photoaging (Kim et al., 2001). Mnich and colleagues (2009) showed that topical application of GTPs on human skin reduced UV-induced p53 expression and decreased the number of apoptotic keratinocytes. Elmets and colleagues (2001) found that topical application of untanned human skin with GTPs prior to UV exposure significantly reduced erythema and sunburn cells when compared to UV-exposed skin that was not treated with GTPs.

UV-induced immunosuppression plays an important role in the development of skin cancers (CA, 1998). Elmets and colleagues (2001) discovered that topical application of GTPs to human skin prevented UV-induced damage of Langerhans cells, which are particularly sensitive to UV radiation. In a human model, topical treatment with GTPs prior to UVB exposure significantly decreased UVB-induced infiltration of inflammatory leukocytes and also decreased myeloperoxidase activity.

Notably, GTPs exhibit considerable antioxidant effects. Topical application of EGCG to human skin before UV exposure significantly reduced UVB-induced production of nitric oxide and hydrogen peroxide by decreasing leukocyte infiltration (Elmets et al., 2001; Katiyar et al., 1999). Katiyar and colleagues (2001) demonstrated that topical treatment of skin with EGCG decreased numbers of hydrogen peroxide-producing and inducible nitric oxide synthase-expressing cells in the epidermis and dermis, natively and after exposure to UVB exposure. In an in vitro model, Silverberg and colleagues (2011) used normal human skin fibroblasts to study the effects of green tea extract (GTE) on hydrogen peroxide-induced necrosis. GTE protected fibroblasts from hydrogen peroxide-induced necrosis in a dose-dependent manner via decreasing intracellular reactive oxygen species (ROS), suggesting that pretreatment with GTE may prevent ROS-induced skin injury. In several studies, topical EGCG significantly prevented UV-induced lipid peroxidation (Elmets et al., 2001; Katiyar et al., 1999). An in vitro study by Jagdeo and Brody (2011) demonstrated that GTPs and caffeine, alone or in combination, inhibited upregulation of hydrogen peroxide-induced free radicals and lipid peroxidation byproducts in human skin fibroblasts. Topical EGCG also protected antioxidant defense enzymes such as glutathione peroxidase and restored total glutathione levels on UV-exposed mouse and human skin (Katiyar et al., 2001; Vayalil et al., 2003).

These studies as well as many others have been a proponent for the use of green tea in various commercial topical applications for the prevention of photoaging and photocarcinogenesis.

Tea Tree Oil (*Melaleuca alternifolia*)

Tea tree oil (TTO) is an essential oil derived from the leaves and crushed twigs of the Australian *Melaleuca alternifolia* tree and has many cosmetic and medical uses. TTO exhibits a wide antimicrobial spectrum against *Propionobacterium acnes, Escherichia coli, Staphylococcus aureus,* herpes simplex, *Candida albicans,* and fungi, among several others (Walton et al., 2004). Several randomized, double-blinded clinical trials have shown that TTO is possibly an effective treatment for acne vulgaris and fungal and yeast infections (Carson et al., 2006; D'Auria et al., 2001).

With the increasing use of TTO, it is important to educate patients that TTO is a major contact allergen (Carson & Riley, 2001). The active compounds in TTO include terpenes, one of the components responsible for the antioxidant activity of TTO. When exposed to air, it auto-oxidizes and forms allergenic compounds (Rudbäck et al., 2012). Additionally, TTO is cytolytic to epithelial cells and fibroblasts and should not be used in the treatment of burns or other inflammatory conditions.

More investigations into the safety and efficacy of TTO should be performed to derive greater understanding of its many effects.

Jojoba Oil (*Simmondsia chinensis*)

Jojoba liquid wax (JLW), also known as jojoba oil, is the clear to light-gold liquid wax derived from the seed of the jojoba shrub (*Simmondsia chinensis*), which is native to the Sonoran Desert of Arizona and Mexico (Meyer et al., 2008). Historically, JLW was used by native Americans to treat sores and wounds (Ranzato et al., 2011). JLW is nonirritating and noncomedogenic and is a popular additive found in many emollients and cosmetics for its moisturizing, wound healing, and anti-inflammatory properties.

JLW is widely known for its moisturizing qualities. At least 97% of JLW is a mix of wax esters of long-chain fatty alcohols and acids, with over 60% containing *cis*-11 eicosenoic (jojobenoic) acid (Miwa, 1984). JLW wax esters closely mimic human sebum, itself composed of 25% wax monoesters (Wertz, 2009). Hydrolyzed JLW effectively penetrates the upper level of human stratum corneum and increases skin hydration (Patzelt et al., 2011), while the JLW fatty acid esters replace missing lipids in dry and damaged stratum corneum (Wertz, 2009). The high viscosity of JLW also results in a smooth feel when applied directly to skin. Additionally, JLW has a stable shelf life due to its innate antioxidant properties (Kampf et al., 1986). These properties make JLW an ideal skin barrier moisturizer.

In vitro experiments have shown that LJW is nontoxic and capable of accelerating wound closures of keratinocyte and fibroblast scratch assays (Ranzato et al., 2011). The mechanism of action is dependent upon calcium and works via activation of PI3K-Akt-mTor pathway and p38 and ERK1/2 MAPK pathway, thus accelerating cell proliferation. Additionally, JLW is able to stimulate synthesis of type I collagen in fibroblasts (Ranzato et al., 2011). In an animal model by Habashy and colleagues (2005), topical application of JLW significantly decreased inflammation of ear skin induced by croton oil. JLW reduced markers of inflammation such as infiltration of neutrophils and polymorphonuclear leukocytes, red blood cell extravasation, and myeloperoxidase activity (Habashy et al., 2005).

Shea Butter (*Butyrospermum parkii*)

Shea butter is an ivory-colored fat extracted from the nut of the African shea tree (*Butyrospermum parkii*, synonymous with *Vitellaria paradoxa*), found in sub-Saharan and East Africa (Masters, 2004). Traditionally, shea butter has been used to treat skin conditions such as atopic dermatitis, psoriasis, burns, and dry skin. It is commonly found in cosmetics and skin care products for its emollient properties due to high levels of triglycerides such as oleic, stearic, and linoleic acids, as well as nonsaponifiable fat constituents (Alander, 2004). The high fat content of liquid fractions is desirable in cosmetic formulations for its smooth texture and excellent skin penetration (Alander, 2002).

The nonsaponifiable constituents of shea fat include the triterpene alcohols α- and β-amyrin, lupeol, and butyspermol, occurring naturally as acetic acid and cinnamic acid esters (Itoh et al., 1974; Peers, 1977). The cinnamic acid of shea fat demonstrates absorbance of UVB radiation and, when added to sunscreens, works synergistically to increase absorbance in the UVB range (Alander, 2002). Additionally, these triterpene alcohols and derivative esters of shea fat demonstrate anti-inflammatory, anticarcinogenic, and antibacterial properties (Akihisa & Yasukawa, 2001; Fernandez et al., 2001).

Shea fat extracts have shown significant anti-inflammatory effects in vitro and in vivo. In an in vitro study by Verma and colleagues (2012), shea fat methanolic extracts significantly reduced levels of pro-inflammatory cytokines in murine macrophages induced by lipopolysaccharides. The pro-inflammatory cytokines included tumor necrosis factor-α (TNF-α) and interleukins 1β (IL-1β) and -12 (IL-12). Expression of pro-inflammatory enzymes inducible nitric oxide synthase and cyclooxygenase-2 was also inhibited by shea fat extracts (Verma et al., 2012).

In a mouse model by Akihisa and colleagues (2010), acetate and cinnamate isolates from shea fat demonstrated significant and rapid anti-inflammatory properties against induced inflammation when applied topically to mouse skin or given orally. These shea fat isolates decreased inflammation to a greater degree when compared to a widely used anti-inflammatory medication, indomethacin (Akihisa et al., 2010). The anti-inflammatory effect of shea isolates was attributable to suppression of skin prostaglandin E_2 (PGE_2) levels via cyclooxygenase-2 (COX-2) expression and its upstream protein kinases (Medeiros et al., 2007).

Shea fat has also exhibited anticarcinogenic effects. In a mouse carcinogenesis model, Akihisa and colleagues (2010) demonstrated that topical application of shea fat significantly inhibited growths of papillomas, as effectively as or more effectively than topical retinoic acid. Quantitative analysis of shea fat by liquid chromatography–mass spectrometry has recently identified eight catechin compounds with a profile comparable to that of green tea (Maranz et al., 2003).

Colloidal Oatmeal (*Avena sativa*)

For centuries, oatmeal (*Avena sativa*) has been used as a natural topical cleanser, emollient, and anti-itch and anti-inflammatory agent for a wide range of dermatologic conditions. In 1945, a ready-to-use colloidal oatmeal was developed by finely milling the oats and then reducing it into a concentrated starch-protein gelatinous material (Franks, 1958). Following the introduction of colloidal oatmeal, several clinical studies demonstrated its benefits as a remedy for inflamed, itchy skin dermatoses (Dick, 1952, 1958; Grais, 1953); many commercial products such as baths, cleansers, and moisturizers containing colloidal oatmeal soon followed (Miller, 1979). In 2003, the FDA approved the use of colloidal oatmeal as a skin protectant (FDA, 2003).

Oat grains contain a large concentration of polysaccharides, most notably starches and beta-glucans. These polysaccharides are capable of holding large amounts of water, thus conferring the high humectant properties of colloidal oatmeal (Paton, 1977; Wood, 1986). The processing of oat grains into a powder results in superfine particles. When mixed with water, as in commercially available colloidal oatmeal baths, these particles form a viscous solution and deposit evenly on skin, creating an occlusive barrier to prevent transepidermal water loss (Kurtz & Wallo, 2007). Additionally, oats contain higher amounts of lipids, mainly unsaturated triglycerides, when compared to other cereal grains (Zhou et al., 1999).

Several studies have supported the efficacy and safety of colloidal oatmeal for the treatment of inflammatory skin disorders. Early studies in pediatric and elderly patients established the safety of colloidal oatmeal in the management of skin disorders (Dick, 1952, 1958). In a pivotal study by Grais (1953), colloidal oatmeal was used as a bath and cleanser for three months in 139 patients aged 21 to 91; over 71% of patients reported complete or significant itch relief. An in vivo model of skin irritation using sodium lauryl sulfate on human skin showed that application of oatmeal extracts significantly reduced irritation when compared to vehicle (Vié et al., 2002).

Oats contain many phenolic compounds, most notably ferulic, hydroxy-cinnamic, p-coumaric, and caffeic acids (Emmons & Peterson, 1999). These compounds, as well as alpha-tocopherol (vitamin E), function as antioxidants to protect oat lipids from oxidation. Additionally, oats contain flavonoids that demonstrate significant absorbance of UVA radiation (Collins, 1986).

Significant anti-inflammatory properties of oats have been demonstrated. An vitro study by Saeed and colleagues (2011) using an extract of *A. sativa* on a bovine model showed significant inhibition of prostaglandin biosynthesis. In a study by Aries and colleagues (2005), oatmeal extract was shown to significantly decrease cytosolic phospholipase-dependent mobilization of arachidonic acid from phospholipids of human keratinocytes, which has been established as a possible mechanism in inflammatory skin disorders.

Avenanthramides, extracted from oat grains, have shown anti-inflammatory and antipruritic properties. In an in vitro study by Sur and colleagues (2008), avenanthramides at concentrations as low as 1 parts per billion significantly inhibited the degradation of nuclear factor-kappa beta in keratinocytes. Additionally, treatment with avenanthramides significantly inhibited TNF-α in a dose-dependent manner, with a subsequent decrease in the pro-inflammatory cytokine IL-8 (Sur et al., 2008). In the same study, topically applied avenanthramides reduced inflammation in murine models of contact hypersensitivity and neurogenic inflammation (Sur et al., 2008).

Ginkgo biloba

The leaves and fruit of *Ginkgo biloba* have been used for centuries in China and Japan to treat a variety of conditions ranging from hypertension to depression and dementia. It is a dioecious tree, having both male and female reproductive organs on separate trees (Mahadevan & Park, 2008). The extract of *G. biloba* leaves (Fig. 5.2) has become the standard extract formulation, EGb 761 (Smith & Luo, 2004). Ginkgo is well known for its free radical scavenging activity and enhancement of microcirculation (Suter et al., 2011). Ginkgo extracts are commonly found in many cosmeceuticals for their purported anti-aging benefits and antioxidant properties.

Ginkgo leaves contain anti-inflammatory and antioxidant polyphenols such as flavone glycosides, terpenoids (ginkgolides, bilobalides), quercetin,

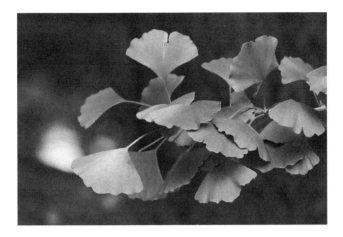

Figure 5.2 *Ginkgo biloba*

and kaempferol derivatives. In vitro experiments on rat hepatocytes demonstrate that ginkgo extract protects against free radical damage and lipid peroxidation (Joyeux et al., 1995). In a study by Ozkur and colleagues (2002), mice were given oral ginkgo extract before UVB irradiation, which conferred a photoprotective effect by significantly decreasing superoxide dismutase and malondialdehyde levels, resulting in decreased UVB-induced sunburn cells when compared to controls. Kwak and colleagues (2002) performed an in vivo study on a murine inflammation model to further elucidate the anti-inflammatory properties of ginkgo. The group showed that ginkgetin, a biflavone from *G. biloba* leaves, demonstrated significant anti-inflammatory activity when applied topically to inflamed mouse skin. Ginkgetin strongly inhibited induction of pro-inflammatory COX-2 and prostaglandin E2 (Kwak et al., 2002).

Ginkgo extracts may also combat aging skin. Kim and colleagues (1997) performed an in vitro assay of normal human fibroblasts incubated with ginkgo extracts, demonstrating enhanced proliferation when compared to controls. The addition of ascorbic acid to ginkgo extracts increased collagen and extracellular fibronectin synthesis (Kim et al., 1997).

There is a paucity of clinical data to support the use of topical *G. biloba,* but it continues to be a popular additive to moisturizers and cosmetics for its antioxidant properties.

Turmeric (*Curcuma longa*)

Curcumin (diferuloylmethane) is a yellow powder derived from the rhizome of the tropical plant turmeric (*Curcuma longa*) (Azuine & Bhide, 1992).

Traditionally, it has been used in Asian cuisine as a spice and coloring agent in curries and mustards, as well as for medicinal purposes. Curcumin is the biologically active component of turmeric, exhibiting many anti-inflammatory, wound healing, anticarcinogenic, and antioxidant pharmacologic properties (Ammon & Wahl, 1991; Sharma, 1976).

Curcumin has demonstrated significant anti-inflammatory effects. In vitro studies have identified various mechanisms by which it suppresses acute and chronic inflammation. Inflammation induced by lipopolysaccharide stimulation of peripheral blood monocytes and alveolar macrophages was significantly diminished by curcumin via inhibition of IL-8, monocyte inflammatory protein-1 (MIP-1), IL-1β, and TNF-α (Abe et al., 1999). Additionally, curcumin has been shown to inhibit lipid peroxide-induced DNA damage (Shalini & Srinivas, 1987). In a mouse model of inflammation, Huang and colleagues (1991) found that topically applied curcumin significantly decreased inflammation via inhibition of arachidonic acid metabolism to prostaglandin compounds.

Curcumin is a potent antioxidant. Studies have shown that it can inhibit lipid peroxidation and oxidation of hemoglobin by scavenging reactive superoxide anion and hydroxyl radicals (Ruby et al., 1995). An in vitro study by Phan and colleagues (2001) established curcumin as a powerful inhibitor of hydrogen peroxide- and hypoxanthine xanthine oxidase-induced damage to cultured human keratinocytes and fibroblasts. This suggested that curcumin would be beneficial in wound healing.

Curcumin has been proven to inhibit tumor formation. A murine model by Azuine and Bhide (1992) demonstrated anticarcinogenic effects of oral curcumin at both the initiation and progression stage of skin carcinogenesis. Further studies have clarified curcumin's mechanism of anticarcinogenesis via inhibition of NF-kappa beta expression. In vitro studies have shown that curcumin inhibits tumors induced by benz(α)pyrine and 7,12-dimethlbenz(α) anthracene, both of which induce NF-kappa beta (Singh & Aggarwal, 1995). Additionally, curcumin can inhibit type 1 human immunodeficiency virus long terminal repeat (HIV-LTR) gene expression and viral replication stimulated by TNF and phorbol ester, which also requires NF-kappa beta (Li et al., 1993). Finally, Singh and Aggarwal (1995) showed that treatment of human myeloid ML-1a cells with curcumin significantly inhibited TNF-α–induced NF-kappa beta expression. These studies have shown curcumin to inhibit tumor progression at the important step of NF-kappa beta phosphorylation.

Considerable investigations have been conducted into the use of curcumin for treatment of psoriasis. Pol and colleagues (2003) showed that low doses of curcumin (10^{-5} M) significantly inhibited keratinocyte proliferation in a human in vitro psoriatic differentiation assay. In a clinical study by Heng and colleagues (2000), topical curcumin 1% in a gel formula demonstrated efficacy in the treatment of psoriasis, comparable to results with commercially available calcipotriol ointment. Assays demonstrated significant inhibition of phosphorylase kinase when psoriatic skin was treated with curcumin. This corresponded with decreased keratinocyte transferrin receptor expression and an accompanying histological decrease in the severity of parakeratosis and the density of epidermal CD8+ T cells (Heng et al., 2000).

Curcumin has shown a plethora of possible pharmacological benefits for the treatment of many conditions ranging from cancer to inflammatory skin conditions such as psoriasis. Many clinical studies are being conducted to investigate curcumin's properties.

Licorice Extract (*Glycyrrhiza glabra* and *inflata*)

The extract of licorice (*Glycyrrhiza glabra* and *inflata*) roots is best known for its use as a sweetener. It is extracted by boiling and evaporating the root, producing a syrup. The main components of licorice extract include flavonoids, isoflavonoids, and triterpene saponins. In dermatology, licorice extract has been used for its anti-inflammatory properties and ability to inhibit melanogenesis, treating a variety of skin disorders from atopic dermatitis and rosacea, to melasma (Yokota et al., 1998). Additionally, alcohol extract of *G. glabra* confers its antimicrobial activity from isoflavonoids and has shown efficacy in vitro against *Propionibacterium acnes, Staphylococcus aureus, Streptococcus mutans,* and *Candida albicans* (Saeedi et al., 2003). Of note, the antibacterial effect of licorice extract does not lead to induction of bacterial resistance when used against *P. acnes* in vitro (Nam et al., 2003).

Licochalcone A (LicA) is a major biologically active component of *G. inflata* (Kolbe et al., 2006). The anti-inflammatory qualities of licorice extract have been established in vitro. Kolbe and colleagues (2006) demonstrated that LicA-rich extracts and synthetic LicA inhibited pro-inflammatory responses in several scenarios: (1) induced granulocyte oxidative burst; (2) human keratinocyte UV-induced PGE2 release; (3) human fibroblast lipopolysaccharide-induced PGE2 release; (4) induced granulocyte LTB4 (an eicosanoid) release; and (5) immature monocytic dendritic cell lipopolysaccharide-induced IL-6/TNF-α release. Barfod and colleagues (2002) also reported similar results: LicA extracts and synthetic LicA inhibited pro-inflammatory cytokines TNF- α, IL-1, IL-6, and I-10 in stimulated human mononuclear cells.

In mouse inflammation models by Kolbe and colleagues (2006), inflammation caused by dry-shave irritation or UV irradiation was treated immediately and five hours later with topical LicA-rich licorice extract; this significantly reduced inflammation when compared to vehicle. A clinical study by Weber and colleagues (2006) evaluated the efficacy of topical LicA for the treatment of mild to moderate erythrotelangiectatic rosacea. Sixty-two patients were treated with a skin care regimen containing LicA for eight weeks; significant improvements in objective redness and subjective quality of life were observed at four and eight weeks (Weber et al., 2006).

The triterpene glycoside glycyrrhizin (also known as glycyrrhizic acid) is the major biologically active component of *G. glabra* and may be useful for the treatment of atopic dermatitis and other anti-inflammatory conditions (Khaksa et al., 1996; Segal & Pisanty, 1987). In an in vitro experiment by Ohuchi and colleagues (1981), glycyrrhizin exhibited a cortisol-like effect by inhibiting pro-inflammatory prostaglandin and leukotriene formation in stimulated rat peritoneal macrophages. In another in vitro experiment, Kolbe and colleagues (2006) induced inflammation in human granulocytes, and then incubated with either LicA or glycyrrhizic acid. Both groups showed dose-dependent inhibition of the oxidative burst, but LicA was more potent than glycyrrhizin by a factor of more than 100 (Kolbe et al., 2006). In a clinical study, Saeedi and colleagues (2003) studied topical licorice gel containing a purified extract of glycyrrhizic acid in a double-blind trial for the treatment of atopic dermatitis. Licorice topical gel was effective in a dose-dependent manner for reducing erythema, edema, and itching over a treatment period of two weeks when compared to controls (Saeedi et al., 2003).

Licorice extract has also been studied for its inhibition of melanogenesis. The hydrophobic fraction contains several flavonoids of which glabridin is the major component. These flavonoids have exhibited inhibition of melanogenesis by via inhibition of tyrosinase. An in vitro study by Yokota and colleagues (1998) showed that low concentrations of glabridin were able to inhibit tyrosinase activity in cultured B16 murine melanoma cells. Additionally, glabridin applied topically to guinea pig skins inhibited UVB-induced pigmentation and erythema (Yokota et al., 1998).

Overall, licorice extract has shown various effects ranging from anti-inflammatory to inhibition of melanogenesis. This is particularly useful for the treatment of inflammatory conditions such atopic dermatitis, rosacea, and melasma.

Lavender (*Lavandula* spp.)

Lavender (*Lavandula* spp.) (Fig. 5.3) is a flowering plant in the *Lamiaciae* family and is found throughout Europe and Asia, cultivated for its beautiful purple flowers and essential oils. Lavender oil has been used for many centuries for

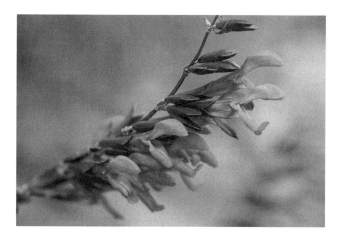

FIGURE 5.3   *Lavandula angustifolia*

a variety of therapeutic and cosmetic purposes and is widely popular for use in aromatherapy. The oil is produced by steam distillation of its flower heads and leaves (McGimpsey, 1993). Lavender oil has demonstrated antibacterial, antifungal, anti-inflammatory, and wound healing properties (Cavanagh & Wilkinson, 2002). In fact, the genus name *Lavandula* is derived from the Latin word *lavare*, meaning "to wash," as lavender has been used for centuries as an antiseptic (Basch et al., 2004). Lavender can be found in many commercial skin care products such as soaps, moisturizers, and hair care products.

An in vitro experiment by Nelson and colleagues (1997) showed that lavender oil (at concentrations less than 1%) showed bactericidal activity against methicillin-resistant *Staphylococcus aureus* and vancomycin-resistant *Enterococcus faecium*, suggesting its potential use as an adjunctive topical antimicrobial. Lavender oil and vapor have also demonstrated significant antifungal activity against *Aspergillus fumigatus, Trichophyton mentagrophytes, Trichophyton rubrum*, and *Candida albicans* (Cavanagh & Wilkinson, 2002). Although lavender oil has been studied for its antimicrobial effects in several in vitro studies, no clinical studies have been conducted yet.

Lavender has exhibited anti-inflammatory properties. In an in vitro experiment, Juergens and colleagues showed that 1,8-cineole, a terpenoid oxide containing 0.5% to 2.5% of *Lavandula angustifolia*, significantly inhibited the formation of pro-inflammatory prostaglandins and cytokines in stimulated human blood monocytes (Juergens et al., 1998). When administered orally, 1,8-cineole significantly decreased inflammation in a rat paw edema model by Santos and Rao (2000). Linalool and linalyl acetate, also major constituents of lavender oil, were shown to decrease inflammation in a similar rat paw edema model by Peana and colleagues (2002).

Lavender has shown some utility in the treatment of childhood atopic dermatitis. In a small eight-week clinical trial by Anderson and colleagues (2000), the use of an essential oil mixture containing lavender oil for massage and addition to bath water resulted in significant improvement in atopic dermatitis symptoms such as skin irritation and nighttime disturbance.

Lavender oil may also show promise in wound healing. Altaei and colleagues (2012) conducted a randomized double-blind, placebo-controlled study on a rabbit model. Aphthous ulcers were induced, and then topical lavender oil or placebo was applied to them. Clinical and histological healing was assessed by measuring the ulceration area and inflammation. Animals treated with lavender oil showed significant reduction in ulcer size and increase in rate of mucosal repair, with rapid healing within three days when compared to placebo. An analogous clinical study was then conducted in human subjects (n = 115) with preexisting aphthous ulcers. Patients treated with topical lavender oil showed a significant decrease in inflammation, ulcer size, and healing time compared to placebo. No side effects were reported (Altaei et al., 2012).

Lavender oil has shown pharmacological benefits, mainly as an antimicrobial and anti-inflammatory. Because there are several varieties of *Lavandula* spp., more studies need to be conducted to differentiate the chemical and biologically active profiles of the different lavenders to isolate the species that demonstrate the most therapeutic potential.

Chamomile (*Chamomilla recutita* or *Matricaria recutita*)

Chamomile (*Chamomilla recutita* or *Matricaria recutita*) is a member of the daisy family *Asteraceae*, with a distinctive yellow floret surrounded by white rays. It is found all over the world. Dried chamomile flowers are commonly taken as an herbal tea and have many purported benefits for the treatment of irritable bowel, stomach pain, and insomnia. Chamomile has also been beneficial as a mouthwash for ameliorating mucositis (Brown & Dattner, 1998). In dermatology, chamomile has shown efficacy as an anti-inflammatory for the treatment of dry and itchy skin and chronic disorders such as atopic dermatitis, and it shows wound healing potential (Jarrahi et al., 2010; Lee et al., 2010).

Chamomile flowers contain 1% to 2% volatile oil (Wichtl, 2000). The active components of chamomile include terpenoids (α-bisabolol, a-bisabolol oxides A and B, matricin, chamazulene) and flavonoids (apigenin, luteolin, and quercetin) (Brown & Dattner, 1998). Chamomile extracts, mainly chamazulene, exhibit anti-inflammatory activity. In an in vitro study by Safayhi and colleagues (1994), chamazulene significantly inhibited the formation of leukotriene B4 and chemical peroxidation of arachidonic acid in stimulated rat peritoneal granulocytes. The flavonoids apigenin and quercetin can inhibit histamine release by stimulated human basophilic polymorphonuclear leukocytes (Middleton & Drzewiecki, 1982).

In a mouse model of atopic dermatitis, Lee and colleagues (2010) showed that daily topical application of chamomile oil clinically improved the symptoms of atopic dermatitis (scratching frequency) by influencing Th2 cell activation by significantly lowering serum IgE, IgG1, and histamine when compared to control. A human study showed that topical chamomile oil was approximately 60% as active as 0.25% hydrocortisone (Albring et al., 1983). One should recall that chamomile could potentially cause allergic contact dermatitis because it is a member of the ragweed family and may cross-react with other members of this family.

Chamomile can also improve wound healing. To study the healing potential of chamomile oil, Jarrahi and colleagues (2010) created linear incisions on the back of rats. The rats were randomized to treatment with topical olive oil (vehicle), chamomile oil, or control (no treatment). Chamomile oil was created from crushed fresh flowers mixed with olive oil. Wounds treated with topical chamomile oil healed significantly faster than those treated with olive oil or control: compared with olive oil, chamomile oil accelerated wound closure by an average of four days (Jarrahi et al., 2010). Jarrahi (2008) conducted a similar experiment by creating second-degree burns on rats and treating the burns with topical chamomile oil, olive oil, or no treatment: the group treated with topical chamomile oil showed the most significant improvement in wound healing when compared with the other groups.

Chamomile has demonstrated beneficial effects as an anti-inflammatory and in wound healing. Further studies on its wound healing effects are warranted, given that wound healing is a remarkably complex process and there are many active compounds in chamomile that could play a major role in wound healing.

Calendula (*Calendula officinalis*)

Calendula (*Calendula officinalis*), also known as pot marigold, is an aromatic perennial plant of the family *Asteraceae*. Its bright-yellow to yellow-orange florets are well recognized. Calendula is native to Europe and is found worldwide due to its easy cultivation. Its aroma is somewhat spicy, and its flowers are commonly added to dishes as a garnish. In medicine, calendula is best known for its anti-inflammatory, wound healing, and soothing effects. It has also been studied for its antioxidant and sun protection factor (SPF) activities;

its antibacterial, antifungal, and antiviral properties (Dumenil et al., 1980; Kasiram et al., 2000); and its antitumorigenic potential (Boucaud-Maitre et al., 1988).

For centuries, calendula has been used to aid wound healing. There are several well-designed studies showing its efficacy. An in vitro assay by Fronza and colleagues (2009) showed that low concentrations of calendula extract stimulated the migration of mouse fibroblasts when added to the growth medium after a scratch assay was performed. Further studies by this group showed that the active components responsible for the anti-inflammatory effects of calendula include its triterpenoids, specifically faradiol monoesters (Fronza et al., 2009). In a rat model by Preethi and Kuttan (2009), surgical wounds were created and then covered with calendula extract. The wounds were examined histologically and it was found that calendula stimulated significantly improved wound healing in the treatment group when compared with control. Interestingly, a significant increase in hydroxyproline and hexoasamine content (the main components of collagen) was noted in the granuloma tissue of treated wounds when compared with control (Preethi & Kuttan, 2009).

In a prospective, randomized controlled clinical trial by Pommier and colleagues (2004), 254 patients with breast cancer applied either topical trolamine or calendula to the irradiated areas after radiation therapy. The primary endpoint was the occurrence of grade 2 acute radiation dermatitis (tender bright erythema with patchy moist desquamation or moderate edema). The use of topical 10% calendula ointment resulted in a significantly lower incidence of grade 2 acute radiation dermatitis when compared with a standard treatment, trolamine. Additionally, the patients who were randomized to the calendula group noted significantly reduced pain, and there was less frequent interruption of radiation therapy (Pommier et al., 2004).

Calendula extract is also a potent anti-inflammatory. In a rat paw edema model by Preethi and colleagues (2009), oral administration of calendula extract significantly inhibited paw edema induced by carrageenan and dextran. Furthermore, calendula extract also significantly inhibited blood levels of pro-inflammatory cytokines IL-1β, IL-6, TNF-α, IFN-γ, and C-reactive protein and significantly decreased COX-2 levels after injection of lipopolysaccharide into the mice (Preethi et al., 2009). Calendula flowers also contain antioxidant compounds such as triterpenoids, flavonoids, and polyphenols.

Calendula extract has shown potential for use as a sunscreen in commercial preparations. In an in vitro study by Mishra and colleagues (2012), fresh calendula petal oil at 5% was determined by UV-visible spectrophotometry to demonstrate an SPF of approximately 15. Studies on its efficacy as a sunscreen have not been performed yet.

Calendula exhibits significant anti-inflammatory, wound healing, and soothing effects and continues to be one of the most popular topical botanicals available today.

Arnica (*Arnica montana*)

Arnica (*Arnica montana*), also known as wolf's bane, is a perennial flowering herb with composite bright-yellow petals and is found indigenously in the meadows and mountains of northern and central Europe. Arnica extract, commonly derived from its flowerheads, is a popular herbal remedy for improvement of bruising, swelling, and inflammation (Stevinson et al., 2003). It is especially popular as a bruising preventive for dermatologic procedures such as dermal fillers and lasers. The active constituents of arnica include sesquiterpene lactones, flavonoids, volatile oils, and others (Cohen et al., 2000).

Oral arnica has been shown to be efficacious in decreasing post-procedure bruising and inflammation. This effect is thought to be secondary to a vasodilatory effect and upregulation of macrophage activity (Cohen et al., 2000). An in vitro study by Puhlmann and colleagues (1991) showed that polysaccharides derived from *A. montana* were able to stimulate macrophages to enhance phagocytosis and release of tumor necrosis factor. The sesquiterpene lactones from the flowerheads of *A. montana* also exert anti-inflammatory effects by inhibiting NF-kappa beta activation and IL-12 production in murine dendritic cells (Lass et al., 2008). This in return reduced the synthesis of pro-inflammatory cytokines, cyclooxygenase, and nitric oxide synthase. In a rat paw edema model by Lussignoli and colleagues (1999), local injection of arnica extract prior to the injection of edema-producing homologous blood significantly inhibited paw edema and increased the speed of wound healing.

Seeley and colleagues (2006) conducted a randomized, double-blind, placebo-controlled clinical trial in which 29 patients undergoing rhytidectomy were treated perioperatively with either *A. montana* or placebo. Using a novel computer photographic analysis model, this group found that *A. montana* given perioperatively resulted in significantly smaller areas of post-procedure ecchymoses compared with placebo.

Contact allergies to *A. montana* may be attributed to its sesquiterpene lactones. As mentioned earlier, these sesquiterpene lactones extracted from *A. montana* flowerheads can also exert anti-inflammatory effects by inhibiting NF-kappa beta activation and IL-12 production. This effect is observed when arnica is applied to murine dendritic cells in high concentrations, but immunostimulatory effects occurred at low concentrations. Contact hypersensitivity could not be induced in a mouse model even when arnica tinctures or sesquiterpene lactones were applied at high concentrations to inflamed skin. Interestingly, arnica tinctures were able to suppress contact hypersensitivity, as measured by ear swelling, when a strong contact sensitizer trinitrochloroben-zene was applied. This experiment by Lass and colleagues (2008) suggested that induction of contact hypersensitivity by arnica was prevented by its inherent anti-inflammatory effect.

A. montana has certainly shown some promise as a potential anti-inflammatory and antibruising remedy. However, further studies are necessary to give merit to its popularity as a bruising preventive for dermatologic procedures.

Conclusion

As topical botanicals continue to gain popularity, dermatologists must continue to learn about these compounds so they can best educate their patients and offer the most complete dermatologic therapy. Although many botanical compounds show promise by providing anti-inflammatory, antimicrobial, and antioxidant properties, there is still a need for more clinical trials and studies to establish the place of botanical compounds in modern dermatologic practice with regards to both efficacy and long-term safety.

REFERENCES

Abe, Y., Hashimoto, S. H. U., & Horie, T. (1999). Curcumin inhibition of inflammatory cytokine production by human peripheral blood monocytes and alveolar macrophages. *Pharmacological Research, 39*, 41–47.

Akihisa, T., & Yasukawa, K. (2001). Antitumor-promoting and anti-inflammatory activities of triterpenoids and sterols from plants and fungi. In *Studies in Natural Products Chemistry, 25*, 43–87.

Akihisa, T., Kojima, N., Kikuchi, T., et al. (2010). Anti-inflammatory and chemopreventive effects of triterpene cinnamates and acetates from shea fat. *Journal of Oleo Science, 59*, 273–280.

Alander, J. A. (2002). The shea butter family—the complete emollient range for skin care formulations. *Cosmetics and Toiletries Manufacture Worldwide*, pp. 28–32.

Alander, J. (2004). Shea butter—a multifunctional ingredient for food and cosmetics. *Lipid Technology, 16*, 202–205.

Albring, M., Albrecht, H., Alcorn, G., et al. (1983). The measuring of the antiinflammatory effect of a compound on the skin of volunteers. *Methods & Findings in Experimental & Clinical Pharmacology, 5*, 575–577.

Altaei, D. T. (2012). Topical lavender oil for the treatment of recurrent aphthous ulceration. *American Journal of Dentistry, 25*, 39–43.

Ammon, H. P. T., & Wahl, M. A. (1991). Pharmacology of *Curcuma longa. Planta Medica, 57*, 1, 7.

Anderson, C., Lis-Balchin, M., & Kirk-Smith, M. (2000). Evaluation of massage with essential oils on childhood atopic eczema. *Phytotherapy Research, 14*, 452–456.

Aries, M. F., Vaissiere, C., Pinelli, E., et al. (2005). *Avena rhealba* inhibits A23187-stimulated arachidonic acid mobilization, eicosanoid release, and cPLA2 expression in human keratinocytes: potential in cutaneous inflammatory disorders. *Biological and Pharmaceutical Bulletin, 28*, 601–606.

Azuine, M. A., & Bhide, S. V. (1992). Chemopreventive effect of turmeric against stomach and skin tumors induced by chemical carcinogens in Swiss mice. *Nutrition and Cancer, 17*, 77–83.

Barfod, L., Kemp, K., Hansen, M., et al. (2002). Chalcones from Chinese liquorice inhibit proliferation of T cells and production of cytokines. *International Immunopharmacology, 2*, 545–555.

Basch, E., Foppa, I., Liebowitz, R, et al. (2004). Lavender (*Lavandula angustifolia* Miller). *Journal of Herbal Pharmacotherapy, 4*, 63–78.

Boucaud-Maitre, Y., Algernon, O., & Raynaud, J. (1988). Cytotoxic and antitumoral activity of *Calendula officinalis* extracts. *Pharmazie, 43*, 220–221.

Brown, D. J., & Dattner, A. M. (1998). Phytotherapeutic approaches to common dermatologic conditions. *Archives of Dermatology, 134*, 1401–1404.

CA, E. (1998). Immune surveillance mechanisms. In S. J. Miller & M. E. Maloney (Eds.), *Cutaneous oncology: pathophysiology, diagnosis, and management* (pp. 39–50). Boston: Blackwell Science.

Carson, C. F., Hammer, K. A., & Riley, T. V. (2006). *Melaleuca alternifolia* (tea tree) oil: a review of antimicrobial and other medicinal properties. *Clinical Microbiology Reviews, 19*, 50–62.

Carson, C. F., & Riley, T. V. (2001). Safety, efficacy and provenance of tea tree (*Melaleuca alternifolia*) oil. *Contact Dermatitis, 45*, 65–67.

Cavanagh, H. M., & Wilkinson, J. M. (2002). Biological activities of lavender essential oil. *Phytotherapy Research, 16*, 301–308.

Charman, C. R., Morris, A. D., & Williams, H. C. (2000). Topical corticosteroid phobia in patients with atopic eczema. *British Journal of Dermatology, 142*, 931–936.

Chithra, P., Sajithlal, G. B., & Chandrakasan, G. (1998). Influence of Aloe vera on collagen characteristics in healing dermal wounds in rats. *Molecular and Cellular Biochemistry, 181*, 71–76.

Cohen, S. M., Rousseau, M. E., & Robinson, E. H. (2000). Therapeutic use of selected herbs. *Holistic Nursing Practice, 14*, 59–68.

Collins, F. (1986). *Oat phenolics: structure, occurrence and function*. American Association of Cereal Chemists, Inc., St. Paul, Minnesota.

D'Auria, F. D., Laino, L., Strippoli, V., et al. (2001). In vitro activity of tea tree oil against *Candida albicans* mycelial conversion and other pathogenic fungi. *Journal of Chemotherapy (Florence, Italy), 13*, 377–383.

Dick, L. A. (1952). Colliodal emollient baths in geriatric dermatoses. *Skin*, pp. 89–91.

Dick, L. A. (1958). Colliodal emollient baths in pediatric dermatoses. *Archives of Pediatrics*, *75*, 506–508.

Draelos, Z. D. (2001). Botanicals as topical agents. *Clinics in Dermatology*, *19*, 474–477.

Dumenil, G., Chemli, R., Balansard, C., et al. (1980). [Evaluation of antibacterial properties of marigold flowers (*Calendula officinalis* L.) and mother homeopathic tinctures of *C. officinalis* L. and *C. arvensis* L. (author's transl)]. *Annales Pharmaceutiques Francaises*, *38*, 493–499.

Elmets, C. A., Singh, D., Tubesing, K., et al. (2001). Cutaneous photoprotection from ultraviolet injury by green tea polyphenols. *Journal of the American Academy of Dermatology*, *44*, 425–432.

Emmons, C. L., & Peterson, D. M. (1999). Antioxidant activity and phenolic contents of oat groats and hulls. *Cereal Chemistry Journal*, *76*, 902–906.

FDA (2003). Skin protectant drug products for over-the-counter human use; final monograph. *Federal Register*, *68*, 33362–33375.

Fenig, E., Nordenberg, J., Beery, E, et al. (2004). Combined effect of aloe-emodin and chemotherapeutic agents on the proliferation of an adherent variant cell line of Merkel cell carcinoma. *Oncology Reports*, *11*, 213–217.

Fernandez, M. A., de las Heras, B., Garcia, M. D., et al. (2001). New insights into the mechanism of action of the anti-inflammatory triterpene lupeol. *Journal of Pharmacy and Pharmacology*, *53*, 1533–1539.

Franks, A. G. (1958). Dermatologic uses of baths. *American Practitioner and Digest of Treatment*, *9*, 1998–2000.

Fronza, M., Heinzmann, B., Hamburger, M., et al. (2009). Determination of the wound healing effect of *Calendula* extracts using the scratch assay with 3T3 fibroblasts. *Journal of Ethnopharmacology*, *126*, 463–467.

Gallagher, J., & Gray, M. (2003). Is aloe vera effective for healing chronic wounds? *Journal of Wound Ostomy & Continence Nursing*, *30*, 68–71.

Gehring, W., Bopp, R., Rippke, F., et al. (1999). Effect of topically applied evening primrose oil on epidermal barrier function in atopic dermatitis as a function of vehicle. *Arzneimittel-Forschung*, *49*, 635–642.

Gensler, H. L., Timmermann, B. N., Valcic, S., et al. (1996). Prevention of photocarcinogenesis by topical administration of pure epigallocatechin gallate isolated from green tea. *Nutrition and Cancer*, *26*, 325–335.

Graham, H. N. (1992). Green tea composition, consumption, and polyphenol chemistry. *Preventive Medicine*, *21*, 334–350.

Grais, M. L. (1953). Role of colloidal oatmeal in dermatologic treatment of the aged. *A.M.A. Archives of Dermatology and Syphilology*, *68*, 402–407.

Habashy, R. R., Abdel-Naim, A. B., Khalifa, A. E., et al. (2005). Anti-inflammatory effects of jojoba liquid wax in experimental models. *Pharmacological Research*, *51*, 95–105.

Heng, M. C. Y., Song, M. K., Harker, J., et al. (2000). Drug-induced suppression of phosphorylase kinase activity correlates with resolution of psoriasis as assessed by clinical, histological and immunohistochemical parameters. *British Journal of Dermatology*, *143*, 937–949.

Huang, M.-T., Lysz, T., Ferraro, T., et al. (1991). Inhibitory effects of curcumin on in vitro lipoxygenase and cyclooxygenase activities in mouse epidermis. *Cancer Research*, *51*, 813–819.

Itoh, T., Tamura, T., & Matsumoto, T. (1974). Sterols, methylsterols, and triterpene alcohols in three Theaceae and some other vegetable oils. *Lipids*, *9*, 173–184.

Jagdeo, J., & Brody, N. (2011). Complementary antioxidant function of caffeine and green tea polyphenols in normal human skin fibroblasts. *Journal of Drugs in Dermatology*, *10*, 753–761.

Jarrahi, M. (2008). An experimental study of the effects of *Matricaria chamomilla* extract on cutaneous burn wound healing in albino rats. *Natural Products Research*, *22*, 422–427.

Jarrahi, M., Vafaei, A. A., Taherian, A. A., et al. (2010). Evaluation of topical *Matricaria chamomilla* extract activity on linear incisional wound healing in albino rats. *Natural Products Research*, *24*, 697–702.

Joyeux, M., Lobstein, A., Anton, R., et al. (1995). Comparative antilipoperoxidant, antinecrotic and scavenging properties of terpenes and biflavones from ginkgo and some flavonoids. *Planta Medica*, *61*, 126, 129.

Juergens, U. R., Stober, M., Schmidt-Schilling, L., et al. (1998). Antiinflammatory effects of euclyptol (1.8-cineole) in bronchial asthma: inhibition of arachidonic acid metabolism in human blood monocytes ex vivo. *European Journal of Medical Research*, *3*, 407–412.

Kampf, A., Grinberg, S., & Galun, A. (1986). Oxidative stability of jojoba wax. *Journal of the American Oil Chemists' Society*, *63*, 246–248.

Kasiram, K., Sakharkar, P., & Patil, A. (2000). Antifungal activity of *Calendula officinalis*. Medknow Publications.

Katiyar, S. K., Afaq, F., Perez, A., et al. (2001). Green tea polyphenol (–)-epigallocatechin-3-gallate treatment of human skin inhibits ultraviolet radiation-induced oxidative stress. *Carcinogenesis*, *22*, 287–294.

Katiyar, S. K., Matsui, M. S., Elmets, C. A., et al. (1999). Polyphenolic antioxidant (-)-epigallocatechin-3-gallate from green tea reduces UVB-induced inflammatory responses and infiltration of leukocytes in human skin. *Photochemistry and Photobiology*, *69*, 148–153.

Khaksa, G., Zolfaghari, M. E., Dehpour, A. R., et al. (1996). Anti-inflammatory and anti-nociceptive activity of disodium glycyrrhetinic acid hemiphthalate. *Planta Medica*, *62*, 326–328.

Kim, J., Jae-Sung, H., Youn-Ki, C., et al. (2001). Protective effects of (-)-epigallocatechin-3-gallate on UVA- and UVB-induced skin damage. *Skin Pharmacology and Physiology*, *14*, 11–19.

Kim, S. J., Lim, M. H., Chun, I. K., et al. (1997). Effects of flavonoids of *Ginkgo biloba* on proliferation of human skin fibroblast. *Skin Pharmacology*, *10*, 200–205.

Klein, A. D., & Penneys, N. S. (1988). Aloe vera. *Journal of the American Academy of Dermatology*, *18*, 714–720.

Kolbe, L., Immeyer, J., Batzer, J., et al. (2006). Anti-inflammatory efficacy of Licochalcone A: correlation of clinical potency and in vitro effects. *Archives of Dermatological Research*, *298*, 23–30.

Kurtz, E. S., & Wallo, W. (2007). Colloidal oatmeal: history, chemistry and clinical properties. *Journal of Drugs in Dermatology, 6*, 167–170.

Kwak, W.-J., Han, C. K., Son, K. H., et al. (2002). Effects of ginkgetin from *Ginkgo biloba* leaves on cyclooxygenases and in vivo skin inflammation. *Planta Medica, 68*, 316, 321.

Lass, C., Vocanson, M., Wagner, S., et al. (2008). Anti-inflammatory and immune-regulatory mechanisms prevent contact hypersensitivity to *Arnica montana* L. *Experimental Dermatology, 17*, 849–857.

Lee, C. K., Han, S. S., Mo, Y. K., et al. (1997). Prevention of ultraviolet radiation-induced suppression of accessory cell function of Langerhans cells by Aloe vera gel components. *Immunopharmacology, 37*, 153–162.

Lee, C. K., Han, S. S., Shin, Y. K., et al. (1999). Prevention of ultraviolet radiation-induced suppression of contact hypersensitivity by Aloe vera gel components. *International Journal of Immunopharmacology, 21*, 303–310.

Lee, S. H., Heo, Y., & Kim, Y. C. (2010). Effect of German chamomile oil application on alleviating atopic dermatitis-like immune alterations in mice. *Journal of Veterinary Science, 11*, 35–41.

Li, C. J., Zhang, L. J., Dezube, B. J., et al. (1993). Three inhibitors of type 1 human immunodeficiency virus long terminal repeat-directed gene expression and virus replication. *Proceedings of the National Academy of Sciences USA, 90*, 1839–1842.

Lussignoli, S., Bertani, S., Metelmann, H., et al. (1999). Effect of Traumeel S, a homeopathic formulation, on blood-induced inflammation in rats. *Complementary Therapies in Medicine, 7*, 225–230.

Maenthaisong, R., Chaiyakunapruk, N., Niruntraporn, S., et al. (2007). The efficacy of aloe vera used for burn wound healing: A systematic review. *Burns, 33*, 713–718.

Mahadevan, S., & Park, Y. (2008). Multifaceted therapeutic benefits of *Ginkgo biloba* L.: Chemistry, efficacy, safety, and uses. *Journal of Food Science, 73*, R14–R19.

Manku, M. S., Horrobin, D. F., Morse, N., et al. (1982). Reduced levels of prostaglandin precursors in the blood of atopic patients: defective delta-6-desaturase function as a biochemical basis for atopy. *Prostaglandins, Leukotrienes, and Medicine, 9*, 615–628.

Maranz, S., Wiesman, Z., & Garti, N. (2003). Phenolic constituents of shea (*Vitellaria paradoxa*) kernels. *Journal of Agricultural and Food Chemistry, 51*, 6268–6273.

Masters, E. T., Yidana, J. A., & Lovett, P. N. (2004). *Vitellaria paradoxa. Unasylva, 219*, 46–52.

McGimpsey, J. A. (1993). *Lavender: a grower's guide for commercial production.* New Zealand Institute for Crop & Food Research, Clyde, N.Z.

Medeiros, R., Otuki, M. F., Avellar, M. C. W., et al. (2007). Mechanisms underlying the inhibitory actions of the pentacyclic triterpene α-amyrin in the mouse skin inflammation induced by phorbol ester 12-O-tetradecanoylphorbol-13-acetate. *European Journal of Pharmacology, 559*, 227–235.

Meyer, J., Marshall, B., Gacula, M., et al. (2008). Evaluation of additive effects of hydrolyzed jojoba (*Simmondsia chinensis*) esters and glycerol: a preliminary study. *Journal of Cosmetic Dermatology, 7*, 268–274.

Middleton, E., Jr., & Drzewiecki, G. (1982). Effects of flavonoids and transitional metal cations on antigen-induced histamine release from human basophils. *Biochemical Pharmacology, 31*, 1449–1453.

Miller, A. (1979). Oat derivatives in bath products. *Cosmetics & Toiletries, 94*, 72–80.

Mishra, A., Mishra, A., & Chattopadhyay, P. (2012). Assessment of in vitro sun protection factor of *Calendula officinalis* L. (Asteraceae) essential oil formulation. *Journal of Young Pharmacists, 4*, 17–21.

Mittal, A., Piyathilake, C., Hara, Y, et al. (2003). Exceptionally high protection of photocarcinogenesis by topical application of (—)-epigallocatechin-3-gallate in hydrophilic cream in SKH-1 hairless mouse model: relationship to inhibition of UVB-induced global DNA hypomethylation. *Neoplasia (New York), 5*, 555–565.

Miwa, T. (1984). Structural determination and uses of jojoba oil. *Journal of the American Oil Chemists' Society, 61*, 407–410.

Mnich, C. D., Hoek, K. S., Virkki, L. V., et al. (2009). Green tea extract reduces induction of p53 and apoptosis in UVB-irradiated human skin independent of transcriptional controls. *Experimental Dermatology, 18*, 69–77.

Morris, G. M., Hopewell, J. W., Harold, M., et al. (1997). Modulation of the cell kinetics of pig skin by the topical application of evening primrose oil or Lioxasol. *Cell Proliferation, 30*, 311–323.

Nam, C., Kim, S., Sim, Y., et al. (2003). Anti-acne effects of Oriental herb extracts: a novel screening method to select anti-acne agents. *Skin Pharmacology and Physiology, 16*, 84–90.

Nelson, R. R. (1997). In-vitro activities of five plant essential oils against methicillin-resistant *Staphylococcus aureus* and vancomycin-resistant *Enterococcus faecium*. *Journal of Antimicrobial Chemotherapy, 40*, 305–306.

Ohuchi, K., Kamada, Y., Levine, L., et al. (1981). Glycyrrhizin inhibits prostaglandin E2 production by activated peritoneal macrophages from rats. *Prostaglandins and Medicine, 7*, 457–463.

Ozkur, M. K., Bozkurt, M. S., Balabanli, B., et al. (2002). The effects of EGb 761 on lipid peroxide levels and superoxide dismutase activity in sunburn. *Photodermatology, Photoimmunology & Photomedicine, 18*, 117–120.

Paton, D. (1977). Oat starch Part 1. Extraction, purification and pasting properties. *Starch—Stärke, 29*, 149–153.

Patzelt, A., Lademann, J., Richter, H., et al. (2011). In vivo investigations on the penetration of various oils and their influence on the skin barrier. *Skin Research and Technology* [E-pub Nov. 14].

Peana, A. T., D'Aquila, P. S., Panin, F., et al. (2002). Anti-inflammatory activity of linalool and linalyl acetate constituents of essential oils. *Phytomedicine, 9*, 721–726.

Peers, K. E. (1977). The non-glyceride saponifiables of shea butter. *Journal of the Science of Food and Agriculture, 28*, 1000–1009.

Phan, T. T., See, P., Lee, S. T., et al. (2001). Protective effects of curcumin against oxidative damage on skin cells in vitro: its implication for wound healing. *Journal of Trauma, 51*, 927–931.

Physicians desk reference for herbal medicines (2nd ed.). (2000). Montvale, NJ: Thomson Medical Economics.

Pol, A., Bergers, M., & Schalkwijk, J. (2003). Comparison of antiproliferative effects of experimental and established antipsoriatic drugs on human kerationocytes, using a simple 96-well-plate assay. *In Vitro Cellular & Developmental Biology—Animal, 39*, 36–42.

Pommier, P., Gomez, F., Sunyach, M. P., et al. (2004). Phase III randomized trial of *Calendula officinalis* compared with trolamine for the prevention of acute dermatitis during irradiation for breast cancer. *Journal of Clinical Oncology, 22*, 1447–1453.

Preethi, K. C., & Kuttan, R. (2009). Wound healing activity of flower extract of *Calendula officinalis*. *Journal of Basic & Clinical Physiology & Pharmacology, 20*, 73–79.

Preethi, K. C., Kuttan, G., & Kuttan, R. (2009). Anti-inflammatory activity of flower extract of *Calendula officinalis* Linn. and its possible mechanism of action. *Indian Journal of Experimental Biology, 47*, 113–120.

Pritchard, R. L. (1990). *Omega-6 essential fatty acids, pathophysiology and roles in clinical medicine*. New York: Alan R. Liss Inc.

Puhlmann, J., Zenk, M. H., & Wagnert, H. (1991). Immunologically active polysaccharides of Arnica montana cell cultures. *Phytochemistry, 30*, 1141–1145.

Puri, B. K. (2004). The clinical advantages of cold-pressed non-raffinated evening primrose oil over refined preparations. *Medical Hypotheses, 62*, 116–118.

Ramesh, G., & Das, U. N. (1998). Effect of evening primrose and fish oils on two stage skin carcinogenesis in mice. *Prostaglandins, Leukotrienes and Essential Fatty Acids, 59*, 155–161.

Ranzato, E., Martinotti, S., & Burlando, B. (2011). Wound healing properties of jojoba liquid wax: An in vitro study. *Journal of Ethnopharmacology, 134*, 443–449.

Rodriguez-Bigas, M., Cruz, N. I., & Suarez, A. (1988). Comparative evaluation of aloe vera in the management of burn wounds in guinea pigs. *Plastic and Reconstructive Surgery, 81*, 386–389.

Ruby, A. J., Kuttan, G., Dinesh Babu, K., et al. (1995). Anti-tumour and antioxidant activity of natural curcuminoids. *Cancer Letters, 94*, 79–83.

Rudbäck, J., Bergström, M. A., Börje, A., et al. (2012). α-Terpinene, an antioxidant in tea tree oil, autoxidizes rapidly to skin allergens on air exposure. *Chemical Research in Toxicology, 25*, 713–721.

Saeed, S. A., Butt, N. M., McDonald-Gibson, W. J., et al. (2011). Inhibitor(s) of prostaglandin biosynthesis in extracts of oat (*Avena sativa*) seeds. *Biochemical Society Transactions, 9*, 444.

Saeedi, M., Morteza-Semnani, K., & Ghoreishi, M. R. (2003). The treatment of atopic dermatitis with licorice gel. *Journal of Dermatological Treatment, 14*, 153–157.

Safayhi, H., Sabieraj, J., Sailer, E. R., et al. (1994). Chamazulene: an antioxidant-type inhibitor of leukotriene B4 formation. *Planta Medica, 60*, 410–413.

Santos, F. A., & Rao, V. S. (2000). Antiinflammatory and antinociceptive effects of 1,8-cineole a terpenoid oxide present in many plant essential oils. *Phytotherapy Research, 14*, 240–244.

Schafer, L., & Kragballe, K. (1991). Supplementation with evening primrose oil in atopic dermatitis: effect on fatty acids in neutrophils and epidermis. *Lipids, 26,* 557–560.

Seeley, B. M., Denton, A. B., Ahn, M. S., et al. (2006). Effect of homeopathic *Arnica montana* on bruising in face-lifts: results of a randomized, double-blind, placebo-controlled clinical trial. *Archives of Facial & Plastic Surgery, 8,* 54–59.

Segal, R., & Pisanty, S. (1987). Glycyrrhizin gel as a vehicle for idoxuridine—I. Clinical investigations. *Journal of Clinical Pharmacy & Therapeutics, 12,* 165–171.

Shalini, V. K., & Srinivas, L. (1987). Lipid peroxide-induced DNA damage: protection by turmeric (*Curcuma longa*). *Molecular and Cellular Biochemistry, 77,* 3–10.

Sharma, O. P. (1976). Antioxidant activity of curcumin and related compounds. *Biochemical Pharmacology, 25,* 1811–1812.

Silverberg, J. I., Jagdeo, J., Patel, M., et al. (2011). Green tea extract protects human skin fibroblasts from reactive oxygen species induced necrosis. *Journal of Drugs in Dermatology, 10,* 1096–1101.

Singh, S., & Aggarwal, B. B. (1995). Activation of transcription factor NF-κB is suppressed by curcumin (diferuloylmethane). *Journal of Biological Chemistry, 270,* 24995–25000.

Smith, J. V., & Luo, Y. (2004). Studies on molecular mechanisms of *Ginkgo biloba* extract. *Applied Microbiology & Biotechnology, 64,* 465–472.

Stevinson, C., Devaraj, V. S., Fountain-Barber, A., et al. (2003). Homeopathic arnica for prevention of pain and bruising: randomized placebo-controlled trial in hand surgery. *Journal of the Royal Society of Medicine, 96,* 60–65.

Sur, R., Nigam, A., Grote, D., et al. (2008). Avenanthramides, polyphenols from oats, exhibit anti-inflammatory and anti-itch activity. *Archives of Dermatological Research, 300,* 569–574.

Suter, A., Niemer, W., & Klopp, R. (2011). A new ginkgo fresh plant extract increases microcirculation and radical scavenging activity in elderly patients. *Advances in Therapy, 28,* 1078–1088.

Syed, T. A., Ahmad, S. A., Holt, A. H., et al. (1996). Management of psoriasis with Aloe vera extract in a hydrophilic cream: a placebo-controlled, double-blind study. *Tropical Medicine & International Health, 1,*505–509.

Thornfeldt, C. (2005). Cosmeceuticals containing herbs: fact, fiction, and future. *Dermatologic Surgery, 31,* 873–881.

Vayalil, P. K., Elmets, C. A., & Katiyar, S. K. (2003). Treatment of green tea polyphenols in hydrophilic cream prevents UVB-induced oxidation of lipids and proteins, depletion of antioxidant enzymes and phosphorylation of MAPK proteins in SKH-1 hairless mouse skin. *Carcinogenesis, 24,* 927–936.

Verma, N., Chakrabarti, R., Das Rakha, H., et al. (2012). Anti-inflammatory effects of shea butter through inhibition of iNOS, COX-2, and cytokines via the NF-Kb pathway in LPS-activated J774 macrophage cells. *Journal of Complementary and Integrative Medicine, 9*(1), 1–11.

Vié, K., Cours-Darne, S., Vienne, M. P., et al. (2002). Modulating effects of oatmeal extracts in the sodium lauryl sulfate skin irritancy model. *Skin Pharmacology and Physiology, 15,* 120–124.

Visuthikosol, V., Chowchuen, B., Sukwanarat, Y., et al. (1995). Effect of aloe vera gel to healing of burn wound a clinical and histologic study. *Journal of the Medical Association of Thailand, 78*, 403–409.

Walton, S. F., McKinnon, M., Pizzutto, S., et al. (2004). Acaricidal activity of *Melaleuca alternifolia* (tea tree) oil: in vitro sensitivity of *Sarcoptes scabiei var hominis* to Terpinen-4-ol. *Archives of Dermatology, 140*, 563–566.

Wang, Z. Y., Agarwal, R., Bickers, D. R., et al. (1991). Protection against ultraviolet B radiation-induced photocarcinogenesis in hairless mice by green tea polyphenols. *Carcinogenesis, 12*, 1527–1530.

Wasserman, L., Avigad, S., Beery, E., et al. (2002). The effect of Aloe Emodin on the proliferation of a new Merkel carcinoma cell line. *American Journal of Dermatopathology, 24*, 17–22.

Weber, T. M., Ceilley, R. I., Buerger, A., et al. (2006). Skin tolerance, efficacy, and quality of life of patients with red facial skin using a skin care regimen containing Licochalcone A. *Journal of Cosmetic Dermatology, 5*, 227–232.

Wertz, P. W. (2009). Human synthetic sebum formulation and stability under conditions of use and storage. *International Journal of Cosmetic Science, 31*, 21–25.

Wichtl, M. (2000). *Herbal drugs and phytopharmaceuticals.* Boca Raton, FL: F.C.P.I.

Wood, P. (1986). *Oat beta-glucan: structure, location and properties.* American Association of Cereal Chemists, Inc., St. Paul, Minnesota.

Wright, S. (1985). Atopic dermatitis and essential fatty acids: a biochemical basis for atopy? *Acta Dermato-Venereologica Supplementum, 114*, 143–145.

Yates, J. E., Phifer, J. B., & Flake, D. (2009). Clinical inquiries. Do nonmedicated topicals relieve childhood eczema? *Journal of Family Practice, 58*, 280–281.

Yokota, T., Nishio, H., Kubota, Y., et al. (1998). The inhibitory effect of glabridin from licorice extracts on melanogenesis and inflammation. *Pigment Cell Research, 11*, 355–361.

Yoon, S., Lee, J., & Lee, S. (2002). The therapeutic effect of evening primrose oil in atopic dermatitis patients with dry scaly skin lesions is associated with the normalization of serum gamma-interferon levels. *Skin Pharmacology and Applied Skin Physiology, 15*, 20–25.

Zhou, M., Robards, K., Glennie-Holmes, M., et al. (1999). Oat lipids. *Journal of the American Oil Chemists' Society, 76*, 159–169.

6

Psychoneuroimmunology in Dermatology

KRISTOPHER DENBY, MD, NANA DUFFY, MD,
AND FRANCISCO TAUSK, MD

Key Concepts

- ♣ The word *psychoneuroimmunology* refers to the study of the interplay between the central nervous and immune systems.
- ♣ Psychological stressors have the potential to alter immune reactions, and the chronicity of the stressor is a major contributing factor.
- ♣ Studies have demonstrated a negative impact of a variety of psychological stressors on wound healing, in terms of duration as well as complications.
- ♣ Stress and anxiety have been shown to increase the perception of itch in atopic dermatitis, with positive benefits of anxiolytic therapy.
- ♣ Stress-reduction techniques such as hypnosis, guided imagery, and mindfulness-based stress reduction can have a significant positive impact on psoriasis.
- ♣ Stress-mediated release of pro-inflammatory cytokines may be the underlying explanation for histopathologic findings in chronic urticaria and may also suggest stress reduction as an adjunctive treatment option.
- ♣ Animal models show that stress plays a role in tumorigenesis and metastasis, suggesting a potential link between stress and skin cancer.

Introduction

The discipline of psychoneuroimmunology (PNI) examines the relationship between the central nervous system (CNS) and the immune system. An interest in the interplay between the mind and body was present as early as the fifth century BCE. At that time, it appears the focus was primarily on how the body altered the mind (Tausk, Elenkov, et al., 2008). Of greater interest to us is how the mind alters the body, specifically the immune system and its implications in the biology of the skin.

During the early 20th century Pavlov described the seminal experiments on dogs that led to the publication of classical conditioning as a concept of associative learning. At that time, Metalnikov and Chorine reported studies showing that immune responses could be modified by similar learning paradigms. This approach remained mostly ignored until the 1970s, when Ader and Cohen (1975) demonstrated that immunosuppressive pharmacotherapy, like salivation, could be behaviorally conditioned. They paired the taste of saccharin with injections of cyclophosphamide in rats. After a period of training (conditioning) the exposure of the rats to saccharin replaced the effects of the cyclophosphamide. At the time, the consequences of these studies were significant, awaking interest in mind–body research and beginning the development of the field of PNI.

Background

The CNS responds to stressors chiefly through two pathways, the sympathetic nervous system and the hypothalamic pituitary axis. The latter exerts its effect through secretion of corticotropin-releasing hormone (CRH) and arginine vasopressin (AVP). In the CNS, CRH acts on the pituitary gland, releasing a variety of peptides created through the cleavage of pro-opiomelanocortin, including adrenocorticotropic hormone (ACTH), which in turn acts on the adrenal cortex to induce the secretion of glucocorticoids. Stimulation of CNS noradrenergic neurons causes the release of epinephrine. Additionally, the stimulation of the locus coeruleus results in release of norepinephrine (NE) by the peripheral nervous system. The end result of this pathway is the classic "fight-or-flight" response (Cannon, 1932). NE-containing autonomic nervous system fibers innervate a wide variety of immune organs, including the skin (Moynihan, Rieder, et al., 2010). The increased levels of cortisol and NE favor T_H2 differentiation over T_H1 (Fig. 6.1) (Tausk, Elenkov, et al., 2008).

Immune cells (including monocytes and both B and T lymphocytes) have receptors to a wide variety of neurohormones and neurotransmitters, which regulate cytokine production and cellular proliferation, among other functions (Chrousos, 1998; Glaser & Kiecolt-Glaser, 2005; Khansari, Murgo, et al., 1990). Furthermore, CRH, among other neurohormones, can be produced by components of the immune system., and CNS cells and T lymphocytes share a variety of surface proteins (Morris & Williams, 1975; Stephanou, Jessop, et al.,

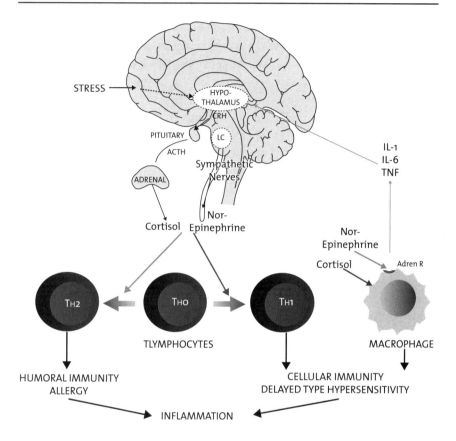

FIGURE 6.1 Stress and Immunity

A threat to the organism's homeostasis is perceived and processed by the brain cortex. The presence of a stressor is subsequently transmitted to the hypothalamus, triggering the activation of the hypothalamic-pituitary-adrenal axis, with the release of corticotropin-releasing hormone (CRH), which reaches the pituitary and in turn mediates the release of adrenocorticotropic hormone (ACTH); the latter induces the systemic secretion of glucocorticosteroids (GC) from the adrenal gland. Additionally, stress activates the locus coeruleus (LC), increasing peripheral norepinephrine (NE) secretion; NE and GC together have a profound effect on immunity through their action on mononuclear cells. GC and NE induce the differentiation of naïve helper T cells (T_H0) toward T_H2 lymphocytes, associated with humoral immunity and allergy, and inhibit the development of the T_H1 lineage, which mediate cellular immunity (delayed-type hypersensitivity). NE binds to adrenergic receptors on macrophages, rapidly inducing the generation of pro-inflammatory cytokines such as interleukin (IL)-1, IL-6, and tumor necrosis factor (TNF)-alpha, through the translocation of nuclear factor-kappa beta to the nucleus. These may reach the hypothalamus through a leaky blood–brain barrier, inducing further activation of the hypothalamic-pituitary-adrenal axis and favoring peripheral inflammation. Subsequently GC reaches macrophages, shutting off the inflammation mediated by nuclear factor-kappa beta. Adren R, Adrenergic Receptor.

1990), further illustrating the connection between the CNS and the immune system. In light of these parallels, it is logical that psychological stressors have the potential to alter immunity via the above-described pathways.

The chronicity of the stressor is one of the factors that determines its immunologic impact (Selye, 1936, 1946; Tausk, Elenkov, et al., 2008). As Selye observed in 1936, stress facilitates adaptations that are advantageous in the acute setting but detrimental over extended periods of stress:

> As much as we see ourselves as evolved and civilized, humans still appear to be superbly adapted to avoid being attacked by wild predators, encounters that fortunately nowadays are relatively infrequent in normal city streets. However, this stress response does not seem to be as appropriate when we are coping with the persistent chronic stressors of our modern daily lives. We have replaced lions with traffic jams, pollution, and over-burdened work environments, but the mechanisms to deal with adversity have not evolved accordingly. As originally described by Selye, the pioneer of stress research, the organism has the ability to adapt to acute homeostatic challenges; however, chronicity leads to exhaustion, distress, and disease. Indeed, chronic stress has been shown to have an adverse effect on health and life expectancy. (Tausk & Nousari, 2001, p. 78)

The importance of PNI to dermatologic disorders cannot be overstated. PNI has already been used to explain the link between psychological stress and a variety of topics, including wound healing and chronic inflammatory conditions (atopic dermatitis, psoriasis). While the precise mechanism has not yet been elucidated, it is possible that PNI will explain the mechanism by which psychological stress exacerbates a variety of dermatologic disorders.

Wound Healing

The initial critical steps of wound healing involve the localized release of chemokines and pro-inflammatory cytokines, including interleukin (IL)-1 (both α and β), IL-6, IL-8, transforming growth factor-β, tumor necrosis factor (TNF)-α, and vascular endothelial growth factor (Hubner, Brauchle, et al., 1996; Werner & Grose, 2003). Interference with this cascade alters the migration and activation of phagocytes, tissue remodeling, re-epithelialization, and angiogenesis, among other things, and ultimately impairs the wound healing process as a whole. IL-6 knockout mice demonstrated markedly decreased re-epithelialization, resulting in slow wound healing (Werner & Grose, 2003). Just as too little IL-6 can inhibit wound healing, too much results in excessive scar tissue formation (Werner & Grose, 2003). Similarly, glucocorticoid-treated mice have been shown to produce less IL-1α, IL-1β, and TNF-α in response to a wound than their untreated counterparts (Hubner, Brauchle, et al., 1996).

It has been shown that anxiety and depression can predispose patients with chronic lower extremity wounds to slow healing (Cole-King & Harding, 2001). Self-reported stress and depression are associated with decreased wound healing (Bosch, Engeland, et al., 2007; Ebrecht, Hextall, et al., 2004). Interestingly, patients who have trouble managing their anger also demonstrated slower wound healing and increased cortisol production compared to their better-adjusted counterparts (Gouin, Kiecolt-Glaser, et al., 2008). Additionally, depressive symptoms also correlate with increased surgical wound infections in cardiac patients (Doering, Moser, et al., 2005). Presumably, the association of depression and increased propensity for surgical site infections also exists in dermatology patients following excisions.

To increase the precision of measured effects on wound healing, punch biopsy, blister formation, and tape stripping have been used to create reproducible standardized wounds. Using these methods it has been demonstrated that a wide variety of stressors delay wound healing. In assessing the impact of caregiver stress, Kiecolt-Glaser and colleagues (1995) performed 3.5-mm punch biopsies on the nondominant forearm of 13 women caring for relatives with Alzheimer's dementia and 13 controls matched for age and socioeconomic status. The authors found that the experimental group took 9 days longer (24% more time) to heal the wounds compared to controls. Additionally, the authors observed that the caregivers' leukocytes had impaired production of IL-1β in response to a lipopolysaccharide challenge. Other psychological stressors shown to decrease wound healing include pain (Graham, Robles, et al., 2006; McGuire, Heffner, et al., 2006), marital turmoil (Muizzuddin, Matsui, et al., 2003), the Trier Social Stress Test (TSST) (a standardized test consisting of a mock job interview and mental arithmetic task) (Altemus, Rao, et al., 2001; Robles, 2007), and even student examinations (Garg, Chren, et al., 2001; Marucha, Kiecolt-Glaser, et al., 1998). Furthermore, it has been shown that discussion of a prior marital disagreement also delayed wound healing, likely through reduced local production of IL-6, IL-1β, and TNF-α (Christian, Graham, et al., 2006; Kiecolt-Glaser, Loving, et al., 2005); greater observed hostility increased the delay in wound healing and resulted in higher systemic levels of TNF-α and IL-6 the following morning (Kiecolt-Glaser, Loving, et al., 2005). The converse, that positive interactions and social support accelerate wound healing, has also been reported (Gouin, Carter, et al., 2010).

In light of these data, it is unsurprising that reducing stress accelerates wound healing. Even brief interventions, such as engaging in the writing of prior traumatic events, stimulate healing (Weinman, Ebrecht, et al., 2008).

In one study, subjects were asked to write on a particular topic for 20 minutes on three consecutive days. Subjects randomized to explore their feelings and thoughts surrounding a personal experience that was traumatic or distressing had markedly improved wound healing compared to those asked to write about time management. In older adults, one hour of physical exercise three times per week has been shown to reduce psychological distress and accelerate wound healing (Emery, Kiecolt-Glaser, et al., 2005; Gouin & Kiecolt-Glaser, 2011). Administration of fluoxetine (a selective serotonin reuptake inhibitor [SSRI]) has been shown to blunt the decrease in wound healing associated with housing isolation and crowding stress in rats (Farahani, Sadr, et al., 2007). As fluoxetine acts by altering neurochemistry, which in turn modulates the immune system, it is likely that other SSRIs would similarly blunt the negative impact that stress and depressive symptoms have on wound healing. Other classes of antidepressants might similarly improve wound healing under psychological stress. Additionally, other methods of reducing stress, anxiety, and depression, whether rooted in pharmacology or behavioral psychology, may contribute to expedite wound healing.

Atopic Dermatitis

The pattern of inflammation seen in atopic dermatitis (AD) is predominantly within the T_H2 immune reaction (Lin, Wang, et al., 2011) driven by Langerhans cells presenting allergens or autoantigens to T cells in draining lymph nodes. Production of prostaglandin E2 and IL-10 by these activated Langerhans cells induces T_H2 differentiation in naïve T cells. Consequently, the cytokine profile seen in AD is composed of IL-4, IL-5, and IL-13.

The interplay between stress and the course of AD has long been known (Gil, Keefe, et al., 1987). A variety of psychological stressors have been linked to increased incidence and exacerbations of AD. These include parental divorce or separation (Bockelbrink, Heinrich, et al., 2006), other more general familial dysfunction (Poot, Antoine, et al., 2011), moving abroad (Anderzen, Arnetz, et al., 1997), parental diagnosis of panic disorder (Slattery, Klein, et al., 2002), and separation anxiety disorder (Slattery, Klein, et al., 2002). Similarly, there is a wealth of evidence indicating that a diagnosis of AD in a child is quite disruptive not only to the affected child but to the family unit as a whole, resulting in more stressful life events, including divorce (Al Shobaili, 2010; Beattie & Lewis-Jones, 2006; Kilpelainen, Koskenvuo, et al., 2002; Lapidus, 2001). These stressful life events can in turn cause an exacerbation of AD. Importantly, consultation with a dermatologist can mitigate this decrease in quality of life (Beattie & Lewis-Jones, 2006). The frustration engendered by the itch–scratch cycle is likely to be at least partly responsible for this increase in stress. As psychological stress has been shown to enhance pruritus (Paus, Schmelz, et al., 2006), it is unsurprising that Oh and colleagues (2010) found that increased anxiety in AD subjects was associated with increased pruritic symptoms. However, they did not find a corresponding increase in objective disease severity as measured by the Eczema Area and Severity Index (EASI).

Given the similarities between chronic itch and chronic pain, it has been suggested that psychobehavioral therapies and anxiolytics/antidepressants may have a place in the treatment of AD (Tran, Papoiu, et al., 2010). Kawana and colleagues (2010) performed a randomized controlled of tandospirone citrate, a serotonin agonist, in AD patients. After four weeks of tandospirone citrate therapy, treated subjects experienced a marked improvement in the Scoring Atopic Dermatitis (SCORAD) rating and anxiety and depressive symptoms. Wolf and colleagues (2008) reported that higher levels of parental perceived stress and parental depression are linked to an increase of two atopy-relevant inflammatory markers, IL-4 and eosinophilic cationic protein (ECP), after a six-month period in children with AD. Buske-Kirschbaum and colleagues (2010) showed that atopic children express a blunted cortisol response to stressors, suggesting that this effect may explain the exacerbation of symptoms during episodes of stress.

Psoriasis

Immune dysregulation plays a pivotal role in the pathophysiology of psoriasis. Psoriasis has long been considered an autoimmune disease with a complex genetic basis (Valdimarsson, 2007). While initial examinations of the immunologic underpinnings of psoriasis focused on T_H1 cells, more recent examinations into its immunopathogenesis implicate the T_H17 inflammatory pathway (Ma, Liang, et al., 2008; Nickoloff, 2007; van Beelen, Teunissen, et al., 2007; Zheng, Danilenko, et al., 2007). Levels of IFN-γ and TNF-α produced by both T_H1 and T_H17 cells are elevated in psoriatic lesions (Lowes, Kikuchi, et al., 2008; Zheng, Danilenko, et al., 2007). A mouse model demonstrated that injection of IL-23, a cytokine produced by keratinocytes and monocyte-derived cells (Langerhans cells, dendritic cells, and macrophages) that induces expansion of T_H17 populations, is sufficient to cause the epidermal changes observed in biopsied psoriatic lesions (Zheng, Danilenko, et al., 2007). Acting in conjunction, IL-6 and TGF-β induce differentiation of CD4+ T cells into T_H17 (Iwakura & Ishigame, 2006).

Psychosocial stressors have been implicated both in increased incidence of psoriasis (Malhotra & Mehta, 2008; Naldi, Peli, et al., 2001; Poot, Antoine, et al.,

2011) and disease flares (Fortune, Richards, et al., 2002, 2005; Malhotra & Mehta, 2008; Poot, Antoine, et al., 2011). When exposed to the acute stressor of the TSST, patients with psoriasis have been shown to have an exaggerated increase in the number of circulating monocytes and CD4+ cells and a concomitant decrease in the percentage of activated T cells (Buske-Kirschbaum, Kern, et al., 2007).

Psoriasis patients whose flares are precipitated by stress have been found to have a blunted HPA axis with low cortisol in response to a stressor (Richards, Ray, et al., 2005). When not selecting for individuals whose psoriasis is precipitated by stress, no difference was seen between subjects and controls in cortisol, ACTH, or catecholamines following the TSST (Buske-Kirschbaum, Ebrecht, et al., 2006). However, the authors did observe that patients with psoriasis had an exaggerated sympathetic nervous system response (increased secretion of NE and epinephrine).

In support of the role played by the nervous system in psoriasis, it has been observed that patients with psoriasis who experienced loss of sensory innervation due to trauma clear their psoriatic plaques in the skin that has been denervated. Furthermore, with the return of sensation, these subjects again developed psoriatic plaques in these regions (Farber, Lanigan, et al., 1990). This finding led to the hypothesis that local cutaneous nerves secrete factors that are essential for the development of psoriatic lesions (Raychaudhuri & Farber, 1993, 2001; Raychaudhuri & Raychaudhuri, 2009). This hypothesis has been strengthened by the increased density of cutaneous nerve fibers and upregulation of calcitonin gene-related peptide, substance P, vasoactive intestinal peptide, and nerve growth factor in active plaques (Raychaudhuri & Raychaudhuri, 2009). Increased nerve growth factor has been shown to induce T-cell and keratinocyte proliferation, attract memory T cells and mast cells, and promote mast cell degranulation (Raychaudhuri & Raychaudhuri, 2009).

As psychological factors play a role in the pathogenesis of psoriasis, it is unsurprising that incorporating psychological interventions into a therapeutic plan can be effective. Ader and colleagues (2010) recently reported a study of classical conditioning in the pharmacotherapy of psoriasis. Patients were treated with 0.1% triamcinolone cream that had a distinct odor and color. Once the psoriatic plaques resolved, subjects were randomized to three groups; the first one (Full Dose) continued to receive the same full dose as before, the second (Dose Control) received one fourth of the dose, and the third (conditioned; Partial Reinforcement) was treated with full dose (one out of four patients) or an identical placebo (the other three), lacking any active drug. The Dose Control group had a higher relapse rate than either the partial or complete reinforcement groups. The ability to use less drug to derive the same benefit is important, particularly given the potential for skin thinning seen with corticosteroids.

Hypnosis has been reported to significantly improve psoriasis (Shenefelt, 2000; Tausk & Whitmore, 1999). Cognitive-behavioral therapy has also been shown to be effective, if not yet in a randomized controlled trial (Fortune, Richards, et al., 2005). Meditation (Gaston, Crombez, et al., 1991) as well as stress reduction and guided imagery also decrease psoriasis symptoms (Zachariae, Oster, et al., 1996). Additionally, patients undergoing photo-therapy cleared in half the time when mindfulness-based stress reduction tapes were supplied during the phototherapy (Benhard, Kristeller, et al., 1988; Kabat-Zinn, Wheeler, et al., 1998).

Urticaria

Chronic idiopathic urticaria (CIU) has also been repeatedly linked with psychi-atric comorbidities, including depression and anxiety (Chung, Symons, et al., 2010; Herguner, Kilic, et al., 2011; Ozkan, Oflaz, et al., 2007; Staubach, Dechene, et al., 2011; Uguz, Engin, et al., 2008). While so far the assumption has been that the psychiatric condition is partially caused by the skin condition, it is conceiv-able that the psychiatric illness precedes the cutaneous manifestations. Stressful life events have also been shown to precipitate flares of CIU (Malhotra & Mehta, 2008) as well as cases of acute urticaria (Deacock 2008). Recently, CIU has been linked to posttraumatic stress disorder (PTSD) (Gupta & Gupta, 2012). In this case series of five patients with CIU and PTSD, the authors discovered that addressing the patients' underlying PTSD resulted in marked or total resolution of the CIU. The authors postulated that the chronic hyperarousal of the auto-nomic nervous system that occurs in PTSD facilitated the development of CIU flares. Additionally, it appears that neuropeptides and CRH play an important role in stress-related degranulation of mast cells in urticaria and other inflam-matory skin diseases (Papadopoulou, Kalogeromitros, et al., 2005; Theoharides, Alysandratos, et al., 2012; Theoharides, Donelan, et al., 2004). As discussed pre-viously, conflict can result in elevated levels of pro-inflammatory cytokines, leading to increased inflammation in tissue. Histopathologic examination of urticaria biopsies reveals dense inflammatory infiltrates. The stress-mediated release of these pro-inflammatory cytokines may be the underlying explanation for the histopathologic findings.

Skin Cancer

A link between malignancy and emotional state has been suspected for cen-turies (Leshan, 1959; Smith, Fuhrmann, et al., 2009). Rodent models have demonstrated that a variety of social stressors can promote tumor growth and metastasis (Azpiroz, De Miguel, et al., 2008; Ben-Eliyahu, 2003; Riley, 1981). Similarly, mice that were chronically stressed through multiple exposures to the scent of fox urine developed squamous cell carcinoma tumors markedly faster than controls when exposed to carcinogenic levels of ultraviolet radiation (Parker, Klein, et al., 2004). A variety of stressors have been shown to decrease the activity of natural killer cells and macrophages, decrease the number of T cells (both overall and within the target tissue), and increase angiogenesis (Antoni, Lutgendorf, et al., 2006). Interestingly, patients who responded to melanoma with hopelessness experienced more rapid progression of their disease as well as worse quality of life than those with more active, adaptive coping strategies (Temoshok, 1985; Temoshok, Heller, et al., 1985).

Other Dermatologic Disorders

Familial dysfunction (Poot, Antoine, et al., 2011) and stressful life events (Diaz-Atienza & Gurpegui, 2011) appear to contribute to exacerbations of alopecia areata. Furthermore, it has been suggested that better coping strategies are associated with increased rates of remission of alopecia areata (Matzer, Egger, et al., 2011). While a causative link between psychological stress and acne has been demonstrated (Yosipovitch, Tang, et al., 2007), no PNI mechanism has yet been articulated. In patients whose acne severity correlates with psychological stressors, sebum production is not altered, indicating this is not a mechanism by which stress contributes to acne severity (Yosipovitch, Tang, et al., 2007). Proposed mechanisms include increased production of pro-inflammatory neuropeptides and hormones such as CRH (Ganceviciene, Graziene, et al., 2009; Tom & Barrio, 2008).

There is some evidence that other autoinflammatory disorders may also carry a worse prognosis when compounded by psychological distress, but the evidence is less extensive than for AD, psoriasis, urticaria, and wound healing. While the health-related quality of life has been found to be worse in patients with systemic lupus erythematosus (Bricou, Taieb, et al., 2006; Hyphantis, Palieraki, et al., 2011), systemic sclerosis (Hyphantis, Tsifetaki, et al., 2007), and Sjögren's syndrome (Hyphantis, Mantis, et al., 2011) who have concomitant psychological distress, this may not be a result of objectively worse disease but rather a decreased ability to tolerate these stressors. In a Swedish study, Strombeck and colleagues (2007) found that 45 minutes of Nordic walking (using specially constructed ski poles) three times per week for 12 weeks improved mood and decreased fatigue (one of the debilitating features of Sjögren's) in women with primary Sjögren's syndrome. A review paper by

Strombeck and Jacobsson (2007) found that patients with mild to moderate lupus experience similar exercise-related improvements in mood and fatigue.

Conclusion

PNI is a field filled with promise for improved patient outcomes. Understanding how an intangible psychological state produces concrete changes in the immune system and ultimately affects the health of the organism may allow us to design effective psychosocial complementary interventions that can be deployed in the clinical setting, such as mindfulness-based stress reduction, exploration of emotions, and antidepressants, and achieve significant clinical benefit while minimizing untoward side effects. Conversely, studies of PNI explain how alexithymia, psychosocial stressors (including chronic caregiver stress), and psychiatric comorbidities exacerbate or precipitate physical diseases. By appropriately addressing underlying psychiatric comorbidities, we maximize our management of patients for a host of dermatologic conditions. Further, we have the opportunity to decrease surgical site infections, thus decreasing the amount of antibiotics that are prescribed. Given the continued evolution of antimicrobial-resistant pathogens, this benefit must not be ignored.

REFERENCES

Ader, R., & Cohen, N. (1975). Behaviorally conditioned immunosuppression. *Psychosomatic Medicine, 37*(4), 333–340.

Ader, R., Mercurio, M. G., et al. (2010). Conditioned pharmacotherapeutic effects: a preliminary study. *Psychosomatic Medicine, 72*(2), 192–197.

Al Shobaili, H. A. (2010). The impact of childhood atopic dermatitis on the patients' family. *Pediatric Dermatology, 27*(6), 618–623.

Altemus, M., Rao, B., et al. (2001). Stress-induced changes in skin barrier function in healthy women. *Journal of Investigative Dermatology, 117*(2), 309–317.

Anderzen, I., Arnetz, B. B., et al. (1997). Stress and sensitization in children: a controlled prospective psychophysiological study of children exposed to international relocation. *Journal of Psychosomatic Research, 43*(3), 259–269.

Antoni, M. H., Lutgendorf, S. K., et al. (2006). The influence of bio-behavioural factors on tumour biology: pathways and mechanisms. *Nature Reviews Cancer, 6*(3), 240–248.

Azpiroz, A., De Miguel, Z., et al. (2008). Relations between different coping strategies for social stress, tumor development and neuroendocrine and immune activity in male mice. *Brain, Behavior, and Immunity, 22*(5), 690–698.

Beattie, P. E., & Lewis-Jones, M. S. (2006). An audit of the impact of a consultation with a paediatric dermatology team on quality of life in infants with atopic eczema and their families: further validation of the Infants' Dermatitis Quality of Life Index and Dermatitis Family Impact score. *British Journal of Dermatology, 155*(6), 1249–1255.

Ben-Eliyahu, S. (2003). The promotion of tumor metastasis by surgery and stress: immunological basis and implications for psychoneuroimmunology. *Brain, Behavior, and Immunity, 17*(Suppl 1), S27–36.

Benhard, J. D., Kristeller, J., et al. (1988). Effectiveness of relaxation and visualization techniques as an adjunct to phototherapy and photochemotherapy of psoriasis. *Journal of the American Academy of Dermatology, 19*(3), 572–574.

Bockelbrink, A., Heinrich, J., et al. (2006). Atopic eczema in children: another harmful sequel of divorce. *Allergy, 61*(12), 1397–1402.

Bosch, J. A., Engeland, C. G., et al. (2007). Depressive symptoms predict mucosal wound healing. *Psychosomatic Medicine, 69*(7), 597–605.

Bricou, O., Taieb, O., et al. (2006). Stress and coping strategies in systemic lupus erythematosus: a review. *Neuroimmunomodulation, 13*(5–6), 283–293.

Buske-Kirschbaum, A., Ebrecht, M., et al. (2006). Endocrine stress responses in TH1-mediated chronic inflammatory skin disease (psoriasis vulgaris)—do they parallel stress-induced endocrine changes in TH2-mediated inflammatory dermatoses (atopic dermatitis)? *Psychoneuroendocrinology, 31*(4), 439–446.

Buske-Kirschbaum, A., Ebrecht, M., et al. (2010). Blunted HPA axis responsiveness to stress in atopic patients is associated with the acuity and severeness of allergic inflammation. *Brain, Behavior, and Immunity, 24*(8), 1347–1353.

Buske-Kirschbaum, A., Kern, S., et al. (2007). Altered distribution of leukocyte subsets and cytokine production in response to acute psychosocial stress in patients with psoriasis vulgaris. *Brain, Behavior, and Immunity, 21*(1), 92–99.

Cannon, W. B. (1932). *The wisdom of the body*. New York: Norton Pubs.

Christian, L. M., Graham, J. E., et al. (2006). Stress and wound healing. *Neuroimmunomodulation, 13*(5–6), 337–346.

Chrousos, G. P. (1998). Stressors, stress, and neuroendocrine integration of the adaptive response. The 1997 Hans Selye Memorial Lecture. *Annals of the New York Academy of Science, 851*, 311–335.

Chung, M. C., Symons, C., et al. (2010). Stress, psychiatric co-morbidity and coping in patients with chronic idiopathic urticaria. *Psychology & Health, 25*(4), 477–490.

Cole-King, A., & Harding, K. G. (2001). Psychological factors and delayed healing in chronic wounds. *Psychosomatic Medicine, 63*(2), 216–220.

Deacock, S. J. (2008). An approach to the patient with urticaria. *Clinical & Experimental Immunology, 153*(2), 151–161.

Diaz-Atienza, F., & Gurpegui, M. (2011). Environmental stress but not subjective distress in children or adolescents with alopecia areata. *Journal of Psychosomatic Research, 71*(2), 102–107.

Doering, L. V., Moser, D. K., et al. (2005). Depression, healing, and recovery from coronary artery bypass surgery. *American Journal of Critical Care, 14*(4), 316–324.

Ebrecht, M., Hextall, J., et al. (2004). Perceived stress and cortisol levels predict speed of wound healing in healthy male adults. *Psychoneuroendocrinology, 29*(6), 798–809.

Emery, C. F., Kiecolt-Glaser, J. K., et al. (2005). Exercise accelerates wound healing among healthy older adults: a preliminary investigation. *Journal of Gerontology A Biological Science & Medical Science, 60*(11), 1432–1436.

Farahani, R. M., Sadr, K., et al. (2007). Fluoxetine enhances cutaneous wound healing in chronically stressed Wistar rats. *Advances in Skin & Wound Care, 20*(3), 157–165.

Farber, E. M., Lanigan, S. W., et al. (1990). The role of cutaneous sensory nerves in the maintenance of psoriasis. *International Journal of Dermatology, 29*(6), 418–420.

Fortune, D. G., Richards, H. L., et al. (2002). Psychological stress, distress and disability in patients with psoriasis: consensus and variation in the contribution of illness perceptions, coping and alexithymia. *British Journal of Clinical Psychology, 41*(Pt 2), 157–174.

Fortune, D. G., Richards, H. L., et al. (2005). Psychologic factors in psoriasis: consequences, mechanisms, and interventions. *Dermatology Clinics, 23*(4), 681–694.

Ganceviciene, R., Graziene, V., et al. (2009). Involvement of the corticotropin-releasing hormone system in the pathogenesis of acne vulgaris. *British Journal of Dermatology, 160*(2), 345–352.

Garg, A., Chren, M. M., et al. (2001). Psychological stress perturbs epidermal permeability barrier homeostasis: implications for the pathogenesis of stress-associated skin disorders. *Archives of Dermatology, 137*(1), 53–59.

Gaston, L., Crombez, J. C., et al. (1991). Psychological stress and psoriasis: experimental and prospective correlational studies. *Acta Dermato-Venereologica Supplementum (Stockh) 156*: 37–43.

Gil, K. M., Keefe, F. J., et al. (1987). The relation of stress and family environment to atopic dermatitis symptoms in children. *Journal of Psychosomatic Research, 31*(6), 673–684.

Glaser, R., & Kiecolt-Glaser, J. K. (2005). Stress-induced immune dysfunction: implications for health. *Nature Review Immunology, 5*(3), 243–251.

Gouin, J. P., Carter, C. S., et al. (2010). Marital behavior, oxytocin, vasopressin, and wound healing. *Psychoneuroendocrinology, 35*(7), 1082–1090.

Gouin, J. P., & Kiecolt-Glaser, J. K. (2011). The impact of psychological stress on wound healing: methods and mechanisms. *Immunology & Allergy Clinics of North America, 31*(1), 81–93.

Gouin, J. P., Kiecolt-Glaser, J. K., et al. (2008). The influence of anger expression on wound healing. *Brain, Behavior, and Immunity, 22*(5), 699–708.

Graham, J. E., Robles, T. F., et al. (2006). Hostility and pain are related to inflammation in older adults. *Brain, Behavior, and Immunity, 20*(4), 389–400.

Gupta, M. A., & Gupta, A. K. (2012). Chronic idiopathic urticaria and post-traumatic stress disorder (PTSD), an under-recognized comorbidity. *Clinical Dermatology, 30*(3), 351–354.

Herguner, S., Kilic, G., et al. (2011). Levels of depression, anxiety and behavioural problems and frequency of psychiatric disorders in children with chronic idiopathic urticaria. *British Journal of Dermatology, 164*(6), 1342–1347.

Hubner, G., Brauchle, M., et al. (1996). Differential regulation of pro-inflammatory cytokines during wound healing in normal and glucocorticoid-treated mice. *Cytokine, 8*(7), 548–556.

Hyphantis, T. N., Tsifetaki, N., et al. (2007). The impact of psychological functioning upon systemic sclerosis patients' quality of life. *Seminare in Arthritis & Rheumatism, 37*(2), 81–92.

Hyphantis, T., Mantis, D., et al. (2011). The psychological defensive profile of primary Sjogren's syndrome patients and its relationship to health-related quality of life. *Clinical & Experimental Rheumatology, 29*(3), 485–493.

Hyphantis, T., Palieraki, K., et al. (2011). Coping with health-stressors and defence styles associated with health-related quality of life in patients with systemic lupus erythematosus. *Lupus, 20*(9), 893–903.

Iwakura, Y., & Ishigame, H. (2006). The IL-23/IL-17 axis in inflammation. *Journal of Clinical Investigation, 116*(5), 1218–1222.

Kabat-Zinn, J., Wheeler, E., et al. (1998). Influence of a mindfulness meditation-based stress reduction intervention on rates of skin clearing in patients with moderate to severe psoriasis undergoing phototherapy (UVB) and photochemotherapy (PUVA). *Psychosomatic Medicine, 60*(5), 625–632.

Kawana, S., Kato, Y., et al. (2010). Efficacy of a 5-HT1a receptor agonist in atopic dermatitis. *Clinical & Experimental Dermatology, 35*(8), 835–840.

Khansari, D. N., Murgo, A. J., et al. (1990). Effects of stress on the immune system. *Immunology Today, 11*(5), 170–175.

Kiecolt-Glaser, J. K., Loving, T. J., et al. (2005). Hostile marital interactions, proinflammatory cytokine production, and wound healing. *Archives of General Psychiatry, 62*(12), 1377–1384.

Kiecolt-Glaser, J. K., Marucha, P. T., et al. (1995). Slowing of wound healing by psychological stress. *Lancet, 346*(8984), 1194–1196.

Kilpelainen, M., Koskenvuo, M., et al. (2002). Stressful life events promote the manifestation of asthma and atopic diseases. *Clinical & Experimental Allergy, 32*(2), 256–263.

Lapidus, C. S. (2001). Role of social factors in atopic dermatitis: the US perspective. *Journal of the American Academy of Dermatology, 45*(1 Suppl), S41–43.

Leshan, L. (1959). Psychological states as factors in the development of malignant disease: a critical review. *Journal of the National Cancer Institute, 22*(1), 1–18.

Lin, Y. T., Wang, C. T., et al. (2011). Skin-homing CD4+ Foxp3+ T cells exert Th2-like function after staphylococcal superantigen stimulation in atopic dermatitis patients. *Clinical & Experimental Allergy, 41*(4), 516–525.

Lowes, M. A., Kikuchi, T., et al. (2008). Psoriasis vulgaris lesions contain discrete populations of Th1 and Th17 T cells. *Journal of Investigative Dermatology, 128*(5), 1207–1211.

Ma, H. L., Liang, S., et al. (2008). IL-22 is required for Th17 cell-mediated pathology in a mouse model of psoriasis-like skin inflammation. *Journal of Clinical Investigation, 118*(2), 597–607.

Malhotra, S. K., & Mehta, V. (2008). Role of stressful life events in induction or exacerbation of psoriasis and chronic urticaria. *Indian Journal of Dermatology, Venereology, & Leprology, 74*(6), 594–599.

Marucha, P. T., Kiecolt-Glaser, J. K., et al. (1998). Mucosal wound healing is impaired by examination stress. *Psychosomatic Medicine, 60*(3), 362–365.

Matzer, F., Egger, J. W., et al. (2011). Psychosocial stress and coping in alopecia areata: a questionnaire survey and qualitative study among 45 patients. *Acta Dermato-Venereologica, 91*(3), 318–327.

McGuire, L., Heffner, K., et al. (2006). Pain and wound healing in surgical patients. *Annals of Behavioral Medicine, 31*(2), 165–172.

Morris, R. J., & Williams, A. F. (1975). Antigens on mouse and rat lymphocytes recognized by rabbit antiserum against rat brain: the quantitative analysis of a xenogeneic antiserum. *European Journal of Immunology, 5*(4), 274–281.

Moynihan, J., Rieder, E., et al. (2010). Psychoneuroimmunology: the example of psoriasis. *Giornale Italiano di Dermatologia e Venereologia, 145*(2), 221–228.

Muizzuddin, N., Matsui, M. S., et al. (2003). Impact of stress of marital dissolution on skin barrier recovery: tape stripping and measurement of trans-epidermal water loss (TEWL). *Skin Research & Technology, 9*(1), 34–38.

Naldi, L., Peli, L., et al. (2001). Family history of psoriasis, stressful life events, and recent infectious disease are risk factors for a first episode of acute guttate psoriasis: results of a case-control study. *Journal of the American Academy of Dermatology, 44*(3), 433–438.

Nickoloff, B. J. (2007). Cracking the cytokine code in psoriasis. *Nature Medicine, 13*(3), 242–244.

Oh, S. H., Bae, B. G., et al. (2010). Association of stress with symptoms of atopic dermatitis. *Acta Dermato-Venereologica, 90*(6), 582–588.

Ozkan, M., Oflaz, S. B., et al. (2007). Psychiatric morbidity and quality of life in patients with chronic idiopathic urticaria. *Annals of Allergy, Asthma, Immunology, 99*(1), 29–33.

Papadopoulou, N., Kalogeromitros, D., et al. (2005). Corticotropin-releasing hormone receptor-1 and histidine decarboxylase expression in chronic urticaria. *Journal of Investigative Dermatology, 125*(5), 952–955.

Parker, J., Klein, S. L., et al. (2004). Chronic stress accelerates ultraviolet-induced cutaneous carcinogenesis. *Journal of the American Academy of Dermatology, 51*(6), 919–922.

Paus, R., Schmelz, M., et al. (2006). Frontiers in pruritus research: scratching the brain for more effective itch therapy. *Journal of Clinical Investigation, 116*(5), 1174–1186.

Poot, F., Antoine, E., et al. (2011). A case-control study on family dysfunction in patients with alopecia areata, psoriasis and atopic dermatitis. *Acta Dermato-Venereologica, 91*(4), 415–421.

Raychaudhuri, S. K., & Raychaudhuri, S. P. (2009). NGF and its receptor system: a new dimension in the pathogenesis of psoriasis and psoriatic arthritis. *Annals of the New York Academy of Science, 1173*, 470–477.

Raychaudhuri, S. P., & Farber, E. M. (1993). Are sensory nerves essential for the development of psoriatic lesions? *Journal of the American Academy of Dermatology, 28*(3), 488–489.

Raychaudhuri, S. P., & Farber, E. M. (2001). Neuroendocrine influences on the pathogenesis of psoriasis. In *Psychoneuroimmunology* (pp. 471–482). San Diego: Academic Press.

Richards, H. L., Ray, D. W., et al. (2005). Response of the hypothalamic-pituitary-adrenal axis to psychological stress in patients with psoriasis. *British Journal of Dermatology*, *153*(6), 1114–1120.

Riley, V. (1981). Psychoneuroendocrine influences on immunocompetence and neoplasia. *Science*, *212*(4499), 1100–1109.

Robles, T. F. (2007). Stress, social support, and delayed skin barrier recovery. *Psychosomatic Medicine*, *69*(8), 807–815.

Selye, H. (1936). A syndrome produced by diverse nocuous agents. *Journal of Neuropsychiatry & Clinical Neuroscience*, *10*(2), 230–231.

Selye, H. (1946). The general adaptation syndrome and the diseases of adaptation. *Journal of Clinical Endocrinology & Metabolism*, *6*, 117–230.

Shenefelt, P. D. (2000). Hypnosis in dermatology. *Archives of Dermatology*, *136*(3), 393–399.

Slattery, M. J., Klein, D. F., et al. (2002). Relationship between separation anxiety disorder, parental panic disorder, and atopic disorders in children: a controlled high-risk study. *Journal of the American Academy of Child & Adolescent Psychiatry*, *41*(8), 947–954.

Smith, N., Fuhrmann, T., et al. (2009). Psychoneuro-oncology: its time has arrived. *Archives of Dermatology*, *145*(12), 1439–1442.

Staubach, P., Dechene, M., et al. (2011). High prevalence of mental disorders and emotional distress in patients with chronic spontaneous urticaria. *Acta Dermato-Venereologica*, *91*(5), 557–561.

Stephanou, A., Jessop, D. S., et al. (1990). Corticotrophin-releasing factor-like immunoreactivity and mRNA in human leukocytes. *Brain, Behavior, and Immunity*, *4*(1), 67–73.

Strombeck, B., & Jacobsson, L. T. (2007). The role of exercise in the rehabilitation of patients with systemic lupus erythematosus and patients with primary Sjogren's syndrome. *Current Opinion Rheumatology*, *19*(2), 197–203.

Strombeck, B. E., Theander, E., et al. (2007). Effects of exercise on aerobic capacity and fatigue in women with primary Sjogren's syndrome. *Rheumatology (Oxford)*, *46*(5), 868–871.

Tausk, F., Elenkov, I., et al. (2008). Psychoneuroimmunology. *Dermatologic Therapy*, *21*(1), 22–31.

Tausk, F. A., & Nousari, H. (2001). Stress and the skin. *Archives of Dermatology*, *137*(1), 78–82.

Tausk, F., & Whitmore, S. E. (1999). A pilot study of hypnosis in the treatment of patients with psoriasis. *Psychotherapy & Psychosomatics*, *68*(4), 221–225.

Temoshok, L. (1985). Biopsychosocial studies on cutaneous malignant melanoma: psychosocial factors associated with prognostic indicators, progression, psychophysiology and tumor-host response. *Social Science & Medicine*, *20*(8), 833–840.

Temoshok, L., Heller, B. W., et al. (1985). The relationship of psychosocial factors to prognostic indicators in cutaneous malignant melanoma. *Journal of Psychosomatic Research*, *29*(2), 139–153.

Theoharides, T. C., Alysandratos, K. D., et al. (2012). Mast cells and inflammation. *Biochimica et Biophysica Acta*, *1822*(1), 21–33.

Theoharides, T. C., Donelan, J. M., et al. (2004). Mast cells as targets of corticotropin-releasing factor and related peptides. *Trends in Pharmacological Science, 25*(11), 563–568.

Tom, W. L., & Barrio, V. R. (2008). New insights into adolescent acne. *Current Opinion Pediatrics, 20*(4), 436–440.

Tran, B. W., Papoiu, A. D., et al. (2010). Effect of itch, scratching and mental stress on autonomic nervous system function in atopic dermatitis. *Acta Dermato-Venereologica, 90*(4), 354–361.

Uguz, F., Engin, B., et al. (2008). Axis I and Axis II diagnoses in patients with chronic idiopathic urticaria. *Journal of Psychosomatic Research, 64*(2), 225–229.

Valdimarsson, H. (2007). The genetic basis of psoriasis. *Clinical Dermatology, 25*(6), 563–567.

van Beelen, A. J., Teunissen, M. B., et al. (2007). Interleukin-17 in inflammatory skin disorders. *Current Opinion Allergy & Clinical Immunology, 7*(5), 374–381.

Weinman, J., Ebrecht, M., et al. (2008). Enhanced wound healing after emotional disclosure intervention. *British Journal of Health Psychology, 13*(Pt 1), 95–102.

Werner, S., & Grose, R. (2003). Regulation of wound healing by growth factors and cytokines. *Physiology Review, 83*(3), 835–870.

Wolf, J. M., Miller, G. E., et al. (2008). Parent psychological states predict changes in inflammatory markers in children with asthma and healthy children. *Brain, Behavior, and Immunity, 22*(4), 433–441.

Yosipovitch, G., Tang, M., et al. (2007). Study of psychological stress, sebum production and acne vulgaris in adolescents. *Acta Dermato-Venereologica, 87*(2), 135–139.

Zachariae, R., Oster, H., et al. (1996). Effects of psychologic intervention on psoriasis: a preliminary report. *Journal of the American Academy of Dermatology, 34*(6), 1008–1015.

Zheng, Y., Danilenko, D. M., et al. (2007). Interleukin-22, a T(H)17 cytokine, mediates IL-23-induced dermal inflammation and acanthosis. *Nature, 445*(7128), 648–651.

7

Traditional Chinese Medicine and Acupuncture in Dermatology

KACHIU C. LEE AND PETER A. LIO

Key Concepts

♣ The history of Traditional Chinese Medicine (TCM) extends back over 2,000 years in Eastern culture but has only recently gained increased recognition in the Western world.

♣ TCM focuses on balancing natural functions and components of the body, composed of five phases: wood, fire, earth, metal, and water.

♣ TCM emphasizes individualized treatments and diagnosis based on a person's yin and yang, using a combination of oral or topical herbal preparations.

♣ Acupuncture, using various locations and methods, is a promising modality of treatment for acne based on observational studies.

♣ The nature of TCM diagnosis precludes easy comparison of treatment methods for the Western conception of these diseases.

Introduction

The history of Traditional Chinese Medicine (TCM) extends back over 2,000 years in Eastern culture but has only recently gained increased recognition in the Western world. Unlike the more standardized Western medicine approach, TCM and acupuncture emphasize individualized treatment plans based on the interplay between a patient's personal characteristics and disease. Thus, a single contributory factor can manifest different responses in different individuals.

TCM focuses on balancing natural functions and components of the body, composed of five phases: wood, fire, earth, metal, and water. Yin and yang also represent two opposite but complementary aspects: dark and light, cold and hot, stillness and movement. The interdependence and balance of yin and yang dictate a person's well-being and general health. Furthermore, an imbalance of these two aspects can act as the root cause of illness and progression. An overabundance of yin can be balanced by introducing yang elements, whether in the form of yang-related herbal medications or food sources. Correspondingly, an overabundance of yang needs to be balanced by yin elements to restore health. TCM emphasizes individualized treatments and diagnosis based on a person's yin and yang, using a combination of oral or topical herbal preparations. Therefore, two people diagnosed with the same condition by Western medicine (e.g., acne, atopic dermatitis, or herpes simplex virus infection) may be treated with completely different therapies based on their yin and yang profile. Because of this more holistic approach, dermatologic diseases do not exist in isolation, with the result being that "acne" or "eczema" may have multiple causes and treatments that do not match up with the Western approach to such diseases (Xu, 2004). Similarly, external contributory factors such as diet, humidity, or environmental influences all exert different influences on people, triggering vastly different disease responses (Zhang et al., 2009).

Analogously, acupuncture is based on the principle that the body is regulated and influenced by vital energy, or *qi*. Through an imbalance of *qi*, disease can manifest. Acupuncture uses needles (and other techniques) to restore the disrupted flow of *qi* via the stimulation of acupuncture points. These points are connected to each other through meridians, or paths of *qi* energy flow. While there is no clear physiological or anatomical correlation with acupuncture meridians and Western understanding of medicine and disease pathology, several papers have suggested some physiological and biochemical differences in tissues at acupuncture points versus control tissues (Hwang, 1992; Ifrim-Chen & Ifrim, 2005; Panasiuk & Zaiachkivs'ka, 1995). There are 12 standard bilateral and 2 midline meridians, corresponding to yin and yang groups and also to one of the five phases (wood, fire, earth, metal, water).

Acne

Acne results from dysfunction of the pilosebaceous unit and manifests as non-inflammatory (open and closed comedones) and inflammatory (papules, pustules, nodules) lesions. *Propionibacterium acnes* bacteria is often implicated as a causative agent. Generally speaking, TCM approaches acne through dietary changes, herbal remedies, and acupuncture. The choice of treatment is largely based on an individual's characteristics and disease severity.

Dietary relationships between acne and TCM have long been acknowledged. In *Plain Questions of Yellow Emperor's Internal Medicine* (*Huangdi Neijing,* 黄帝内经), a foundational classic of TCM, diet was acknowledged as causing facial lesions remarkably similar to acne (Ming, 2001). In one cross-sectional study examining the association of food with the occurrence of acne, subjects were divided into yin and yang classifications, a prime principle of TCM. Yin individuals consuming yang-rich foods (fatty, deep fried goods) were less likely to have clinical acne. Yang individuals consuming yang-rich foods (sweets, desserts, juices) had exacerbation of acne, thought to be related to an overabundance of yang. Yang individuals consuming yin-rich foods (dairy or soy) had improvement in their acne thought secondary to a balancing of the yin and yang entities (Cai, 1987). The results of this study appeared to support the basic principles of TCM—that yin and yang must be balanced to prevent disease. However, the poorly described methodology and significant limitation of recall bias limits interpretation of this study.

Bactericidal activity against *P. acnes* using TCM herbal medications has been demonstrated. An in vitro experiment demonstrated that Keigai-rengyo-to has activity against *P. acnes* compared to control colonies. The production of *P. acnes* was suppressed with 1 mg/mL Keigai-rengyo-to, compared to 0.1 µg/mL minocycline, a conventional antibiotic. Keigai-rengyo-to is a Kampo (the Japanese study and adaptation of TCM) formulation created by powdered extracts of 17 Kampo crude drugs and is a systemic medicine used in TCM (Higaki et al., 2004). Similarly, other Kampo formulations have been found to suppress the production of propionic acid and butyric acid by *P. acnes* in laboratory conditions (Higaki et al., 1995, 1996, 1997, 1998, 2000). Clinically, Kampo formulations may decrease symptoms of acne, although a lack of clinical trials prevents evidence-based assessment of these observations (Higaki et al., 2002).

Acupuncture, using various locations and methods, is a promising modality of treatment for acne based on observational studies. There is a lack of randomized, placebo-controlled trials on acupuncture and acne, perhaps complicated by the fact that each person's acupuncture points vary based on his or her individual composition and disease severity. Nie and Wang (2008) conducted an extensive review of the Chinese literature, describing various acupuncture and other methods used to successfully treat acne. While vastly informative on the acupuncture variations used for acne treatment, the major limitation lies in the fact that most of the referenced published studies are observational and conducted by a single practitioner. Other observational studies demonstrating successful treatment of acne with acupuncture suffer from the same limitations (Liu, 2008).

Multiple limitations to studying TCM for acne exist. First, since each TCM herbal remedy is individualized based on a person's balance of yin, yang, and the five elements, it is difficult to examine a single specific combination of medications for a disease state. Second, many TCM studies are observational and draw on the experience of one practitioner who may have significant practice variations from other practitioners. Third, numerous TCM studies are conducted and published in non-English languages and journals, making them less accessible to most English-speaking clinicians and researchers.

Two notable trials of acupuncture are worth considering. In one, 68 subjects were randomized to Helium-Neon (He-Ne) laser auricular irradiation for 3 to 5 minutes plus acupuncture at a minimum of six points or acupuncture alone. The group receiving combination therapy demonstrated a 78% cure rate versus a 47% cure rate in the control group (Lihong, 2006). In another controlled trial, 36 subjects were randomized to a double-blinded study, receiving acupuncture in either general acupuncture points (control group) versus general acupuncture points plus *ah shi* points (experimental group). There was a significant reduction in inflammatory acne lesions as well as improvement in the quality of life measured by the Skindex-29 in the experimental group (Son et al., 2010). The lack of a placebo group (receiving either no acupuncture or acupuncture at sham points) deters from the validity of both studies.

Atopic Dermatitis

Multiple controlled studies have examined the effectiveness of TCM for atopic dermatitis (AD). Notably, Sheehan and colleagues treated 40 adults with TCM herbal medications for 2 months, with the experimental group showing decreased objective disease severity and subjective improvement in sleep and pruritus sensation (Sheehan et al., 1992). Hon and colleagues (2007) treated 85 children in a randomized, placebo-controlled trial. At the end of 12 weeks, experimental subjects demonstrated improvement compared to control subjects. Experimental subjects also had decreased use of corticosteroids and antihistamines, even 4 weeks after stopping TCM herbal therapy.

A Cochrane review on TCM examined several English- and Chinese-language studies on AD. While the majority of herbal medications lacked sufficient sample sizes to draw definitive conclusions, Zemaphyte, made from a combination of multiple herbal medications, was thoroughly examined. Zemaphyte has been shown in vitro to decrease levels of CD23; CD23 acts as a low-affinity IgE receptor, and levels are often elevated in AD subjects. However, the clinical effectiveness of this medication is mixed, with some studies showing marked improvement and others showing no difference compared to placebo. Therefore, additional studies of TCM herbal concoctions are necessary before firm conclusions can be made (Zhang et al., 2005).

Acupuncture can also be an effective therapy for control of AD, possibly via modulation of pruritus. Notable trials on acupuncture have demonstrated that one session of acupuncture (Quchi and Xuehai points) can effectively decrease artificially induced wheal-and-flare responses in patients with AD. Itch sensation, as measured by the validated Eppendorf Itch Questionnaire, was also significantly decreased in experimental groups compared to control and placebo groups (Pfab et al., 2010). A pilot study by the same group also noted decreased in vitro allergen-induced CD63 basophil activation in AD patients (Pfab et al., 2011).

Another double-blinded, randomized controlled pilot trial in adults with AD examined the effect of self-applied acupressure at Quchi three times weekly for 4 weeks. In the acupressure group there was a statistically significant decrease in itch and in lichenification compared to the control group (Lee et al., 2012), further supporting the possibility that stimulation of certain points on the body can lead to improvement in AD symptoms.

TCM in combination with acupuncture has been studied for AD. In one study, children with AD were treated with the following regimen: TCM (drinking Erka Shizheng herbal tea twice daily), herbal bath soaks for 20 minutes daily, application of an herbal cream three times daily, and acupuncture for 3 months. At the end of the study, SCORAD reduction ranged from 60% to 90% in 13 of 14 subjects treated. Quality-of-life scores were also improved by 50% in all subjects, and a reduction in usage of topical corticosteroids and antihistamines was also noted. However, the complexity of such a regimen makes it difficult for researchers and individuals to reproduce, and the potential cost and complexity make it impractical for some patients (Wisniewski et al., 2009). Based on these studies, acupuncture and TCM hold significant promise for AD, but more work must be done to identify key aspects of therapy and further standardization must be sought so that the treatments can be used more generally.

Herpes Simplex Virus

In vitro studies of traditional herbal medications have demonstrated effectiveness at inhibiting herpes simplex virus (HSV) replication without apparent cytotoxicity (Hsiang et al., 2001; Khan et al., 2005; Li et al., 2004; Xiong et al., 2011). Experiments on mice have further shown decreased mortality in HSV-1–infected mice, as well as decreased body surface area affected (Nagasaka et al., 1995).

Kuo and colleagues have performed extensive basic science research on the effect of herbal medications on HeLa cells infected with HSV, investigating the mechanism of action of TCM. Notably, antiviral action appears to be mediated primarily through inhibition of early transcription in HSV-infected cells, arresting HSV-1 viral DNA synthesis, and inhibition of formation of protein complexes necessary for replication (Kuo et al., 2001, 2002, 2005, 2006). Chiang and colleagues have also examined the antiviral effects of herbal medications on various DNA viruses, including HSV-1 and HSV-2. This research also suggests a promising role for these medications in inhibiting DNA replication in HSV (Chiang, Chang, et al., 2003; Chiang, Cheng, et al., 2003; Chiang, Ng, et al., 2005). The results of these in vitro studies are promising and offer a basis for additional clinical investigations.

Lichen Simplex (Neurodermatitis)

Lichen simplex is a condition caused and exacerbated by repeated scratching or rubbing. This chronic skin problem frequently presents with thickened skin and accentuation of skin lines. The initial stimulus setting off the itch–scratch cycle may be unrecognized but can range from stress to underlying eczema or insect bites.

Evidence-based review of TCM reveals reports on successful treatment of lichen simplex with plum-blossom needle usage from the 1980s (Zhong, 1984). In another study comparing TCM and conventional methods, 141 subjects with neurodermatitis were randomized into three groups (plum-blossom needle tapping plus oral herbal medications, oral herbal medications only, oral diphenhydramine plus topical 10% urea ointment). Subjects receiving plum-blossom needle tapping plus oral herbal medications did better at the 1-month follow-up than subjects in the other two groups (Weiying et al., 2006). Plum-blossom needles were used to gently tap the skin, inserting to approximately the dermal layer. The name "plum-blossom" comes from the configuration of five needles bound together in a bundle similar to the appearance of a plum blossom in bloom. Observational case series have also reported the success of acupuncture in treating lichen simplex when inserted near the affected areas (Yang, 1997).

Pruritus

Pruritus, or itch, can accompany most inflammatory skin conditions or occur as a result of underlying illness. In Eastern medicine, pruritus can be treated with both oral medications and acupuncture. One herbal preparation, Unsei-in, can reduce itch through inhibition of nitric oxide synthase 1 in mice after repeated administration of high dosages (300 mg/kg) (Andoh et al., 2004).

Acupuncture, through stimulation of Aδ or C fibers and release of vasoactive mediators from inflammatory cells, can also reduce pruritus. The main target for this technique in itchy skin is likely sensory cutaneous innervation. Several small-scale studies have investigated and found beneficial results of acupuncture for treatment of uremic pruritus. Che-Yi and colleagues (2005) examined 40 subjects randomized to acupuncture at real points versus acupuncture at sham points located 2 cm away. Experimental group subjects reported a significant decrease in itch compared to control group subjects. However, a systemic review on the subject found a high risk of bias in these small studies, leaving the current evidence insufficient to support the use of acupuncture in subjects with uremic pruritus (Kim et al., 2010).

Similarly, in skin-related literature, notable small-scale studies have found a positive effect of acupuncture on pruritus, although these may be influenced by bias as well. Histopathologically, skin biopsies taken before and 3 to 6 days after acupuncture showed a decreased number of calcitonin-gene related peptide immunoreactive nerve fibers per biopsy section (Carlsson et al., 2006). One notable clinical study of 80 subjects showed significant reduction in nasal itch after acupuncture at four points. The control group received sham acupuncture at sites 1 to 1.5 cm away from the experimental group's actual insertion points. Study investigators applying the acupuncture were not blinded during the study, however, leading to the possibility of bias (Xue et al., 2007). A clinical review of the use of acupuncture in skin-related illnesses concluded that additional studies are needed prior to drawing conclusions on the effectiveness of acupuncture for pruritus (Carlsson et al., 2010).

Psoriasis

In TCM, psoriasis is most commonly categorized into blood-heat syndrome, blood-dryness syndrome, or blood-stasis syndrome, with disease features attributed to an imbalance in these characteristics. In those with the most common syndrome, blood-heat syndrome, the most frequently used herbal medications are Radix Rehmanniae, Radix Arnebiae seu Lithospermi, and Cortex Moutan (Tan et al., 2011; Tse, 2003). These herbs, and others, may have anti-inflammatory effects, ability to induce apoptosis, and immunomodulating properties. Side effects range from mild gastrointestinal symptoms of nausea and vomiting to severe liver enzyme disturbances. Temporary suppression of white blood cell counts has also been reported in subjects orally using Indigo compounds (Bartosinska et al., 2011).

Radix Angelicae pubescentis is a Chinese herbal medicine that has been compared to psoralen when administered in combination with UVA radiation. One study of 204 subjects randomized subjects to receive either Radix

Angelicae pubescentis or traditional oral psoralen. After exposure to UVA, both groups demonstrated beneficial clearing of psoriatic lesions. There was no statistical significance between the groups when comparing degree of clearance, but subjects in the TCM group noted fewer side effects than those in the psoralen group (Koo & Arain, 1998).

In a randomized, placebo-controlled study of topical usage of indigo naturalis, 42 subjects with chronic plaque psoriasis applied either indigo naturalis cream or placebo cream to two large psoriatic areas. At 12 weeks of follow-up, significant reductions in redness, scaling, and induration were noted in experimental-group subjects. Body surface area affected was also significantly reduced, with 74% experiencing clearance or near-clearance of psoriasis in the areas treated with indigo ointment. Patient blinding was not complete, however, as the indigo ointment is a natural blue whereas the placebo ointment was yellow (Lin et al., 2008). Case reports of children treated with topical indigo naturalis after failing to respond to conventional alternatives suggest a possible role for this medication in pediatrics (Lin et al., 2006). No severe side effects were reported in either study. Skin biopsies of subjects using indigo naturalis daily for 8 weeks have also shown decreased Ki-67 expression (a marker of proliferation) and CD3 expression (an inflammatory marker) (Lin et al., 2007).

The efficacy of TCM was examined against conventional medicine in a randomized, placebo-controlled trial of TCM versus methotrexate. A total of 50 subjects with moderate to severe plaque psoriasis completed the 6-month study, receiving TCM, placebo, or methotrexate. All other conventional medications (topical corticosteroids, phototherapy, systemic therapies) were stopped. Dropout rates were most significant in the TCM group (33%) compared to the patients receiving placebo (10%) and methotrexate (1%). Mean improvement in psoriasis area severity index was worst in the TCM group (15.1%) compared to placebo (32%) and methotrexate (74%) groups, suggesting that the TCM herbals used in this study might actually worsen psoriasis. Elevation in liver enzymes was a common side effect of methotrexate, and gastrointestinal side effects with some abnormalities in liver function were found in the TCM group (Ho et al., 2010).

Acupuncture is uncommonly used for the treatment of psoriasis, and one study examining this subject found no clinical effectiveness. A Swedish study examined 56 subjects with plaque psoriasis, randomized to receive electrostimulation and auricular acupuncture, or placebo (minimal acupuncture) for 10 weeks. On follow-up, mean psoriasis area severity index decreased from 9.6 to 8.3 in the experimental group, and from 9.2 to 6.9 in the placebo group. Both of these effects were less than the usual considered placebo effect of 30% change. At 3 months, there was no difference in outcomes between groups either subjectively or objectively as measured by the psoriasis area severity index (Jerner et al., 1997).

Urticaria

While acupuncture has long been used to treat urticaria in Eastern medicine, few evidence-based, controlled English-language studies are available. In Eastern medicine, urticaria is sometimes thought to be due to pathogenic wind, perhaps because this condition can come and spread quickly just like the wind itself. Acute urticaria is commonly treated with acupuncture at four acupuncture points (LI11: Quchi, Sp10: Xuehai, Sp6: Sanyinjiao, S36: Zusanli). In one observational study of 114 subjects with acute urticaria, 90% experienced relief after one session of acupuncture (Lu, 1993).

In contrast, chronic urticaria is significantly more difficult to treat. Numerous acupuncture methods have been employed with varying results: ordinary acupuncture, acupuncture point bleeding, ordinary plus auricular acupuncture, acupuncture point injection with herbal medications, and acupuncture in combination with cupping (Chen & Yu, 2003). Using ordinary acupuncture, approximately 30% to 50% of subjects experienced relief from urticaria in an observational study of 2,300 subjects (Chen & Yu, 1998). In a randomized study of 40 subjects with chronic urticaria, experimental-group subjects were treated at real acupuncture points while control subjects were treated at sham points for 3 weeks. At the end of the study, experimental subjects reported a 25% reduction in number of urticarial episodes, as well as a decrease in the duration of episodes (Iraji et al., 2006).

Acupuncture point bleeding, in which a peripheral vein is purposely punctured and bled, is used to adjust and balance the flow of vital energy in the subject. This method may be more effective than ordinary acupuncture (approximately 83% response in a study of 36 patients). However, patients, and even some acupuncturists, may not be able to tolerate this bloodletting method (Chen & Yu, 1998).

Ordinary acupuncture with point injection has also been reported with good results. In one study of 64 patients with chronic urticaria, 32 received acupuncture plus point injections of herbal medications. Control-group participants were treated with antihistamines only and showed significantly less improvement than the experimental group. Experimental-group subjects also had a lower relapse rate than their counterparts (Zhao, 2006). Acupuncture point injections with thiamine hydrochloride (vitamin B1) also yielded relief in 40 subjects with chronic urticaria. Approximately 31 of these patients were cured of chronic urticaria, and only 4 patients experienced relapse during a 2-year follow-up period (Chen & Yu, 1998).

While ordinary acupuncture and its variations have been successfully used for centuries in Eastern medicine, these methods still lack adequate evidence-based studies in comparison to conventional medications.

Conclusion

TCM and acupuncture have long been used in Eastern cultures for treatment of dermatologic conditions. However, the nature of TCM diagnosis precludes easy comparison of treatment methods for the Western conception of these diseases. Because three patients with urticaria may have three very distinct underlying TCM diagnoses, within the context of TCM it may be invalid to ask "What is the treatment for urticaria?" This fundamental difference in approach may explain some of the difficulties in performing studies that satisfy the stringent constraints of evidence-based medicine, and the general paucity of data for most dermatologic conditions.

Until such epistemological issues are resolved, there remain tempting morsels from many studies that may lead to improved integrative approaches and possibly better understanding of dermatologic diseases.

REFERENCES

Andoh, T., Al-Akeel, A., Tsujii, K., et al. (2004). Repeated treatment with the traditional medicine Unsei-in inhibits substance P-induced itch-associated responses through downregulation of the expression of nitric oxide synthase 1 in mice. *Journal of Pharmacological Sciences, 94*, 207–210.

Bartosinska, J. P., Pietrzak, A., Szepietowski, J., et al. (2011). Traditional Chinese medicine herbs—are they safe for psoriatic patients? *Folia Histochemica et Cytobiologica, 49*, 201–205.

Cai, J. F. (1987). Toward a comprehensive evaluation of alternative medicine. *Social Science & Medicine, 25*, 659–667.

Carlsson, C. P., Sundler, F., & Wallengren, J. (2006). Cutaneous innervation before and after one treatment period of acupuncture. *British Journal of Dermatology, 155*, 970–976.

Carlsson, C. P., & Wallengren, J. (2010). Therapeutic and experimental therapeutic studies on acupuncture and itch: review of the literature. *Journal of the European Academy of Dermatology and Venereology, 24*, 1013–1016.

Chen, C. J., & Yu, H. S. (1998). Acupuncture treatment of urticaria. *Archives of Dermatology, 134*, 1397–1399.

Chen, C. J., & Yu, H. S. (2003). Acupuncture, electrostimulation, and reflex therapy in dermatology. *Dermatologic Therapy, 16*, 87–92.

Che-Yi, C., Wen, C. Y., Min-Tsung, K., & Chiu-Ching, H. (2005). Acupuncture in haemodialysis patients at the Quchi (LI11) acupoint for refractory uraemic pruritus. *Nephrology, Dialysis, Transplantation, 20*, 1912–1915.

Chiang, L. C., Chang, J. S., Chen, C. C., et al. (2003). Anti-Herpes simplex virus activity of *Bidens pilosa* and *Houttuynia cordata*. *American Journal of Chinese Medicine, 31*, 355–362.

Chiang, L. C., Cheng, H. Y., Liu, M. C., et al. (2003). Antiviral activity of eight commonly used medicinal plants in Taiwan. *American Journal of Chinese Medicine, 31*, 897–905.

Chiang, L. C., Ng, L. T., Cheng, P. W., et al. (2005). Antiviral activities of extracts and selected pure constituents of *Ocimum basilicum*. *Clinical and Experimental Pharmacology & Physiology, 32*, 811–816.

Higaki, S., Hasegawa, Y., Morohashi, M., et al. (1995). The correlation of Kampo formulations and their ingredients on anti-bacterial activities against *Propionibacterium acnes*. *Journal of Dermatology, 22*, 4–9.

Higaki, S., Kitagawa, T., Kagoura, M., et al. (2000). Relationship between *Propionibacterium acnes* biotypes and Jumi-haidoku-to. *Journal of Dermatology, 27*, 635–638.

Higaki, S., Morimatsu, S., Morohashi, M., et al. (1997). Susceptibility of *Propionibacterium acnes, Staphylococcus aureus* and *Staphylococcus epidermidis* to 10 Kampo formulations. *Journal of International Medical Research, 25*, 318–324.

Higaki, S., Morimatsu, S., Morohashi, M., et al. (1998). The anti-lipase activity of shiunko on *Propionibacterium acnes*. *International Journal of Antimicrobial Agents, 10*, 251–252.

Higaki, S., Nakamura, M., Morohashi, M., et al. (1996). Activity of eleven kampo formulations and eight kampo crude drugs against *Propionibacterium acnes* isolated from acne patients: retrospective evaluation in 1990 and 1995. *Journal of Dermatology, 23*, 871–875.

Higaki, S., Nakamura, M., Morohashi, M., et al. (2004). *Propionibacterium acnes* biotypes and susceptibility to minocycline and Keigai-rengyo-to. *International Journal of Dermatology, 43*, 103–107.

Higaki, S., Toyomoto, T., & Morohashi, M. (2002). Seijo-bofu-to, Jumi-haidoku-to and Toki-shakuyaku-san suppress rashes and incidental symptoms in acne patients. *Drugs Under Experimental and Clinical Research, 28*, 193–196.

Ho, S. G., Yeung, C. K., & Chan, H. H. (2010). Methotrexate versus traditional Chinese medicine in psoriasis: a randomized, placebo-controlled trial to determine efficacy, safety and quality of life. *Clinical and Experimental Dermatology, 35*, 717–722.

Hon, K. L., Leung, T. F., Ng, P. C., et al. (2007). Efficacy and tolerability of a Chinese herbal medicine concoction for treatment of atopic dermatitis: a randomized, double-blind, placebo-controlled study. *British Journal of Dermatology, 157*, 357–363.

Hsiang, C. Y., Hsieh, C. L., Wu, S. L., et al. (2001). Inhibitory effect of anti-pyretic and anti-inflammatory herbs on herpes simplex virus replication. *American Journal of Chinese Medicine, 29*, 459–467.

Hwang, Y. C. (1992). Anatomy and classification of acupoints. *Problems in Veterinary Medicine, 4*, 12–15.

Ifrim-Chen, F., & Ifrim, M. (2005). Acupoints [corrected] and meridians: a histochemical study. *Italian Journal of Anatomy and Embryology, 110*, 51–57.

Iraji, F., Saghayi, M., Mokhtari, H., et al. (2006). Acupuncture in the treatment of chronic urticaria: a double-blind study. *Internet Journal of Dermatology, 3*(2); DOI: 10.5580/491

Jerner, B., Skogh, M., & Vahlquist, A. (1997). A controlled trial of acupuncture in psoriasis: no convincing effect. *Acta Dermato-Venereologica, 77*, 154–156.

Khan, M. T., Ather, A., Thompson, K. D., et al. (2005). Extracts and molecules from medicinal plants against herpes simplex viruses. *Antiviral Research, 67*, 107–119.

Kim, K. H., Lee, M. S., & Choi, S. M. (2010). Acupuncture for treating uremic pruritus in patients with end-stage renal disease: a systematic review. *Journal of Pain and Symptom Management, 40*, 117–125.

Koo, J., & Arain, S. (1998). Traditional Chinese medicine for the treatment of dermatologic disorders. *Archives of Dermatology, 134*, 1388–1393.

Kuo, Y. C., Chen, C. C., Tsai, W. J., et al. (2001). Regulation of herpes simplex virus type 1 replication in Vero cells by *Psychotria serpens*: relationship to gene expression, DNA replication, and protein synthesis. *Antiviral Research, 51*, 95–109.

Kuo, Y. C., Kuo, Y. H., Lin, Y. L., et al. (2006). Yatein from *Chamaecyparis obtusa* suppresses herpes simplex virus type 1 replication in HeLa cells by interruption of the immediate-early gene expression. *Antiviral Research, 70*, 112–120.

Kuo, Y. C., Lin, L. C., Tsai, W. J., et al. (2002). Samarangenin B from *Limonium sinense* suppresses herpes simplex virus type 1 replication in Vero cells by regulation of viral macromolecular synthesis. *Antimicrobial Agents and Chemotherapy, 46*, 2854–2864.

Kuo, Y. C., Lin, Y. L., Liu, C. P., et al. (2005). Herpes simplex virus type 1 propagation in HeLa cells interrupted by *Nelumbo nucifera*. *Journal of Biomedical Science, 12*, 1021–1034.

Lee, K. C., Keyes, A., Hensley, J. R., et al. (2012). Effectiveness of acupressure on pruritus and lichenification associated with atopic dermatitis: a pilot trial. *Acupuncture in Medicine: Journal of the British Medical Acupuncture Society, 30*, 8–11.

Li, Y., Ooi, L. S., Wang, H., et al. (2004). Antiviral activities of medicinal herbs traditionally used in southern mainland China. *Phytotherapy Research, 18*, 718–722.

Lihong, S. (2006). He-Ne laser auricular irradiation plus body acupuncture for treatment of acne vulgaris in 36 cases. *Journal of Traditional Chinese Medicine, 26*, 193–194.

Lin, Y. K., Chang, C. J., Chang, Y. C., et al. (2008). Clinical assessment of patients with recalcitrant psoriasis in a randomized, observer-blind, vehicle-controlled trial using indigo naturalis. *Archives of Dermatology, 144*, 1457–1464.

Lin, Y. K., Wong, W. R., Chang, Y. C., et al. (2007). The efficacy and safety of topically applied indigo naturalis ointment in patients with plaque-type psoriasis. *Dermatology, 214*, 155–161.

Lin, Y. K., Yen, H. R., Wong, W. R., et al. (2006). Successful treatment of pediatric psoriasis with Indigo naturalis composite ointment. *Pediatric Dermatology, 23*, 507–510.

Liu, Z. (2008). Clinical observation on the effect of earlobe-bleeding plus body acupuncture in 85 cases of common acne. *Journal of Traditional Chinese medicine, 28*, 18–20.

Lu, S. (1993). Acupuncture and moxibustion in the treatment of dermatoses. *Journal of Traditional Chinese Medicine, 13*, 69–75.

Ming, Z. (2001). *The medical classic of the yellow emperor*. Beijing: Foreign Language Press.

Nagasaka, K., Kurokawa, M., Imakita, M., et al. (1995). Efficacy of kakkon-to, a traditional herb medicine, in herpes simplex virus type 1 infection in mice. *Journal of Medical Virology, 46*, 28–34.

Nie, Y., & Wang, C. (2008). A survey of treatment of acne by acupuncture. *Journal of Traditional Chinese Medicine, 28,* 71–74.

Panasiuk, I. M., & Zaiachkivs'ka, O. S. [The clinico-physiological characteristics of biologically active points]. *Fiziologicheskii Zhurnal, 41,* 117–121.

Pfab, F., Athanasiadis, G. I., Huss-Marp, J., et al. (2011). Effect of acupuncture on allergen-induced basophil activation in patients with atopic eczema: a pilot trial. *Journal of Alternative & Complementary Medicine, 17,* 309–314.

Pfab, F., Huss-Marp, J., Gatti, A., et al. (2010). Influence of acupuncture on type I hypersensitivity itch and the wheal and flare response in adults with atopic eczema—a blinded, randomized, placebo-controlled, crossover trial. *Allergy, 65,* 903–910.

Sheehan, M. P., Rustin, M. H., Atherton, D. J., et al. (1992). Efficacy of traditional Chinese herbal therapy in adult atopic dermatitis. *Lancet, 340,* 13–17.

Son, B. K., Yun, Y., & Choi, I. H. (2010). Efficacy of ah shi point acupuncture on acne vulgaris. *Acupuncture in Medicine: Journal of the British Medical Acupuncture Society, 28,* 126–129.

Tan, Y. Q., Liu, J. L., Bai, Y. P., et al. (2011). Literature research of Chinese medicine recipes for the treatment of psoriasis vulgaris with blood-heat syndrome type. *Chinese Journal of Integrative Medicine, 17,* 150–153.

Tse, T. W. (2003). Use of common Chinese herbs in the treatment of psoriasis. *Clinical and Experimental Dermatology, 28,* 469–475.

Weiying, L., Yuanjiang, D., & Baolian, L. (2006). Treatment of the localized neurodermatitis by plum-blossom needle tapping and with the modified yangxue dingfeng tang—a clinical observation of 47 cases. *Journal of Traditional Chinese Medicine, 26,* 181–183.

Wisniewski, J., Nowak-Wegrzyn, A., Steenburgh-Thanik, E., et al. (2009). Efficacy and safety of traditional Chinese medicine for treatment of atopic dermatitis (AD). *Journal of Allergy & Clinical Immunology, 123*(2), S37.

Xiong, H. R., Luo, J., Hou, W., et al. (2011). The effect of emodin, an anthraquinone derivative extracted from the roots of *Rheum tanguticum*, against herpes simplex virus in vitro and in vivo. *Journal of Ethnopharmacology, 133,* 718–723.

Xu, Y. (2004). *Dermatology in traditional Chinese medicine.* New York: Elsevier Science.

Xue, C. C, An, X., Cheung, T. P., et al. (2007). Acupuncture for persistent allergic rhinitis: a randomised, sham-controlled trial. *Medical Journal of Australia, 187,* 337–341.

Yang, Q. (1997). Acupuncture treatment of 139 cases of neurodermatitis. *Journal of Traditional Chinese Medicine, 17,* 57–58.

Zhang, G. Z., Wang, J. S., Wang, P., et al. (2009). Distribution and development of the TCM syndromes in psoriasis vulgaris. *Journal of Traditional Chinese Medicine, 29,* 195–200.

Zhang, W., Leonard, T., Bath-Hextall, F., et al. (2005). Chinese herbal medicine for atopic eczema. *Cochrane Database of Systematic Reviews.*

Zhao, Y. (2006). Acupuncture plus point-injection for 32 cases of obstinate urticaria. *Journal of Traditional Chinese Medicine, 26,* 22–23.

Zhong, M. Q. (1984). Neurodermatitis treated by plum-blossom needle. *Journal of Traditional Chinese Medicine, 4,* 265–268.

8

Herbal Medicine in Dermatology

PHILIP D. SHENEFELT

Key Concepts

♣ Herbal medicines have been used effectively for many centuries for skin disorders. The types of herbs used depend not only on their efficacy, but on their local availability or their availability through trade—thus, different cultures tend to use the ethnobotanicals available to their particular area.

♣ Western herbal medicines are often used singly, while Eastern herbal medicines such as in Chinese traditional medicine and Japanese folk medicine are often used in extensive combination, with mixtures containing from a few to a dozen or more specific herbs.

♣ Two traditions that continue to use herbal medicines extensively are the Indian Ayurvedic system and the Chinese traditional medicine system. In Western culture, the popularity of herbal medicines waned as purified and synthesized compounds became available, but recently there has been a trend toward using herbal medicines extensively again in the West.

♣ Herbal medicines may be less potent than pharmaceutical preparations at treating skin diseases, but often the herbal medicines have fewer and gentler side effects. Integrative dermatology can utilize the best of both to help the patient.

Introduction

Herbal medicines for skin disorders have been used since antiquity and, from archeological evidence, even before recorded history. African great apes have also used herbal medicines (Huffman 2001). In various parts of the world, uses of specific herbs and combinations developed regionally based on plants available locally and through trade into ethnobotanical medicines for that region. More elaborate systems of herbal use developed regionally in Europe, the Middle East (Ghazanfar, 1994), Africa, India (Behl & Srivastava, 2002; Khan & Khanum, 2009), China, Japan, Australia, and the Americas. Two well-established Eastern medicine systems still using specific herbs or combinations of herbs as part of their medical treatments are the Ayurvedic system in India (Kapoor, 1990) and traditional Chinese medicine (TCM) in China (Xu, 2004).

In Western medicine, herbal medicine began as folk medicine in Europe. In the United States, it began in the colonial days with homemade botanicals prepared and used by women in the home (Winslow & Kroll, 1998). European settlers also benefited from Native American knowledge and use of botanical remedies that greatly influenced the further development of herbal medicine in the United States. Iroquois medical botanicals in the northeastern United States became well known to the colonists (Herrick, 1995). In the 19th century a group of physicians known as the Eclectics used and expanded these Old World European and Native American herbal traditions. As herbal medicine continued to develop in the United States, it was further influenced by European and Chinese practices (Winston & Dattner, 1998). Herbal medicine use then declined in Europe and the United States as purified extracts and synthetic chemical drugs became available. Recently patients have become more active again in initiating self-therapy with herbal medicines as the side effects and limitations of synthetic drugs have become better known, and also as a part of the return-to-nature philosophy. The use of herbal medicine, including for skin disorders, is currently increasing among patients; to a lesser degree it is being recommended by physicians as part of an integrative approach to care.

In India, records of Ayurvedic medicine date back to about 3000 B.C. Ayurvedic medicine combines physiological and holistic principles and is based on the concept that the human body consists of five energy elements that also make up the universe: earth, water, fire, air, and space. The interactions of these five elements gives rise to the three *doshas* (forces), seven *dhatus* (tissues), and three *malas* (waste products). All diseases are attributed to an imbalance between the three *doshas* (Bedi & Shenefelt, 2002). Ayurvedic diagnosis is made using an elaborate system that includes examining the physical findings, the pulse, and the urine, and an eight-fold detailed examination to evaluate both the physical and mental aspects of the condition. Treatment often includes herbal medicine and is individually tailored based on the findings (Routh & Bhowmik, 1999).

TCM records date back about 4,000 years. TCM also is aimed at treating the whole person and is based on the complementary forces of yin and yang. In healthy individuals, the yin and yang are in balance, and illness occurs when there is inequality between them. The Chinese also recognize five elements: earth, water, fire, air, and metal, each related to specific organs. They also recognize a flow of energy called *chi* or *qi* through the body in 12 bilateral and two central major meridians that have numbered associated acupuncture points. TCM evaluates the exchange between the environment and the body, such as food, drink, and air into the body and waste leaving the body. Special attention is given to the physical examination of the tongue, iris, and pulses of the individual to determine the cause of the imbalance and then to determine the appropriate individual treatment. TCM treatment is usually a combination of herbs, massage, and acupuncture (Latchman et al., 1994). An entire textbook on dermatology in TCM is available that includes many herbal formulations (Xu, 2004).

Herbal treatments that have been used for centuries are now being studied scientifically, with many randomized control trials being published yearly. The regulatory Commission E in Germany oversees recommended uses and quality of herbal preparations there (Blumenthal et al., 1998). By contrast, the United States does not currently regulate herbal products except as dietary supplements, with no standardization of accepted usage, active ingredients, purity, or concentration. Included in this review of herbal medications are those that show scientific evidence of clinical efficacy, as well as the more common herbs shown to be useful in the treatment of dermatologic disorders. The safety of each herb when available has been included to better enable the physician and patient to know which herbal therapies they may want to begin to use. Common drug interactions and side effects of herbal medicines used for dermatologic conditions are also included. Many other herbs too numerous to cover in this chapter have also been used to treat skin disorders around the world.

Use of herbal medicine has increased in the past two decades among patients seeking alternative treatments to conventional Western allopathic medicine. Visits to alternative medicine practitioners in the United States grew so rapidly that by 1997, the number of visits to alternative practitioners was estimated to be 629 million, surpassing the number of visits to all primary care physicians (Neldner, 2000). Approximately $27 billion was spent for these alternative therapies in 1997, of which $3.24 billion was spent on herbal medicine (Klepser & Klepser, 1999). About 50% of the population has used some form of alternative medicine. Many patients choose not to tell this information to their physicians. Persons most likely to use unconventional treatment modalities, according to a previous survey, were non-black, college-educated, between the ages of 25 and 49 years, and with an annual income greater than $35,000 (Eisenburg et al., 1993). Most patients seek alternatives because conventional therapy has failed to help them sufficiently or because they feel there are fewer side effects with the natural products. The recent increase in the use of alternative medicine has led to more research regarding alternatives and has required education of physicians on the subject so they can better inform and care for their patients. Some physicians and other medical providers have chosen to integrate alternative practices including herbal medicines into their practices and practice integrative medicine.

Herbal remedies in the United States currently continue to be sold as dietary supplements, with standards of potency and efficacy not required. The Dietary Supplement Health and Education Act of 1994 did set purity standards for some commonly used herbs. By contrast, in Germany Commission E has extensively reviewed common European botanicals. Commission E has evaluated the quality of evidence for clinical efficacy, safety, and uses of 300 herbal preparations (Bisset & Wichtl, 2001; Blumenthal et al., 1998). This information has led to the standardization of herbal medicines in Germany. A number of herbal medicines have stood the test of time for their efficacy for dermatologic conditions, and some have significant scientific evidence of their usefulness.

Individuals frequently self-treat themselves, family members, and friends with herbal medicines, many times without first seeking high-quality professional advice. Information for individuals to consider about the safe use of herbal therapies includes identification of health goals, information about efficacy, safety, interactions, and usages, selecting therapies that are likely to achieve those goals, having a correct diagnosis before using the therapy, consulting reputable practitioners, informing the practitioners about all of the remedies they are using, monitoring the effects of the remedies, both positive and negative, being patient for effects to become noticeable, and adjusting doses as needed to accommodate surgery, illness, or changes in conventional therapy (Dunning, 2003). Product labeling information that the patient should look for includes the name and composition of the product, including the parts of the plant and quantity of raw material used, daily dosage and timing of dosages, allergy and other warning statements, quality and safety testing, expiration date, manufacturer, country of manufacture, claims and indications for use, and how to store the product (Kron, 2002). The *Botanical Safety Handbook* (McGuffin et al., 1997) places herbs in classes of safety, with Class 1 safe to consume appropriately, Class 2 with restrictions (2a for external use only, 2b not for use in pregnancy, 2c not for use while nursing, 2d other specific restrictions), Class 3 restricted only to use supervised by an expert, and Class 4 herbs with insufficient data for classification of safety. It often is wise for individuals to consult with integrative practitioners to obtain the full benefits of both conventional and alternative medicine approaches.

Herbal Medicines that May Be Integrated with Conventional Therapies for Dermatologic Disorders

ACNE

Fruit Acids

Fruit acids, such as citric, gluconic, gluconolactone, glycolic, malic, and tartaric acids, used topically have exfoliative properties that have shown some effectiveness in treating acne. In one study gluconolactone was as effective in clearing inflamed and noninflamed acne lesions as 5% benzoyl peroxide and more effective than placebo (Hunt et al., 1998). Irritation is the main adverse effect, especially in higher concentrations. When contained in the fruit, the fruit acids are botanical safety Class 1.

Tannins

Tannins have natural astringent protein precipitant properties and are used topically to treat acne. Witch hazel (*Hamamelis virginiana*) bark extract can be prepared and used as a home remedy by making a decoction from 5 to 10 g bark in 1 cup (0.24 L) water. Witch hazel is considered very safe to use topically and is Class 1 (McGuffin et al., 1997, p. 59; Peirce et al., 1998). Commercially available preparations of witch hazel are not astringent, as the tannins are lost in the distillation process (Buchness, 1998). Similar tannin astringents can be made from white oak tree bark or the English walnut tree bark. These preparations should be strained before use and can be used two or three times per day.

Tea Tree Oil

Tea tree oil is an essential oil extracted from the leaves of *Melaleuca alternifolia*, a small tree indigenous to Australia. Tea tree oil contains approximately 100 compounds, mainly plant terpenes and their corresponding alcohols (Swords & Hunter, 1978). An acne study in 1990 compared 5% tea tree oil in a water-based gel with 5% benzoyl peroxide in 124 patients. Although the tea tree oil did not act as rapidly as benzoyl peroxide, it did show statistical improvement in the number of acne lesions at the end of 3 months. The tea tree oil had a significantly lower incidence of adverse effects such as dryness, irritation, itching, and burning (44%) compared with benzoyl peroxide (79%) (Peirce et al., 1998, p. 629). Allergic contact dermatitis to tea tree oil has been reported (de Groot & Weyland, 1993; Knight & Hansen, 1994; Selvaag et al., 1994), as well as poisoning if taken internally (Elliot, 1993; Moss, 1994). It is the degradation products of monoterpenes in the tea tree oil that actually appear to be the allergic contact sensitizing agents (Hausen, 1999).

Vitex

Oral vitex (*Vitex agnus-castus*) or chasteberry has been shown to be effective in treating premenstrual acne. The whole-fruit extract has an amphoteric hormone-regulating effect thought to act on follicle-stimulating hormone and luteinizing hormone levels in the pituitary to increase progesterone levels and reduce estrogen levels. It is Class 2b, 2c, and 2d and may counteract the effectiveness of oral contraceptives. The German Commission E monographs recommend 40 mg/d. The main adverse effects reported are gastrointestinal tract upset and rash. It should not be taken by pregnant or nursing women (Fleming, 2000, p. 176).

Other Herbs

Bitter herbs that stimulate digestive function, including acid secretion, may improve acne (Yarnell & Abascal, 2006). The German Commission E also approved topical bittersweet nightshade (*Solanum dulcamara*) (Fleming, 2000, p. 88) and orally administered brewer's yeast (*Saccharomyces cerevisiae*) (Fleming, 2000, p. 118) for the treatment of acne because of their antimicrobial effects. Topical duckweed (*Lemna minor*) is used in China to treat acne (Fleming, 2000, p. 258). Herbal mixtures are also used in China both internally and externally to treat acne (Xu, 2004, pp. 260–263).

ALOPECIA AREATA

Essential Oils

A mixture of essential oils, including thyme, rosemary, lavender, and cedarwood, in carrier oils, grapeseed, and jojoba (a liquid wax) was massaged into the scalp daily in a randomized controlled double-blind study of 86 patients with alopecia areata (Hey et al., 1998). The control group massaged only the carrier oils into the scalp. Evaluation on the basis of sequential photographs by both a 6-point scale and a computerized analysis of areas of alopecia revealed that the treatment group had a statistically significant improvement over the control group (44% vs. 15%). There were no adverse effects. Other TCM herbal mixtures have been used for alopecia areata (Xu, 2004, pp. 541–543).

ANDROGENIC ALOPECIA

Chinese Herbal Medicine

The topical use of a Chinese herbal formula, Dabao (manufactured by Engelbert & Vialle, Venlo, the Netherlands), was evaluated for the treatment of androgenic alopecia in a double-blind study that lasted 6 months and in which 396 patients participated (Kessels et al., 1991). The ingredients of Dabao include 50% ethanol, 42% water, and 8% Chinese herbal extracts, including saffron flowers, mulberry leaves, stemona root, fruits of the pepper plant, sesame leaves, the skin of the Szechuan pepper fruit, ginger root, Chinese angelica root, pseudolarix bark, and hawthorn fruit. The ingredients of the placebo included 50% ethanol, 48% water, and 2% odor and coloring agents consisting of cherry laurel water, cinnamon water, licorice syrup, sugar syrup, and a solution of burned sugar. In both groups there was an increase in non-vellus hairs. The cosmetic improvement in both groups was minimal but the Dabao group was statistically superior to the placebo group in number of new non-vellus hairs. There were no reported adverse effects.

BACTERIAL AND FUNGAL INFECTIONS OF THE SKIN

Garlic

Garlic (*Allium sativum*) contains ajoene, which has been shown to have antifungal activity. Of 34 patients treated topically with 0.4% ajoene cream once a day for tinea pedis, 79% noted clearing within 7 days and the remainder had clearing within 14 days. At a 3-month follow-up, all participants remained free of fungus (Ledezma et al., 1996). Contact dermatitis has occasionally been reported with frequent topical exposure to garlic (Fleming, 2000, p. 328). Oral administration of garlic should be avoided while breastfeeding, Class 2c (McGuffin et al., 1997, p. 6). Prolonged bleeding may occur when garlic is taken orally (Fleming, 2000, p. 328).

Tea Tree Oil

Tea tree oil (see above under "Acne") has been applied topically for the treatment of bacterial and fungal infections. Tea tree oil has shown in vitro activity against a wide variety of microorganisms, including *Propionibacterium acnes, Staphylococcus aureus, Escherichia coli, Candida albicans, Trichophyton mentagrophytes*, and *Trichophyton rubrum* (Beylier, 1979; Williams et al., 1988). Topical tea tree oil 10% cream was compared in a randomized double-blind trial of 104 patients with 1% tolnaftate cream and placebo cream. Although symptomatic relief was comparable in the tea tree oil and the tolnaftate groups, there was significantly greater mycologic cure in the tolnaftate group (85%) than the tea tree oil group (30%), while cure rates between the tea tree oil and placebo groups were not statistically different (Tong et al., 1992). Another randomized double-blind study of 117 patients compared a solution of 100% tea tree oil with 1% clotrimazole solution in the treatment of onychomycosis. The two groups showed comparable results after 6 months of treatment on the basis of mycologic cure (11% for clotrimazole and 18% for tea tree oil) and clinical assessment and subjective rating of appearance and symptoms (61% for clotrimazole and 60% for tea tree oil) (Buck et al., 1994). Tea tree oil may be used for at least symptomatic treatment of tinea pedis and onychomycosis and other superficial wounds. However, tea tree oil should not be used on burns because of its cytolytic effect on epithelial cells and fibroblasts (Faoagali el al., 1997).

Other Herbs

Thyme oil from the herb thyme (*Thymus vulgaris*) has been used topically as an antibacterial and an anticandidal agent (van Wyk et al., 2004) and is Class 1 (McGuffin et al., 1997 p. 116). A methanol extract of the Korean traditional antifungal herb *Galla rhois* was found to be active against *Candida albicans* (Seong, 2007). TCM herbal mixtures for bacterial and fungal infections of the skin are extensively discussed by Xu (2004, pp. 405–470).

CHRONIC VENOUS INSUFFICIENCY

Chronic venous insufficiency (CVI) occurs in at least 10% to 15% of men and 20% to 25% of women (Callam, 1994) and can result in great cost and morbidity. Compliance with wearing of compression stockings is poor, leading many to seek alternative therapies (Abascal & Yarnell, 2007).

Butcher's Broom and Sweet Clover

The German Commission E has approved oral butcher's broom (*Ruscus acuteatus*) and sweet clover (*Melilotus officinalisis*) for assistance in relief of pain, heaviness, pruritus, and swelling associated with venous insufficiency. Butcher's broom has been demonstrated in animal studies to increase venous tone and also has diuretic properties, while sweet clover has been shown to increase venous reflux, better termed venous return (Fleming, 2000, p. 132). Butcher's broom, which is Class 1, and sweet clover appear to be safe when used as recommended (Fleming, 2000, p. 132; McGuffin et al., 1997, p. 100).

Ginkgo

Ginkgo (*Ginkgo biloba*) has been used orally in China for centuries and more recently in Europe and the United States for numerous conditions. Research indicates that ginkgo promotes vasodilation, thereby improving blood flow in cerebral insufficiency and claudication. It may be more useful for these arterial disorders than for CVI (Hadley & Petry, 1999; Peirce et al., 1999, p. 293). When ginkgo is taken orally there have been reports of subarachnoid and intracerebral hemorrhage, as well as increased bleeding time (Fleming, 2000, p. 344), but it is Class 1 (McGuffin et al., 1997, p. 57).

Grapeseed

Double-blind trials have studied the effects of grapeseed (*Vinus vinifera*) extract on CVI. Grapeseed extract contains oligomeric proanthocyanidins, which are bioflavonoids shown to help strengthen capillaries. Dosages in the studies varied from 50 mg orally once a day to 100 mg three times per day. No serious adverse effects have been reported (Fleming, 2000, pp. 363–364).

Horse Chestnut

Horse chestnut (*Aesculus hippocastanum*) contains plant compounds known as *terpenes* with the main active component identified as aescin (Peirce et al., 1999, p. 343). The mechanism of action appears to be related to inhibiting leukocyte activation, an important pathophysiological mechanism contributing to CVI. Aescin is also thought to reduce vascular leakage by inhibiting elastase and hyaluronase, which are involved in proteoglycan degradation at the capillary endothelium (Pittler & Ernst, 1998). Double-blind randomized trials of oral horse chestnut seed extract (HCSE) have been conducted for patients with CVI, and it has been shown that HCSE decreases lower-leg volume as well as calf and ankle circumference. Patients also had decreased symptoms such as fatigue, tenderness, and pruritus. HCSE has been shown to be as effective as grade II compression stockings for treatment of CVI (Diehm, 1996). Most of the studies achieved statistically significant results for treatment of CVI with doses of HCSE containing 100 to 150 mg aescin per day, most often taken as 50 mg twice a day. Adverse effects reported were minimal and included gastrointestinal tract symptoms, dizziness, headache, and pruritus. Rates of adverse effects were from 0.9% to 3.0% and in several studies were not statistically different from rates of adverse effects with placebo. HCSE has also been used in Europe topically as a gel, lotion, or ointment to reduce inflammation and discomfort associated with varicose veins, phlebitis, and hemorrhoids (Peirce et al., 1999, p. 344). The horse chestnut seeds are poisonous and must be specially prepared by a reputable manufacturer to remove all toxins before being taken orally. There is one case report of drug-induced lupus attributed to Venocuran (manufactured by Knoll AG, Ludwigshafen, Germany), a drug for venous insufficiency containing HCSE (Peirce et al., 1999, pp. 344–345). Contact dermatitis has occasionally been reported when HSCE was used topically (Bisset & Wichtl, 2001, p. 269).

Witch Hazel

Witch hazel (*Hamamelis virginiana*) contains tannins (see details of preparation above under "Acne" tannins), making it a useful astringent topically to soothe inflammation of the skin and mucous membranes in such disorders as varicose veins and hemorrhoids. Animal research indicates that witch hazel extract has local styptic and vasoconstrictive effects. The alcohol fluid extract has also been shown to cause venous constriction in rabbits. Witch hazel is often used orally for CVI in Europe. Although it appears safe when taken orally and is Class 1, its efficacy has not been well studied in humans (Blumenthal et al., 1998, pp. 670–672; McGuffin et al., 1997, p. 59).

Other Herbs

TCM herbal mixes for stasis dermatitis are listed in Xu (2004, pp. 132–133).

DERMATITIS

Arnica

Arnica is derived from the dried flowers of *Arnica montana* or other arnica species. Although toxic orally, external preparations appear to be very safe and effective. Arnica has been used for centuries as a topical anti-inflammatory for sore muscles and joints, bruises, insect bites, boils, inflamed gums, acne eruptions, and hemorrhoids. It is also included in many seborrheic dermatitis and psoriasis preparations. It is approved by the German Commission E for topical treatment of skin inflammation (Blumenthal et al., 1998). When used as a compress, 1 tbsp (15 mL) tincture is mixed with 0.5 L water. As an infusion, 2 g dried arnica is mixed with 100 mL water. Cream or ointment preparations should contain a maximum of 15% arnica oil or 20% to 25% tincture (Bisset & Wichtl, 2001, p. 85; Peirce et al., 1999, p. 45). The active ingredients of arnica are the sesquiterpene lactones such as helanalin, 11α,13-dihydrohelenalin, chamissonolid, and their ester derivatives. They reduce inflammation by inhibiting the transcription factor nuclear factor-κB (NF-κB), which controls the transcription of many genes, including cytokines such as interleukin (IL)-1, IL-2, IL-6, IL-8, and tumor necrosis factor α, as well as adhesion molecules intercellular adhesion molecule 1, vascular cellular adhesion molecule 1, and endothelial leukocyte adhesion molecule 1. NF-κB inhibition also inhibits many genes responsible for antigen presentation and for cyclooxygenase II (Lyss et al., 1997). Contact dermatitis to arnica has been reported. Irritation may also occur when arnica is used at stronger concentrations or for longer periods than are recommended. Topical arnica is not recommended for use on open wounds or broken skin and is Class 2d (McGuffin et al., 1997, p. 14). Arnica is a protected species in some countries and other plants have been substituted fraudulently in some preparations, so it is important to purchase it from a reputable source.

Chamomile

German chamomile (*Matricaria recutita*), a member of the daisy family, has been used for centuries for many conditions, especially gastrointestinal symptoms and dermatitis. A tea made by using 2 to 3 tsp (10–15 mL) dried flowers per cup of water is taken internally or used as a compress. Topical chamomile creams and ointments bases have also been used in Germany (Bisset & Wichtl, 2001, p. 324). Topical chamomile has been demonstrated in studies to be comparable with 0.25% hydrocortisone in improving a sodium lauryl sulfate–induced contact dermatitis (Brown & Dattner, 1998). Chamomile significantly decreased the surface area of wounds in small double-blind trial, and in animal studies chamomile reduced healing time. Chamomile also has in vitro antimicrobial activities (Peirce et al., 1999, p. 157). The anti-inflammatory, wound-healing, and antimicrobial effects are attributed to a blue essential oil that contains sesquiterpene alcohol, α-bisabolol, chamazulene, and flavonoids, due in part to the inhibition of cyclooxygenase and lipoxygenase in vitro. The flavonoids also act by inhibiting histamine release from antigen-stimulated human basophilic polymorphonuclear leukocytes (Brown & Dattner, 1998). α-Bisabolol has also been demonstrated to promote granulation tissue in wound healing (Peirce et al., 1999, p. 157). The main adverse effect is allergic contact dermatitis. Chamomile is considered safe to use topically and orally and is Class 1 (McGuffin et al., 1997, p. 74).

Chinese Herbal Medicine

In TCM, the body is treated as a whole and the aim of therapy is to restore harmony to the functions of the body (Atherton et al., 1992). Traditional Chinese herbal medicine derived from TCM for the treatment of atopic dermatitis has been reported effective. In TCM mixtures of various herbs usually are individually formulated for each patient (Sheehan et al., 1992), making randomized controlled trials difficult to undertake. However, two randomized placebo-controlled crossover trials were performed in England to study the effects of a standardized oral herbal TCM-type treatment of atopic dermatitis cases where traditional Western therapy had failed (Armstrong et al., 1999; Sheehan & Atherton, 1992; Sheehan et al., 1992). A Chinese physician created a standardized mixture of 10 herbs to be used in treating atopic dermatitis characterized by erythema, lichenification, and plaques of dermatitis in the absence of active exudation or clinical infection. The 10 herbs used were *Potentilla chinensis* Class 1, *Tribulus terrestris, Rehmannia glutinosa* Class 2d, *Lophatherum gracile, Clematis armandii* Class 1, *Ledebouriella saseloides* Class 1, *Dictamnus dasycarpus, Paeonia lactiflora* Class 1, *Schizonepeta tenuifolia,* and *Glycyrrhizia glabra* Class 1 (McGuffin et al., 1997; Sheehan & Atherton, 1992). These herbs were placed in sachets and boiled to make a tea-like infusion that was orally administered daily. The placebo consisted of a tea-like infusion made from several herbs with no known efficacy for treating atopic dermatitis but with similar smells and tastes to that of the active ingredients tea-like infusion. A study with 37 children demonstrated a median decrease in erythema score of 51.0% in the treatment group versus only a 6.1% improvement in the placebo group. The percentage surface involvement decreased by 63.1% and 6.2% for the treatment and placebo groups, respectively. No serious adverse effects were found. These 37 children were offered continued treatment with the TCM herbal mixture and then were followed up for 1 year (Sheehan & Atherton, 1994). Eighteen children completed the year of treatment and showed 90% reduction in eczema activity scores. Those children who withdrew from the study did so because of lack of further response to treatment, dislike of the taste of the tea-like infusion, or difficulty in preparing the treatment. Seven patients were able to discontinue therapy after 1 year without relapse. In two patients, asymptomatic elevation of the aspartate aminotransferase level occurred, with reversion to normal after discontinuing treatment. No serious adverse effects were observed. The design was similar in a study of 31 adult patients with atopic dermatitis (Sheehan et al., 1992). Decreases in erythema and surface damage were statistically superior in the treatment group versus the placebo group. There was also subjective improvement in itching and sleep. These patients were followed for a year, with continued improvement and no serious adverse effects, whereas the patients who discontinued treatment had a relapse in their condition (Sheehan & Atherton, 1994). Although no serious adverse effects were noted in this study, careful monitoring of complete blood cell count and liver function is recommended, as reports of liver failure and even death have been reported with these TCM herbs when baseline laboratory values were not followed up (Graham-Brown, 1991; Koo & Arain, 1998; Mostefa-Kara et al., 1992). Specific herbs used in these studies are known to have anti-inflammatory, antibacterial, antifungal, antihistaminic, immunosuppressant, and corticosteroid-like effects. Several studies have attempted to elucidate the mechanism of action of this group of 10 herbs (Zemophyte, manufactured by Phytotech Limited, Godmanchester, England) in treating atopic dermatitis. Patients with atopic dermatitis are known to have elevated levels of the low-affinity IgE receptor CD23 expressed on circulating monocytes. In studies of IL4-induced CD23 expression on monocytes, there was a reduction of the CD23 expression when the cells were exposed to the aqueous herb extracts (Latchman et al., 1994, 1996). A study examined immunological markers for T cells, macrophages, Langerhans cells, and low-affinity and high-affinity IgE receptors in biopsy specimens of lesional skin treated with Zemophyte compared with biopsy specimens of nonlesional skin (Xu et al., 1997). The researchers found clinical improvement associated with a statistically significant reduction in CD23 antigen-presenting cells. However, an attempt to replicate the Zemophyte double-blind randomized placebo-controlled study in Hong Kong failed to achieve a statistically significant effect of Zemophyte over placebo (Fung et al., 1999). A different TCM-derived standardized herbal mix called PentaHerbs formula with *Paeonia suffruticosa* root bark Class 1, *Phellodentron chinensis* bark Class 2b, *Lonicera japonica* flower Class 1, *Mentha haplocalux* aerial part Class 1, and *Atractylodes lancea* rhizome Class 1 at a ratio of 2:2:2:1:2 known clinically to be useful for atopic dermatitis was tested on rat peritoneal mast cells, and it suppressed histamine release and prostaglandin D2 synthesis (Chan et al., 2008). Bark of the birch tree (*Betula platyphylla* var. *japonica*) used to treat atopic dermatitis was studied in NC/Nga mice. It decreased scratching and skin inflammation in the mice as well as decreasing IgE and IL4 mRNA levels, suggesting that it suppresses the T-helper 2 cellular response (Kim et al., 2008). Other TCM herbal mixes for dermatitis are listed in Xu (2004, pp. 103–131).

Jewelweed

Jewelweed (*Impatiens biflora*) is alleged in folklore to be useful topically for treating poison ivy contact dermatitis, but research results are conflicting. Treatment with jewelweed in one study was comparable with standard treatment for poison ivy contact dermatitis, and in 108 of 115 patients symptoms cleared within 2 to 3 days (Lipton, 1958), but in another study jewelweed extract failed to reduce symptoms of poison ivy dermatitis (Guin & Reynolds,1980). In an additional study there was no prophylactic effect of jewelweed in poison ivy dermatitis (Long et al., 1997). Jewelweed has been said to be most helpful if applied to the area the poison ivy touched as soon after contact as possible, but this was not addressed in the above studies. There have been no reports of topical jewelweed causing adverse effects (Peirce et al., 1999, p. 365).

Mucilage-Containing Herbs

Several herbs contain a substance called mucilage that is useful topically to soothe and act as an emollient on skin. Heartsease (*Viola tricolor*) Class 1, marsh mallow (*Althea officinalis*), English plantain (*Plantago lanceolata*) Class 1, fenugreek (*Trigonella foenum-gaecum*) Class 2b, mullein (*Verbascum thapsus*) Class 1, slippery elm (*Ulmus fulva*) Class 1, and flax (*Linum usitatissimum*) contain mucilages. Mucilage quickly swells into a gooey mass when exposed to water, moisturizing and coating dry or mildly inflamed skin. Mucilage also is a mild adhesive and can be used as an herbal bandage adhesive for minor wounds (Fleming, 2000; McGuffin et al., 1997; Peirce et al., 1999).

Oats

Oats (*Avena sativa*) have been used topically in baths for their soothing and antipruritic properties for hundreds of years, and they are approved for this use by the German Commission E and are listed as Class 1 (Bisset & Wichtl, 2001, p. 97; Fleming, 2000, p. 552; McGuffin et al., 1997, p. 18). Colloidal oatmeal turns to a gooey sticky mass, attributed to the gluten content, when mixed with liquid, thereby coating the skin and sealing in moisture. This can be beneficial for atopic dermatitis as well as for idiopathic pruritus of the elderly.

Pansy Flower

Pansy flower (*Viola tricolor* hybrids) infusion is recommended as a nontoxic treatment for seborrheic dermatitis, especially in infants. The infusion is made by mixing 1 to 2 tsp of the flowers per cup of water and is used as a wet dressing. Salicylic acid in concentrations of about 0.3% appears to be the active ingredient. The infusion also contains saponins and mucilage, which have softening and soothing actions. No adverse effects have been reported with topical use, and it is Class 1 (McGuffin et al., 1997, p. 123; Peirce et al., 1999, p. 480).

Tannins

Agrimony (*Agrimonia eupatoria*) Class 1, jambolan bark (*Syzygium cumini*) Class 1, oak bark (*Quercus robur*) Class 2d, English walnut leaf (*Juglans regia*) Class 2d, Labrador tea (*Ledum groenlandicum*), goldenrod (*Solidago* spp.) Class 2d, lady's mantle (*Alchemilla* spp.) Class 1, lavender (*Lavandula angustifolia*) Class 1, mullein (*Verbascum thapsus*) Class 1, rhatany (*Krameria* spp.) Class 1, Chinese rhubarb (*Rheum officinale*) Class 2b, 2c, 2d, yellow dock (*Rumex crispus*) Class 2d, witch hazel bark (*Hamamelis virginiana*) Class 1, and St. John's wort (*Hypericum montana*) Class 2d contain tannins and act as astringents. Oat straw (*Avena sativa*) Class 1 is also approved for its sooth-ing and antipruritic qualities (Bisset & Wichtl, 2001; Blumenthal et al., 1998; Fleming, 2000; McGuffin et al., 1997; Peirce et al., 1999). Topically applied tannins treat dermatitis by coagulating surface proteins of cells and exudates, reducing permeability and secretion and forming a protective layer on the skin (Brown & Dattner, 1998). Tannins may also have antimicrobial properties. However, one study showed that a witch hazel extract in a phosphatidyl cho-line base was less effective in reducing erythema from UV radiation and cel-lophane tape stripping in 24 healthy patients than 1% hydrocortisone (Korting et al., 1993). Another clinical trial compared witch hazel extract with control in a group with atopic dermatitis (n = 36) and another group with contact dermatitis (n = 80). In the atopic group, the witch hazel was slightly superior in reducing inflammation and itching; this matches anecdotal reports of witch hazel's usefulness in treating atopic dermatitis (Brown & Dattner, 1998).

HERPES SIMPLEX

Balm

Balm (*Melissa officinalis*) is a lemon-scented member of the mint family. Topical uses of an essential oil steam distilled from the cut leaves include treating herpes simplex and minor wounds. In a randomized double-blind trial of 116 patients with herpes simplex lesions, 96% had complete clear-ing of lesions at day 8 after using 1% balm extract cream five times a day (Wobling & Leonhardt, 1994). In another trial where balm extract was placed on lesions within 72 hours of onset of symptoms, the size of the lesions and healing time were statistically better in the group treated with balm extract (Brown & Dattner, 1998). Tannin and polyphenols appear to be responsible for its antiviral effect (Peirce et al., 1999, p. 58). Balm is Class 1 and appears very safe to use both topically and orally (McGuffin et al., 1997, p. 75; Peirce et al., 1999, p. 58).

Other Herbs

Other herbal preparations that have shown in vitro activity against herpes simplex include *Echinacea* spp., sweet marjoram, peppermint, and propolis, but clinical studies for the latter three have not yet been performed (Peirce et al., 1999, p. 702). A small randomized placebo-controlled crossover clinical trial found no statistically significant differences between Echinacea extract 800 mg twice a day for 6 months and placebo controls for recurrent genital herpes (Basch et al., 2005). TCM herbal mixtures for herpes simplex are listed by Xu (2004, pp. 372–374).

HERPES ZOSTER

Capsaicin

Capsaicin, the main ingredient in the spice cayenne pepper derived from the pod of *Capiscum frutescens*, is Class 1 internally and Class 2d externally (McGuffin et al., 1997, p. 23) and is available as a cream for the treatment of postherptic neuralgia. It is applied four or five times a day over the painful area and initially causes a burning sensation. With continued use it depletes substance P in the regional peripheral nerves, reducing pain.

Hibiscus

In China, herpes zoster is commonly treated topically with hibiscus (*Hibiscus sabdariffa*) (Fleming, 2000, p. 394). Hibiscus has been shown to be very safe and is Class 1 topically and orally (McGuffin et al., 1997, p. 61). TCM herbal mixtures for herpes zoster are listed by Xu (2004, pp. 379–382).

Licorice

Herpes zoster and postherpetic neuralgia have been treated with a topical licorice (*Glycyrrhiza glabra, Glycyrrhiza uralensis*) Class 1 gel preparation (Lininger, 2000, pp. 155–156). Glycyrrhizen, one of the active components of licorice, has been demonstrated to inhibit replication of varicella zoster in vitro (Baba & Shigeta, 1987). There have so far been no clinical trials to support the in vitro findings of inhibition of replication of the virus. Topical use appears to be very safe, but care should be used when it is taken orally as it is Class 2b and 2d (McGuffin et al., 1997, p. 58).

HYPERHIDROSIS

Tannins

Topical tannins can reduce sweat duct openings by precipitating surface proteins and thus reduce sweating locally. These astringents also have antimicrobial properties that help to reduce odorous bacterial byproducts (van Wyk, 2004, p. 368). See above at Tannins under the "Dermatitis" section for information about specific sources of tannins. Black tea also contains tannins.

HYPERPIGMENTATION (DARK SPOTS)

Fruit Acids

Lemon juice contains a high level of citric acid, which when applied topically to the skin has the ability to lighten superficial pigmentation in the epidermis.

Deeper hyperpigmentation in the dermis will be less affected by the topical application. Woods light ultraviolet examination of the skin in a darkened room can help to distinguish between superficial hyperpigmentation, which appears darker, and deeper hyperpigmentation, which does not contrast much with the surrounding skin. Lemon juice can also lighten hair: after applying lemon juice, sit in direct sunlight for 30 minutes. Do not substitute lime juice, because lime juice is photosensitizing and can cause more hyperpigmentation. The flavone glycosides in an unripe Japanese *Citrus hassaku* extract have also been reported experimentally to inhibit melanogenesis (Itoh et al., 2009).

Other Herbs

Both curcumin and neem have been used for hyperpigmentation associated with photodamage. Curcumin is extracted from the spice turmeric, which is the dried and ground rhizome of *Curcuma longa*. See details about curcumin below under the "Psoriasis" heading. Neem, powdered leaves from *Azadirachta indica*, contains flavones and other compounds (Khan & Khanum 2009) that may help to correct photodamage, including the associated hyperpigmentation of solar lentigines (often called "liver spots" because they are the color of cut liver).

LICHEN PLANUS

Aloe vera mouthwash was compared with triamcinolone acetonide 0.1% for oral lichen planus in a randomized double-blind study of 45 patients for 4 weeks. Both treatments significantly and equally reduced visible oral lichen planus lesions, pain, and burning. (Mansourian et al., 2011).

PRURITUS
Camphor

Camphor is derived from a distillate of the wood of the camphor tree (*Cinnamomum camphora*) Class 2b, 2d (McGuffin et al., 1997, p. 30). It is toxic in large doses. As an antipruritic it can be added to lotions or creams at 0.5% concentration.

Menthol

Menthol is derived from Japanese mint (*Mentha arvensis*) Class 1 (McGuffin et al., 1997, p. 75). It has a cooling antipruritic and antibacterial effect. Lotions and creams typically contain 1% to 5% essential oil.

Oats

See "Dermatitis" section above.

Tars Derived from Trees

Tars are antipruritic and antiproliferative and are derived from birch (*Betula* spp.), beech (*Fagus* spp.), or juniper (*Juniperus* spp.) trees (van Wyk, 2004, p. 367). They are used in a 5% to 10% concentration in creams, gels, or soaps. They can stain skin and clothing. They are photosensitizing, and judicious exposure to sunlight can be beneficial.

PSORIASIS

A survey of patients with psoriasis at a large university dermatology practice revealed that 51% of psoriasis patients used one or more alternative therapeutic modalities (Fleischer et al., 1996). This is consistent with previous Norwegian surveys of patients with psoriasis (Jensen, 1990). Herbal therapy is one of the most frequently chosen alternative therapies. Psoriasis has been treated for centuries with herbal preparations, both topical and oral.

Aloe Vera

Aloe vera (*Aloe vera*) has been used for centuries for wound healing and has recently been shown to be a potential treatment for psoriasis. It is Class 1 internally and Class 2d externally (McGuffin et al., 1997, p. 7). In a double-blind placebo-controlled study, 60 patients with slight to moderate plaque psoriasis were treated topically with either 0.5% hydrophilic aloe cream or placebo. The aloe-treated group showed statistically significant improvement (83.3%) compared with placebo (6.6%). There were no adverse effects in the treatment group (Syed et al., 1996).

Capsaicin

Capsaicin, the main ingredient in the cayenne pepper pod spice (*Capiscum frutescens*), is Class 1 internally and Class 2d externally (McGuffin et al., 1997, p. 23) and has also been studied for the treatment of psoriasis. Capsaicin has been shown to inhibit phorbol-ester–induced activation of transcription factors NF-κB and AP-1 in vitro (Surh et al., 2000). Two trials have shown that 0.025% capsaicin cream used topically is effective in treating psoriasis. One clinical trial showed a significant decrease in scaling and erythema during a 6-week period in 44 patients with moderate and severe psoriasis (Bernstein et al., 1986). The other was a double-blind study of 197 patients with psoriasis treated with the capsaicin cream four times daily for 6 weeks; they had a significant decrease in scaling, thickness, erythema, and pruritus (Ellis et al., 1993). The main adverse effect reported was a brief burning sensation at the application site. Capsaicin is contraindicated on injured skin or near the eyes, and the German Commission E suggests it not be used for more than 2 consecutive days, with a 14-day rest interval between applications.

Chinese Herbal Medicine

Furanocoumarins derived from *Ammi majus* and related plants that produce 8-methoxy-psoralin when applied topically or taken orally intercalate with DNA. Subsequent exposure to UVA from the sun or from a lightbox results in photoactivation that causes cross-linkages with the thymine in the DNA, inducing cell death (van Wyk, 2004, p. 367). This in turn inhibits the hyperproliferation in psoriatic lesions. There are many photosensitizing herbal preparations composed of furocoumarins that act as psoralens when combined with UVA (320–400 nanometers). One commonly used in TCM, Radix Angelicae dahurica Class 1 (McGuffin et al., 1997, p. 10), contains the furocoumarins imperatorin, isoimpertorin, and alloimperatorin. A study involving 300 patients with psoriasis showed that this TCM, taken orally and combined with UVA therapy, had equivalent efficacy when compared with standard treatment of psoralen–UVA with methoxypsoralen. However, there were fewer adverse effects such as nausea and dizziness in the group treated with the TCM and UVA (Koo & Arain, 1998). Some other TCM products made from herbs have shown systemic efficacy against psoriasis but are too toxic when given systemically and can be used in topical preparations (Ng, 1998). A topical TCM product of the plant *Camptotheca acuminata*, in an open trial including 92 patients with psoriasis, found that this treatment was statistically more effective than 1% hydrocortisone, but allergic contact dermatitis was noted in 9% to 15% of the patients in the TCM group. Comparison of TCM mixtures in clinical trials is difficult because the mixture of herbs prescribed varies individually depending on the subtype of psoriasis ("blood-heat" type, "blood deficiency dryness" type, and "blood-stasis" type), which is determined in TCM by many findings, including the lesions of psoriasis, the pulse, and the condition of the tongue (Koo & Arain, 1998). Some TCM products may act in part on the microcirculation of the psoriatic lesion (Zhang & Gu, 2007). Additional TCM herbal mixtures for psoriasis are listed in Xu (2004, pp. 172–191).

Curcumin

Curcumin comprises about 5% of turmeric (*Curcuma longa*) Class 2b, 2d (McGuffin et al., 1997, p. 39). Turmeric has been used for centuries in India to provide glow and luster to the skin. It has antimicrobial, antioxidant, astringent, and other useful effects to help heal wounds and reduce scarring

(Chaturvedi, 2009). In vitro, the purified turmeric extract curcumin has been shown to inhibit phorbol-ester–induced activation of transcription factors NF-κB and AP-1 (Surh et al., 2000). The resulting suppression of phosphorylase kinase activity correlates with the resolution of psoriasis when curcumin is applied topically in a gel to the lesions (Heng et al., 2000).

Tars Derived from Trees

Tars derived from birch (*Betula* spp.), beech (*Fagus* spp.), or juniper (*Juniperus* spp.) trees (van Wyk, 2004, p. 367) are antipruritic and antiproliferative. Tars have been used for centuries to treat psoriasis. They are used in a 5% to 10% concentration in creams, gels, or soaps. They are photosensitizing, and judicious exposure to sunlight can be beneficial, or they can be used in conjunction with UVB (250–320 nanometers) or narrow-band UVB (311 nanometers).

PSYCHOSOMATIC
Kava Kava

Kava kava (*Piper methysticum*) is moderately anxiolytic, but its use is not recommended due to its potential hepatotoxicity. It is Class 2b, 2c, 2d (McGuffin et al., 1997, p. 86).

Lavender Oil

Lavender oil aromatherapy (*Lavendula* spp.) has been demonstrated to produce a significant reduction in anxiety. It is important that the first exposure to lavender oil be a pleasant and relaxing one, as this may in part be a conditioned response. It is Class 1 (McGuffin et al., 1997, p. 68).

Lemon Balm

Lemon balm (*Melissa officinalis*) is approved by the German Commission E for nervousness and insomnia. It is Class 1 (McGuffin et al., 1997, p. 75).

Magnolia Bark

Magnolia bark (*Magnolia obovata*) is moderately anxiolytic. It contains honokiol and magnolol, which are also antioxidant and anti-inflammatory (Kuribara et al., 1998). It is Class 2b (McGuffin et al., 1997, p. 72).

Passionflower

Passionflower (*Passiflora incarnata*) is approved by the German Commission E for nervousness and insomnia. It is Class 1 (McGuffin et al., 1997, p. 82).

St. John's Wort

St. John's wort (*Hypericum perforatum*) is approved by the German Commission E for depression. It can improve mild to moderate depression but not severe depression (Linde et al., 1996). It significantly interacts with the metabolism of a number of other drugs by inducing cytochrome P450 isoform 3A4 and is Class 2d (McGuffin et al., 1997, p. 62).

Valerian

Valerian (*Valariana* spp.) is approved by the German Commission E for insomnia caused by nervousness. It is Class 1 (McGuffin et al., 1997, p.120).

SCABIES

Aloe Vera

Comparison of *Aloe vera* crude gel in an open-label nonrandomized study in 16 patients with benzyl benzoate in 14 patients with two courses of treatment for scabies showed clearing in all patients, with some residual pruritus in two patients in the *Aloe vera* group and three patients in the benzyl benzoate group (Oyelami et al., 2009). There were no significant side effects.

Anise

Anise (*Pimpinella anisum*) seeds contain an essential oil that has displayed antibacterial and insecticidal activity in vitro and has been used topically to treat scabies and head lice. It should not be used in pregnancy and is Class 2b (McGuffin et al., 1997, p. 86).

Neem

Neem (*Azadirachta indica*) is indigenous to India, and every part of the plant has been used medicinally. A paste of neem and turmeric applied topically was reported to treat chronic ulcers and scabies in a study on more than 800 villagers in India (Peirce et al., 1999, p. 452). Neem appears safe in adults but can be poisonous to children (Peirce et al., 1999, p. 453). Numerous other herbs have been used for centuries in India and China to treat scabies (Fleming, 2000).

SCARS

Aloe Vera

A scar is the result of the body's repair of damage to the dermal leathery layer of the skin. The stages of scar tissue healing include an early inflammatory and often crusted phase that lasts from 2 days to about a week. Lay terminology includes the word "scab" for this phase. *Aloe vera* gel can be a useful antiseptic and anti-inflammatory at this early stage of wound healing (Heggers et al., 1996).

Curcumin

Next comes the red proliferative phase of producing collagen and new capillaries. Curcumin (see above under "Psoriasis" section) can help to inhibit microorganisms and promote healing that lessens the appearance of the scar.

Onion Extract

Finally, there is the maturation phase, in which the body produces more collagen and slowly remodels the scar so that the excess collagen is removed and the scar becomes less noticeable. Over the next 6 to 18 months the wound transforms from red and raised to flat and white. Scars often do not reach their final appearance for up to 2 years. If the body builds excess collagen, a hypertrophic thickened scar results, and if the excess collagen building extends beyond the site of the original wound it is called a keloid. An extract of onion from *Allium cepa* has been reported as useful in reducing the neoangiogenesis in hypertrophic scars and keloids with clinical improvement (Campanati et al., 2010).

Other Herbs

Other anecdotally used herbal treatments include olive oil rubbed on. Olive oil (*Olea europa*) contains polyphenols, which are antioxidants including catechins and flavonoids. Olives contain a high level of polyphenols, which when applied topically to a scar increases the amount of beneficial antioxidants to the area. Gotu kola from *Centella asiatica* is a traditional herb used for centuries in China, India, and Indonesia to heal wounds. The active ingredients in gotu kola are called triterpenoids, which inhibit the overproduction of collagen in scar tissue and raise the antioxidant level. Sage essential oil is distilled from the leaves of the perennial sage plant *Salvia officinalis*. It is an antiseptic, an antimicrobial, and a rich source of antioxidants. Sage essential oil works to improve circulation, soften, heal, and regenerate the skin, and break down scar tissue. Sage essential oil should be used in small amounts because it contains thujone, a chemical that can be toxic in a high quantity. Cocoa butter has been used to moisturize and sooth scars. Coconut oil is said to lighten the appearance of old scars. Tea tree oil has been used for old acne scars, as have green tea and neem.

SKIN CANCER

Ginseng

Red ginseng (*Panax ginseng*) is a classic TCM. Red ginseng extracts used topically in a study appeared to inhibit chemically induced skin tumors in mice, thought to be due to immune-modulating properties of the red ginseng (Xiaoguang et al., 1998). It is Class 2d (McGuffin et al., 1997, p. 81).

Propolis

Propolis is a resinous material gathered by honeybees from the buds and bark of certain plants and trees. Propolis has been used for centuries for antimicrobial, anti-inflammatory, analgesic, and antitumor effects, likely due to the flavonoid and related phenolic acids components. A tumoricidal component, clerodane diterpenoid, has also been isolated and was studied topically for its effects on skin tumorigenesis in mice. Clerodane diterpenoid reduced the incidence of chemically induced dysplastic papillomas, likely by inhibiting the synthesis of DNA in a de novo pathway and by suppressing the growth of tumors by decreasing DNA synthesis in a salvage pathway (Mitamura et al., 1996).

Rosemary

Rosemary (*Rosmarinus officinalis*) extract has been said to have antioxidant activity. A methanol extract of the leaves applied topically inhibited the induction and promotion of skin tumors in mice treated with known chemical carcinogens. It appears that several components of the extract are important in this process, suggesting that it was not the antioxidant properties alone that were beneficial in the prevention of skin tumors (Huang et al., 1994). Rosemary should not be used in pregnancy and is Class 2b (McGuffin et al., 1997, p. 99).

Silymarin

Silymarin is a flavonoid isolated from milk thistle (*Silybum marianum*) and is approved by the German Commission E for liver disease because of its antioxidant properties. Topically applied silymarin also appears to protect against chemically induced skin tumor promotion in mice. It may inhibit promoter-induced edema, hyperplasia, and proliferation as well as the oxidant state (Lahiri-Chatterjee et al., 1999). Silymarin appears to be safe to use topically and orally and is Class 1 (McGuffin et al., 1997, p. 107).

Tea

Tea is manufactured from the leaf and bud of *Camellia sinensis*. The majority of tea consumed worldwide is in the form of black tea, which is Class 2d (McGuffin et al., 1997, p. 22). In Asia, green tea is most commonly consumed, and oolong tea is popular in China. Teas contain polyphenolic compounds that have antioxidant properties. The oxidative states of these compounds vary among the different tea formulations. Green tea is produced from the fresh leaves, and preparation is aimed at avoiding oxidation and polymerization of the polyphenols. Black tea production involves a controlled fermentation process. Oolong tea is intermediate between green and black tea. Tea also contains tannins. Green tea has been shown in several mouse models to have anti-inflammatory and antitumorigenic properties. The polyphenolic constituent (−)-epigallocatechin-3-gallate is thought to be the primary active ingredient. Numerous studies of green tea and skin cancer were reviewed by Katiyar and colleagues (2000), and topical application or oral consumption of green tea was found to protect against inflammation, chemical carcinogenesis, and photocarcinogenesis. Green tea has been demonstrated to block many mediators in the inflammatory process important in the early steps of skin tumor promotion It also inhibits biochemical markers of chemical carcinogenesis, inhibits UV-induced oxidative stress, and prevents UV-induced immunosuppression (Katiyar et al., 2000). Green tea also protects against psoralen–UVA–induced photochemical damage to the skin (Zhao et al., 1999). Black tea may also play a role in the prevention of skin tumors, with the theaflavins being the active components in chemoprevention (Nomura et al., 2000). Topical application of constituents in black tea can decrease UVB-induced erythema, inhibit tumor initiation, and act as an antitumor promoter (Javed et al., 1998; Zhao et al., 1999). Oral administration of black tea also appears to inhibit tumor proliferation and promotes tumor apoptosis in nonmalignant and malignant skin tumors (Lu et al., 1997). There was a lower risk of squamous cell carcinoma in patients who consumed hot black tea than in nonconsumers (Hakim et al., 2000). Studies comparing the effectiveness of black and green teas in protecting against UV-induced skin tumors are conflicting as to which is more beneficial (Huang et al., 1997; Lou et al., 1999; Record & Dreosti, 1998; Wang et al., 1994). Caffeinated teas appear to be more protective than decaffeinated teas, and caffeine alone has some inhibitory effects on UVB-induced carcinogenesis (Huang et al., 1997; Lou et al., 1999; Wang et al., 1994).

VERRUCA VULGARIS AND CONDYLOMATA ACUMINATA
Podophyllin

Podophyllin is extracted from the root of the American May apple (*Podophyllum peltatum*) and is used to treat condylomata acuminata (Fleming, 2000, p. 510). It should not be used during pregnancy and is Class 2b externally and toxic internally (McGuffin et al., 1997, p. 89).

Sinecatechins

Sinecatechins 15% ointment (Veregen) extracted from green tea is approved for prescription use in treating condylomata acuminata. The polyphenolic sinecatechins inhibit enzymes related to viral replication and inhibit inflammatory mediators (Tyring, 2012).

Other Herbs

The German Commission E has approved bittersweet nightshade (*Solanum dulcamara*) Class 2b, 2c and oat straw (*Avena sativa*) Class 1 for the treatment of common warts (Fleming, 2000, pp. 88,552; McGuffin et al., 1997, p. 18). Calotropis (*Calotropis procera*) is used in India, and greater celandine (*Chelidonium majus*) Class 2b, 2c, 2d (McGuffin et al., 1997, p. 28) is used in China for the treatment of warts (Fleming, 2000, pp. 142, 170). Bittersweet nightshade and celandine should be avoided in pregnancy and while breastfeeding (Fleming, 2000, pp. 88, 170).

VITILIGO

Ginkgo

Ginkgo (*Ginkgo biloba*) was found to be effective in treating limited, slowly spreading vitiligo (Parsad et al., 2003). Caution should be used when ginkgo is taken orally, as there have been reports of subarachnoid and intracerebral hemorrhage, as well as increased bleeding time (Fleming, 2000, p. 344), but it is Class 1 (McGuffin et al., 1997, p. 57).

Psoralens

See discussion of "Psoriasis" above. By reducing inflammatory cells while stimulating melanogenesis from melanocytes in hair follicles, the treatment often will induce repigmentation of vitiliginous skin.

WOUNDS AND BURNS

Aloe Vera

Aloe vera leaves produce a gel obtained from the central core of the leaf that has been used topically for centuries for the treatment of wounds and burns. There is also an aloe juice or latex that is a bitter yellow fluid extracted from the inner leaf skin that has very potent laxative effects (Peirce et al., 1999, p. 31). Aloe vera gel reduces burning, itching, and scarring associated with radiation dermatitis (Klein & Penneys, 1988). Aloe vera gel has also been shown to accelerate healing of chronic leg ulcers, surgically induced wounds, and frostbite. The aloe vera gel decreases levels of thromboxane A_2, thromboxane B_2, and prostaglandin 2α, which cause vasoconstriction and platelet aggregation. Decreasing these vasoconstrictors and platelet aggregators increases dermal perfusion, reducing tissue loss from ischemia (Klein & Penneys, 1988). With respect to pain reduction, in vitro studies have also demonstrated a carboxypeptidase that inactivates bradykinin, decreasing pain at the treatment site (Fujita & Shosike, 1976). Salicylic acid present in aloe vera also acts as an analgesic and anti-inflammatory by inhibiting prostaglandin production (Robinson et al., 1982). Magnesium lactate is also present in aloe vera and is thought to be anti-pruritic by inhibiting histidine decarboxylase, which controls the conversion of histidine to histamine in mast cells (Klein & Penneys, 1988). Reduction in inflammation is thought to be due also to the immunomodulatory properties of the gel polysaccharides present, especially the acetylated mannans (Reynolds & Dweck, 1999). Aloe vera has also demonstrated bactericidal, anticandidal, and antifungal activity in vitro. Allergic contact dermatitis is the main adverse effect of topical aloe vera gel. Oral and topical aloe vera is considered very safe when used properly. It is Class 1 internally and Class 2d externally (McGuffin et al., 1997, p. 7).

Honey

Honey used topically on wounds, including burns, decubitus ulcers, and infected wounds, has assisted healing for centuries (Greenwood, 1993). In vitro it has antibacterial and antifungal activity to organisms that commonly infect surgical wounds (Efam & Udoh, 1992). Honey was used in a study of nine infants with large, open, culture-positive postoperative wound infections where standard treatment consisting of appropriate intravenous antibiotics and cleansing with chlorhexidine for more than 14 days failed. When the wounds were treated with 5 to 10 mL fresh unprocessed honey twice a day, there was marked clinical improvement by day 5, and by day 21, the wounds were all closed, clean, and sterile (Vardi et al., 1998). In a randomized controlled trial, honey-impregnated gauze was compared with a polyurethane film (OpSite, manufactured by Smith & Nephew, North Humberside, England) for partial-thickness burns. The honey-treated wounds healed statistically earlier with a mean of 10.8 days versus 15.3 days with the polyurethane film–treated wounds and with equal numbers of complications such as infection, excessive granulation, and contracture (Subrahmanyam, 1993). The wound-healing properties of honey are believed to result from the debriding properties of the enzyme catalase, absorption of edema due to honey's hygroscopic properties, its ability to promote granulation and re-epithelialization from the wound edges, and its antimicrobial properties (Efam, 1988). Other than rare reports of contact dermatitis to honey there have been no reports of significant adverse effects (Efam, 1988).

Marigold

Marigold (*Calendula officinalis*) topically has been used since ancient times and is currently approved by the German Commission E as an antiseptic and for wound healing (Bisset & Wichtl, 2001, p. 119). Topical marigold preparations continue to be recommended for the treatment of wounds, ulcers, burns, boils, rashes, chapped hands, herpes zoster, and varicose veins. Marigold gargles are also used for mouth and throat inflammation (Peirce, 1999, p. 129). Marigold is also widely used as a topical treatment for diaper dermatitis and other mild skin inflammations (Brown & Dattner, 1998). Treatment consists of an application several times a day of an ointment or cream made by mixing 2 to 5 g of the flower heads with 100 g ointment. A gargle or lotion is made by mixing 1 to 2 tsp (5–10 mL) of tincture with 0.25 to 0.5 L water (Peirce, 1999, p. 130). The anti-inflammatory effects of marigold are ascribed to the triterpenoids. In animal studies *Calendula* appears to stimulate granulation and increase glycoproteins and collagen at wound sites (Brown & Dattner, 1998). Marigold also shows in vitro antimicrobial and immune-modulating properties (Peirce, 1999, p. 130). Allergic contact dermatitis is the main adverse event. It is considered safe to use both topically and orally and is Class 1 (McGuffin et al., 1997, p. 22).

Tannins

Many herbs contain tannins that act as astringents, helping to dry oozing and bleeding wounds. Tannin-containing herbs that may be helpful for the topical treatment of wounds include English walnut leaf, goldenrod, Labrador tea, lavender, mullein, oak bark, rhatany, Chinese rhubarb, St. John's wort, and yellowdock (see Tannins above under "Dermatitis" for a list of scientific plant names and ratings of toxicity) (Peirce, 1999, p. 709).

Risks Associated with Oral Herbs and Dermatologic Surgery

BLEEDING

Some medicinal herbs contain coumarin, salicylate, or other platelet-inhibiting substances that can increase the risk of intraoperative and postoperative bleeding. Coumarin-containing herbs include danshen (*Salvia miltiorrhiza*), dong quai (*Angelica sinensis*), horse chestnut bark (*Aesculius hippocastanum*), sweet clover (*Melilotus officianalis*), sweet vernal (*Anthoxanthum odoratum*), sweet-scented bedstraw (*Galium triflorum*), tonka beans (*Dipteryx odorata*), vanilla leaf (*Trilisa odoratissima*), and woodruff (*Asperula odorata*). Salicylate-containing herbs include black cohosh (*Cimifuga racemosa*), meadowsweet (*Spirea ulmaria*), poplar bark (*Populus* spp.), sweet birch bark (*Betula* spp.), willow bark (*Salix* spp.), and wintergreen (*Gaultheria procumbens*). Other platelet function inhibitors include bromelain (*Ananas comosus*), cayenne (*Capiscum frutescens*), Chinese skullcap (*Scutullaria baicalensis*), feverfew (*Tanacetum parthenium*), garlic (*Allium sativum*), ginger (*Zingiber officinale*), ginkgo (*Ginkgo biloba*), ginseng (*Panex ginseng*), onion (*Allium cepa*), papain (*Carica papaya*), reishi fruit (*Ganoderma lucidum*), and turmeric (*Curcuma longa*) (Pribitkin, 2005).

BLOOD PRESSURE

Plants that may induce hypertension include black cohosh (*Cimifuga racemosa*), ephedra or ma huang (*Ephedra* spp.), licorice (*Glycyrrhiza glabra*), and yohimbe (*Pausinystalia yohimbe*). Hypertension increases the risk of bleeding. Plants that may induce hypotension include garlic (*Allium sativum*) (Pribitkin, 2005).

Other Potential Adverse Effects of Herbal Medicines

Some herbal medicines are very safe and may be consumed as foods, while others are highly biologically active and toxic and must be used very carefully. Many cutaneous reactions to herbal preparations have been reported. The most common cutaneous adverse reaction to herbal preparations is allergic contact dermatitis, but more serious cutaneous reactions have been reported. Two patients developed erythroderma after using topical herbal medicines for psoriasis and atopic dermatitis, and one patient developed Stevens-Johnson syndrome after taking "Golden Health Blood Purifying Tablets," which contained multiple herbs, including red clover, burdock, queen's delight, poke root, prickly ash, sassafras bark, and *Passiflora* (Monk, 1986). Bullous and nodular lichen planus have been reported following ingestion of native African herbal medicines (Soyinka, 1973). A leukemia-related Sweet syndrome was also described in a young woman, elicited by a pathergic response to topical arnica cream (Delmonte et al., 1998). Serious systemic adverse effects have been reported with the use of TCM herbal mixtures for the treatment of dermatologic disorders, with the most common being hepatotoxic effects. Although most patients recover without serious consequences after the medication is stopped, there have been reports of patients with acute liver failure and death. Additionally there are reports of renal failure and agranulocytosis (Graham-Brown, 1992; Koo & Arain, 1998; Mostefa-Kara et al., 1992). One patient had adult respiratory distress syndrome after administration of a TCM, Kamisyoyo-san, for seborrheic dermatitis (Shota et al., 1961). A patient developed reversible dilated cardiomyopathy after treatment with a Chinese herbal tea for her atopic dermatitis (Ferguson et al., 1997). A few Chinese and

Indian herbal medicines have also been reported to contain heavy metals, such as lead, arsenic, and mercury as contaminants. Prescription drugs have also been found as unlabeled ingredients in some over-the-counter herbal formulations from other countries. Some herbs themselves are mislabeled or misidentified. Many possible drug interactions can also occur between herbs and prescription medications. Patients should share with their physician information about what herbs and supplements and other over-the-counter remedies they are taking orally or applying to their skin. Immune-upmodulating effects of *Echinacea, Astragalus*, licorice, alfalfa sprouts, vitamin E, and zinc may decrease the efficacy of corticosteroids and immunosuppressants (Miller, 1998). Herbs that have been shown to cause hepatic damage should not be used in combination with medications such as methotrexate. These potentially hepatotoxic herbs include many of the ingredients in the TCM preparations, as well as *Echinacea*, chaparral, germander, ragwort, and life root (Borins, 1998; Ferguson et al., 1997). Herbs containing gamma-linolenic acid, such as evening primrose oil used for dermatitis, psoriasis, and xerosis, lower the seizure threshold, so anticonvulsant dosages may need to be increased (Ferguson et al., 1997). Rue (*Ruta graveolens*) and other herbs containing psoralens can cause phototoxic reactions externally on the skin (Eickhorst et al., 2007).

Conclusion

Patients taking prescription oral medications should consult their physician or other provider before self-medicating with herbs. Patients should also be counseled on the relative lack of regulation for herbal medicines in the United States and in many other areas of the world. Currently in the United States there are only minimal quality-control requirements to ensure the purity, concentration, or safety of herbal supplements. Herb manufacturers are restricted from making efficacy statements, but there are no regulations on claims of what symptoms these herbal medicines can alleviate. There are also minimal regulations on which herbs can be restricted in formulations (Shaw, 1998).

REFERENCES

Abascal, K., & Yarnell, E. (2007). Botanicals for chronic venous insufficiency. *Alternative and Complementary Therapy, 13*(6), 304–311.

Armstrong, N. C., & Ernst, E. (1999). The treatment of eczema with Chinese herbs, a systematic review of randomized clinical trials. *British Journal of Clinical Pharmacology, 48*, 262–264.

Atherton, D. J., Sheehan, M. P., Rustin, M. H. A., et al. (1992). Treatment of atopic eczema with traditional Chinese medicinal plants. *Pediatric Dermatology, 9*, 373–375.

Baba, M., & Shigeta, S. (1987). Antiviral activity of glycyrrhizen against varicella zoster virus in vitro. *Antiviral Research, 7*, 99–107.

Basch, E., Ulbricht, C., Basch, S., et al. (2005). An evidence-based systemic review of Echinacea (E. angustifolia DC, E. pallida, E. purpurea) by the natural standard research collaboration. *Journal of Herbal Pharmacotherapy, 5*(2), 57–88.

Bedi, M. K., & Shenefelt, P. D. (2002). Herbal therapy in dermatology. *Archives of Dermatology, 138*, 232–242.

Behl, P. N., & Srivastava G. (2002). *Herbs useful in dermatological therapy* (2nd ed.). New Delhi, India: CBS Publishers.

Bernstein, J. E., Parish, L. C., Rapaport, M., et al. (1986). Effects of topically applied capsaicin on moderate and severe psoriasis vulgaris. *Journal of the American Academy of Dermatology, 14*, 504–507.

Beylier, M. F. (1979). Bacteriostatic activity of some Australian essential oils. *Perfumes and Flavorings, 4*(2), 23–25.

Bisset, N. G., & Wichtl, M. (Eds.) (2001). *Herbal drugs and phytopharmaceuticals* (2nd ed.). Boca Raton, FL: CRC Press.

Blumenthal, M., Gruenwald, J., Hall, T., & Rister, R. S. (Eds.) (1998). *The complete German Commission E monographs, therapeutic guide to herbal medicine*. Boston, Mass: Integrative Medicine Communications.

Borins, M. (1998). The dangers of using herbs, what your patients need to know. *Postgraduate Medicine, 104*, 91–100.

Brown, D. J., & Dattner, A. M. (1998). Phytotherapeutic approaches to common dermatological conditions. *Archives of Dermatology, 1*, 15–17.

Buchness, M. R. (1998). Alternative medicine and dermatology. *Seminars in Cutaneous Medicine and Surgery, 17*, 284–290.

Buck, D. S., Nidorf, D. M., & Addini, J. G. (1994). Comparison of two topical preparations for the treatment of onychomycosis, *Melaleuca alternifolia* (tea tree) oil and clotrimazole. *Journal of Family Practice, 38*, 601–605.

Callam, M. J. (1994). Epidemiology of varicose veins. *British Journal of Surgery, 81*, 167–173.

Campanati, A., Savelli, A., Sandroni, L., et al. (2010). Effect of allium cepa-allantoin-pentaglycan gel on akin hypertrophic scars, clinical and video-capillaroscopic results of an open-label, controlled, nonrandomized clinical trial. *Dermatologic Surgery, 36*, 1439–1444.

Chan, B. C., Hon, K. L., Leung, P. C., et al. (2008). Traditional Chinese medicine for atopic eczema, PentaHerbs formula suppresses inflammatory mediators release from mast cells. *Journal of Ethnopharmacology, 120*(1), 85–91.

Chaturvedi, T. P. (2009). Uses of turmeric in dentistry, an update. *Indian Journal of Dental Research, 20*(1), 107–109.

de Groot, A. C., & Weyland, J. W. (1993). Contact allergy to tea tree oil. *Contact Dermatitis, 28*, 309.

Delmonte, S., Brusati, C., Parodi, A., et al. (1998). Leukemia-related Sweet's syndrome elicited by pathergy to arnica. *Dermatology, 197*, 195–197.

Diehm, C. (1996). Comparison of leg compression stocking and oral horse-chestnut seed extract therapy in patients with chronic venous insufficiency. *Lancet, 347*, 292–294.

Dunning, T. (2003). Complementary therapies and diabetes. *Complementary Therapy in Nursing and Midwifery, 9*, 74–80.

Efam, S. E. (1988). Clinical observations on the wound healing properties of honey. *British Journal of Surgery, 75*, 679–681.

Efam, S. E., & Udoh, K. T. (1992). The antimicrobial spectrum of honey and its clinical significance. *Infection, 29*, 527–529.

Eickhorst, K., Deleo, V., & Csaposs, J. (2007). Rue the herb, *Ruta graveolens*-associated phytotoxicity. *Dermatitis, 18*(1), 52–55.

Eisenburg, D. M., Kessler, R. C., Foster, C., et al. (1993). Unconventional medicine in the United States, prevalence, costs and pattern uses. *New England Journal of Medicine, 328*, 246–252.

Elliot, C. (1993). Tea tree oil poisoning. *Medical Journal of Australia, 159*, 830–831.

Ellis, C. N., Berberian, B., Sulica, V. I., et al. (1993). A double-blind evaluation of topical capsaicin in pruritic psoriasis. *Journal of the American Academy of Dermatology, 29*, 438–442.

Faoagali, J., George, N., & Leditschke, J. F. (1997). Does tea tree oil have a place in the topical treatment of burns? *Burns, 23*, 349–351.

Ferguson, J. E., Chalmers, R. J. G., & Rowlands, D. J. (1997). Reversible dilated cardiomyopathy following treatment of atopic eczema with Chinese herbal medicine. *British Journal of Dermatology, 136*, 592–593.

Fleischer, A. B., Feldman, S. R., Rapp, S. R., et al. (1996). Alternative therapies commonly used within a population of patients with psoriasis. *Cutis, 58*, 216–220.

Fleming, T. (Ed.) (2000). *PDR for herbal medicines* (2nd ed.). Montvale, NJ: Medical Economics Co.

Fujita, K., & Shosike, I. (1976). Bradykinase activity of aloe extract. *Biochemical Pharmacology, 25*, 205.

Fung, A. Y., Look, P. C., Chong, L. Y., et al. (1999). A controlled trial of traditional Chinese herbal medicine in Chinese patients with recalcitrant atopic dermatitis. *International Journal of Dermatology, 38*(5), 387–392.

Ghazanfar, S. A. (1994). *Handbook of Arabian medicinal plants*. Boca Raton, FL: CRC Press.

Graham-Brown, R. (1992). Toxicity of Chinese herbal remedies [letter]. *Lancet, 340*, 673.

Greenwood, D. (1993). Honey for superficial wounds and ulcers. *Lancet, 341*, 90–91.

Guin, J. D., & Reynolds R. (1980). Jewelweed treatment of poison ivy dermatitis. *Contact Dermatitis, 6*, 287–288.

Hadley, S. K., & Petry, J. J. (1999). Medicinal herbs, a primer for primary care. *Hospital Practice, 34*(6), 105–123.

Hakim, I. A., Harris, R. B., & Weisgerber, U. M. (2000). Tea intake and squamous cell carcinoma of the skin, influences of type of tea beverages. *Cancer Epidemiology Biomarkers and Prevention, 9*, 727–731.

Hausen, B. M., Reichling, J., & Harkenthal, M. (1999). Degradation products of monoterpenes are sensitizing agents in tea tree oil. *American Journal of Contact Dermatitis, 10*(2), 68–77.

Heggers, J. P., Kucukcelebi, A., Listengarten, D., et al. (1996). Beneficial use of aloe on wound healing in an excisional wound model. *Journal of Alternative and Complementary Medicine, 2*(2), 271–277.

Heng, M. C., Song, M. K., Harker, J., et al. (2000). Drug-induced suppression of phosphorylase kinase activity correlates with resolution of psoriasis as assessed by clinical, histological and immunohistochemical parameters. *British Journal of Dermatology, 143*(5), 937–949.

Herrick, J. W. (1995). *Iroquois medical botany.* Syracuse, NY: Syracuse University Press.

Hey, I. C., Jamieson, M., & Ormerod, A. D. (1998). Randomized trial of aromatherapy. *Archives of Dermatology, 134*, 1349–1352.

Huang, M. T., Ho, C. T., Wang, Z. Y., et al. (1994). Inhibition of skin tumorigenesis by rosemary and its constituents carnosol and ursolic acid. *Cancer Research, 54*, 701–708.

Huang, M. T., Xie, J. G., Wang, Z. Y., et al. (1997). Effects of tea, decaffeinated tea, and caffeine on UVB light–induced complete carcinogenesis in SKH-1 mice, demonstration of caffeine as a biologically important constituent of tea. *Cancer Research, 57*(13), 2623–2629.

Huffman, M. A. (2001). Self-medicative behavior in the African great apes, an evolutionary perspective into the origins of human traditional medicine. *Bioscience, 51*(8), 651–661.

Hunt, M. J., & Barnston, R. S. (1992). A comparative study of gluconolactone versus benzoyl peroxide in the treatment of acne. *Australasian Journal of Dermatology, 33*, 131–134.

Itoh, K., Hirata, N., Masuda, M., et al. (2009). Inhibitory effects of Citrus hassaku extract and its flavanone glycosides on melanogenesis. *Biological and Pharmacological Bulletin, 32*(3), 410–415.

Javed, S., Mehrotra, N. K., & Shukla, Y. (1998). Chemopreventive effects of black tea polyphenols in mouse skin model of carcinogenesis. *Biomedical and Environmental Science, 11*, 307–313.

Jensen, P. (1990). Use of alternative medicine by patients with atopic dermatitis and psoriasis. *Acta Dermatologica et Venereologica, 70*, 421–424.

Kapoor, L. D. (1990). *CRC handbook of Ayurvedic medicinal plants.* Boca Raton, FL: CRC Press.

Katiyar, S. K., Ahmad, N., & Mukhtar, H. (2000). Green tea and skin. *Archives of Dermatology, 136*, 989–994.

Kessels, A. G. H., Cardynaals, R. L. L. M., Borger, R. L. L., et al. (1991). The effectiveness of the hair restorer "Dabao" in males with alopecia androgenetica, a clinical experiment. *Journal of Clinical Epidemiology, 44*, 439–447.

Khan, I. A., & Khanum, A. (2009). *Herbal therapy for skin afflictions.* Hyderabad, India: Ukaaz Publications.

Kim, E. C., Lee, H. S., Kim, S. K., et al. (2008). The bark of Betula platyphylla var. japonica inhibits the development of atopic dermatitis-like skin lesions in NC/Nga mice. *Journal of Ethnopharmacology, 116*, 270–278.

Klein, A. D., & Penneys, N. S. (1988). Aloe vera. *Journal of the American Academy of Dermatology, 18*, 714–720.

Klepser, T. B., & Klepser, M. E. (1999). Unsafe and potentially safe herbal therapies. *American Journal of Health Systems Pharmacy, 56*, 125–138.

Knight, T. E., & Hansen, B. M. (1994). Melaleuca oil (tea tree oil) dermatitis. *Journal of the American Academy of Dermatology, 30*, 423–427.

Koo, J., & Arain, S. (1998). Traditional Chinese medicine for the treatment of dermatologic disorders. *Archives of Dermatology, 134*, 1388–1393.

Korting, H. C., Schafer-Korting, M., Hart, H., et al. (1993). Anti-inflammatory activity of hamamelis distillate applied topically to the skin. *British Journal of Clinical Pharmacology, 44*, 315–318.

Kron, J. (2002). Herbalism. *Complementary Medicine, 1*(2), 27–31.

Kuribara, H., Stavinoha, W. B., & Maruyama, Y. (1998). Behavioral characteristics of honkiol, an anxiolytic agent present in extracts of magnolia bark, evaluated by an elevated plus-maze test in mice. *Journal of Pharmacy and Pharmacology, 50*, 819–826.

Lahiri-Chatterjee, M., Katiyar, S. K., Mohan, R. R., et al. (1999). A flavonoid antioxidant, silymarin, affords exceptionally high protection against tumor promotion in the SENCAR mouse skin tumorigenesis model. *Cancer Research, 59*, 622–632.

Latchman, Y., Banerjee, P., Poulter, L. W., et al. (1996). Association of immunological changes with clinical efficacy in atopic eczema patients treated with traditional Chinese herbal therapy (Zemaphyte). *International Archives of Allergy & Immunology, 109*(3), 243–249.

Latchman, Y., Whittle, B., Rustin, M., et al. (1994). The efficacy of traditional Chinese herbal therapy in atopic eczema. *International Archives of Allergy and Immunology, 104*, 222–226.

Ledezma, E., DeSousa, L., & Jorquera, A. (1996). Efficacy of ajoene, an organosulphur derived from garlic, in the short-term therapy of tinea pedis. *Mycoses, 39*, 393–395.

Linde, K., Ramirez, G., Mulrow, C., et al. (1996). St. John's wort for depression, an overview and meta-analysis of randomized clinical trials. *British Medical Journal, 313*, 253–258.

Lininger, S. W. (Ed.) (2000). *The natural pharmacy* (2nd ed.). Montvale, NJ: Medical Economics Co.

Lipton, R. A. (1958). Comparison of jewelweed and steroid in the treatment of poison ivy contact dermatitis. *Annals of Allergy, 16*, 526–567.

Long, D., Ballentine, N. H., & Marks, J. G. Jr. (1997). Treatment of poison ivy/oak allergic contact dermatitis with an extract of jewelweed. *American Journal of Contact Dermatitis, 8*, 150–153.

Lou, Y. R., Lu, Y. P., Xie, J. G., et al. (1999). Effects of oral administration of tea, decaffeinated tea, and caffeine on the formation and growth of tumors in the high-risk

SKH-1 mice previously treated with ultraviolet B light. *Nutrition and Cancer, 33,* 146–153.

Lu, Y. P., Lou, Y. R., Xie, J. G., et al. (1997). Inhibitory effect of black tea on the growth of established skin tumors in mice, effects on tumor size, apoptosis, mitosis, and bromodeoxyuridine incorporation into DNA. *Carcinogenesis, 18,* 2163–2169.

Lyss, G., Schmidt, T. J., Merfort, I., et al. (1997). Helenalin, an anti-inflammatory sesquiterpene lactone from arnica, selectively inhibits transcription factor NF-κB. *Biological Chemistry, 378,* 951–961.

Mansourian, A., Momen-Heravi, F., Saheb-Jamee, M., et al. (2011). Comparison of aloe vera mouthwash with triamcinolone acetonide 0.1% on oral lichen planus, a randomized double-blinded clinical trial. *American Journal of Medical Science, 342*(6), 447–451.

McGuffin, M., Hobbs, C., Upton, R., et al. (Eds.) (1997). *Botanical safety handbook.* Boca Raton, FL: CRC Press.

Miller, L. G. (1998). Herbal medicinals. *Archives of Internal Medicine, 158,* 2200–2208.

Mitamura, T., Matsuno, T., Sakamoto, S., et al. (1996). Effects of a new clerodane diterpenoid isolated from propolis on chemically induced skin tumors in mice. *Anticancer Research, 16,* 2669–2672.

Monk, B. (1986). Severe cutaneous reactions to alternative remedies. *British Medical Journal, 293,* 665–666.

Moss, A. (1994). Tea tree oil poisoning [letter]. *Medical Journal of Australia, 160,* 236.

Mostefa-Kara, N., Pauels, A., Pines, E., et al. (1992). Fatal hepatitis after herbal tea. *Lancet, 340,* 674.

Neldner, K. H. (2000). Complementary and alternative medicine. *Dermatologic Clinics, 18,* 189–193.

Ng, S. K. (1998). Topical traditional Chinese medicine. *Archives of Dermatology, 134,* 1395–1396.

Nomura, M., Ma, W. Y., Huang, C., et al. (2000). Inhibition of ultraviolet B–induced AP-1 activation by theaflavins from black tea. *Molecular Carcinogenesis, 28,* 148–155.

Oyelami, O. A., Onayemi, A., Oyedeji, O. A., et al. (2009). Preliminary study of effectiveness of aloe vera in scabies treatment. *Phytotherapy Research, 23*(10), 1482–1484.

Parsad, D., Pandhi, R., & Juneja, A. (2003). Effectiveness of oral Ginkgo biloba in treating limited, slowly spreading vitiligo. *Clinical and Experimental Dermatology, 28*(3), 285–287.

Peirce, A., Fargis, P., & Scordato, E. (Eds.) (1999). *The American Pharmaceutical Association practical guide to natural medicines.* New York: Stonesong Press Inc.

Pittler, M. H., & Ernst, E. (1998). Horse-chestnut seed extract for chronic venous insufficiency. *Archives of Dermatology, 143,* 1356–1360.

Pribitkin, E. D. (2005). Herbal medicine and surgery. *Seminars in Integrative Medicine, 3,* 17–23.

Record, I. R., & Dreosti, I. E. (1998). Protection by black tea and green tea against UVB and UVA+B induced skin cancer in hairless mice. *Mutation Research, 422,* 191–199.

Reynolds, T., & Dweck, A. C. (1999). Aloe vera leaf gel, a review update. *Journal of Ethnopharmacology, 68,* 3–37.

Robinson, M. C., Heggers, J. P., & Hagstrom, W. J. (1982). Myth, magic, witchcraft, or fact? Aloe vera revisited. *Journal of Burn Care Rehabilitation*, *3*, 157–162.

Routh, H. B., & Bhowmik, K. R. (1999). Traditional Indian medicine in dermatology. *Clinics in Dermatology*, *17*, 41–47.

Selvaag, E., Eriksen, B., & Thure, P. (1994). Contact allergy due to tea tree oil and cross-sensitization to colophony. *Contact Dermatitis*, *31*, 124–125.

Seong, I. (2007). Antifungal activity of the extracts from Galla rhois against Candida albicans. *Korean Journal of Medical Mycology*, *12*(4), 175–179.

Shaw, D. (1998). Risks or remedies? Safety aspects of herbal remedies in the UK. *Journal of the Royal Society of Medicine*, *91*, 294–296.

Sheehan, M. P., & Atherton, D. J. (1992). A controlled trial of traditional Chinese medicinal plants in widespread non-exudative atopic eczema. *British Journal of Dermatology*, *126*, 179–184.

Sheehan, M. P., & Atherton, D. J. (1994). One-year follow up of children treated with Chinese medicinal herbs for atopic eczema. *British Journal of Dermatology*, *130*, 488–483.

Sheehan, M. P., Rustin, M. H. A., Atherton, D. J., et al. (1992). Efficacy of traditional Chinese herbal therapy in adult atopic dermatitis. *Lancet*, *340*, 13–17.

Shota, Y., Wilson, J. G., Matsumoto, H., et al. (1961). Adult respiratory distress syndrome induced by a Chinese medicine, kamisyoyo-san. *Internal Medicine*, *65*, 494–496.

Soyinka, F. (1973). Atypical lichen planus induced by native medicine. *British Journal of Dermatology*, *88*, 341–345.

Subrahmanyam, M. (1993). Honey-impregnated gauze versus polyurethane film (Op-Site®) in the treatment of burns, a prospective randomised study. *British Journal of Plastic Surgery*, *46*, 322–323.

Surh, Y. J., Seoung, S. H., Keum, Y. S., et al. (2000). Inhibitory effects of curcumin and capsaicin on phorbol ester-induced activation of eukaryotic transcription factors, NF-κB and AP-1. *Biofactors*, *12*, 107–112.

Swords, G., & Hunter, G. L. K. (1978). Composition of Australian tea tree oil. *Journal of Agriculture and Food Chemistry*, *26*, 734–737.

Syed, T. A., Ahmad, S. A., Holt, A. H., et al. (1996). Management of psoriasis with aloe vera extract in a hydrophilic cream, a placebo-controlled, double-blind study. *Tropical Medicine and International Health*, *1*, 505–509.

Tong, M. M., Altman, P. M., & Barnetson, R. (1992). Tea tree oil in the treatment of tinea pedis *Australasian Journal of Dermatology*, *33*, 145–149.

Tyring, S. K. (2012). Sinecatechins, effects on HPV-induced enzymes involved in inflammatory mediator generation. *Journal of Clinical and Aesthetical Dermatology*, *5*(1), 19–26.

van Wyk, B., & Wink, M. (2004). *Medicinal plants of the world*. Portland, Oregon: Timber Press.

Vardi, A., Barzilay, Z., Linder, N., et al. (1998). Local application of honey for the treatment of neonatal postoperative wound infections. *Acta Paediatrica*, *87*, 429–432.

Wang, Z. Y., Huang, M. T., Lou, Y. R., et al. (1994). Inhibitory effects of black tea, green tea, decaffeinated black tea, and decaffeinated green tea on ultraviolet B light–induced skin carcinogenesis in 7,12-dimethybez[a]anthracene–initiated SKH-1 mice. *Cancer Research, 54,* 3428–3435.

Williams, L. R., Home, V. N., & Zang, X. (1988). The composition and bactericidal activity of oil of Melaleuca alternifolia. *International Journal of Aromatherapy, 1*(3), 15–17.

Winslow, L. C., & Kroll, D. J. (1998). Herbs as medicine. *Archives of Internal Medicine, 158,* 2192–2199.

Winston, D., & Dattner, A. (1999). The American system of medicine. *Clinics in Dermatology, 17,* 53–56.

Wobling, R. H., & Leonhardt, K. (1994). Local therapy of herpes simplex with dried extract of Melissa officinalis. *Phytomedicine, 1,* 25–31.

Xiaoguang, C., Hongyan, L., Xiaohong, L., et al. (1998). Cancer chemopreventive and therapeutic activities of red ginseng. *Journal of Ethnopharmacology, 60,* 71–78.

Xu, X. J., Banerjee, P., Rustin, M. H. A., et al. (1997). Modulation by Chinese herbal therapy of immune mechanisms in the skin of patients with atopic eczema. *British Journal of Dermatology, 136,* 54–59.

Xu, Y. (2004). *Dermatology in traditional Chinese medicine.* St. Albans, UK: Donica Publishing Ltd.

Yarnell, E., & Abascal, K. (2006). Herbal medicine for acne vulgaris. *Alternative and Complementary Therapy, 12*(6), 303–309.

Zhang, H., Gu, J. (2007). Progress of experimental study on treatment of psoriasis by Chinese medicinal monomer and single or compound recipe in Chinese material medica. *Chinese Journal of Integrative Medicine, 13*(4), 312–316.

Zhao, J., Jin, X., Yaping, E., et al. (1999). Photoprotective effect of black tea extracts against UVB-induced phototoxicity in skin. *Photochemistry and Photobiology, 70,* 637–644.

Zhao, J. F., Zhang, Y. J., Jin, X. H., et al. (1999). Green tea protects against psoralen plus ultraviolet A–induced photochemical damage to skin. *Journal of Investigative Dermatology, 113,* 1070–1075.

9

An Ayurvedic Perspective on Dermatology

VASANT LAD

Key Concepts

♣ Philosophical foundations of Ayurveda completely accept the principles of *Sankhya* philosophy. Creation occurs from the unmanifest to manifestation into physical substance. Cosmic consciousness moves into creation through universal principles, which include intelligence and the three *gunas* (qualities) manifesting into the mind, the cognitive and motor organs, and organic and inorganic substances that are further differentiated into the five elements, both gross and subtle.

♣ The five elements govern the structural makeup of the body, which is functionally governed by the three organizations called *vata, pitta*, and *kapha*. These three *doshas* are responsible for the biological and energetic functioning of the body, the proportions of which are established at conception. Each *dosha* has characteristic qualities and functions specific to its role and the three have functional integrity between them.

♣ The human body is made up of seven bodily tissues, called *dhatus*, which have functional integrity. These tissues have a cyclical relationship of nutrition and maintenance of the body, beginning with *rasa* and *rakta*'s role of transforming food by carrying it throughout the body and nourishing each subsequent tissue.

♣ Ayurveda understands the skin as having seven layers that have a correlation to the seven tissues of the body, so the health of the seven tissues is shown in the health of the skin. Each layer of the skin has

(continued)

a role that corresponds to the characteristics of the tissue layer. Skin plays a role in immunity as well.

♣ The functions of the skin, as defined by modern science, are protection, temperature, cognitive perception, excretion, synthesis, secretion, lactation, absorption, and sweat.

♣ Ayurveda defines the skin a doorway to healing. Touch therapy can stimulate adjustments in the biochemical balances of the body, while medicated oils and pastes, absorbed through the skin, can further support these desired changes.

♣ The skin parallels the characteristics of the *doshic* constitution of each individual.

♣ Ayurveda states that increase of the *doshas* will cause typical signs and symptoms that indicate which *dosha* is out of balance. These skin diseases and disorders are known as *kushta*, which means skin diseases.

♣ The etiology or causes of *kushta* include physical contact, skin to skin or with shared items such as clothing or utensils, incompatible food combinations, a heavy meal followed by hard work, overheating in the sun, exposure to chemicals, sugar, salt, or alcohol, sex after a meal, and sleep during the daytime. Psychological factors could be fear, anxiety, irritability, and frustration.

♣ Chronic skin conditions respond well to the Ayurvedic detoxification program known as *panchakarma*. A series of treatments typically repeated for 7 or more days, it is followed by rejuvenation treatments that support the continued balance of the *doshas*.

♣ Specific skin conditions are defined in the classic Ayurvedic texts. These conditions are described here and their modern names are included. Classical herbal formulas to treat these conditions are explained. The benefits of the application of leeches in skin conditions are outlined.

♣ Ayurvedic medicine has an extensive pharmacopoeia of herbal medications for skin conditions. These include herbal combinations taken orally and applied directly to the skin.

♣ Medicated oils comprise herbs or herbal compounds combined with specific oils boiled together in a concoction. These are applied to the skin over a period of time. Herbal pastes are composed of herbs and oil or another substance that is applied to the skin. Herbal baths are a preventive and treatment technique.

Introduction

In this chapter, we summarize some of the basic philosophies and framework of Ayurveda. This includes the origins of creation, the human being, and his/her manifestation as a being of body, mind, and spirit. These fundamental points are essential to an understanding of Ayurveda, since Ayurveda aims to balance these parts of human existence in order to maintain health. Then we discuss the relationship of skin with the seven tissues of the body, the skin's functions from the modern viewpoint, and the types of skin defined by Ayurveda. Finally, we will cover the causes of skin problems and a range of skin conditions and their treatment, as defined by the ancient texts of Ayurveda.

Ayurveda is the traditional medicine of India. The oral tradition extends back thousands of years, and some authorities estimate that the first written texts arose approximately 1,000 B.C.E.[1] (Sharma, 1981, Introduction). These classical texts are the basis of Ayurveda as it is practiced today. They were written in Sanskrit, but modern scholars have translated them into English. The oldest texts are credited to Charaka, Sushruta, Vagbhata, and Madhava. While often arising from the same Sanskrit verses, each text provides its unique perspective on the topics.[2]

Ayurveda is a Sanskrit word derived from two roots: *ayuh* means life, and *veda* means knowledge. Systematized knowledge is science, so Ayurveda is the science of life. What is life? Life is our daily existence, which is an expression of pure consciousness. Ayurveda accepts *Sankhya* philosophy as the premise for its understanding of existence. According to *Sankhya* philosophy, every life is a divine and unique expression of cosmic consciousness, called *Purusha*. *Purusha* is pure, choiceless, passive awareness that does not take part in creation, while *Prakruti* is primordial matter, creative will that expresses herself through the form, shape, and attribute of every object. *Purusha* is passive; *Prakruti* is active. *Purusha* is the male aspect of energy and *Prakruti* is the female aspect, and they both lie behind the creation of this universe.

The first expression of universal creation, *Prakruti*, is *Mahad*, cosmic intelligence. This intelligence permeates all of creation. Then *Mahad* manifests into *ahamakar*, the awareness of one's own existence, the "I am." The sense of "I am," of identity, is *ahāmkār*. This feeling of "I am" is expressed into three qualities (*gunas*) that encompass all of creation and are used to describe *Prakruti*. *Sattva* is the principle of equilibrium and light; *tamas* is the principle of inertia, darkness, and manifestation; and *rajas* is the principle of movement. These are known as the three *gunas* and creation can be described according to these attributes. One example is observation: *sattva* gives clarity of perception; *rajas* is the movement of that perception; and *tamas* is the object of perception.

The three *gunas* move further into manifestation. *Sattva guna* generates the mind, the five cognitive organs, and five motor organs, expressing itself in the organic universe. The sensory faculties have cognitive organs that perceive sound, touch, sight, taste, and smell. *Tamas guna* produces the inorganic universe, including the five gross elements and their corresponding subtle elements. The five elements are Space[3], Air, Fire, Water, and Earth, and they correspond to sound, touch, vision, taste, and smell. *Rajas guna* is expressed as the interaction between *sattva* and *tamas,* linking the mind and the cognitive and motor organs with the five gross and subtle elements. For example, when one puts a substance on the tongue, the organ of perception, the action of taste is *sattva*. The movement of information about the taste is *rajas* and the object of perception, the substance, is *tamas.*

The Five Elements and Their Manifestation in the Body

Ancient Vedic philosophy of India attributes the origins of the universe to the vibration of the cosmic sound, *aum*, somewhat like the modern theory of creation, the big bang theory. This first element to arise, sound, becomes cosmic space, showing the connection between Space and the subtle element, sound. Sequentially, each element brings on the next, so within Space, the pulsation of the Air element is created. The corresponding subtle element of Air is touch. This pulsation generates heats heat or the Fire element, whose subtle element is vision. The energy of consciousness liquefies into Water, which crystallizes into Earth. Water corresponds to taste and Earth to smell.

The five elements govern the structural aspects of the human body, but the functional aspects are governed by the three energies or organizations: *vata, pitta,* and *kapha. Vata* is the biological combination of primarily ether and air elements; *pitta* is predominantly fire and water elements; *kapha* is mainly water and earth elements. These three *doshas* are present in every cell, tissue, organ, and system and energetically they are present in every gene. According to Ayurveda, every biological substance has certain qualities and functions. So *vata, pitta,* and *kapha* have definite qualities and, because of these attributes, they have particular functions.

Vata is dry, light, cold, mobile, rough, subtle, and clear and it has astringent taste. We can see how these qualities manifest as certain functions at the cellular level. Due to dry quality, *vata* separates cells from one another. Light quality makes the cells and tissues light, so they can move. Cold quality helps to maintain optimal body temperature. Mobile quality governs all biological movement. Rough quality ensures that the muscle cells and bone cells do not stick together. Astringent helps mineral absorption and binds the stools.

Vata is primarily present in the colon, pelvic cavity, bones, ears, and skin and governs the physiological functions of movement, ingestion, ejection, circulation, and respiration, as well as the sensory functions of touch, pain, and temperature.

Pitta is a biological combination of fire and water, so it is hot, sharp, light, oily, liquid, sour, and slightly pungent, and it has a strong smell. The hot quality of *pitta* helps to maintain body temperature and creates appetite, thirst, hunger, and digestion. Because of its sharp quality, pitta penetrates into the subtle molecules of food and governs molecular digestion. *Pitta* is closely related to bile, which is oily, and this quality keeps the colon soft and lubricated and allows regular bowel movements. Its liquid quality allows *pitta* to have a medium for digestive juices and enzymes. Hence, *pitta* people rarely get constipation whereas *vata* types tend to be constipated easily. The sour attribute maintains the acid pH of the body and governs the digestive enzymes, most of which are acidic. *Pitta* is also pungent, so it does digestion of fats and protein. *Pitta* has a strong smell and this makes the *pitta* person sensitive to strong smells.

Pitta is present particularly in the stomach, intestines, liver, spleen, sweat, sebaceous secretions, blood, eyes, and gray matter of the brain. *Pitta* governs digestion, metabolic activity, understanding, and comprehension. *Pitta* maintains luster, color complexion, vision and color perception, and normal body color and temperature.

Kapha is a biological combination of earth and water. It is heavy, dull, slow, cool, oily, liquid, slimy, dense, and sticky and has sweet and salty tastes. Heavy quality creates growth. As it is dull and slow, *Kapha* creates relaxation. The cool quality of *Kapha* protects the stomach lining from burning, and the oily quality lubricates the joints, muscles, bones, and tendons. The liquid quality manifests in mucus and saliva. Because of its slimy quality, *Kapha* makes the body flexible, while the dense attribute gives solidity and firmness. The sticky quality keeps things together in the body. The sweet characteristic regulates blood sugar and gives energy, while the salty attribute bestows vigor and helps to maintain the water–electrolyte balance.

Kapha is present primarily in the stomach, chest, lungs, sinuses, blood plasma and lymphatic system, vitreous humor, white matter of the brain, and synovial fluid. Among other things *Kapha* governs gastric mucus secretions, bronchial secretions, sinus secretions, and lubrication of the joints.

Vata, *Pitta*, and *Kapha* have collective functional integrity. However, all bodily movements and catabolic functions are governed by *Vata*; all biochemical changes, thermodynamics, and metabolic functions are governed by *Pitta*;

and all building and anabolic functions, lubrication, and protection are governed by *Kapha*.

Ayurvedic Anatomy and Physiology

The human anatomy comprises seven bodily tissues, called *dhatus*.

- *Rasa* (plasma and lymph) *dhatu* governs nutrition of the body.
- *Rakta* (blood cells) *dhatu* governs oxygenation, which is the function of bestowing life.
- *Mamsa* (muscles, including skeletal, smooth, sphincter, cardiac, and hamstring muscles) *dhatu* covers and protects the vital organs and governs bodily locomotion.
- *Meda* (adipose or fatty tissue) *dhatu* has the function of lubrication of the skin, joints, and muscles, plus storage of energy and regulation of body temperature.
- *Asthi* (bones, cartilage, and teeth) *dhatu* gives the body form and support.
- *Majja* (bone marrow and the nervous system) *dhatu* has two main functions. As bone marrow it fills space (in the bones), and as nerve tissue it enables communication within the synaptic spaces.
- *Shukra* (male reproductive tissue) and *artava* (female reproductive tissue) *dhatus* have the primary function of procreation.

These seven tissues also have functional integrity. For instance, physical and mechanical movements happen because of the integration between *majja*, *mamsa*, and *asthi dhatus*. The nervous system carries a message to the muscles and they move the bones.

The Ayurvedic Understanding of Skin

Skin in the Sanskrit language is called *twag*[4], which means the outermost covering of the body acts as a protective covering. It minimizes the loss of water from the bodily tissues. Various sensory nerve endings on the skin help to protect the body from injury by evoking appropriate responses to noxious stimuli. Skin is like the cream of embryonic plasma. One could compare embryonic plasma to hot milk; when whole milk cools down it forms a layer of cream on the surface. So skin is the cream of *rasa dhatu*. Ayurveda says that the skin is the *upadhatu* (byproduct) of *rasa dhatu*.

Twag Sara = Excellence of Skin

Charaka provides a definition of superior skin in *Vimanasthana*, Chapter 8, Verse 103, p. 378:

In persons who are *twagsara*,... the skin is unctuous, smooth, soft, clear with fine, sparse, deep-rooted and delicate hairs and is lustrous. This essence indicates happiness, good fortune, power, enjoyment, intelligence, learning, health, cheerfulness and longevity.

An embryo has three germ layers: ectoderm, mesoderm, and endoderm. The outermost layer of the embryo is the ectoderm, which eventually develops into the epidermis, nervous tissue, pituitary gland, and the epithelium of the nasal cavity, mouth, salivary glands, bladder, and urethra. This embryonic development of the ectoderm shows the functional relationship of the skin with the tonsils, nervous system, and even the endocrine system in the form of the pituitary gland.

THE SEVEN LAYERS OF THE SKIN

Ayurveda considers the skin to have seven layers that correspond to the seven *dhatus* (Fig. 9.1) (Bhishagratna, 1991 [Sharirasthana 4:3–23, 166–171]). The topmost or outer layer is called *avabhasini*, which relates to the *rasa dhatu*. It covers the entire body and holds the hair, nails, feathers, or scales. In humans, it becomes thick at the soles of the feet and palms and is very thin at the nipple areola and the lips. It is the pure essence of *rasa dhatu*. One function of *rasa dhatu* is nutrition.

Seven Layers of the Skin and the Seven Dhatus

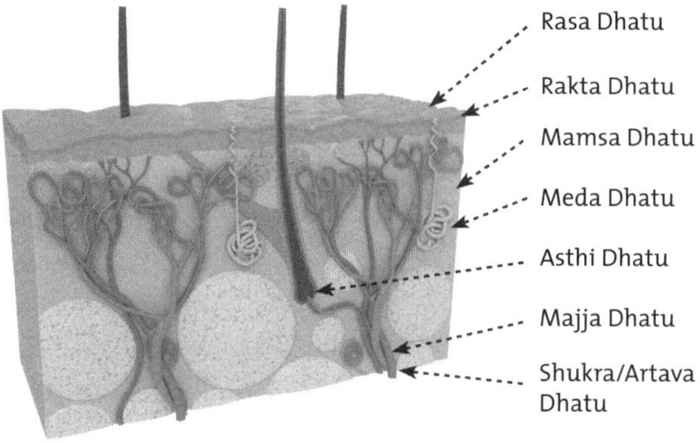

Rasa Dhatu
Rakta Dhatu
Mamsa Dhatu
Meda Dhatu
Asthi Dhatu
Majja Dhatu
Shukra/Artava Dhatu

FIGURE 9.1 Skin anatomy. © Sebastian Kaulitzki, Eraxion@istockphoto.com

Underneath is *sveta*, the white skin. If you press on the skin, you will see a white patch, displaced capillaries or *rasa/rakta dhatu*. When you lift the fingers, the skin becomes pink, so that is the red zone. *Sveta*, the white skin, is related to the lymphatic system and *tamara*, the red skin, is related to the capillaries and the hematopoietic systems. A function of *rakta dhatu* is oxygenation, and the skin helps with oxygenation of the fat and other tissues through cutaneous breathing.

Mamsa dhara kala,[5] the third layer, is composed of arrector pili muscles, an elastic tissue near the root of the hair. When one is startled or frightened, this muscle contracts and the hair of the skin stands upright. This layer is related to *mamsa dhatu*. When muscles are stiff, the skin becomes stiff; when they are relaxed, the skin relaxes. The texture of the skin is governed by the muscular layer. *Mamsa dhatu* serves to do the plastering and covering in the body, in the form of muscles. When we massage medicated oils into the skin, it helps to relax the muscles.

Meda dhara kala is the subcutaneous tissue, the fat, where the sweat and sebaceous glands reside. They secrete sebaceous secretions and sweat, which maintain the moisture of the skin. The nervous systems pass through this cutaneous layer and, through them, the skin can perceive touch, pain, and temperature. *Meda dhatu* provides lubrication and perspiration, keeping the skin moist. The fat under the skin acts as an insulating material to retain heat in the body.

The fifth layer relates to *asthi dhatu*, the bones and cartilage. The roots of the hair are sourced in this *dhatu*. According to Ayurveda, hair and nails are the waste products of *ashti dhatu*. The skin helps to grow hair and support the root of the nails through this layer, the *asthi dhara kala* layer. *Asthi dhatu* structurally supports the vital organs with this layer.

Lastly, *shukra dhara kala* (or *artava dhara kala* for females) occupies the deepest layer of the skin. This layer is predominantly present in the muco-cutaneous junction of the lips and in the areola, clitoris, and glans penis, all of which are related to sexual energy. Communication is one function of the interplay between the skin and procreation. The skin absorbs externally applied medicine and hormones through this layer.

Skin is also the organ of *ojas, tejas,* and *prana. Ojas* supports the immunity of the skin, the immune function. *Tejas* maintains the color, complexion, and glowing characteristics of the skin, while *prana* maintains subcutaneous respiration. Oil massaged into the skin penetrates the superficial fascia, deep fascia, and nerve endings. There it stimulates the secretion of neuropeptides. Some neuropeptides are released in the nervous system, which maintains psycho-neuroimmunological response. Skin is an organ of immunity.

THE FUNCTIONS OF SKIN

Modern science defines the functions of the skin as follows.

- Skin's most important function is protection. It protects capillaries, nerve endings, and neuropeptides as well as plasma, serum, and most of the vital organs.
- Its second function is regulation of body temperature. When exposed to the heat, the cutaneous blood vessels dilate and perspiration occurs, lowering the body temperature. When exposed to cold weather, the capillaries constrict, preventing heat from leaving the body.
- Thirdly, skin governs the cognitive functions of touch, pain, and temperature. Skin also has three-dimensional perception called stereognosis. Everyone—even a blind person—can recognize, through the tactile perception of touch, objects such as a chair, table, coin, pencil, etc. Hair on the skin also plays a role in touch sensation. Even a little insect sitting on the skin causes the hair follicles to send that message.
- Skin has the function of excretion as well. Through sweating and perspiration, the skin excretes nitrogenous waste, salt, and metabolites.
- The next function is synthesis. When exposed to the ultraviolet rays of sunlight, skin synthesizes vitamin D and, because vitamin D promotes healthy bone growth, skin nourishes bone. Without sufficient exposure to sunlight, a person can develop deficiency of vitamin D, resulting in osteoporosis. Hence, skin has nutritive and synthesis functions.
- Skin secretes, through the subcutaneous gland, a fatty substance rich in cholesterol called sebum. This sebum prevents dryness of the skin and helps with the cooling and warming of the skin. Skin is both a secretory and excretory organ.
- Skin serves in the nourishment of one's child through lactation. The mammary gland is a modified sweat gland. In a lactating female, lactation is stimulated by the cry or touch of a child.
- Absorption is another function of skin. If one applies ointment to the skin, it is apparent that the skin is not waterproof. Skin can absorb ointment, medicated oils, and herbal pastes. It is one of the primary delivery systems of Ayurvedic medicine: the absorption of medicated substances through the skin. This absorption happens because of a subtype of *Pitta* in the skin called *ranjaka Pitta*. Another subtype of *Pitta, bhrajaka Pitta*, maintains color complexion of the skin, while a subtype of *Vata, prana vayu*, is responsible for tactile sensation and touch through the skin.

- Skin sustains water–electrolyte balance through sweat. The skin governs acid–base equilibrium. Sweat is acidic and, when people sweat, they remove the acid. Skin also performs the function of storage. The dermis and subcutaneous layers store fat, water, salt, and hormones. Additionally, skin carries out gaseous exchange. It absorbs oxygen and releases carbon dioxide in what is called "cutaneous breathing." Skin helps breathing.

SKIN IS THE DOORWAY OF HEALING

Ayurveda uses a touch therapy with specific energy points called *marma* points. They are somewhat similar to the points used in acupuncture and acupressure therapies. Ayurvedic *marma* energy points are accessed in the deep layer of the skin called *vedini*[6] and are considered the pathways to the inner pharmacy. By using gentle pressure to the *marma* point at the level of *vedini*, you are sending a message to the body. *Vedini* is functionally related to neuropeptides and nerve endings. When we apply medicated oils or pastes to the skin, they penetrate and influence neuropeptides. This technique can change the brain chemistry, stimulating whatever chemical substances are required at the time to achieve balance. Of course, all of this happens through the medium of the skin. The human body is a complex universal chemical lab. It can produce endorphins (pain relief), antibiotics (immune function), and even steroids and other hormones, as needed. *Marma* therapy provides a safe, effective means to balance these complex systems. Skin has the capacity to convey feelings and emotions through a touch of love or a healing touch.

CONSTITUTIONAL TYPES OF SKIN

Just as there are seven types of constitutions, there are seven types of skin. There are mono-*doshic* types predominated by a single *dosha*: Vata, Pitta, or *Kapha*. Dual-doshic types are a combination of two *doshas*: Vata-Pitta, Pitta-Kapha, or Vata-Kapha. There can also be skin that is equally influenced by all three *doshas*. Each type will display characteristics of the main *dosha* or a combination of the *doshas* (Table 9.1).

Ayurveda divides the span of life into three milestones: child age, adult age, and old age. The skin reflects these ages. Child age is the age of *Kapha* and the skin has baby fat and is soft, smooth, and touchable. *Pitta* time starts in the teenage years and continues through middle age. *Pitta* skin tends to be hot, flushed, and prone to acne. Elevated *Pitta* is why you'll see acne more in the teenage years, because of the hot, oily, and spreading qualities of *Pitta*. During

Table 9.1. Doshic Characteristics of the Skin, Hair, and Nails

	Vata Characteristics	*Pitta Characteristics*	*Kapha Characteristics*
Skin	Thin, dry, cold, rough, dark, brown, easily cracked	Smooth, oily, warm, rosy, red, yellow, sensitive to sunlight	Thick, oily, cool, white, pale, retains water
Hair	Dry brown, black, knotted, brittle, scarce	Straight, oily, blond, prematurely gray, red, bald	Thick, curly, oily, wavy, luxuriant
Nails	Dry, rough, brittle, break easily into the cuticles	Sharp, flexible, pink, lustrous	Thick, oily, smooth, polished

the *Vata* time of life, skin becomes dry, rough, scaly, and wrinkled, with freckles and brownish discolorations that we call age spots or liver spots.[7]

ETIOLOGICAL FACTORS OF SKIN DISEASES

When *Vata* in the colon is high, this produces constipation, gas, bloating, and *ama*[8] in the colon. These conditions will affect the skin and it will appear dry and wrinkled, with a dark discoloration. These are typical signs of increased *Vata* in the body.

Pitta's "home" is in the small intestine. It is also present in the liver and the skin (via *ranjaka Pitta*). When *Pitta* is elevated, a person will have multiple moles, acne, hives, rash, and urticaria. These kinds of *Pitta* disorders of the skin have their origin in the small intestine.

Seats of Vata, Pitta, Kapha

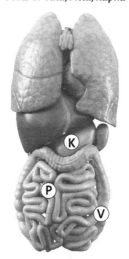

FIGURE 9.2 Internal organs. © cosmin4000, cosmin4000@istockphoto.com

The seat of *Kapha* is in the lungs and the fundus of the stomach (Fig. 9.2). Increased *Kapha* makes the skin cold and clammy and prone to fungal and yeast infections. It can manifest as cysts, cutaneous tumors, skin tags, transparent moles, bumps, and fatty deposits under the skin.

Because of long-lingering *dosha* (*Vata, Pitta, Kapha*) in the colon, the *doshas* move into the *rasa* and *rakta dhatus* and the *doshas* remain in the skin (Sharma, 1981 [Cikitsitasthana 7:9–10, 125]). From this, the skin undergoes irritation, inflammation, infection, dryness, and scaliness. These disturb the texture, color, and complexion of the skin. This effect is called *kushta*.[9] *Kushta* is that which disturbs the color complexion of the skin. The whole skin health is affected by this *kushta* quality, so we could say that *kushta* is the broad term for all skin diseases. *Kushta* also means fermentation, putrefaction, and rottenness, and in the advanced stages of skin disorders, these qualities show up as necrosis of the skin.

While not as much of a concern today, the ancient texts also say that many skin diseases arise because of *prasanga*, too much physical contact. Even today, we are cautious about touching other people's hands during flu season. Other forms of physical contact include sleeping in the same bed, having contact with another person's clothing that may be contaminated, and sharing eating utensils. Even viruses like herpes can be transmitted by any skin-to-skin contact. Sexually transmitted diseases fall into this category.

Incompatible food combinations can cause skin disorders. Eating too much fatty, fried food or oily or greasy food will increase *Kapha dosha* and the skin will suffer from this. Eating fermented foods, old yogurt, and pickles, especially at night or on cloudy days, reduces the immune function of the skin.[10]

Eating a heavy meal and working hard immediately afterward can cause skin disorders. One should wait at least 2 hours after a heavy meal to do work outside. The texts say that one cause of eczema and psoriasis is doing heavy work after food. This pushes *ama* from the gastrointestinal tract into the skin.

Pratap means overheating under the sun. This can happen from exposure to sunlight or working in the hot sun or dry weather, like the desert of New Mexico, and can cause skin problems. Other causes include detergents and exposure to chemicals such as deodorant and chemical fragrances. Working in environments with chemicals like manufacturing can be causative factors. Bathing every day can help skin problems.

Eating too much sugar, alcohol, or salt affects skin conditions. Having sex after a heavy meal and sleeping during the daytime can cause skin disorders. A nap should last for only a half an hour.

Psychological factors of skin diseases include fear, anxiety, irritability, frustration, and deadline situations. Having a stressful job can be one of the factors for skin diseases. Repressed anger and hatred can adversely affect the skin as well.

Overview of Ayurvedic Treatment Protocols[11]

In Ayurveda, disease is defined as an aggravated *dosha* that leaves its site, enters into general circulation, and lodges in a *dhatu* (tissue), disturbing the nature, function, and/or structure of that tissue. Skin is one of the first places that you will see *dhatu* and *doshic* disorders because the increased *dosha* travels first to the *rasa* then *rakta dhatu* and manifests according to the *dosha* that is entering the *dhatu*. *Vata* will cause dry, rough, scaly skin; *Pitta* causes inflammation, irritation, and itching and burning conditions; and *Kapha* shows up as swelling, discharges, and even patchy changes on the skin.

Many skin diseases are chronic, such as eczema and psoriasis. Most skin diseases are mono-*doshic* or dual *doshic*. However, eczema, psoriasis, and leprosy are tri-*doshic* diseases. Briefly, the treatment protocol for such conditions would be the Ayurvedic detoxification program known as *panchakarma*. Because the *doshas* are stuck in the *rasa* and *rakta dhatu* under the skin, the client would need *abhyanga* (massage), *snehana* (medicated oil treatment), and *svedana* (medicated steam treatment). This would lubricate the *doshas* and bring them back to the gastrointestinal tract. The *Vata dosha* under the skin should come back to the colon, *Pitta dosha* should come back to the intestines, and *Kapha dosha* should come back to the stomach. Then *vamana* (therapeutic vomiting) is done for *Kapha dosha, virechana* (laxatives) for *Pitta dosha*, and *basti* (enema) for *Vata dosha*. Rejuvenation therapies and herbal combinations to maintain *doshic* balance would follow these specific treatments. Ayurvedic protocol calls for treatments that are *vyadhi pratyanik, dosha pratyanik*, and *ubhaya pratyanik* specific to the overall condition, *dosha,* and skin disorder. These include *swayambhu guggulu, bakuchi, guduchi*, and *shilajit* (Sharma, 1981 [Cikitsitasthana 7:39–49, 128–129).

Classical treatments for specific conditions are shown in Table 9.2. The herbs described are listed in the Appendix with their binomials or scientific botanical names.

SPECIFIC CONDITIONS AND THEIR TREATMENT

Ayurvedic literature speaks about *maha kushta*. These are descriptions of symptoms that the physician may observe. One type is *kapala kushta. Kapala* means a piece of broken clay pot. This describes the skin as looking like the surface of a broken clay pot: dry, rough, and cracked. Next is *udhumbara*, skin that looks like the skin of overripe figs. It would be reddish-brown, wrinkled and bumpy, and very thin so that when you touch it, it bleeds underneath the surface. The next category is *mandala*. This condition is patches on the skin, as with a fungus. Another description is *rushya jihva*. In this case, skin

Table 9.2. Classical Treatments for Specific Conditions

Condition[12]	Sanskrit Name	Description	Internal Herbs	External Applications
Eczema	*Pama, Isaba*	*Vata* type: dry	*Dashamula, Guduchi, Guggulu,* neem, turmeric	*Dashamula* in a sesame oil base
Eczema	*Pama*	*Pitta* type: angry red	*Shatavari, Gulvel sattva, Kama dudha,* neem, camphor	Neem oil Sandalwood paste
Eczema	*Pama*	*Kapha* type: weeping, oozing	*Punarnava, Kutki, Chitrak,* neem, turmeric	Nutmeg essential oil in a base of corn or olive oil
Pustular dermatitis	*Vicharchika*	With discharge	*Sukshma triphala*	*Tikta ghrita* ghee
Eczema	*Pama*	General remedies	Leaves of *Tephrossia purpurea* orally *Mahamanjistha qwath*[13]	*Chakramarda* oil *Karanja* oil
Eczema	*Rakasa*	Lesion looks like dry ashes	*Tikta ghrita* ghee	Neem oil Black currant seed oil *Karanja* oil Paste of the pulp of fresh sweet basil leaves
Dandruff (1)	*Darunaka*	Crust or flakes of skin on the scalp	*Dashamula, Kaishore guggulu*	Apply to scalp a mixture of *dashamula*, neem, and sandalwood oil combined with 8 ounces of lemon juice.
Dandruff (2)	*Darunaka*			Combine egg whites and fresh lime juice. Apply to whole scalp and leave on for 1 hour. Wash this off.

Condition	Sanskrit name	Herbs	Treatment
Dry, cracked feet	*Vipadika, Padadari*		Before bed, soak feet in warm water. Apply neem oil or *tikta ghrita* ghee and wear socks in bed. *Padadari malam*
Seborrhea dermatitis	*Arunsika*	*Shatavari, Guduchi*, neem	Neem oil Turmeric oil *Bakuchi* oil
Ringworm	*Dadru*		Lemongrass oil in a base of coconut oil. Combine senna, *chakramardra* oil, and coconut oil.
Itching Scabies	*Kandu*	*Sukshma triphala, Tikta ghrita* ghee	*Karanja* oil *Nirgundi* oil
Acne	*Pitika*	*Arogya vardhini, Kaishore guggulu*	Seed oil of *bonduc* nut and nutmeg paste Rose petals, turmeric, and red sandalwood paste
Prickly heat	*Sarvanga Dhara*	*Guduchi*	Make a cold infusion of sandalwood, coriander, turmeric, and *musta*. Wash the area with this tea. Sandalwood oil
Psoriasis	*Padma Kushta*	*Arogya vardhini, Kaishore guggulu*, neem, and *Manjistha*	Combine *vidanga, chitrak*, and neem into a paste.
Leukoderma Vitiligo	*Svitra*	*Amalaki, Vidanga, Chitrak*, neem, *Bakuchi*	*Bakuchi* oil

looks rough, red, and sandy, like the tongue of a bull. *Pundarika* compares the skin to the petals of a lotus flower, which would be long striations and red patches on the skin. Each of these is a type of *kushta*, skin disease (Sharma, 1981 [Cikitsitasthana, Chapter 7, pp. 125–142).

- *Kapala kushta* is chronic eczema with *Vata dosha* dominant. The skin is dry, rough, and cracked. To treat this, classical recommendations include *swayambhu guggulu, bakuchi, guduchi, shilajit*, and mint oil topically.
- With *udhumbara kushta* there is a burning sensation. This is a *Pitta* disorder and we can use *shatavari, guduchi, kama dudha*, neem, turmeric, and topical sandalwood and coconut oil.
- *Mandala kushta*, a *Kapha* disorder, has patches of skin that are light at the center and red on the periphery. There is itching, burning, and some oozing. For that, you can use a combination of *arogya vardhini, kama dudha, punarnava, manjistha*, and milk applied topically.
- *Rushya jihva kushta* skin looks hard, rough, and like sandpaper. This condition is *Vata-Pitta* predominant. Use *gulvel sattva, kama dudha*, and *haridra* (turmeric) and *tikta*, bitter herbs. *Tikta ghrita* ghee can be taken orally and applied topically and will eradicate this condition.
- *Pundarika* is a *Kapha-Pitta* disorder where the skin looks like lotus flower petals. Classically, we would apply leeches to the skin and they would suck the toxic blood from the area, healing this condition (Fig. 9.3). Today the person could donate blood to remove some of the toxins from the blood, but this would not be as specific as leeches applied directly to the skin (Sharma, 1981 [Sutrasthana 19:2, 134).

Kshudra Kushta

Herbal treatments specific to *kshudra* (simple) *kushta* skin diseases are *kadhira, haridra* (turmeric), neem, *vidanga, amalaki*, and *haritaki*. These are general remedies for skin conditions. There are many skin diseases caused by bacteria or parasites (*krumi*). Anthelmintics and antibacterial substances include ginger, black pepper, *Piper longum*, cayenne pepper, *vidanga, nirgundi, gokshura*, and *shigru*. These are specifically for parasites and bacteria. When there is pain and a burning sensation, anti-inflammatory herbs are needed. One can use camphor, blue lotus, then sandalwood or *guduchi* oil. Rejuvenating tonics that protect and nourish the skin include *sariva*, neem, coconut, *bhringaraj, triphala, haridra*, and camphor. *Manjistha* is specifically good for all skin conditions because of its beneficial tri-*doshic* action. It is *vyadhi pratyanika*, specific to skin disease (Bhishagratna, 1991 [Cikitsitasthana 10:4–36, 523–530).

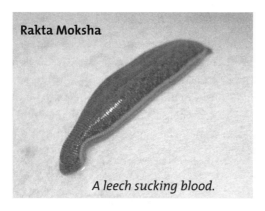

Rakta Moksha

A leech sucking blood.

FIGURE 9.3 Medicinal leech—*Hirudo medicinalis.* © D.Copy, Photocrea@istock-photo.com

MEDICATED OILS FOR THE SKIN

With skin diseases, Ayurveda uses a variety of medicated oils. To make a medicated oil concoction, take one part of the herb or herbal compound and 16 parts of water and mix together in a pot and cook on medium heat. Powdered herbs are best, but you can use the whole herb. Stir occasionally so the mixture does not burn. Boil this down until only one fourth of the concoction remains. Then, add to the concoction the same quantity of oil or ghee. Stirring as necessary, simmer over low heat until no water remains. In this slow, time-consuming process, the qualities of the herbs are yielded into the oil or ghee. Strain this mixture, leaving behind the solid residue.

Specific Medicated Oils for the Skin

Medicated mustard oil: Use *nirgundi*, turmeric, and mustard oil as the oil in this mixture. Use equal parts each of *nirgundi* and turmeric with 16 parts oil and four parts water. Applied topically, it prevents and cures many *Vata* skin conditions. Eczema, psoriasis, and acne respond well to this medicated oil (Babu, 2005, Chapter 52, p. 404).

Medicated coconut oil: Use *nirgundi, brahmi,* and seed of *gunja* in equal proportions with 16 parts oil and four parts water. This is good for *Pitta* disorders.

Medicated olive or corn oil: Use one of the following herbs: *trikatu*, ginger, black pepper, *Piper longum*, neem, turmeric, or *musta* for *Kapha* disorders. Proportions are olive oil 16 parts, four parts of the water, and one part of the herb.

HERBAL PASTES FOR THE SKIN

For *Vata* types of skin diseases, we can use *dashamula, guggulu,* and *vidari* oil paste on the skin. That will take care of the dry, rough, scaly skin. For *Pitta* conditions, make a paste of red sandalwood, turmeric, and camphor for inflammatory conditions. For *Kapha,* use nutmeg and *vacha* (calamus root) with mustard oil topically to help swelling or stagnant circulatory issues.

These are examples of medicated oils and herbal pastes for the skin according to *doshic* imbalance.

Herbal Baths for the Skin

To prevent skin diseases, Ayurveda recommends herbal baths. Make a tea that you will apply all over the skin. Take a gallon of water and one ounce of powdered herb, and then boil these together to make the herbal tea. Cool this mixture, then get into the bathtub. With a washcloth, apply the tea over your whole body. Leave it on for a while, and then rinse it off. Then wash with a good-quality herbal soap such as sandalwood or neem. Use one of these herbs to wash the skin: neem, *haridra, manjistha,* sandalwood, or licorice (Sharma, 1981 [Cikitsitasthana 7:92, 134]).

Avoid chemical detergents, shampoos, and soaps as they create dry skin conditions. To help this, apply a light layer of oil to the skin such as sesame oil for *Vata,* sunflower oil for *Pitta,* or corn oil for *Kapha.*

A simple herbal bath that will clean the *dosha* from the skin is ginger powder and baking soda. Baking soda is anti-inflammatory and ginger improves circulation and detoxifies the deeper layers of the skin. Run a bath and put ½ cup of each in the water. Soak for about ½ hour. It is a heating bath but very cleansing. If you get too hot, then get out of the bath. Rinse off well after this bath and apply oil as directed above.

REFERENCES

Babu, S. S. (2005). *The principles and practice of Kaya Chikitsa.* Varanasi: Chaukhamba Orientalia.

Bhishagratna, K. K. (trans.) (1991). *Sushruta Samhita.* Varanasi: Chaukhamba Orientalia.

Chinmayananda, S. (commentator) (1992). *The Holy Geeta* (2nd ed.). Mumbai: Central Chinmaya Mission Trust.

Murthy, K. R. S. (trans.) (1991). *Vaghbata's Ashtanga Hridaya.* Varanasi, India: Chaukhamba Orientalia.

Murthy, K. R. S. (trans.) (1993). *Madhava Nidanam*. Varanasi, India: Chaukhamba Orientalia.

Sharma, P. V. (trans.) (1981). *Charaka Samhita*. Varanasi, India: Chaukhamba Orientalia.

Appendix: Herbs Used

Amalaki (*Embelica officinalis*)
Arogya vardhini (compound)
Bakuchi (*Psoralea corylifolia*)
Bhringaraj (*Eclipta alba*)
Bibhitaki (*Terminalia belerica*)
Black currant oil (*Ribes nigrum*) (seed)
Black pepper (*Piper nigrum*)
Blue lotus (*Nymphaea caerulea*)
Bonduc nut (*Caesalpinia bonduc*) [Sanskrit *putikaranja*]
Camphor (*Cinnamomum camphora*)
Cayenne (*Capsicum annuum*)
Chakramarda oil (from *Cassia tora*)
Chitrak (*Plumbago zeylanica*)
Coriander (*Coriandrum sativum*)
Dashamula [ten roots] (compound)
Ginger (*Zingiberis officinalis*)
Gokshura (*Tribulus terrestris*)
Guduchi (*Tinospora cordifolia*)
Guggulu (*Commiphora mukul*)
Gulvel sattva (compound)
Gunja seed (*Abrus precatorius*)
Haridra (see "turmeric")
Haritaki (*Terminalia chebula*)
Kadhira (*Acacia catechu*)
Kaishore guggulu (compound)
Kama dudha (compound)
Karanja (*Millettia pinnata*)
Kutki (*Picrorhiza kurroa*)
Licorice (*Glycyrrhiza glabra*)
Long pepper (see "*pippali*")
Manjistha (*Rubia cordifolia*)
Mint (*Mentha*)
Musta (*Cyperus rotundus*)
Neem (*Azadiracta indica*)

Nirgundi (*Vitex negundo*)
Nutmeg (*Myristica fragrans*)
Pippali [long pepper] (*Piper longum*)
Punarnava (*Boerhaavia diffusa*)
Sandalwood (*Santalum album*)
Sariva (*Hemidesmus indicus*)
Senna (*Cassia angustifolia*)
Shatavari (*Asparagus racemosus*)
Shigru [drum stick] (*Moringa pterygosperma*)
Shilajit (*Asphaltum*)
Sukshma triphala tablets (compound)
Swayambhu guggulu (compound)
Sweet basil (*Ocimum basilicum*)
Tephrossia purpurea
Tikta ghrita ghee (compound)
Trikatu (compound of ginger, black pepper, *pippali*)
Triphala (compound of *amalaki*, *bibhitaki*, *haritaki*)
Turmeric (*Curcuma longa*)
Vacha (*Acorus calamus*)
Vidanga (*Embelia ribes*)
Vidari (*Ipomoea digitata*)

Notes

[1] The ancient texts on Ayurveda were written in Sanskrit verses called *sutras* that the students memorized. The verses represent the essence of the knowledge on the topic. Students were expected to learn the further details from the teacher. Many times, a short verse refers to a vast amount of information on the topic and its recitation would trigger these deeper memories for the physician. Over time, famous clinicians would write their own commentaries on the texts, expanding upon the knowledge from their own experiences.

[2] For more information on the classical texts, see the article at this link: http://www.ayurveda.com/online_resource/ancient_writings.html

[3] Traditionally called Ether.

[4] It is also called *tvacha*, which is a Hindi and Marathi word.

[5] *Kala* is the membranous structure that holds a tissue, separating one from the other; it also lines all organs and cavities in the body.

[6] *Vedini* is close to *majja dhara kala*, the layer related to *majja dhatu*, the nerve and bone tissue.

[7] These brown spots are technically known as solar lentigines and are caused by sun damage.

[8] *Ama* is a toxic, morbid metabolic waste substance that accumulates in the colon and other tissues (Murthy, 1991, 1993 [Sutrasthana 13:25–26, 187]).

[9] In Ayurveda, skin diseases and disorders are categorized under *kushta*. *Twag roga* is another name for skin diseases.

[10] For more information on incompatible food combinations, see the article at this link: http://www.ayurveda.com/pdf/food_combining.pdf

[11] **Please Note:** The herbs and compounds mentioned in this chapter for the formulas are traditional combinations used in Ayurveda and the ancient texts. Some of these are unavailable or very difficult to obtain for a variety of reasons. Some have problems with contamination of heavy metals, others are endangered species, some are prevented from export by the government of India, others are not approved by the U.S. Food and Drug Administration for consumption, and some are simply not available in the United States.

[12] Sharma, 1981 (Cikitsitasthana, Chapter 8, pp. 97–107)

[13] *Qwath* is a fermented concoction with self-generated alcohol. *Mahamanjistha* is a classical formula.

10

Hypnosis, Hypnoanalysis, and Mindfulness Meditation in Dermatology

PHILIP D. SHENEFELT

Key Concepts

- ♣ Hypnosis and meditation both utilize the natural trance state. Hypnosis is Western culture centered, has many induction methods, and has the Western "let's fix it" approach. Meditation is Eastern culture oriented, often uses breath induction, and is more concerned about centering and balance.

- ♣ Hypnosis and meditation do require training and effort but have minimal side effects and can sometimes help when other approaches have failed.

- ♣ Obtaining lasting effects from hypnosis or meditation can often require that the patient do at least 20 to 40 repetitions to rewire the synapses in the nervous system.

- ♣ Hypnosis for relaxation for dermatologic procedures has strong randomized controlled trial evidence supporting its efficacy, as does hypnosis for treating warts. Hypnosis for atopic dermatitis has good nonrandomized controlled trial evidence for efficacy. For most other dermatologic conditions, randomized control trials have yet to be performed. Similarly, psychosomatic hypnoanalysis has only case series and case reports to support its use in dermatology.

- ♣ Mindfulness meditation has strong supporting evidence as an adjunct in treating psoriasis. For most other dermatologic conditions, randomized controlled trials have yet to be performed.

Introduction

Hypnosis, hypnoanalysis, and mindfulness meditation utilize the natural trance state. During the waking state the mind tends to cycle through ultradian rhythms about every 90 minutes, consisting of alternating alertness with dominant beta brainwave activity followed by relaxation with dominant alpha brainwave activity (Rossi 1982). During the trance state the mind shifts out of conscious awareness with dominant low alpha and high theta activity (Freeman et al., 2000). The trance state occurs spontaneously several times daily when the conscious mind is quieted. Daydreaming, being absorbed in a book or movie or TV show, or focusing on spontaneous thoughts while driving and suddenly realizing that you have traveled a distance without consciously being aware of it are all everyday spontaneous trance experiences. Clear objective evidence of the trance state has been reported recently through detection of specific changes in eye movement in the trance state related to the so-called "trance stare" (Kallio et al., 2011). These eye movements are distinctly different and cannot be replicated by persons attempting to simulate trance. The other mind states are rapid eye movement (REM) sleep, which is different from the trance state and has dominant lower theta brainwave activity, and deep sleep, which has dominant delta wave activity. Of the four primary states of mind— alert consciousness, trance, REM sleep, and deep sleep—it the trance state that will be the focus of this chapter. Just as an individual can resist or cooperate with entering the sleep state, the individual can resist or cooperate with entering the trance state. The trance state allows access to capabilities and memories that often are not accessible in the conscious state.

While everyone can and does transition through alert consciousness, trance, REM sleep, and deep sleep states daily, some individuals have a natural trait of being able to shift into trance easily, while others have a natural trait of less ability to shift into trance. This trait correlates in part with the genetic alleles that code for production of the catechol-o-methyl-transferase (COMT) enzyme that degrades dopamine, an important neurotransmitter. The COMT enzyme with valine at the single nucleotide polymorphism 158 position degrades dopamine at about four times the rate that the COMT enzyme with methionine does. Those individuals homozygous in genetic coding to produce the COMT enzyme with methionine at the 158 position tend to be lower hypnotizable than those that are heterozygous for methionine and valine and who tend to be medium hypnotizable, while those who are homozygous for valine at the 148 position on the COMT enzyme tend to be more highly hypnotizable (Szekely et al., 2010)—that is, less able to enter into trance readily. About one quarter of individuals are homozygous for producing the COMT enzyme with methionine at the 158 position, about one half of individuals are heterozygous, and about one quarter of individuals are homozygous to produce the COMT enzyme with valine (Szekely et al., 2010). This roughly corresponds to the proportions of individuals who are low, medium, and high hypnotizable. Hypnotizability is to a large extent hardwired into individuals' brains and tends to be consistent over time as measured by the Hypnotic Induction Profile (HIP) (Spiegel & Spiegel, 2004). The trance state can be induced more easily in high and medium hypnotizables, but even low hypnotizables can often obtain some benefit from trance. Children can respond to hypnotic induction from about age 4 years and older, and hypnotic ability peaks at about ages 7 to 11 years (Morgan & Hilgard, 1973), then declines a little for adolescents and adults.

In trance, the left prefrontal cortex regional cerebral blood flow decreases as demonstrated on positron emission tomography (PET) scanning when compared with the alert conscious state (Rainville et al., 2002). There is an associated suspension of judgment, suspension of time sense, and often a feeling of connectedness or unity with the universe. Associated with this are higher suggestibility and openness to changing behavior patterns. Suggestions given in the trance state are also more able to alter autonomic function, blood flow, and immune responsiveness. There is also a better ability to block reaction to pain in trance, associated with the anterior cingulate cortex. Some individuals with the high hypnotizable trait are able to shift deeply into trance and undergo major surgical procedures with no anesthesia other than hypnosis and are able to control blood loss through decreased blood flow at surgical sites. For most other purposes, light to medium levels of trance are sufficient to promote effectiveness of suggestions, calming and balancing of the autonomic nervous system and of immune responsiveness, and increasing comfort.

With the conscious mind quieted in trance, there is greater access to both the higher authentic self and the lower vegetative self. The latter operates at roughly the level of a 5- or 6-year-old, with concrete interpretation of language, and often ignores negatives. Hence, the suggestion to not think of an elephant results in thinking of an elephant. Using the word "pain" will be clearly understood and often elicits a negative harmful reaction, a nocebo response, while using the word "discomfort" will often be heard as "comfort," eliciting a positive beneficial reaction, a placebo response. Patients who have just been injured or who are overwrought with anxiety may shift spontaneously into trance and be more highly suggestible to anything positive or negative that they hear. Even patients under general anesthesia or who are comatose can still hear and subconsciously store the memory of what they heard (Cheek, 1964). Careful selection of words with awareness of their potential effect can be as potent as a drug and have strong positive (placebo) or negative (nocebo) side effects. Often when drugs are tested the placebo does almost as well as the active drug, indicating the power of the mind to influence the body. As Dr. David Spiegel has said, it is not mind over matter, but mind matters (Spiegel, 2011).

Stress is epidemic in modern society, with excessive and chronic activation of the sympathetic nervous system and stress hormones and with eventual negative effects on the immune system. Stress can also trigger or aggravate many inflammatory skin diseases, as illustrated in the Griesemer index (Griesemer, 1978) (Table 10.1). Stress and anxiety or anger can feed on each other in a harmful positive feedback loop of increasing distress. Neuropeptides released by the sensory nerve fibers activate neuropeptide receptors on skin cells to induce inflammatory activities. The central nervous system (CNS) also mediates hormone release through the hypothalamus with its actions on the pituitary and other endocrine glands. Stress hormones influence the immune system, affecting inflammatory processes in the skin. Many inflammatory skin diseases such as acne, alopecia areata, aphthous stomatitis, atopic dermatitis, herpes simplex recurrences, lichen planus, rosacea, psoriasis, seborrheic dermatitis, telogen effluvium, vitiligo, and others are exacerbated by excessive stress (Zane, 2003). The interactions of the CNS and the immune system were well reviewed by Kiecolt-Glaser and colleagues (2002). This interaction permits interventions such as relaxation, hypnosis, and meditation to have positive impacts on many cutaneous diseases. Reducing chronic stress through nonpharmacologic methods can help calm inflammatory skin disorders and rebalance the immune response without the adverse side effects often associated with drugs.

The appearance of the skin and hair can have a significant impact on self-image (in the CNS) and social interactions, leading to stress. Skin diseases also affect self-image, social interactions, and behavior. Chronic skin disorders such as acne, alopecia areata, atopic dermatitis, or psoriasis can induce or aggravate depression in susceptible individuals (Gupta & Gupta, 2003). There is a significant psychosomatic or behavioral component to many skin disorders.

Stress in patients can be detected by asking them about their stress level on a 0 to 10 subjective units of distress scale (SUDS) where 0 is none and 10 is the worst imaginable stress. Patients can be asked to give a global SUDS rating for their overall stress level and then to rate the stress levels separately for their job/occupation/student situation, their financial situation, their health situation, their family/social situation, and any other significant area of stress.

Relaxation, hypnosis, hypnoanalysis, and meditation can help calm and rebalance the inflammatory immune response in inflammatory skin disorders that are exacerbated by stress. The relaxation response assists in rebalancing immune functioning. Hypnosis can help decrease inflammation and discomfort in a number of skin disorders and can improve the patient's attitude about

Table 10.1. Griesemer Index of Emotional Triggering of
Dermatoses in 4,576 Patients

Diagnosis	% Triggered	Time elapsed
Hyperhidrosis	100.0	Seconds
Lichen simplex chronicus	98.5	Days–2 weeks
Neurotic excoriations	97.5	Seconds
Alopecia areata	96.4	2 weeks
Warts, multiple & spreading	94.9	Days
Rosacea	94.1	2 days
Pruritus	85.7	Seconds
Lichen planus	81.8	Days–2 weeks
Dyshidrotic hand dermatitis	75.8	2 days
Atopic dermatitis	70.2	Seconds
Factitial dermatosis	69.2	Seconds
Urticaria	68.1	Minutes
Psoriasis	62.3	Days–2 weeks
Traumatic dermatitis	55.6	Seconds
Dermatitis not otherwise specified	55.6	Days
Acne vulgaris	55.3	2 days
Telogen effluvium	54.7	2–3 weeks
Nummular dermatitis	51.8	Days
Seborrheic dermatitis	40.6	Days–2 weeks
Herpes simplex/zoster	35.7	Days
Vitiligo	33.3	2–3 weeks
Pyoderma/bacterial infection	29.1	Days
Nail dystrophy	28.5	2–3 weeks
Cysts	27.0	2–3 weeks
Warts, single/multiple	17.4	Days
Contact dermatitis	15.3	2 days
Fungal infections	8.7	Days–2 weeks
Basal cell carcinoma	0	N/A
Keratoses	0	N/A
Nevi	0	N/A

Modified from Shenefelt (2000). *Archives of Dermatology, 136*, 393–399, Table 1, p. 394.

having the condition. Autogenic training is a specialized form of hypnosis. Psychocutaneous hypnoanalysis permits diagnostic evaluation of whether psychosomatic issues are initiating, triggering, or exacerbating specific skin disorders. When psychosomatic issues are present, hypnosis allows reframing of the initiating event in a way that defuses the negative emotions associated with it. Rapid induction hypnosis followed by deepening and then self-guided imagery can be effective in alleviating the anxiety and discomfort associated with dermatologic procedures. Mindfulness meditation enhances the response of psoriasis to ultraviolet light treatments. These will be further discussed in the sections below.

Breath relaxation has been practiced for centuries. It has been an aspect of some yoga traditions such as prana yoga and has been used in the Lamaze method of natural childbirth. The basic method is to focus attention on the breath and to intentionally slow and deepen breathing, shifting from more shallow and rapid chest-centered breathing to deeper and slower diaphragmatic abdominal breathing with longer exhalations. Breath relaxation can induce trance. It is more commonly used to induce meditative trance but also can be used as a hypnotic induction. Focusing attention on the sensation of air flowing in and out of the nostrils or focusing on the diaphragmatic movements of deep abdominal breathing helps to induce trance. The resulting calming effect can improve the psychosomatic aspects of skin disorders.

Progressive muscular relaxation was developed by Edmund Jacobson (Jacobson, 1929). He also developed biofeedback instrumentation and found that excess muscular tension was present in many psychosomatic disorders. Intentionally tensing and then relaxing the muscles decreased emotional distress and the resulting calmness and relaxation reduced psychosomatic symptoms. The basic method is to sit or lie recumbent and start at the hands, head, or toes with intentional muscle tensing followed by relaxation. The adjacent body part muscles are then tensed and relaxed, followed by those of the next adjacent body area until all areas of the body have been covered. Progressive muscular relaxation can be used by itself for treatment and prophylaxis of psychosomatic components of skin disorders. It may induce a meditative trance and is a frequently used method of hypnotic trance induction. The relaxation should be maintained for 5 to 25 minutes for optimal benefit. The sitting position is preferred if the patient desires to return to alertness after the progressive muscular relaxation, while the recumbent position is preferred if the patient desires to drift off to sleep for a nap or at bedtime.

For patients who have difficulty with hypnosis or meditation, there are alternatives. Biofeedback of muscle tension via electromyography (EMG) can enhance teaching of relaxation. Biofeedback-assisted relaxation can have a positive effect on inflammatory and emotionally triggered skin conditions such as acne (Hughes et al., 1983), atopic dermatitis, dyshidrotic dermatitis (Koldys & Meyer, 1979), hyperhidrosis (Duller & Gentry, 1980), lichen planus, neurodermatitis, psoriasis (Benoit & Harrell, 1980), and urticaria. The most common mechanism is through influencing immunoreactivity (Tausk, 1998). Patients who have low hypnotic ability may be especially suitable for this type of relaxation training utilizing EMG biofeedback. Other biofeedback devices for relaxation include the simple temperature sensor card. Alfred A. Barrios, a clinical psychologist, is the inventor of the Stress Control Card (Barrios, 1985), with a heat-sensitive color-changing biofeedback thermometer placed on a credit card-sized card having color indications from colder black through red and green to warmer blue, similar in function to the well-known mood ring. It measures ranges of finger temperatures, giving biofeedback of vasoconstriction versus vasodilatation associated with autonomic activity. Heart rate variability hand-held devices for promoting relaxation include the em-Wave Personal Stress Reliever and the StressEraser. A device that coaches slowing respirations to music is the RespeRate. Simply slowing the breaths to six per minute suffices to induce relaxation and shift from sympathetic to parasympathetic dominance.

Hypnosis

We all experience spontaneous mild trances daily while absorbed in watching television or a movie, reading a book or magazine, or other focused activity. After appropriate training, we may intensify this trance state and use this heightened focus to induce mind–body interactions that help to alleviate suffering or to promote healing. We may induce the trance state using guided imagery, relaxation, deep breathing, hypnosis induction techniques, self-hypnosis, or meditation techniques.

Hypnosis is the intentional induction, deepening, maintenance, and termination of the trance state for a specific purpose. Trance has been used since antiquity to assist the healing process. In ancient times and even today shamans, medicine men and women, and other healers have entered trance states themselves and induced trance in their patients to assist with healing. Hypnosis was developed in Europe as a Western approach to utilizing trance. It is a goal-oriented approach to use trance to attempt to improve or fix something. The purpose of medical hypnotherapy is to reduce suffering, to promote healing, or to help the person alter a destructive behavior. Some people are more highly hypnotizable, others less so, but most can obtain some benefit from hypnosis.

Defining hypnosis is still somewhat controversial. Marmer (1959) defined hypnosis as a psychophysiological tetrad of altered consciousness consisting of narrowed awareness, restricted and focused attentiveness, selective wakefulness, and heightened suggestibility. Discussions on definitions of hypnosis are available in Crasilneck and Hall (1985) or Barabasz and Watkins (2005). Many myths about hypnosis distort, overrate, or underrate its true capabilities. Evidence from electroencephalography (EEG) studies and PET studies comparing brain activity in the same individual when alert and when in trance supports the theory that hypnosis is a describable altered state of consciousness rather than simply a social compliance with expectations. This altered state is confirmed by a study on "trance stare" that showed that simulators of hypnosis could not produce the same changes in ocular movements as that produced in actual trance (Kallio et al., 2011). Quantitative EEG findings by Freeman and colleagues (2000) in a study of hypnosis versus distraction effects on cold pressor pain showed significantly greater high theta (5.5–7.5 Hz) activity for high hypnotizables (based on Stanford Hypnotic Susceptibility Scale, Form C [SHSS:C] scores) compared with low hypnotizables at parietal and occipital sites during hypnosis and also during waking relaxation. PET subtraction studies by Faymonville and colleagues (2000) demonstrated specific areas of the cerebral cortex with higher blood flow during hypnosis and others with lower blood flow, presumably related to cerebral activity. In their study, pain reduction mediated by hypnosis localized to the mid-anterior cingulate cortex.

How hypnosis produces improvement in symptoms and in skin lesions is not yet fully understood. Hypnosis can help regulate blood flow and other autonomic functions not usually under conscious control. Stress reduction through the relaxation response that accompanies hypnosis alters the neurohormonal systems that in turn regulate many body functions (Tausk, 1998).

Hypnosis can help induce the resolution of some skin diseases, including verruca vulgaris (warts). Hypnosis may also help to reduce stress, skin pain, pruritus, or psychosomatic aspects of skin diseases. Suggestion without formal trance induction may be sufficient in some cases. Bloch (1927) and Sulzberger (1934) used suggestion to treat verrucae successfully.

Hypnosis is a tool, not a therapy in and of itself. It has many useful dermatologic applications, including stress reduction. Hypnosis involves guiding the patient into a trance state for a specific purpose such as relaxation, pain or pruritus reduction, or habit modification. Hypnosis may be used to help control stress-exacerbated harmful habits such as scratching. Hypnosis may also facilitate improvement or clearing of numerous skin disorders. Skin diseases responsive to hypnosis are described in the relatively old book by Scott (1960) and in the chapter on the use of hypnosis in dermatologic problems in Crasilneck and Hall (1985). Koblenzer (1987) also mentions some of the uses of hypnosis in common dermatologic problems. Grossbart and Sherman (1992) include hypnosis as recommended therapy for a number of skin conditions in an excellent resource book for patients. Examples include acne excoriée, alopecia areata, atopic dermatitis, congenital ichthyosiform erythroderma, dyshidrotic dermatitis, erythromelalgia, furuncles, glossodynia, herpes simplex, hyperhidrosis, ichthyosis vulgaris, lichen planus, neurodermatitis, nummular dermatitis, post-herpetic neuralgia, pruritus, psoriasis, rosacea, trichotillomania, urticaria, verruca vulgaris, and vitiligo (Shenefelt, 2000) (Box 10.1). Hypnosis can also reduce stress, anxiety, and pain associated with dermatologic procedures. It can also be used to provide immediate and long-term analgesia, improve recovery from surgery, and facilitate the mind–body connection to

Box 10.1 Skin Disorders Responsive to Hypnosis

Randomized controlled trials (representing strong evidence of effectiveness)
- Hypnotic relaxation during dermatologic procedures
- Verruca vulgaris
- Psoriasis

Nonrandomized controlled trials
- Atopic dermatitis

Case series
- Alopecia areata
- Urticaria

Single or few case reports (representing weak evidence of effectiveness)
- Acne excoriée
- Congenital ichthyosiform erythroderma
- Dyshidrotic dermatitis
- Erythema nodosum
- Erythromelalgia
- Furuncles
- Glossodynia
- Herpes simplex
- Hyperhidrosis
- Ichthyosis vulgaris
- Lichen planus
- Neurodermatitis
- Nummular dermatitis
- Post-herpetic neuralgia
- Pruritus
- Rosacea
- Trichotillomania
- Vitiligo

Table 10.2. Suggestion Approach Based on Hypnotizability
as Measured by HIP or SHSS-C

Hypnotizability	
High	Dissociative type—encourage dissociation
	Fantasy type—encourage fantasy
Medium	Distortion, distancing, displacement of time and discomfort
Low	Distraction and redirection
	Biofeedback

promote healing. The type of suggestions used for a given individual may be modified based on his or her level of hypnotizability (Table 10.2). Skin disorders that have responded to hypnotherapy are discussed below. Hypnosis integrates very well with both conventional and alternative therapies and often has a synergistic effect with them in promoting healing and health.

MEDICAL HYPNOTHERAPY

Hypnosis can be used to reduce stress and to reduce psychological or behavioral impediments to healing. Hypnosis facilitates supportive therapies that promote ego-strengthening and self-efficacy and improvements through autogenic training, direct suggestion, symptom substitution, and hypnoanalysis (Hartland 1969; Scott, 1960, 1963, 1964). Observing the patient's response when mentioning hypnosis will allow the practitioner to gauge the patient's receptiveness to this treatment modality. The time needed to screen patients, educate them about realistic expectations for results from hypnosis, and actually perform the hypnotherapy is similar to or less than those for screening, preparing, and educating patients about cutaneous surgery and then actually performing the surgery. Practitioners who prefer to refer patients to hypnotherapists or who desire further information about training in hypnotherapy may obtain referrals or training information from the American Society of Clinical Hypnosis at www.asch.net or similar professional organizations.

Some advantages of medical hypnotherapy for skin diseases include nontoxicity, cost-effectiveness, ability to obtain a response where other treatment modalities have failed, and ability of patients to self-treat and gain a sense of control when taught self-hypnosis. The self-hypnosis can be reinforced by using recordings that they can play back in the form of CDs or MP3s. Disadvantages include the practitioner training required, the low hypnotizability of some patients, the negative social attitudes still prevalent about hypnosis, and the lower reimbursement rates for cognitive therapies such as hypnosis when compared with procedural therapies such as cutaneous surgery. Patient selection

Table 10.3. Hypnotic Trance Sequence During Medical Hypnotherapy

Trance induction
Rapid—Eye roll Slow—Progressive relaxation or other method
Trance deepening
Trance work (one or more)
Ego-strengthening—self-efficacy Autogenic training Direct suggestion Indirect suggestion Hypnoanalysis Relaxation for procedures
Trance termination

is an important aspect of successful medical hypnotherapy. With proper selection of disease process, patient, and provider, hypnosis can decrease suffering and morbidity from skin disorders with minimal side effects.

The hypnotic state can be induced in adults by methods that focus attention, soothe, and/or produce monotony or confusion (Barabasz & Watkins, 2005; Crasilneck & Hall, 1985). Adults usually appear somewhat sedated when in trance. The hypnotic state may be induced in children by having the child make-believe that he or she is watching television, a movie, or a play or by using some other distractive process that employs the imagination, such as imagining doing a favorite thing (Olness, 1986). Younger children are often more animated when in trance. Following induction, trance work can be performed, followed by realerting (Table 10.3).

Ego-strengthening and self-efficacy–promoting therapies include positive suggestions and posthypnotic suggestions for self-worth and effectiveness. Reinforcement can be achieved by recording a CD or MP3 that the patient can use subsequently for repeated self-hypnosis. The strengthened ego with self-belief in self-efficacy is then better able to deal with psychological elements that inhibit healing.

Autogenic training is a specialized type of hypnosis developed by Johann Heinrich Schultz, a German who first trained in dermatology and then in neurology. He became fascinated with hypnosis and developed a formula for relaxation in trance that became known as autogenic training (Linden, 1990). It may be performed lying supine or sitting. The formula is to close the eyes, find a comfortable body position, and allow yourself to concentrate on what is going on inside of you. First concentrate on your arms and legs and repeat six times that "my arms and legs are very heavy" (muscular relaxation). Next concentrate on your hands and feet and repeat six times that "my hands and feet are very warm" (vasodilation). Then repeat six times that "my heartbeat is calm and strong" (regulation and slowing of heartbeat). Next repeat six times that "it breathes me" (shift from thoracic to abdominal breathing). Then repeat six times that "warmth radiates over my abdomen" (calming of visceral gut activity). Finally, repeat six times that "my forehead is cool" (mental relaxation). Research has shown autogenic training to be helpful for stress reduction and for Raynaud's disease. Autogenic training was demonstrated to be superior to standard dermatologic care for treatment of atopic dermatitis (Ehlers et al., 1995).

Direct suggestion during hypnosis may be used to decrease stress, skin discomfort from pain, pruritus, burning sensations, anxiety, and insomnia. Posthypnotic suggestion and repeated use of a CD or MP3 by the patient for self-hypnosis helps to reinforce the effectiveness of direct suggestion. In highly hypnotizable individuals, direct suggestion may produce sufficiently deep anesthesia to permit cutaneous surgery. Direct suggestion can also reduce compulsive acts of skin scratching or picking, nail biting or manipulating, and hair pulling or twisting (Scott, 1960). Autonomic responses in hyperhidrosis, blushing, and some forms of urticaria can also be controlled by direct suggestion. Verrucae can be induced to resolve using direct suggestion (see below).

Symptom substitution replaces a negative habit pattern with a more constructive one (Scott, 1960). For example, another physical activity, such as grasping something and holding it so tightly for a half-minute that it almost hurts, can be substituted for scratching. Other activities that can be substituted for scratching include athletics, artwork, journaling of feelings, meditation, or verbal expression of feelings.

Change in response to hypnosis often does not happen instantly, especially if ingrained habits are involved. Just as in most instances one should not expect one dose of medicine to correct a chronic problem, one should not expect one session of hypnosis to correct a chronic problem. It typically takes 20 to 40 repetitions of doing something differently to change a behavior. Occasionally one session of hypnosis or hypnoanalysis (see below) will produce significant and permanent change, but usually several sessions of hypnosis along with the patient's use of self-hypnosis are necessary to obtain permanent change.

MEDICAL HYPNOTHERAPY FOR TREATING SPECIFIC SKIN DISORDERS

Most reports of the effectiveness of hypnosis on specific dermatologic conditions were until recently based on one or a few uncontrolled cases. The trend toward controlled trials has produced more reliable information (Kaschel et al., 1991), although randomized controlled trial results are still not available for most skin disorders (see Box 10.1).

Acne tends to flare under stress in some individuals. Picking associated with acne excoriée also intensifies with stress. Posthypnotic suggestion was successful in reducing or stopping the picking associated with acne excoriée in two reported cases (Hollander, 1959). One patient was instructed to remember the word "scar" whenever she wanted to pick her face and to refrain from picking by saying "scar" instead. The author has had similar success in one case (Shenefelt, 2004). Hypnosis may be an appropriate treatment for the picking habit aspect of acne excoriée in conjunction with standard treatments for the acne itself.

Alopecia areata commonly flares with stress in some individuals. In a small clinical trial of medical hypnotherapy with five patients having extensive alopecia areata, only one patient showed a significant increase in hair growth. Hypnosis did improve stress and psychological parameters in these five patients, although three patients had only a slight increase in hair growth and one had no change (Harrison & Stepanek, 1991). In a larger clinical trial (Willemsen et al., 2006), all 21 patients with severe alopecia areata had improvement of anxiety and depression with hypnotherapy. Nine patients had total regrowth of scalp hair, and another three patients had better than 75% regrowth. Hypnosis is appropriate as a supportive treatment for the psychological impact of having alopecia areata and may sometimes have a positive effect on the condition itself.

Stress can exacerbate **atopic dermatitis**. A number of case reports describe improvement of atopic dermatitis in both children and adults as a result of hypnotherapy (Twerski & Naar, 1974). In a nonrandomized controlled clinical trial. Stewart and Thomas (1995) treated 18 adults with extensive atopic dermatitis who had been resistant to conventional treatment with hypnotherapy that included relaxation, stress management, direct suggestion for non-scratching behavior, direct suggestion for skin comfort and coolness, ego strengthening, posthypnotic suggestions, and instruction in self-hypnosis. The results were statistically significant ($p < 0.01$) for reductions in itch, scratching, sleep disturbance, and tension. Topical corticosteroid use decreased by 40% at 4 weeks, 50% at 8 weeks, and 60% at 16 weeks. For atopic dermatitis, hypnosis can be a very useful therapy that can decrease the needed amount of other treatments.

Clearing of **congenital ichthyosiform erythroderma of Brocq** in a 16-year-old boy was reported following direct suggestion for clearing under hypnosis (Mason, 1952). Similar though less spectacular results were confirmed with two sisters aged 8 and 6 (Wink, 1961), with a 20-year-old woman (Schneck, 1966), and with a 34-year-old father and his 4-year-old son (Kidd, 1966). Based on these case reports, hypnosis may be potentially very useful as a therapy in addition to emollients.

Stress is a common trigger factor for **dyshydrotic dermatitis**, to the point where some individuals can use the flaring of their dyshidrotic dermatitis as a barometer of their stress levels. Reduction in the severity of dyshidrotic dermatitis has been reported with hypnosis (Tobia, 1982).

The author reported a case of **erythema nodosum** that had failed to resolve with medical treatment for 9 years but that resolved following hypnoanalysis (Shenefelt, 2007).

There is one case report of successful treatment of **erythromelalgia** in an 18-year-old woman using hypnosis alone followed by self-hypnosis (Chakravarty et al., 1992). Permanent resolution occurred.

A 33-year-old man with a negative self-image and recurrent multiple *Staphylococcus aureus*-containing **furuncles** occurring since age 17 was unresponsive to multiple treatment modalities. Hypnosis and self-hypnosis with imagined sensations of warmth, cold, tingling, and heaviness brought about dramatic improvement over 5 weeks, with full resolution of the recurrent furuncles (Jabush, 1969). The patient also had substantial mental improvement. Conventional antibiotic therapy is the first line of treatment for furuncles, but in unusually resistant cases with significant psychosomatic overlay, use of hypnosis may help to end the chronic susceptibility to recurrent infection.

Oral pain such as **glossodynia** may respond well to hypnosis as a primary treatment if there is a significant psychological component (Golan, 1997). With organic disease, hypnosis may give temporary relief from pain.

Discomfort relief from **herpes simplex** is similar to that for post-herpetic neuralgia (see below). Reduction in the frequency of recurrences of herpes simplex following hypnosis has also been reported (Bertolino, 1983). In cases with an apparent emotional stress trigger factor, hypnotic suggestion may be useful as a therapy for reducing the frequency of recurrence.

Hypnosis or autogenic training may be useful as adjunctive therapy for **hyperhidrosis** (Hölzle, 1994). Stress is a common trigger or exacerbator of hyperhidrosis.

A 33-year-old man with **ichthyosis vulgaris** that was better in summer and worse in winter began hypnotic suggestion therapy in the summer and was able to maintain the summer improvement throughout the fall, winter, and spring (Schneck, 1954).

Stress is a definite exacerbating factor in **lichen planus**. Pruritus and lesions of lichen planus may be reduced in selected cases using hypnosis (Scott, 1960; Tobia, 1982).

Some cases of **neurodermatitis** or psychogenic dermatitis have resolved and stayed resolved with up to 4 years of follow-up using hypnosis as an alternative therapy (Collison, 1965; Kline, 1953; Lehman, 1978; Sacerdote, 1965).

Stress is a major factor in increasing scratching or picking of the skin in these patients.

Reduction of pruritus and resolution of lesions of **nummular dermatitis** has been reported with the use of hypnotic suggestion (Scott, 1960; Tobia, 1982).

Pain from herpes zoster and **post-herpetic neuralgia** can be reduced by hypnosis (Scott, 1960; Tobia, 1982). Hypnosis may be useful as a therapy for post-herpetic neuralgia. The author had one patient who for 6 years had had post-herpetic neuralgia that greatly limited his enjoyment of life. He had been a highly successful attorney and had retired before anticipated at age 65 due to the post-herpetic neuralgia. After he learned self-hypnosis he regained a sense of control over his life. He could diminish the pain, and it no longer ruled his activities.

Pruritus typically increases with stress. Hypnosis can modify and lessen the intensity of pruritus (Scott, 1960). A man with chronic myelogenous leukemia had intractable pruritus that was much improved with hypnotic suggestion (Ament & Milgram, 1967).

Stress is a common exacerbating factor in **psoriasis**. Hypnosis and suggestion have been demonstrated to have a positive effect on psoriasis (Kantor, 1990; Winchell & Watts, 1988; Zachariae et al., 1996). A 75% clearing of psoriasis was reported in one case using a hypnotic sensory-imagery technique (Kline, 1954). A patient with extensive severe psoriasis of 20 years' duration had marked improvement using sensory imagery to replicate the feelings in the patient's skin that he had experienced during sunbathing (Frankel & Misch, 1973). Another case of severe psoriasis of 20 years' duration resolved fully with a hypnoanalytic technique (Waxman, 1973). Tausk and Whitmore (1999) performed a small randomized controlled trial using hypnosis as adjunctive therapy in psoriasis and found significant improvement only in the highly hypnotizable subjects and not in the moderately hypnotizable subjects. Hypnosis can be quite useful as a therapy for resistant psoriasis, especially if there is a significant emotional factor in the triggering of the psoriasis.

The vascular blush component of **rosacea** has been reported to improve in selected cases of resistant rosacea where hypnosis has been added (Scott, 1960; Tobia, 1982). Stress can increase blushing.

Several reports of successful adjunctive treatment of **trichotillomania** have been published (Barabasz, 1987; Galski, 1981; Rowen, 1981). Stress is an exacerbating factor. Hypnosis may be a useful therapy for trichotillomania.

Two cases of **urticaria** with stress as a trigger factor responded to hypnotic suggestion in one study. An 11-year-old boy who had an urticarial reaction to chocolate could have the hives blocked by hypnotic suggestion so that they appeared on one side of his face but not the other (Perloff & Spiegelman, 1973). In 15 patients with chronic urticaria with an average duration of 7.8 years, hypnosis with relaxation therapy resulted within 14 months in six patients being cleared and another eight patients improved, with decreased medication requirements reported by 80% of the subjects (Shertzer & Lookingbill, 1987).

Bloch (1927) and Sulzberger and Wolf (1934) reported on the efficacy of suggestion in treating **verruca vulgaris (warts)**. This has been confirmed numerous times to a greater or lesser degree (Dudek, 1967; Obermayer & Greenson, 1949; Sheehan, 1978; Ullman, 1959) and failed to be confirmed in a few studies (Clarke, 1965; Stankler, 1967). A study that showed negative results was criticized for using a negative suggestion of not feeding the warts rather than a positive suggestion about having the warts resolve (Felt et al., 1998). Many reports have confirmed the efficacy of hypnosis in treating warts (Clawson & Swade, 1975; Dreaper, 1978; Ewin, 1974, 1992; Gottlieb et al., 1972; Johnson & Barber, 1978; McDowell, 1949; Morris, 1985; Noll, 1988, 1994; Spanos et al., 1988, 1990; Straatmeyer & Rhodes, 1983; Surman et al., 1977; Tasini & Hackett, 1977; Ullman & Dudek, 1960; Vickers, 1961). One study (Tenzel & Taylor, 1969) that tried to replicate the remarkable success reported in *Lancet* (Sinclair-Gieben & Chalmers, 1959) of using hypnotic suggestion to cause warts to disappear from one hand but not the other in persons with bilateral hand warts was unsuccessful. A well-conducted randomized controlled study resulted in 53% of the experimental group having improvement of their warts 3 months after the first of five hypnotherapy sessions, while none of the control group had improvement (Surman et al., 1973). Hypnosis has been proved to be helpful as a therapy for warts.

Having **vitiligo** can be very stressful to some individuals, especially those with a naturally dark skin tone. Vitiligo has been improved using hypnotic suggestion as supportive therapy (Scott, 1960; Tobia, 1982), but it is unclear whether the recovery was simply spontaneous. Hypnosis may be appropriate as a supportive treatment for the psychological impact of having vitiligo.

MEDICAL HYPNOTHERAPY FOR REDUCING PROCEDURAL STRESS AND ANXIETY

Hypnosis can reduce stress, anxiety, needle phobia, and pain during cutaneous surgery, as well as reduce postoperative discomfort and enhance postoperative healing. Fick and colleagues (1999) used self-guided imagery content during nonpharmacologic analgesia to help 56 nonselected patients referred for percutaneous interventional procedures in the radiology procedure suite. A standardized protocol and script was used to guide patients into a state of self-hypnotic relaxation followed by suggestion to go where they would rather be. All 56 patients developed an imaginary scenario. The imagery they chose was highly individualistic. The authors concluded that average patients can engage in imagery, but the topics patients chose were highly individualistic, making recorded suggested scenarios or provider-directed imagery likely to be less effective than self-directed imagery. The author has used this technique with good success in dermatology patients (Shenefelt, 2003).

Lang and colleagues (2000) conducted a larger randomized trial of adjunctive nonpharmacologic analgesia for invasive percutaneous vascular radiologic procedures consisting of three groups: standard care (control group), structured attention, and self-hypnotic relaxation. Pain increased linearly with time in the standard and the attention group but remained flat in the hypnosis group. Anxiety decreased over time in all three groups, but more so with hypnosis. Conscious sedation drug use was significantly higher in the standard group than in the structured attention and self-hypnosis groups. The hemodynamic stability was significantly higher in the hypnosis group than in the attention and standard groups. Procedure times were significantly shorter in the hypnosis group than in the standard group, with the attention group intermediate. A cost analysis of this study (Lang & Rosen, 2002) showed that the cost associated with standard conscious sedation averaged $638 per case, while the cost for sedation with adjunct hypnosis was $300 per case, making the latter considerably more cost-effective.

The author conducted a randomized controlled trial of hypnotically induced relaxation with self-guided imagery with 39 patients undergoing dermatologic surgery. They were randomly assigned to live induction, recorded induction, and control groups. The live induction group had significantly less anxiety by 20 minutes than the controls, with the recorded induction group being close to the controls in response (Shenefelt, 2013).

A meta-analysis of hypnotically induced analgesia found that hypnosis can significantly relieve pain in patients with headache, burn injury, heart disease, cancer, dental problems, eczema, and chronic back problems (Montgomery et al., 2000). For most purposes light and medium trance is sufficient, but deep trance is required for hypnotic anesthesia for surgery (Barabasz & Watkins, 2005). Pain reduction mediated by hypnosis localized to the mid-anterior cingulate cortex in a study by Faymonville and colleagues (2000) using PET.

In general, for hypnosis to be of benefit, patients must be mentally intact, not psychotic nor heavily intoxicated; motivated, not resistant; and preferably medium or high hypnotizable as rated by the Hypnotic Induction Profile (HIP; Spiegel & Spiegel, 2004) or Stanford Hypnotic Susceptibility Scale and its variants. However, for self-guided imagery a moderate or high degree of hypnotizability is not critical to success. Letting patients choose their own self-guided imagery allows most individuals to reach a state of relaxation during procedures. Both the patient and the physician can benefit from a more pleasant experience attended by fewer complications during the procedure.

HYPNOANALYSIS

Hypnoanalysis may help patients with skin disorders unresponsive to other simpler approaches. Using hypnoanalysis, results may also occur much more quickly than with standard psychoanalysis (Scott, 1960). Psychologists and psychiatrists have focused primarily on the mind and the emotions and have used hypnoanalysis to speed therapeutic results. Nonpsychiatrist physicians and others have focused on the body and how the mind interacts with the body. To differentiate this from the type of hypnoanalysis used by psychologists and psychiatrists, the author has coined the term "psychosomatic hypnoanalysis" (Shenefelt, 2007). Seven key factors have been identified by Cheek and LeCron (1968) associated with psychosomatic issues. The author has slightly modified their naming to create a mnemonic. The key issues are **C**onflict, **O**rgan language, **M**otivation or secondary gain, **P**ast experiences or traumatic conditioning, **A**ctive identification, **S**uggestion, and **S**elf-punishment. The C.O.M.P.A.S.S. method of identifying seven trigger or exacerbating psychosomatic root causes is well described in Ewin and Eimer (2006) (Table 10.4). Ideomotor signaling is used for nonverbal communication (Ewin & Eimer, 2006; Shenefelt, 2011). Uncovering the initiating or trigger or exacerbating factors and neutralizing the associated negatively charged emotion often leads to the resolution of the psychosomatic aspects of the problem. Dr. Ewin used psychosomatic hypnoanalysis on a series of 41 patients with recalcitrant warts that had failed to respond to ordinary hypnotic suggestion and had resolution in 33 of the 41 patients (Ewin, 1992). In these cases a psychological blocking factor had inhibited the delayed cellular immune system from eliminating the warts until the negative emotional blockage was removed. One of the author's patients who had persistent erythema nodosum for 9 years with no apparent physical trigger factors had resolution of the lesions after hypnoanalysis (Shenefelt, 2007). Another patient had resolution of resistant neurodermatitis on the face (Shenefelt, 2010). This C.O.M.P.A.S.S. method can be used for screening for psychosomatic factors. Although not empirically demonstrated,

Table 10.4. C.O.M.P.A.S.S. Method of Psychosomatic Hypnoanalysis for Root Causes

Conflict between "want to" and "ought to"
Organ language
Motivation or secondary gain
Past experiences, especially traumatic
Active identification with similar issue in a significant person
Self-punishment
Suggestion from a significant person

experience has taught that if all of the C.O.M.P.A.S.S. factors are negative, there is likely not a psychosomatic component to the disease process. If one or two factors are positive, appropriate neutralizing suggestions may be sufficient. If three or more factors are positive, referral to an appropriate psychologist or psychiatrist or other experienced mental health worker would be appropriate (Shenefelt, 2007).

Mindfulness Meditation

Meditation has been used since antiquity and is an efficient and effective means of reducing stress. Meditation may broadly be divided into concentrative meditation, where the focus is on one object such as a candle flame or mandala, image, sound, word, or mantra, and mindfulness meditation, where the focus is on emotional nonattachment but broad awareness of many objects, sounds, other sensations, or thoughts. With concentrative meditation, the focus is on a single item, while with mindfulness meditation the focus is open to the flow of all stimuli. Mindfulness meditation involves focusing on the moment and accepting things as they are. Both involve entering a trance state. The concentrative trance reduces external awareness, similar to an internally focused hypnotic trance, while the mindfulness trance maintains external awareness while remaining calmly centered, similar to an alert awake hypnotic trance.

The Western scientific paradigm for healing generally evaluates the "how" of disease, examining the subsystems involved and the means to repair and cure or control the problem with a short-term focus, while the Eastern paradigm for healing looks more at the "what" of disease, examining the systems and supersystems involved and the means to restore or rebalance the system with a long-term focus (Otani, 2003). Although intentional utilization of the trance state doubtless existed in prehistory, hypnosis as we know it arose in the Western cultural milieu in Europe, while meditation as we know it arose in the Eastern cultural milieu, primarily in India, with spread throughout Asia. They both use the trance phenomenon, but with different conceptual approaches and different types of emphasis. Table 10.5 compares hypnosis with mindfulness meditation.

The relaxation response, a form of concentrative meditation, was introduced by Herbert Benson (1975). It involves sitting in a quiet place, closing your eyes, letting your muscles loosen and relax, starting at your feet and working upward with progressive muscular relaxation trance induction, breathing evenly through your nose, and becoming aware of the breath as breath trance induction. With each exhalation, say the word "one" to yourself as a concentrative mantra meditation trance induction. Maintain a passive attitude. Let any distracting thoughts or sensations drift away, ignored, like clouds in the sky.

Table 10.5. Contrasting Hypnosis with
Mindfulness Meditation

Hypnosis	*Mindfulness Meditation*
Western "fix it"	Eastern "balance"
Rapport	Independent
Suggestion	Let everything pass by
Concentration inward	Concentration with awareness
Focused on past and future	Focused on present
High theta deeper trance	Low alpha lighter trance
Deep reflection	Nonattachment
Introspection	Open to the universe

Maintain the concentrative meditation for 10 to 15 minutes. When you finish, remain sitting quietly for a few minutes, first with your eyes closed, then with your eyes open. The health benefits of the relaxation response have been extensively researched, with positive results in areas such as cardiovascular health.

Mindfulness meditation has also been used. Originally associated with Buddhism and in particular Zen, it has been adapted for medical use for stress reduction. Jon Kabat-Zinn (1990, 1994) has been a major proponent of this methodology, employing mindfulness meditation and hatha yoga stretching. He developed the Mindfulness-Based Stress Reduction program. The 8-week course comprised weekly 2-hour classes involving techniques of breath, awareness of body sensations, and stretching yoga. He combined that with a half-day of meditation and daily homework of 45 minutes of taped guided meditation or 30 minutes of meditation on their own. Gentle coaching helped patients to develop nonjudgmental, moment-to-moment awareness, attention monitoring, and acceptance. He also performed a study (Kabat-Zinn, 1998) with randomization of psoriasis patients undergoing ultraviolet B (UVB) or psoralen plus ultraviolet A (PUVA) light treatments into two groups, those listening to mindfulness meditation tapes and those who were controls. Patients in the mindfulness meditation tape group reached the halfway point in clearing and the clearing point significantly more rapidly than the controls for both UVB and PUVA treatments. The mindfulness meditation worked synergistically with the UVA or PUVA to promote healing.

REFERENCES

Ament, P., & Milgram, H. (1967). Effects of suggestion on pruritus with cutaneous lesions in chronic myelogenous leukemia. *New York State Journal of Medicine, 67,* 833–835.

Barabasz, A., & Watkins, J. G. (2005). *Hypnotherapeutic techniques* (2nd ed.). New York: Brunner-Routledge.

Barabasz, M. (1987). Trichotillomania, a new treatment. *International Journal of Clinical and Experimental Hypnosis, 35*, 146–154.

Barrios, A. A. (1985). *Towards greater freedom and happiness.* Los Angeles: SPC Press.

Benoit, J., & Harrell, E. H. (1980). Biofeedback and control of skin cell proliferation in psoriasis. *Psychological Reports, 46*, 831–839.

Benson, H. (1975). *The relaxation response.* New York: Morrow.

Bertolino, R. (1983). L'ipnosi in dermatologia. *Minerva Medica, 74*, 2969–2973.

Bloch, B. (1927). Über die heilung der warzen durch suggestion. *Klinische Wochenschrift, 6*, 2271–2275, 2320–2325.

Chakravarty, K., Pharoah, P. D. P., Scott, D. G. I., et al. (1992). Erythromelalgia—the role of hypnotherapy. *Postgraduate Medical Journal, 68*, 44–46.

Cheek, D. B. (1964). Further evidence of persistence of hearing under chemo-anesthesia, detailed case report. *American Journal of Clinical Hypnosis, 7*, 55–59.

Cheek, D. B., & LeCron, L. M. (1968) *Clinical hypnotherapy.* Orlando: Grune & Stratton.

Clarke, G. H. V. (1965). The charming of warts. *Journal of Investigative Dermatology, 45*, 15–21.

Clawson, T. A., & Swade, R. H. (1975). The hypnotic control of blood flow and pain, the cure of warts and the potential for the use of hypnosis in the treatment of cancer. *American Journal of Clinical Hypnosis, 17*, 160–169.

Collison, D. R. (1965). Medical hypnotherapy. *Medical Journal of Australia, 1*, 643–649.

Crasilneck, H. B., & Hall, J. A. (1985). *Clinical hypnosis* (2nd ed.). Orlando, FL: Grune & Stratton.

Dreaper, R. (1978). Recalcitrant warts on the hand cured by hypnosis. *Practitioner, 220*, 305–310.

Dudek, S. Z. (1967). Suggestion and play therapy in the cure of warts in children, a pilot study. *Journal of Nervous and Mental Diseases, 145*, 37–42.

Duller, P., & Gentry, W. D. (1980). Use of biofeedback in treating chronic hyperhidrosis, a preliminary report. *British Journal of Dermatology, 103*, 143–146.

Ehlers, A., Stangier, U., & Gieler, U. (1995). Treatment of atopic dermatitis, a comparison of psychological and dermatological approaches to relapse prevention. *Journal of Consulting and Clinical Psychology, 63*, 624–635.

Ewin, D. (1974). Condyloma acuminatum, successful treatment of four cases by hypnosis. *American Journal of Clinical Hypnosis, 17*, 73–78.

Ewin, D. M. (1992). Hypnotherapy for warts (verruca vulgaris), 41 consecutive cases with 33 cures. *American Journal of Clinical Hypnosis, 35*, 1–10.

Ewin, D. M., & Eimer, B. N. (2006). *Ideomotor signals for rapid hypnoanalysis, a how-to manual.* Springfield, IL: Charles C. Thomas.

Faymonville, M. E., Laurys, S., Degueldre, C., et al. (2000). Neural mechanisms of antinociceptive effects of hypnosis. *Anesthesiology, 92*, 1257–1267.

Felt, B. T., Hall, H., Olness, K., et al. (1998). Wart regression in children, comparison of relaxation-imagery to topical treatment and equal time interventions. *American Journal of Clinical Hypnosis, 41*, 130–138.

Fick, L. J., Lang, E. V., Logan, H. L., et al. (1999). Imagery content during nonpharmacologic analgesia in the procedure suite, where your patients would rather be. *Academic Radiology, 6,* 457–463.

Frankel, F. H., & Misch, R. C. (1973). Hypnosis in a case of long-standing psoriasis in a person with character problems. *International Journal of Clinical and Experimental Hypnosis, 21,* 212–130.

Freeman, R., Barabasz, A., Barabasz, M., et al. (2000). Hypnosis and distraction differ in their effects on cold pressor pain. *American Journal of Clinical Hypnosis, 43,* 137–148.

Galski, T. J. (1981). The adjunctive use of hypnosis in the treatment of trichotillomania, a case report. *American Journal of Clinical Hypnosis, 23,* 198–201.

Golan, H. P. (1997). The use of hypnosis in the treatment of psychogenic oral pain. *American Journal of Clinical Hypnosis, 40,* 89–96.

Griesemer, R. D. (1978). Emotionally triggered disease in a dermatological practice. *Psychiatric Annals, 8,* 49–56.

Grossbart, T. A., & Sherman, C. (1992). *Skin deep, a mind/body program for healthy skin* (rev. ed.). Santa Fe, NM: Health Press.

Gupta, M. A., & Gupta, A. K. (2003). Depression and dermatological disorders. In J. Y. M. Koo & C. S. Lee (eds.), *Psychocutaneous medicine* (pp. 233–249). New York: Marcel Dekker.

Harrison, P. V., & Stepanek, P. (1991). Hypnotherapy for alopecia areata [letter]. *British Journal of Dermatology, 124,* 509–510.

Hartland, J. (1969). Hypnosis in dermatology. *British Journal of Clinical Hypnosis, 1,* 2–7.

Hollander, M. B. (1959). Excoriated acne controlled by post-hypnotic suggestion. *American Journal of Clinical Hypnosis, 1,* 122–123.

Hölzle, E. (1994). Therapie der hyperhidrosis. *Hautarzt, 35,* 7–15.

Hughes, H., Brown, B. W., Lawlis, G. F., et al. (1983). Treatment of acne vulgaris by biofeedback relaxation and cognitive imagery. *Journal of Psychosomatic Research, 3,* 185–191.

Jabush, M. (1969). A case of chronic recurring multiple boils treated with hypnotherapy. *Psychiatric Quarterly, 43,* 448–455.

Jacobson, E. (1929). *Progressive relaxation.* Chicago: University of Chicago Press.

Johnson, R. F. Q., & Barber, T. X. (1978). Hypnosis, suggestions, and warts, an experimental investigation implicating the importance of "believed-in efficacy". *American Journal of Clinical Hypnosis, 20,* 165–174.

Kabat-Zinn, J. (1990). *Full catastrophe living: Using the wisdom of your body and mind to face stress, pain and illness.* New York: Delacorte.

Kabat-Zinn, J. (1994). *Wherever you go, there you are: Mindfulness meditation in everyday life.* New York: Hyperion.

Kabat-Zinn, J. (1998). Influence of a mindfulness meditation-based stress reduction intervention on rates of skin clearing in patients with moderate to severe psoriasis undergoing phototherapy (UVB) and photochemotherapy (PUVA). *Psychosomatic Medicine, 60,* 625–632.

Kallio, S., Hyona, J., Revonsuo, A., et al. (2011). The existence of a hypnotic state revealed by eye movements. *PLOS One, 6*(10), e26374.

Kantor, S. D. (1990). Stress and psoriasis. *Cutis, 46,* 321–322.

Kaschel, R., Revenstorf, D., & Wörz, B. (1991). Hypnose und haut, trends und perspecktiven. *Experimentalische und Klinische Hypnose, 7,* 65–82.

Kidd, C. B. (1966). Congenital ichthyosiform erythroderma treated by hypnosis. *British Journal of Dermatology, 78,* 101–105.

Kiecolt-Glaser, J. K., McGuire, L., Robles, T. F., et al. (2002). Psychoneuroimmunology and psychosomatic medicine, back to the future. *Psychosomatic Medicine, 64,* 15–28.

Kline, M. (1953). Delimited hypnotherapy, the acceptance of resistance in the treatment of a long standing neurodermatitis with a sensory-imagery technique. *International Journal of Clinical and Experimental Hypnosis, 1,* 18–22.

Kline, M. V. (1954). Psoriasis and hypnotherapy, a case report. *International Journal of Clinical and Experimental Hypnosis, 2,* 318–322.

Koblenzer, C. S. (1987). *Psychocutaneous disease.* Orlando, (FL: Grune & Stratton.

Koldys, K. W., & Meyer, R. P. (1979). Biofeedback training in the therapy of dyshidrosis. *Cutis, 24,* 219–221.

Lang, E. V., Benotsch, E. G., Fick, L. J., et al. (2000). Adjunctive non-pharmacological analgesia for invasive medical procedures, a randomised trial. *Lancet, 355,* 1486–1490.

Lang, E. V., & Rosen, M. P. (2002). Cost analysis of adjunct hypnosis with sedation during outpatient interventional radiologic procedures. *Radiology, 222,* 375–382.

Lehman, R. E. (1978). Brief hypnotherapy of neurodermatitis, a case with four-year follow-up. *American Journal of Clinical Hypnosis, 21,* 48–51.

Linden, W. (1990). *Autogenic training, a clinical guide.* New York: Guilford Press.

Marmer, M. J. (1959). *Hypnosis in anesthesiology.* Springfield, IL: Charles C. Thomas.

Mason, A. A. (1952). A case of congenital ichthyosiform erythroderma of Brocq treated by hypnosis. *British Medical Journal, 2,* 422–423.

McDowell, M. (1949). Juvenile warts removed with the use of hypnotic suggestion. *Bulletin of the Menninger Clinic, 13,* 124–126.

Montgomery, G. H., DuHamel, K. N., & Redd, W. H. (2000). A meta-analysis of hypnotically induced analgesia, how effective is hypnosis? *International Journal of Clinical and Experimental Hypnosis, 48,* 138–153.

Morgan, A. H., & Hilgard, E. R. (1973). Age differences in susceptibility to hypnosis. *International Journal of Clinical and Experimental Hypnosis, 21,* 78–85.

Morris, B. A. P. (1985). Hypnotherapy of warts using the Simonton visualization technique, a case report. *American Journal of Clinical Hypnosis, 27,* 237–240.

Noll, R. B. (1988). Hypnotherapy of a child with warts. *Journal of Developmental and Behavioral Pediatrics, 9,* 89–91.

Noll, R. B. (1994). Hypnotherapy for warts in children and adolescents. *Journal of Developmental and Behavioral Pediatrics, 15,* 170–173.

Obermayer, M. E., & Greenson, R. R. (1949). Treatment by suggestion of verrucae planae of the face. *Psychosomatic Medicine, 11,* 163–164.

Olness, K. N. (1986). Hypnotherapy in children. *Postgraduate Medicine*, *79*(4), 95–100, 105.

Otani, A. (2003). Eastern meditative techniques and hypnosis, a new synthesis. *American Journal of Clinical Hypnosis*, *46*, 97–108.

Perloff, M. M., & Spiegelman, J. (1973). Hypnosis in the treatment of a child's allergy to dogs. *American Journal of Clinical Hypnosis*, *15*, 269–272.

Rainville, P., Hofbauer, R. K., Bushnell, M. C., et al. (2002). Hypnosis modulates activity in brain structures involved in the regulation of consciousness. *Journal of Cognitive Neuroscience*, *14*(6), 887–901.

Rossi, E. (1982). Hypnosis and ultradian cycles, a new state(s) theory of hypnosis? *American Journal of Clinical Hypnosis*, *25*, 21–32.

Rowen, R. (1981). Hypnotic age regression in the treatment of a self-destructive habit, trichotillomania. *American Journal of Clinical Hypnosis*, *23*, 195–197.

Sacerdote, P. (1965). Hypnotherapy in neurodermatitis, a case report. *American Journal of Clinical Hypnosis*, *7*, 249–253.

Schneck, J. M. (1954). Ichthyosis treated with hypnosis. *Diseases of the Nervous System*, *15*, 211–214.

Schneck, J. M. (1966). Hypnotherapy for ichthyosis. *Psychosomatics*, *7*, 233–235.

Scott, M. J. (1960). *Hypnosis in skin and allergic diseases*. Springfield, IL: Charles C. Thomas.

Scott, M. J. (1963). Hypnosis in dermatology. In J. M. Schneck (ed.), *Hypnosis in modern medicine* (3rd ed., pp. 122–142). Springfield, IL: Charles C. Thomas.

Scott, M. J. (1964). Hypnosis in dermatologic therapy. *Psychosomatics*, *5*, 365–368.

Sheehan, D. V. (1978). Influence of psychosocial factors on wart remission. *American Journal of Clinical Hypnosis*, *20*, 160–164.

Shenefelt, P. D. (2000). Hypnosis in dermatology. *Archives of Dermatology*, *136*, 393–399.

Shenefelt, P. D. (2003). Hypnosis-facilitated relaxation during self-guided imagery during dermatologic procedures. *American Journal of Clinical Hypnosis*, *45*, 225–232.

Shenefelt, P. D. (2004). Using hypnosis to facilitate resolution of psychogenic excoriations in acne excoriée. *American Journal of Clinical Hypnosis*, *46*(3), 239–245.

Shenefelt, P. D. (2007). Psychocutaneous hypnoanalysis, detection and deactivation of emotional and mental root factors in psychosomatic skin disorders. *American Journal of Clinical Hypnosis*, *50*, 131–136.

Shenefelt, P. D. (2010). Hypnoanalysis for dermatologic disorders. *Journal of Alternative Medicine Research*, *2*(4), 439–445.

Shenefelt, P. D. (2011). Ideomotor signaling, from divining spiritual messages to discerning subconscious answers during hypnosis and hypnoanalysis, a historical perspective. *American Journal of Clinical Hypnosis*, *53*(3), 157–167.

Shenefelt, P. D. (2013) Anxiety reduction using hypnotic induction and self-guided imagery for relaxation during dermatologic procedures. *International Journal of Clinical and Experimental Hypnosis*, *61*(3), 305–318.

Shertzer, C. L., & Lookingbill, D. P. (1987). Effects of relaxation therapy and hypnotizability in chronic urticaria. *Archives of Dermatology*, *123*, 913–916.

Sinclair-Gieben, A. H. C., & Chalmers, D. (1959). Evaluation of treatment of warts by hypnosis. *Lancet, 2,* 480–482.

Spanos, N. P., Stenstrom, R. J., & Johnston, J. C. (1988). Hypnosis, placebo, and suggestion in the treatment of warts. *Psychosomatic Medicine, 50,* 245–260.

Spanos, N. P., Williams, V., & Gwynn, M. I. (1990). Effects of hypnotic, placebo, and salicylic acid treatments on wart regression. *Psychosomatic Medicine, 52,* 109–114.

Spiegel, D. (2011). Mind matters in cancer survival. *Journal of the American Medical Association, 305*(5), 502–503.

Spiegel, H., & Spiegel, D. (2004). *Trance and treatment, clinical uses of hypnosis* (2nd ed., pp. 51–92). Washington DC: American Psychiatric Publishing.

Stankler, L. (1967). A critical assessment of the cure of warts by suggestion. *Practitioner, 198,* 690–694.

Stewart, A. C., & Thomas, S. E. (1995). Hypnotherapy as a treatment for atopic dermatitis in adults and children. *British Journal of Dermatology, 132,* 778–783.

Straatmeyer, A. J., & Rhodes, N. R. (1983). Condyloma acuminata, results of treatment using hypnosis. *Journal of the American Academy of Dermatology, 9,* 434–436.

Sulzberger, M. B., & Wolf. J. (1934). The treatment of warts by suggestion. *Medical Record, 140,* 552–556.

Surman, O. S., Gottlieb, S. K., & Hackett, T. P. (1972). Hypnotic treatment of a child with warts. *American Journal of Clinical Hypnosis, 15,* 12–14.

Surman, O. S., Gottlieb, S. K., Hackett, T. P., et al. (1973). Hypnosis in the treatment of warts. *Archives of General Psychiatry, 28,* 439–441.

Szekely, A., Kovacs-Nagy R., Bányai, E. I., et al. (2010) Association between hypnotizability and the catechol-o-methyltansferase (COMT) polymorphism. *International Journal of Clinical and Experimental Hypnosis, 58*(3), 301–315.

Tasini, M. F., & Hackett, T. P. (1977). Hypnosis in the treatment of warts in immunodeficient children. *American Journal of Clinical Hypnosis, 19,* 152–154.

Tausk, F., & Whitmore, S. E. (1999). A pilot study of hypnosis in the treatment of patients with psoriasis. *Psychotherapeutics and Psychosomatics, 495,* 1–9.

Tausk, F. A. (1998). Alternative medicine: is it all in your mind? *Archives of Dermatology, 134,* 1422–1425.

Tenzel, J. H., & Taylor, R. L. (1969). An evaluation of hypnosis and suggestion as treatment for warts. *Psychosomatics, 10,* 252–257.

Tobia, L. (1982). L'ipnosi in dermatologia. *Minerva Medica, 73,* 531–537.

Twerski, A. J., & Naar, R. (1974). Hypnotherapy in a case of refractory dermatitis. *American Journal of Clinical Hypnosis, 16,* 202–205.

Ullman, M. (1959). On the psyche and warts, I. Suggestion and warts, a review and comment. *Psychosomatic Medicine, 21,* 473–488.

Ullman, M., & Dudek, S. (1960). On the psyche and warts, II. Hypnotic suggestion and warts. *Psychosomatic Medicine, 22,* 68–76.

Vickers, C. F. H. (1961). Treatment of plantar warts in children. *British Medical Journal, 2,* 743–745.

Waxman, D. (1973). Behaviour therapy of psoriasis—a hypnoanalytic and counter-conditioning technique. *Postgraduate Medical Journal, 49,* 591–595.

Willemsen, R., Vanderlinden, J., Deconinck, A., et al. (2006). Hypnotherapeutic management of alopecia areata. *Journal of the American Academy of Dermatology, 55,* 233–237.

Winchell, S. A., & Watts, R. A. (1988). Relaxation therapies in the treatment of psoriasis and possible pathophysiologic mechanisms. *Journal of the American Academy of Dermatology, 18,* 101–104.

Wink, C. A. S. (1961). Congenital ichthyosiform erythroderma treated by hypnosis. *British Medical Journal, 2,* 741–743.

Zachariae, R., Oster, H., Bjerring, P., et al. (1996). Effects of psychologic intervention on psoriasis, a preliminary report. *Journal of the American Academy of Dermatology, 34,* 1008–1015.

Zane, L. T. (2003). Psychoneuroendocrinimmunodermatology: Pathophysiological mechanisms of stress in cutaneous disease. In J. Y. M. Koo & C. S. Lee (eds.), *Psychocutaneous medicine* (pp. 65–95). New York: Marcel Dekker.

11

Energy Medicine in Dermatology

PHILIP D. SHENEFELT

Key Concepts

- ♣ Energy medicine involves the nonpharmacologic concept of using energy flow for the treatment of disorders, including skin conditions. Its use is derived from a number of cultures ranging from Chinese with their emphasis on acupuncture meridians, to Russian with their emphasis on electrical phenomena, to Peruvian shamans with their emphasis on light refined versus heavy energy. These approaches contrast with the usual Western European focus on biochemical treatments based on pharmacology.
- ♣ Acupuncture point tapping with or without muscle testing is a simple, nontoxic, and easily learned method that has been reported effective for certain skin conditions but does not yet have randomized controlled trial evidence.
- ♣ Biofeedback has been shown to be useful for skin conditions with autonomic aspects and for relaxation training.
- ♣ Cranial electrotherapy stimulation has produced significant improvement in patients with neurodermatitis and atopic dermatitis, including less scratching.
- ♣ Eye movement desensitization and reprocessing has helped to improve atopic dermatitis and psoriasis.
- ♣ Qigong may benefit those with atopic dermatitis or psoriasis.

Introduction

Energy medicine covers a range of nonpharmacologic methods that involve the concept of using energy flow for treatment. A much more extensive discussion is available in Shealy (2011). Most of these methods do not yet have good evidence-based scientific validation. Some are based on the concept of energy stagnating or being blocked in some part of the body with deleterious health effects, and with treatments restoring the free flow of energy.

An example is the Chinese acupuncture techniques that help to restore the normal flow of stagnant, blocked, or excessive *chi* or *qi* energy (see Chapter 7). With acupressure, firm pressure may be used instead of needles at acupuncture points. Tapping on specific acupuncture points similarly helps to rebalance energy. Tapping on acupuncture points has been developed into several systems, including Thought Field Therapy, Emotional Freedom Technique, Be Set Free Fast, and others (see below for references). Another example is Cosmic Freedom Qigong (CFQ; see below), with its focus on loosening and releasing stuck energy through slow exercises and meditation.

The metaphor used by the Peruvian Andean Q'ero *paqo* (shaman) is that the life force energy that animates everything, called *kawsay* in Quechua, when it is not flowing properly in the body becomes thick, congealed, and heavy, termed *hucha*, especially in the area centered near the navel (*poq'po*) when the person fails to live in attuned reciprocity. There is no value judgment that the heavy dense energy is "bad" or "evil," only that it is harmful in obstructing natural flow and can eventually cause disease. Fear, anger, grief, shame, and resentment from unresolved traumas can leave the person drained of life force energy and filled with toxic emotions and patterns that set him or her up for rewounding or remaining stuck. In some instances, this can manifest as a skin disease. With proper use of intention, the heavy energy can be digested and cleansed (*mikhuy*), making room for light refined energy (*sami*) that restores proper flow (Wilcox, 1999). The *paqo* shaman apprentice learns to do this first for himself and then to assist others. Villoldo (2000) describes additional aspects of Peruvian shamanism in more detail. Levi-Strauss (1963) describes how individual cognitions may be shaped by cultural assumptions during the process. The shaman reorganizes the chaotic and painful experience for the patient through processes of abreaction and transference and fits it into a comprehensible familiar mythical system. This reorganization on the psychospiritual level also affects the emotional and physical levels. Frequently relatives and other community members are present during the process and lend support before, during, and after the shamanic session. One criticism of modern Western healing is that it often lacks the integrative community support aspects that are helpful adjuncts to shamanic healing. Harner (1980, 2013) describes many aspects of shamanism in greater detail.

In India the body energy system is metaphorically described as seven chakras, wheels of light or energy vortices, that likewise can become impaired or blocked by stagnant energy and can be cleared by meditation with proper intention. Each chakra is associated with specific aspects of bodily function, including an endocrine gland, and with a specific musical note and a specific color of light. Chakra clearing can be done through meditation, toning of musical notes, or experiencing associated colors of light.

Various other systems involving subtle energy transfer from one person to another have been developed but not scientifically verified beyond the placebo effect. Such methods include Reiki, Therapeutic Touch, and many others. Therapeutic massage such as neurolymphatic massage and Mayan abdominal massage are other nonverified methods. Electronic devices such as the Alpha-Stim using a weak alternating current of specific design (see details below) can be used regionally for pain relief in conditions such as post-herpetic neuralgia, or as cranial electrotherapy stimulation for altering anxiety and picking behaviors in neurodermatitis. The Alpha-Stim has been relatively well researched. Biofeedback devices that help train a person to alter heart rate variability, such as the emWave Personal Stress Reliever or StressEraser, are also available and can help a person attain relaxation. The word "energy" (Ancient Greek: ἐνέργεια [energeia], meaning "activity, operation") describes an abstract concept of an indirectly observed quantity that is often understood as the ability of a physical system to do work on other physical systems. Since work is defined as a force acting through a distance (a length of space), energy is always equivalent to the ability to exert pulls or pushes against the basic forces of nature, along a path of a certain length. The joule (J) is a derived unit of energy equivalent to (kilogram $\times$ meter^2)/second^2 in the International System of Units. This applies to kinetic energy and physical potential energy as well as electromagnetic light energy. Visible light is also measured in lumens, which relates to luminous flux that can be perceived by the eye. Chemical energy in food is more commonly expressed in kilocalories, usually just called "calories," representing about 4.2 kilojoules per (kilo)calorie. Electrical energy is usually expressed in watts per second, equivalent to passing an electric current of one ampere through a resistance of one ohm for one second, which is equivalent to one joule. Electrical energy is also expressed in kilowatt hours equivalent to 3.6 megajoules per kilowatt hour. As a reminder of electrical relationships, a volt equals amperes times resistance, which equals watts divided by amperes, which equals joules divided by (amperes $\times$ seconds). Voltage is electrical potential difference, while amperage is electrical current flow. The subtle energies discussed in this chapter are on the order of microwatts per second or microjoules. Biological systems are sensitive to small amounts of energy. The heart electrocardiogram is in the millivolt range, and the brain electroencephalogram (EEG) is weaker but also in the millivolt range.

The placebo effect is a factor in all treatment modalities, both conventional and alternative. Positive expectations and a positive doctor–patient relationship affect the patient's experience of treatment, can reduce pain, and may influence outcome. Negative expectations can produce negative (nocebo) results (Spiegel, 2004). Care must be taken in selecting language that will have a positive rather than a negative effect on the patient. Research on the placebo effect illustrates that the natural healing capacities of individuals can be enhanced and nurtured (Di Blasi & Reilly, 2005). The placebo effect for some common dermatologic conditions such as acne and urticaria is about 30% (Gupta & Gupta, 1996). The Griesemer index (Griesemer, 1978, also see Table 10.1 in Chapter 10) rates dermatologic disorders on a percentage scale from 100% to 0% based on emotional triggering of the condition. Those skin disorders higher on the Griesemer scale are likely to be influenced more by the placebo effect. Adults exercise varying degrees of judgment and have varying beliefs and expectations, both conscious and unconscious, that interact with the placebo effect. Younger children are often easily influenced, while adolescents may resist influence by physicians and parents. Ethical considerations often limit the application of the placebo in clinical practice.

Suggestion in the usual alert conscious state can also be used to change subjective perceptions and to reduce pain and may influence outcome. Reports on the efficacy of suggestion in treating verruca vulgaris have since been confirmed numerous times to a greater or lesser degree (Ullman, 1959). Adults exercise varying degrees of judgment and have varying beliefs and expectations that interact with conscious and subconscious acceptance or rejection of the suggestion. Younger children often are in a hypnoid state of consciousness as they play imaginatively and often readily accept suggestions. Resistant toddlers can sometimes be directed to do the opposite to get the desired effect. Resistant adolescents are more difficult to reach except through peers. Physician or provider interactions with the patient have metaphorically been called a symphony in four hemispheres, with the left and right hemispheres of each person interactive on a conscious and subconscious level. Linguistic, cultural, and individual factors all play a role in communication, expectations and beliefs, trust and faith, and a multitude of other factors that can influence treatment outcome.

Specific Energy Medicine Options for Integrative Medicine

ACUPUNCTURE POINT TAPPING WITH OR WITHOUT MUSCLE TESTING

Acupuncture point meridian tapping and holding techniques and muscle testing techniques include Applied Kinesiology (Goodheart, 1975), Behavioral

Kinesiology (Diamond, 1979), Thought Field Therapy (TFT) (Callahan, 1985), Emotional Stress Release (Goodheart, 1987), Visual/Kinesthetic Dissociation, which is a NeuroLinguistic Programming technique (Bandler & Grinder, 1979), Eye Movement Desensitization and Reprocessing (EMDR) (Shapiro, 1995), Traumatic Incident Reduction (Gerbode, 1989), Emotional Freedom Techniques (EFT) (Craig and Fowlie, 1995), Be Set Free Fast (Nims, 2002), Touch for Health (Thie, 1973), Clinical Kinesiology (Beardall, 1995), Educational Kinesiology (Dennison & Dennison, 1989), Tapas Acupressure Technique (Fleming, 1996), Healing From the Body Up (Swack, 2002), Frontal/Occipital Holding as part of Three-in-One Concepts or One Brain (Stokes and Whiteside, 1984), Neuro-Emotional Technique (Walker, 1996), Seemorg Matrix Work (Clinton, 2002), Energy Diagnostic and Treatment Methods (Gallo 2000), Negative Affect Releasing Method (Gallo and Vincenzi, 2000), Neuro-Energetic Sensory Technique (Gallo, 2005), and Healing Energy Light Process (Gallo, 2000). Some consider the tapping and holding techniques to be trance-inducing. They deserve consideration for a place in the therapeutic toolbox despite scanty solid scientific corroboration of their effectiveness at this time. These methods do not lend themselves well to evaluation by the logical positivist first-order linear scientific randomized controlled trial method, similar to Newtonian physics, where the observer is considered external to the system and is not influencing the system. Second-order "cybernetics of cybernetics" methods similar to quantum physics, which include the observer in the system and influencing the system, are more appropriate for studying the efficacy of the above methods but are currently less developed and accepted by our society (Becvar & Becvar, 2009). The muscle testing is performed to gain responses from the subconscious without having to induce trance. It is a form of ideomotor signaling. A study on highly efficient therapies compared four therapeutic modalities for post-traumatic stress disorder (PTSD). Visual/Kinesthetic Dissociation (Bandler & Grinder, 1979), EMDR (Shapiro, 1995), Traumatic Incident Reduction (Gerbode, 1989), and TFT (Callahan, 1985) were compared in a study by Carbonell and Figley (1999) for effectiveness in terms of time required and preintervention and postintervention subjective units of distress scale scores, with TFT being more time efficient. These methods may also be used to reduce chronic excessive stress and specific traumatic issues, with the potential for improvement of inflammatory skin diseases such as atopic dermatitis and psoriasis.

ENERGY DIAGNOSTIC AND TREATMENT METHODS
WITH MUSCLE TESTING

Gallo described this method in the first edition of *Energy Psychology* (Gallo, 1998), in *Energy Diagnostic and Treatment Methods* (Gallo, 2000), and in the second edition of *Energy Psychology* (Gallo, 2005). He also has coauthored *The Neurophysics of Human Behavior* (Furman & Gallo, 2000), *Energy Psychology and EMDR* (Hartung et al., 2003), *Energy Tapping* (Gallo & Vincenzi, 2000, 2008), and *Energy Tapping for Trauma* (Gallo & Robbins, 2007) and edited *Energy Psychology in Psychotherapy* (Gallo, 2002). The second edition of *Energy Psychology* (Gallo, 2005) laid the conceptual and historical background and then described the process. "Scientific Theaters" discusses various paradigms or lenses through which psychotherapy can be viewed. These include psychodynamic, behavioral-environmental, cognitive, system-cybernetic, biochemical, neurologic, and energy paradigms. "The Energy Paradigm (Or the Electric Patterns of Life)" describes acupuncture with its energy meridians and points and morphogenetic fields. "Origins of Energy Psychology (Or Adding Muscle to Therapy)" relates the historical development of manual muscle testing (strong or weak), neurolymphatic reflexes, and neurovascular reflexes as Applied Kinesiology (Goodheart, 1975), Touch for Health (Thie, 1973), Clinical Kinesiology (Beardall, 1995), Educational Kinesiology (Dennison & Dennison, 1989), One Brain/Three-in-One Concepts (Stokes & Whiteside, 1984), Neuro-Emotional Technique (Walker, 1996), Behavioral Kinesiology (Diamond, 1979), and TFT (Callahan, 1985). "The Diamond Method to Cantillation" describes Behavioral Kinesiology in more depth. Diamond applied the manual muscle testing (strong or weak) in Behavioral Kinesiology while the client touched a specific acupuncture point called an alarm point and concluded that each of the 12 acupuncture meridians is associated with specific negative and positive emotions. He also discovered energy "morality" reversal and emphasized the importance of the thymus, a major gland of the immune system. "Thought Field Therapy" relates how with TFT (Callahan, 1985) developed diagnostic and treatment algorithms based on manual muscle testing (strong or weak) and 14 key meridian points (one for each of the 12 bilateral meridians and one for each of the two central meridians). He also emphasized treating psychological reversal and had ancillary treatments such as nine gamut, eye roll, and collarbone breathing. "The Energy Therapist's Manual" is the core chapter in Gallo (2005). It describes TFT techniques followed by algorithms for specific psychological problems, listed in alphabetical order. Following this are descriptions of related treatment methods, including Frontal/Occipital Holding (Stokes & Whiteside, 1894), EFT (Craig & Fowlie, 1995), Tapas Acupressure Technique (Fleming, 1996), Energy Diagnostic and Treatment Methods (Gallo, 2000), Negative Affect Releasing Method (Gallo & Vincenzi, 2000), Healing Energy Light Process (Gallo, 2000), and Neuro-Energetic Sensory Technique (Gallo, 2005). "Beginnings" further discusses research in energy psychology, further clinical issues, and standard algorithms such as in EFT versus energy diagnostics such as in TFT. The appendix "Manual Muscle Testing Uses and

Abuses" describes appropriate uses of manual muscle testing and also times when it is not necessary, such as when using EFT. Muscle testing can also be thought of as ideomotor signaling without formal trance induction. The glossary includes several methods not previously mentioned in the book, including Be Set Free Fast (Nims, 2002), Energy Consciousness Therapy (Gallo, 2005), Healing From the Body Up (Swack, 2002), and Seemorg Matrix Work (Clinton, 2002), now renamed Advanced Integrative Therapy.

So what is one to make of this group of techniques? Is there fire in the energy medicine paradigm or just smoke (the placebo effect)? Viewed from the logical positivist first-order approach of Newtonian physics-type external observer science, research thus far is not very objective and it all looks rather suspect. Viewed from the second-order approach of quantum physics-type involved observer science, however, subjectivity and interconnectedness and uncertainty make the energy paradigm harder to reject. At the pragmatic level, empowering the patient or client to self-soothe through learned tapping or holding routines, rather than relying on the physician or provider for soothing, promotes self-reliance and increased resilience in the face of life's traumas and stressors. These tapping and holding techniques can be used to increase efficacy in the fields of psychology and psychiatry. They can be equally helpful for the many psychosomatic issues that are prevalent in medicine and its specialty areas, including dermatology.

EMOTIONAL FREEDOM TECHNIQUE
WITHOUT MUSCLE TESTING

EFT (Craig, 2008) tapping points are related to acupressure. EFT starts with selecting a negatively emotionally charged memory or problem area, focusing intently on that thought or memory or condition, pressing on the subclavicular "sore spot," and repeating an affirmation such as "Even though I have this problem with _____, I deeply and completely accept myself" while progressively tapping with the finger on a series of up to 14 specific acupuncture sites on the head, chest, and hand. For infants, toddlers, and preschoolers, this tapping process can be done for them, either directly on them or on a surrogate. Older children, adolescents, and adults can be taught to use the technique themselves. EFT can neutralize negative emotionally charged memories or problem areas, reducing anxiety and enhancing performance (Craig, 2008). Tapping on all 14 of the acupressure sites obviates the need for muscle testing. Anecdotally reported improvements or resolution of skin conditions on www.EFTuniverse. com (accessed August 28, 2011) include acne, allergic contact dermatitis, atopic dermatitis, herpes simplex recurrences, lupus erythematosus, needle phobia, procedure anxiety, post-herpetic neuralgia, psoriasis, and warts.

A controlled comparison of EFT with EMDR (see below) in a study that included older adolescents and adults showed that for PTSD both produced significant therapeutic gains (Karatzias et al., 2011). Some patients do develop PTSD as a result of life events that were overwhelmingly traumatic to them, including hospitalizations and medical procedures. A lay-oriented book, *The Tapping Cure* (Temes, 2006), is an easily accessible quick read for understanding EFT. Reducing emotional distress often results in improvement of inflammatory skin conditions such as acne, atopic dermatitis, and psoriasis.

BIOFEEDBACK

Biofeedback involves the use of instruments to provide real-time visual or auditory feedback about specifically measureable biological activities. The focus here will be on biofeedback of electrical activities. Biofeedback training can improve skin problems that have an autonomic nervous system component such as biofeedback of galvanic skin resistance for hyperhidrosis. For children, incorporating a game or some play aspect into the biofeedback can help to maintain the child's interest and motivation. Biofeedback may result in some improvement in atopic dermatitis (Haynes et al., 1979). Hypnosis may enhance the effects obtained by biofeedback (Dikel & Olness, 1980; Shenefelt, 2003). Quantitative EEG biofeedback has been used to alter behaviors and rewire the brain through promoting neuroplasticity. Heart rate variability biofeedback with hand-held electronic devices such as the emWave Personal Stress Reliever or StressEraser can promote relaxation, improving skin conditions worsened by stress. Relaxation can benefit most inflammatory skin disorders, including atopic dermatitis and psoriasis.

CHAKRA CLEARING AND BALANCING

Chakras are conceived as deeper energy centers in the body. Seven main chakras are perceived in both the Hindu and the Incan descriptions. The root chakra at the base of the spine in the pudendal area is associated with survival and procreation, fear, the adrenals, the color red, and the musical note C. The sacral chakra below the navel in the abdomen is connected to sexuality, guilt, the ovaries and testes, the color orange, and the musical note D. The solar plexus chakra above the navel in the abdomen is associated with power, shame, the pancreas, the color yellow, and the musical note E. The heart chakra in mid-chest is connected with love, grief, the thymus, the color green, and the musical note F. The throat chakra at the throat is associated with psychic expression, lies, the thyroid and parathyroid, the color sky blue, and the musical note G. The third eye chakra mid-forehead is connected with truth, illusion, the pituitary, the color indigo blue, and the musical note A. The crown chakra is associated with universal ethics, attachment, the pineal gland, the color violet, and the musical note B. The solar plexus chakra is said to influence the skin, while the heart chakra influences immunity and the skin. The sacral chakra can affect the skin through the sex hormones. The root and crown chakras can also be associated with skin diseases. The throat chakra can affect the skin through the thyroid and the third eye chakra through the pituitary. Meditative visualizing or otherwise sensing each chakra in turn can pinpoint blockages that can be cleared through meditation or toning of the appropriate musical note. Perceived weak chakras can be strengthened and the chakras balanced. Metaphorically by extension, chakras can also connote geographic healing places (Grover & Lakasing, 2009). Inflammatory skin diseases such as atopic dermatitis and psoriasis are the most likely to respond. Whether this process achieves more than placebo effect has not yet been established through scientific study.

CRANIAL ELECTROTHERAPY STIMULATION

Cranial electrotherapy stimulation (CES) was first developed in Russia and then transferred via Japan to the United States. Kirsch (2002) developed the Alpha-Stim, first focusing on its use for chronic pain as a milder and more effective method than the transepidermal nerve stimulation electrical devices developed by Shealy. The Alpha-Stim was also used for CES and was found to be effective in reducing anxiety and depression (Kirsch, 2002; Kirsch & Smith, 2007). In describing the historical development of CES, Smith (2002) noted the differences in basic reference framework for scientists in different cultures. The Russians who first developed CES as electrosleep (a misnomer) had a theoretical science of the nervous system built on Pavlov's research, conceptualized in terms of inhibition, disinhibition, neural excitation, and conditioning. There was more focus in Russia on the electrical aspects of the nervous system compared with Western medicine, where brain activity is conceptualized mostly in terms of neurochemical reactions at the presynaptic and postsynaptic neural junctures. The Western emphasis for treatment has been primarily on drugs that can affect the nervous system, such as antidepressants and antipsychotics. The Chinese emphasis has been on *qi* energy flow, and treatment has been with acupuncture and herbal medicine combinations, while in India the emphasis has been on chakra energy flow treated with yoga, diet, balancing of the *doshas*, and herbal medicines. The Alpha-Stim, when used with earclips, measurably affects the brain, normalizing the EEG and inducing predominant alpha rhythm using 10 to 600 microamperes of rectangular-wave spiked alternating current at low voltage and at 0.5 hertz and 50% duty cycle powered by a nine-volt battery and applied usually for 20 minutes per session. For chronic problems, usually 30 or more sessions are needed to effect permanent change. As a rule of thumb, it typically takes 20 to 40 repetitions of doing something different to change a habit or a reactive pattern. Use of the Alpha-Stim CES has excellent supportive research documenting reduced anxiety and depression (Kirsch, 2002). CES has produced significant improvement of atopic dermatitis and neurodermatitis, including reduction in scratching behavior (Turaeva, 1967).

EYE MOVEMENT DESENSITIZATION AND REPROCESSING

EMDR involves selecting a negatively emotionally charged memory or problem area, focusing on that thought, and doing an alternating bilateral activity such as following a finger from side to side with the eyes (Shapiro, 2001), hearing alternating left and right tones through headphones, feeling alternating left and right vibrations in handheld paddles, or alternately tapping left and right distal thighs or upper arms. It is slightly more effective than EFT in producing positive benefits in PTSD (Karatzias et al., 2011). The efficacy of EMDR in children has been evaluated in a meta-analysis. The post-treatment effect size was medium and significant (Rodenburg et al., 2009). When combined with the EFT affirmations it becomes a hybrid known as Wholistic Hybrid derived from EMDR and EFT (WHEE), reducing anxiety and enhancing performance (Benor et al., 2009). EMDR has been reported to be effective for improving atopic dermatitis and psoriasis (Gupta & Gupta, 2002).

QIGONG

CFQ (Cosmic Freedom Qigong or Chaoyi Fanhuan Qigong) healing is an approach to releasing stuck energy from prior trauma or stress through repetition of a set of releasing movements and through meditation. Developed by Yap Soon Yeong in Malaysia and propagated in the west by Chok C. Hiew, PhD, a retired professor of psychology at the University of New Brunswick in Fredericton, New Brunswick, CFQ is a method that may enhance release work for stuck energy. The relaxing repetitive movements of CFQ can induce an active alert trance. A set of seven slow CFQ movements called the hexagram dance (after the *I Ching* hexagram patterns) typically takes about 12 to 15 minutes to complete. Three sets per day are recommended. These gentle releasing movements are well described and photographically illustrated in *Dynamics of Qigong Healing* (Hiew & Yeong, 2005). The first third of the book briefly describes the theoretical and practical underpinnings of the process.

This is dealt with in much more detail in their earlier book, *Energy Medicine in CFQ Healing* (Yeong & Hiew, 2002). The remaining two thirds of the book *Dynamics of Qigong Healing* describes and illustrates step by step the movements of the hexagram dance and other complementary movements. The hexagram dance consists of seven sets of movement sequences followed by affirmations and resilient breathing. It is said to promote release of heavy, sticky, unhealthy energy that blocks the natural flow of lighter healthy energy in the body. Dissolving the heavy energy permits recovery of natural homeostatic physical, emotional, mental, and spiritual balance and facilitates healing and resilience.

Western medicine and psychology are analogous to classical Newtonian physics, based on deterministic science thought models where a known cause produces an expected predictable effect. Eastern energy medicine offers a different approach that is comparable to quantum physics thought models in which matter is condensation of energy. The observer affects the observed. All energy and matter are interconnected. Energy is primal, and matter is secondary. Particle and wave are descriptive manifestations of the same quantum of energy. Probability rather than certainty defines location. Humans manifest as energy as well as matter. Because there is an inverse effect with small amounts of matter manifesting large energy components, and large amounts of matter manifesting small energy components, manifestation of human energy is subtle. With proper training and skill development, it is possible for the healer to tune into the subtle human energies and diagnose and treat through evaluating them and having an influence on them. Many systems of energy medicine, such as Reiki and traditional qigong, have complex rules and hierarchies of mastery, requiring accumulation of skills and energy. CFQ focuses on simplicity and release, the opposite of accumulation. Awareness is centered in the abdomen rather than in the head, and wisdom is of the heart rather than of the head.

Natural healing occurs once heavy, sticky energy impediments to healing are dissolved through the relaxed sets of movements and alert mindful releasing meditations. CFQ uses integrative rather than sequential steps to achieve downward release followed by outward radiation of "gold body" ninth chakra energy that promotes healing. The main focus is on the physical mechanics of the movements. CFQ meditation is covered in *Qigong Healing Meditation* (Yeong & Hiew, 2007). The information is again summarized in *Chaoyi Fanhuan Qigong Healing* (Yeong & Hiew, 2009). Further information is available at www.cfqatlantic.ca.

Advantages of CFQ healing are that it is inexpensive and safe, promotes self-help, and may be effective when other measures fail. Disadvantages of CFQ healing include its basis in Buddhist/Taoist philosophies that are not commonly accepted in the West and the experiential learning curve for the practitioner. The commitment required from the patient/client to practice movements and meditation for almost an hour a day is also an issue in a Western culture that prefers quick, easy fixes. There is also the lack of financial support for promoting CFQ because it in many ways is the antithesis to the capitalist system that highly values acquisition and devalues release and true letting go. Fibromyalgia has been reported to improve with qigong in a randomized controlled trial (Astin et al., 2003). CFQ has been shown effective in a pilot trial for fibromyalgia (Lynch et al., 2009). Any stress-aggravated skin disease such as atopic dermatitis or psoriasis may improve or resolve with this CFQ process of gentle releasing movements and meditations.

THERAPEUTIC TOUCH

Oschman (2000) believes that the phenomena of energy medicine can be studied, measured, and explained scientifically without invoking any mysterious life forces or unmeasurable subtle energies. Oschman remarks that "In the past, the most remarkable success stories of complementary therapists (as well as healings in the religious context) were often dismissed because there was no logical explanation." He assumes without support that complementary therapists have had a greater success rate than can be explained by placebo, natural course of disease, and chance, and that dismissal is not simply due to insufficient evidence. Oschman accepts kinds of evidence that most scientists would not. He also believes that some electrotherapy devices of the early 1900s may have been effective, saying there was no evidence for or against them. His core argument begins with the fact that electromagnetic aspects can be detected for all body functions. The heart generates an electrical signal that can be recorded by an electrocardiograph and by magnetocardiography. Electrical aspects of brain function can be monitored on an EEG. Magnetomyograms detect magnetic pulses when muscles contract. Medical uses of x-ray and magnetic resonance imaging, pacemakers, external and internal defibrillators, deep brain pacemakers to inhibit tremor in Parkinson's patients, gastric pacemakers to simulate fullness to help reduce obesity, lasers for treating skin and internal conditions, and blue light for treating acne are all examples of the conventional use of electromagnetic phenomena for diagnosis and treatment. Becker and Selden (1985) demonstrated that alternating magnetic fields applied for 8 to 10 hours a day helps heal broken bones. From these examples, Oschman assumes that application of hands can also heal. Interaction of the patient's and therapist's biomagnetic fields could explain polarity therapy, Therapeutic Touch, and other types of energy healing. He believes that energy healers can perceive electromagnetic fields and can adjust them to optimize health. Oschman takes as evidence a couple of experiments.

A Japanese research group (Seto et al., 1992) measured magnetic fields from the palms of 37 subjects who were believed capable of emitting external *qi* energy. In three of the 37, they detected magnetic fields of 2 to 4 milligauss in the frequency range of 4 to 10 Hz, 1,000 times greater than had been previously measured in humans. In one subject, they attempted to measure the corresponding bioelectric current but were unable to detect it. The experiment so far has not been replicated. Zimmerman(1990) used a superconducting quantum interference device (SQUID) to detect a large biomagnetic field emanating from the hands of a practitioner during Therapeutic Touch so large it could not be quantified by the SQUID device and varying in frequency from 0.3 to 30 Hz, with most of the activity in the 7- to 8-Hz range. Cells are interconnected through molecules in the cell membrane called integrins that regulate most functions of the body and play a role in arthritis, heart disease, stroke, osteoporosis, skin diseases, and cancer. Oschman describes the entire body as being one interconnected organism, a living matrix of communication analogous to the nervous system. "Each fiber of the living matrix, both outside and inside cells and nuclei, is surrounded by an organized layer of water that can serve as a separate channel of communication and energy flow" (Oschsman 2000, p. 56). He claims that communication also occurs through solid-state biochemistry, crystalline arrays, piezoelectricity, and a living tensegrity network that forms a mechanical and vibratory continuum that absorbs healing energies and converts them into acoustic signals. "Each molecule, cell, tissue, and organ has an ideal resonant frequency that coordinates its activities" (Oschsman 2000, p. 58). The perineural tissue forms a distinct communication system that regulates nerve function; acupuncture accesses this network. Energetic bodywork somehow opens and balances the information channels to prevent disease and maintain health. Acupuncture, acupressure, Shiatsu, massage, and structural integration all activate tissue repair processes, possibly by simulating injury. Communication also occurs when changes in collagen density form somatic "memories." Application of therapeutic pressure can release a vivid recollection of trauma, as well as releasing toxins that have accumulated in connective tissues. Structural integration can be achieved through Rolfing, osteopathy, chiropractic, Feldenkrais, yoga, Alexander, craniosacral, myofascial release, and similar methods. Body shape and patterns of movement are said to tell our evolutionary history, the history of our personal traumas, and the story of our present emotional state. Heart rate variability correlates to emotions. With training, it is possible to achieve a state of internal coherence with a heart rate variability of almost zero. This is a calm state where the person is aware of his or her electrical body. It promotes health. DNA acts as a resonant antenna to receive and transmit information coded in the heart's electrical rhythms and in the oscillations of the DNA molecules themselves. Rossi (2002) describes how mind–body interactions can help activate or deactivate transcription of DNA in genes in the cells in a process known as epigenetics. According to Oschman, "A sensitive individual can begin to tune in to these phenomena by focusing on any body rhythm" such as heart rate or cerebrospinal fluid pulsations or breathing. Oschman also invokes quantum theory, which says that strange things can happen, but the risk is that it may provide a convenient excuse for believing ideas that don't make sense to science. He uses the concept of scalar potentials from quantum theory where when two waves cancel each other out, residual information is still available. He then argues that physics allows for action at a distance and instantaneous propagation of scalar waves not bound by the limit of light velocity, proposes that this has biological effects, and claims the only way to study this is to observe electromagnetically sensitive individuals. He also believes in subtle actions at a distance, Jung's synchronicity, transference of evoked brainwaves to another subject in an electromagnetic field-shielded room, and telepathic experiences correlated with calm periods of global geomagnetic activity. Oschman concludes that energy medicine was discovered before its time, but now the time has come to integrate it into scientific knowledge. There is probably no single "life force" or "healing energy." Instead, there is an interaction of many electrical, magnetic, elastic, acoustic, thermal, gravitational, and photonic energies, and possibly other subtle energies that remain to be discovered. He claims that there is a growing body of evidence for energy healing, but that even carefully controlled studies have been dismissed, simply because science does not recognize their rationale. There is much speculation contained in this synthesis. There are anecdotal stories of inflammatory skin conditions such as psoriasis and atopic dermatitis improving or clearing with the use of Therapeutic Touch, but so far no reliable research with respect to skin diseases.

REFERENCES

Astin, J. A., Berman, B. M., Bausell, B., et al. (2003). The efficacy of mindfulness meditation plus Qigong movement therapy in the treatment of fibromyalgia: a randomized controlled trial. *Journal of Rheumatology, 30*(10), 2257–2262.

Bandler R., & Grinder J. (1979). *Frogs into princes*. Moab, UT: Real People Press.

Beardall, A. G. (1995). *Clinical kinesiology laboratory manual*. Portland, OR: Human Biodynamics, Inc.

Becker, R. O., & Selden, G. (1985). *The body electric: Electromagnetism and the foundation of life*. New York: Harper.

Becvar, D. S., & Becvar, R. J. (2009). *Family therapy, a systemic integration* (7th ed.). Boston: Allyn & Bacon.

Benor, D. J., Ledger, K., Toussaint, L., et al. (2009). Pilot study of emotional freedom techniques, wholistic hybrid derived from eye movement desensitization and reprocessing and emotional freedom technique, and cognitive behavioral therapy for treatment of test anxiety in university students. *Explore, 5*, 338–340.

Callahan, R. J. (1985). *Five minute phobia cure: Dr. Callahan's treatment for fears, phobias and self-sabotage*. Wilmington: Enterprise Publishing.

Carbonell, J. L., & Figley, C. (1999). A systematic clinical demonstration project of promising PTSD treatment approaches. *Traumatology-e*, 5(1), article 4, available at www.fsu.edu/~trauma/

Clinton, A. N. (2002). Seemorg Matrix Works, the transpersonal energy psychotherapy. In F. Gallo (Ed.), *Energy psychology in psychotherapy* (pp. 93–115). New York: Norton.

Craig, G. (2008). *The EFT manual*. Santa Rosa, CA: Energy Psychology Press.

Craig, G., & Fowlie, A. (1995). *Emotional freedom techniques: the manual*. The Sea Ranch, CA: author, available at http://www.emofree.com/

Dennison, P. E., & Dennison, G. (1989). *Brain Gym handbook*. Ventura, CA: Educational Kinesiology Foundation.

Di Blasi, Z., & Reilly, D. (2005). Placebos in medicine: medical paradoxes need disentangling [letter]. *British Medical Journal, 330*, 45.

Diamond, J. (1979). *Behavioral kinesiology*. New York: Harper and Row.

Dikel, W., & Olness, K. (1980). Self-hypnosis, biofeedback, and voluntary peripheral temperature control in children. *Pediatrics, 66*, 335–340.

Fleming, T. (1996). *Reduce traumatic stress in minutes: The Tapas Acupressure Technique (TAT) workbook*. Torrance, CA: Author.

Furman, M. E., & Gallo, F. P. (2000). *The neurophysics of human behavior*. Boca Raton, FL: CRC Press.

Gallo, F. P. (1998). *Energy psychology* (1st ed.). Boca Raton, FL: CRC Press.

Gallo, F. P. (2000). *Energy diagnostic and treatment methods*. New York: W.W. Norton & Company.

Gallo, F. P. (Ed.) (2002). *Energy psychology in psychotherapy: a comprehensive sourcebook*. New York: W.W. Norton & Company.

Gallo, F. P. (2005). *Energy psychology: Explorations at the interface of energy, cognition, behavior, and health* (2nd ed.). Boca Raton, FL: CRC Press.

Gallo, F. P., & Robbins, A. (2007). *Energy tapping for trauma*. Oakland, CA: New Harbinger Publications.

Gallo, F. P., & Vincenzi H. (2000, 2nd ed., 2008). *Energy tapping*. Oakland, CA: New Harbinger Publications.

Gerbode, F. (1989). *Beyond psychology: an introduction to metapsychology*. Palo Alto, CA: IRM Press.

Goodheart, G. J. (1975). *Applied kinesiology 1975 workshop procedure manual* (11th ed.). Detroit: Author.

Goodheart, G. J. (1987). *You'll be better*. Geneva, OH: Author.

Griesemer, R. D. (1978). Emotionally triggered disease in a dermatological practice. *Psychiatric Annals, 8*, 49–56.

Grover, S., & Lakasing, E. (2009).The Incas: a journey through history and spirituality. *British Journal of General Practice, 59*(559), 134–135.

Gupta, M. A., & Gupta, A. K. (1996). Psychodermatology: an update. *Journal of the American Academy of Dermatology, 34*, 1030–1046.

Gupta, M. A., & Gupta, A. K. (2002). Use of eye movement desensitization and repro-cessing (EMDR) in the treatment of dermatologic disorders. *Journal of Cutaneous Medicine and Surgery, 6*, 415–421.

Harner, M. (1980). *The way of the shaman: a guide to power and healing.* San Francisco, CA: Harper and Row.

Harner, M. (2013). *Cave and cosmos: shamanic encounters with another reality.* Berkeley, CA, North Atlantic Books.

Hartung, J. G., Galvin, M. D., & Gallo, F. P. (2003). *Energy psychology and EMDR.* New York: W.W. Norton & Company.

Haynes, S. N., Wilson, C. C., Jaffe, P. G., et al. (1979). Biofeedback treatment of atopic dermatitis: controlled case studies of eight cases. *Biofeedback and Self-Regulation, 4*, 195–209.

Hiew, C. C., & Yeong, Y. S. (2005). *Dynamics of qigong healing.* North Charleston, SC: BookSurge Publishing.

Karatzias, T., Power, K., Brown, K., et al. (2011). A controlled comparison of the effec-tiveness and efficiency of two psychological therapies for posttraumatic stress disorder: eye movement desensitization and reprocessing vs. emotional freedom techniques. *Journal of Nervous and Mental Diseases, 199*, 372–378.

Kirsch, D. L. (2002). *The science behind cranial electrotherapy stimulation* (2nd ed.). Edmonton, Alberta: Medical Scope Publishing.

Kirsch, D. L., & Smith, R. B. (2007). Cranial electrotherapy stimulation for anxiety, depression, insomnia, cognitive dysfunction, and pain. In P. J. Rosch & M. Markov (Eds.), *Bioelectromagnetic medicine* (pp. 727–740). New York: Informa Healthcare.

Lynch, M. E., Sawynok, J., & Bouchard, A. (2009). A pilot trial of CFQ for treatment of fibromyalgia. *Journal of Alternative and Complementary Medicine, 15*(10), 1057–1058.

Nims, L. (2002). Be Set Free Fast: an advanced energy therapy. In F. Gallo (Ed.), *Energy psychology in psychotherapy* (pp. 77–92). New York: Norton.

Oschman, J. L. (2000). *Energy medicine: the scientific basis.* London: Churchill Livingstone, an imprint of Harcourt Publishers Limited.

Rodenburg, R., Benjamin, A., de Roos, C., et al. (2009). Efficacy of EMDR in chil-dren: a meta-analysis. *Clinical Psychology Review, 29*, 599–606.

Rossi, E. L. (2002). *The psychobiology of gene expression.* New York: W. W. Norton & Company.

Seto, A., Kusaka, C., Nakazato, S., et al. (1992). Detection of extraordinary large bio-magnetic field strength from human hand during external Qi emission. *Acupuncture and Electrotherapy Research, 17*(2), 75–94.

Shapiro, F. (1995). *Eye movement desensitization and reprocessing: basic principles, pro-tocols, and procedures.* New York: Guilford.

Shapiro, F. (2001). *Eye movement desensitization and reprocessing (EMDR): basic prin-ciples, protocols, and procedures* (2nd ed.). New York: Guilford Press.

Shealy, C. N. (2011). *Energy medicine: practical applications and scientific proof.* Virginia Beach, VA: 4th Dimension Press.

Shenefelt, P. D. (2003). Biofeedback, cognitive-behavioral methods, and hypnosis in dermatology: is it all in your mind? *Dermatological Therapy, 16*, 114–122.

Smith, R. B. (2002). Introduction. In D. L. Kirsch, *The science behind cranial electrotherapy stimulation* (2nd ed.). Edmonton, Alberta: Medical Scope Publishing.

Spiegel, D. (2004). Placebos in practice [editorial]. *British Medical Journal, 329,* 927–928.

Stokes, G., & Whiteside, D. (1984). *Basic one brain, dyslexic learning correction and brain integration.* Burbank, CA: Three-in-One Concepts.

Swack, J. A. (2002). Healing from the Body Level Up. In F. Gallo (Ed.), *Energy psychology in psychotherapy* (pp. 59–76). New York: Norton.

Temes, R. (2006). *The tapping cure.* New York: Marlowe & Company.

Thie, J. F. (1973). *Touch for health.* Pasadena, CA: T. H. Enterprises.

Turaeva, V. A. (1967). Treatment of eczema and neurodermatitis by electrosleep. In F. M. Wageneder & S. T. Schuy (Eds.), *Electrotherapeutic sleep and electroanaesthesia* (pp. 203–204). Amsterdam, Netherlands, Excerpta Medical Foundation.

Ullman, M. (1959). On the psyche and warts: I. Suggestion and warts: a review and comment. *Psychosomatic Medicine, 21,* 473–488.

Villoldo, A. (2000). *Shaman, healer, sage: how to heal yourself and others with the energy medicine of the Americas.* New York: Harmony Books.

Walker, S. (1996). *Neuro Emotional Technique: N.E.T. basic manual.* Encinitas, CA: NET Inc.

Wilcox, J. P. (1999). *Keepers of the Ancient Knowledge: The Mystical World of the Q'ero Indians of Peru.* Rockport, MA, Element Books Ltd.

Yeong, Y. S., & Hiew, C. C. (2002). *Energy medicine in CFQ healing.* New York: Writers Club Press.

Yeong, Y. S., & Hiew, C. C. (2007). *Qigong healing meditation: Coming home awakening into light.* North Charleston, SC: BookSurge Publishing.

Yeong, Y. S., & Hiew, C. C. (2009). *Chaoyi Fanhuan Qigong healing: healing self, healing others.* Bloomington, IN: iUniverse.

Zimmerman, J. (1990). Laying-on-of-hands healing and therapeutic touch: a testable theory. *Newsletter of the Bio-Electro-Magnetics Institute, 2*(1), 8–17.

12

Integrative Management of Acne

WHITNEY P. BOWE AND JAIMIE B. GLICK

Key Concepts

- ♣ As oxidative stress has been implicated in acne, antioxidants such as zinc, vitamin C, and nicotinamide may play a role in acne prevention and management.
- ♣ Botanicals that have shown efficacy in acne include tea tree oil, green tea, and resveratrol.
- ♣ Dietary modifications, including the avoidance of high-glycemic-index foods and skim milk, and the addition of probiotics to the diet, are worthy of discussion with acne patients.
- ♣ As stress hormone receptors are present in and near the pilosebaceous unit, stress reduction should be emphasized to help reduce acne flares.

Introduction

Acne vulgaris is the most prevalent skin condition, affecting more than 80% of adolescents and commonly continuing into adulthood (White, 1998). Our understanding of the pathophysiology of acne continues to evolve, leading to new therapeutic targets and the development of advanced treatment regimens. Some of the most recent advances in acne therapy include new drug combinations, novel formulations, and innovative vehicle technologies. Additionally, interest in the use of integrative therapies for acne is increasing as dermatologists are learning more about the important roles of inflammation, oxidative stress, and diet on acne initiation and progression. Botanicals, herbs, antioxidants, and light- and heat-based therapies provide additional options for patients and providers in cases where standard therapies have proven insufficient, intolerable, or undesirable.

This chapter begins with a discussion of recent updates into the pathophysiology of acne. New directions for acne therapy, including novel drug combinations and formulations as well as advanced vehicle technologies, are subsequently addressed. The remainder of the chapter will be devoted to the role of integrative therapies in acne treatment, including the use of botanicals, herbs, antioxidants, and probiotics as well as the influence of diet and procedural therapies on acne treatment.

Pathophysiology of Acne

The pathogenesis of acne is traditionally attributed to four pathogenic factors: hyperkeratinization, excess sebum production, colonization by *Propionibacterium acnes*, and inflammation (Harper & Thiboutot, 2003; Jeremy et al., 2003). It was previously believed that hyperkeratinization and colonization by *P. acnes* preceded inflammation in the progression of the acne comedo. However, recent evidence suggests that subclinical inflammatory events may actually precede hyperkeratinization (Holland & Jeremy, 2005; Jeremy et al., 2003).

In addition to the above four pathogenic factors, it is believed that oxidative stress likely plays a key role in the development of acne. In fact, it is thought that cutaneous lipid peroxidation may be the match that lights the inflammatory cascade (Bowe & Logan, 2010; Bowe et al., 2012). The idea that lipid peroxidation is the initial event in acne is not a new one and rather constitutes a 50-year-old theory of acne (Lorincz, 1965). Acne patients have increased sebum production, with squalene lipids being overproduced. The breakdown products of oxidized squalene are highly comedogenic. Additionally, squalene peroxides diminish glutathione, a key antioxidant present in the skin (Chiba et al., 2001). The presence of peroxidated squalene in keratinocytes may lead to an inflammatory cascade of cytokine production and enhance lipoxygenase activity (Ottaviani et al., 2006). The oxygen-scavenging capabilities of squalene also serve to decrease oxygen tension in the pilosebaceous unit, creating an ideal environment for the survival of *P. acnes* (Saint-Leger et al., 1986). In a recent study, adult acne patients were found to have 43% higher levels of the reactive oxygen species hydrogen peroxide compared to healthy controls (Akamatsu et al., 2003). Furthermore, it has been reported that markers of oxidative stress, including malondialdehyde, are higher in patients with acne (Arican et al., 2005), while levels of antioxidants like superoxide dismutase are lower in patients with acne (Bowe & Logan, 2012).

New insights into the role of the androgen receptor and sebum production have also been proposed. It is known that androgenic hormones stimulate androgen receptors and lead to increased sebum production. Melnik (2010a, b, c) has proposed a theory that the removal of the polypeptide nuclear transcription factor Foxo1 "opens" the androgen receptor so that it can be stimulated by androgenic agonists. It is believed that increased levels of IGF-1 and insulin mediate the phosphorylation of Foxo1, resulting in its destruction (Melnik, 2010b). Dairy products and high-glycemic diets have been implicated in this cascade as they increase IGF-1, thereby potentially compromising Foxo1's protective role (see below) (Melnik & Schmitz, 2009).

It has been suggested that the sebaceous gland is regulated by neuropeptides and can act as an independent neuroendocrine organ (Bellew et al., 2011). Recent studies demonstrate that corticotropin-releasing hormone (CRH) and the CRH receptor are present in human sebaceous glands in situ, and this CRH/CRH-receptor system was subsequently confirmed via a human sebocyte culture system (SZ95 sebocytes) in vitro (Kono et al., 2001; Zouboulis et al., 2002). It is also known that CRH is activated by proinflammatory cytokines in response to stress (Slominiski et al., 2000), suggesting a relationship between acne, stress, and neuroendocrine function. Additionally, melanocortins and their receptors have been identified in human skin and likely play a role in sebogenesis (Bohm et al., 2002; Gancevicience et al., 2007; Zhang et al., 2011).

The relationship of the skin, neuroendocrine function, and stress is an evolving concept in acne and has led to bench studies investigating neuroendocrine targets for acne therapy. Recently, a study demonstrated the effectiveness of a CRH-receptor antagonist in blocking the effects of CRH on the SZ95 sebocyte (Krause et al., 2007). Additionally, results of a study investigating a novel MCR1 and MCR5 antagonist (JNJ-10229570) demonstrated a reduction in sebum gland size and sebum-specific lipid production in human skin transplanted onto severe combined immunodeficiency mice (Eisinger et al., 2011). In addition to these basic science studies, dermatologists have begun to clinically explore the role of stress in acne (see below).

New Directions for Acne Therapy

Acne treatment involves the use of several medications in order to address the multifactorial nature of the disorder. Common topical medications include retinoids (adapalene, tazarotene, tretinoin), salicylic acid, benzoyl peroxide (BP), and antibiotics such as clindamycin and erythromycin. Although effective, topical medications can be associated with unpleasant side effects like dryness, erythema, and scaling. These adverse effects often limit patient compliance and lead to decreased therapeutic efficacy. New topical treatment combinations and formulations as well as enhanced delivery systems have been developed to improve the efficacy and side-effect profile of topical medications.

NOVEL FORMULATIONS

Several new formulations involve combining a traditional acne therapy such as an antibiotic or retinoid with a "natural" product. For example, azelaic acid, an organic compound found in wheat, rye, and barley, has anti-inflammatory and antimicrobial properties. Recently, a new acne medication complexing azelaic acid with niacinamide and glycerin has come to the market. Niacinamide, a derivative of vitamin B, enhances treatment effects while glycerin acts as an emollient. Another unique formulation referred to as APDDR-0901 comprises a 0.03% retinol mixed with 0.7% rose extract and a 0.05% hexamidine diisethionate cream. A double-blind randomized controlled trial (RCT) showed similar efficacy between the novel formulation and adapalene gel. Moreover, the APDDR-0901 demonstrated an improved side-effect profile, with fewer cases of erythema, scaling, and burning than adapalene gel (Lee et al., 2011).

Integrative Therapies

Finding both an effective and well-tolerated therapy for acne treatment can be a difficult task. Often patients will turn to complementary and alternative medicine (CAM) to treat this chronic skin condition. In the United States it is estimated that $34 billion is spent annually on the use of CAM therapies (MacLennan et al., 2002). Additionally, it was found that 6.7% of people with a skin disease claim to have used CAM therapy sometime over a 12-month period (Eisenberg, 1998). In a recent study, patients using CAM therapies for acne reported that the CAM treatments were more efficacious than "mainstream" topical therapies but likely less to be effective than oral isotretinoin and oral antibiotics. Moreover, patients believed that the "natural" therapies were safer (Magin et al., 2006). In a time where antibiotic resistance is increasing and Western interest in alternative medicine is growing, integrative treatments for acne are becoming more and more attractive.

ANTIOXIDANTS

As discussed previously, increasing evidence suggests the importance of oxidative stress in the pathogenesis of acne. Another study supporting the link between oxidative stress and acne investigated the levels of glutathione (GSH), an essential antioxidant present in the human body. The results showed that GSH was present in lower concentrations in acne-prone areas of the face. Moreover, glutathione levels were also found in lower concentrations in acne patients even in non-acne-prone areas such as the upper arm, suggesting that GSH levels are systemically decreased in patients with acne (Ikeno et al., 2011). We will focus here on some of the best-studied antioxidants in the treatment of acne, including zinc, vitamin C, nicotinamide, and fullerene.

ZINC

Zinc is a metallic element that supports antioxidant pathways and shows promise in the treatment of acne. It has been shown to improve the efficacy of topical antibiotics (Iinuma et al., 2011) and has been shown to decrease plasma markers of oxidative stress as well as inflammatory cytokines (Prasad, 2008). In a recent study, a daily dose of 30 mg oral zinc gluconate was found to be effective for the treatment of acne, reducing inflammatory lesions over 2 months (Dreno et al., 2005). A 2010 preliminary study evaluated the efficacy of an oral methionine-based zinc antioxidant complex containing zinc, vitamin C, mixed carotenoids, d-alpha-tocopherol acetate, and chromium. The oral nutrition supplement was taken three times a day for 3 months. Results showed significant improvement in acne lesions (Sardana & Garg, 2010).

VITAMIN C

Vitamin C (ascorbic acid) is known to have antioxidant and anti-inflammatory properties (Perricone, 1993). However, ascorbic acid is unstable in its free form, and its modification to sodium ascorbyl phosphate (SAP) enhances its stability for use in topical acne formulations. Several studies have reported the efficacy of SAP in the treatment of acne. In one open-label study of 60 acne patients, 5% SAP was found to be more effective than 5% BP after 12 weeks of treatment (Klock et al., 2005). In another open-label study, 5% SAP proved to be more efficacious than 1% clindamycin in reducing total and inflammatory lesion counts (Ikeno & Nishikawa, 2008). In a recent RCT, 5% SAP and 5% SAP in combination with 0.2% retinol was found to significantly reduce acne lesions (Ruamrak et al., 2009). In the most recent RCT, 5% SAP lotion (compared to vehicle) was found to significantly improve Investigators Global Assessment Score and Subjects Global Assessment Score (Woolery-Lloyd et al., 2010).

NICOTINAMIDE

Nicotinamide is a B3 vitamin with antioxidant (Otte et al., 2005) and anti-inflammatory effects. Nicotinamide is known to inhibit *P. acnes*-induced production of interleukin (IL)-8 through the MAPK and NF-κB pathways (Grange et al., 2009). In a randomized, double-blind, placebo-controlled trial by Shalita and colleagues (1995), 4% nicotinamide gel was found to be more effective in the treatment of moderate inflammatory acne than 1% clindamycin. The authors suggested nicotinamide as an alternative treatment for acne because, unlike clindamycin, it has not been associated with antibiotic resistance (Shalita et al., 1995). A unique formulation of 4% nicotinamide emulsified with 1% linoleic acid-rich phosphatidylcholine and enhanced by chitin nanofibrils was compared to 1% clindamycin gel and placebo. Although both medications were effective, the nicotinamide phosphatidylcholine emulsion was superior to the clindamycin gel (Morganti et al., 2011).

FULLERENE

Fullerene is a spherical carbon that is known to possess significant antioxidant capacity and thus has potential for acne treatment. In a recent open trial of 11 acne patients, fullerene gel, when applied twice daily, was found to significantly reduce the number of inflammatory lesions. The authors also examined the in vitro effects of fullerene on hamster sebocytes and found that fullerene inhibits sebum production (Inui et al., 2011).

The studies above indicate that although the exact role of oxidative stress in acne pathogenesis remains unclear, acne appears to improve with antioxidant therapy. Many other agents, including several botanicals (discussed below), are effective in acne therapy largely because of their antioxidant properties.

Botanicals

Botanicals refer to derivatives of herbs, spices, roots, and stems (Reuter et al., 2010). These plant-based agents have been used for centuries for the treatment of inflammatory skin conditions, promotion of wound healing, and beauty enhancement (Bowe & Logan, 2012). Botanicals provide antioxidant, anti-inflammatory, and antimicrobial effects. While numerous botanicals and herbs are used for the treatment of acne, we will focus here on those with the best evidence.

TEA TREE OIL

Tea tree oil is an essential oil derived from the distillation of the leaves of *Melaleuca alternifolia,* a tree native to Australia. It is known to have antibacterial (Raman et al., 1995) and antifungal (D'Auria et al., 2011) activity. In a study comparing 5% BP to 5% tea tree oil, both treatments significantly reduced the number of inflamed and noninflamed acne lesions, although the onset of action was slower for tea tree oil. Of note, patients treated with tea tree oil had fewer side effects (Bassett et al., 1990). The most recent RCT compared tea tree oil to placebo in 60 patients with mild to moderate acne vulgaris. Results showed tea tree oil gel significantly improved total lesion counts and acne severity index compared to placebo (Enshaieh et al., 2007). It is important to note that tea tree oil has been reported to cause an allergic contact dermatitis in some patients (Rutherford et al., 2007).

GREEN TEA

Green tea is derived from the leaves of the tea plant, *Camellia sinensis,* through a process of steam drying (which does not involve fermentation) to preserve the polyphenolic compounds of the leaves. Epigallocaetechin-3-gallate (EGCG) is the most abundant and likely the most biologically active catechin present in green tea. Green tea's usefulness in acne therapy is multifactorial as its catechins possess antioxidant, anti-inflammatory, and antimicrobial (Lee et al., 2009) properties. Green tea may be able to contend with the lipid peroxidation in acne as it contains antioxidants that are able to prevent local and systemic declines in superoxide dismutase and GSH activity (Li et al., 2020; Xu et al., 2010). Research has also suggested that green tea is able to reduce sebum production by inhibition of 5-alpha reductase (Liao & Hiipakka, 1995). In a recent study of healthy males, a 3% green tea emulsion was found to significantly reduce sebum production (Mahmood et al., 2010). Furthermore, in an open label study of patients with mild to moderate acne, twice-daily applications of topical 2% green tea lotion reduced total acne lesions counts by 58% after 6 weeks (Elsaie et al., 2009).

RESVERATROL

Resveratrol is a phytoalexin (3,4,5-trihydroxy-transtilbene) produced by spermatophytes (plants that produce seeds) such as grapes, peanuts, mulberries, spruce, and eucalyptus. Resveratrol is thought to have antioxidant and anti-inflammatory properties (Donnelly et al., 2004) and is known to be cardioprotective. Additionally, in vitro studies of resveratrol have demonstrated bactericidal effects against *P. acnes* (Docherty et al., 2007). In a single-blind, vehicle-controlled study of 20 patients with acne, resveratrol-containing hydrogel was found to significantly decrease acne lesions (Fabbrocini et al, 2011).

GLUCONOLACTONE

Gluconolactone is a polyhydroxy acid derived from *Saccharomyces bulderi*. In a double-blind clinical study of 150 patients, 14% topical gluconolactone was found to be effective in the treatment of inflammatory acne. The gluconolactone showed similar efficacy to 5% BP with fewer adverse effects (Hunt & Barnetson, 1992).

Although the botanicals described above have the most evidence supporting their potential role as acne therapies to date, large numbers of basic science studies have begun to assess the use of other botanicals for the treatment of acne. One study demonstrated the ability of *Echinacea* to reverse increased cytokine levels produced by *P. acnes* (Sharma et al., 2010). A study of several Thai herbal extracts reported anti-inflammatory and antimicrobial activity against *P. acnes* (Niyomkam et al., 2009). In a recent animal study, nobiletin, a citrus polymethoxy flavonoid, was found to inhibit sebum production and augment sebum excretion from mature sebocytes (Sato et al., 2007). Although many botanicals and herbal extracts show promise in the treatment of acne in the laboratory setting, clinical studies are needed to better evaluate the true value of these extracts in acne therapy.

Diet

The relationship between diet and acne has long been a controversial one. However, research over the past few years has begun to uncover important links, especially in regards to high-glycemic-load (HGL) diets and dairy products (Bowe et al., 2010). Glycemic index has to do with a food's potential to increase blood glucose and insulin levels. An important study by Cordain and colleagues (2002) reported the apparent absence of acne in Papua New Guinea and Paraguay, locations in which individuals do not consume HGL diets. Several RCTs have provided evidence for the positive effects of low-glycemic-load (LGL) diets on acne (Smith et al., 2007a, b, 2008). The most recent RCT not only demonstrated an improvement in acne lesions with LGL diets but also evaluated the histopathology of subjects' skin. Results showed that LGL diets reduced sebaceous gland size and decreased inflammation, two of the key factors in the pathogenesis of acne (Kwon et al., 2012). Ingestion of high-glycemic-index foods triggers a cascade of endocrine responses that may promote acne through androgens, growth hormones, and cell-signaling pathways.

Several studies by Adebamowo and colleagues (2005, 2006, 2008) indicate an association between acne and dairy products, especially skim milk. Conversely, one study based on traditional Chinese medicine reported that the intake of dairy was associated with a lower incidence of acne (Law et al., 2010).

It is thought that HGL diets and dairy products result in increased levels of IGF-1 and ultimately increase sebum production (Adebamowo et al., 2005; Smith et al., 2007a). The hormonal factors present in dairy products are also thought to contribute to its comedogenicity (Adebamowo et al., 2005; Darling et al., 1974; Hartmann et al., 1998).

The consumption of omega-3 fatty acids may also be important in the reduction of acne, specifically inflammatory lesions. Intake of omega-3 fatty acids such as those in fish may suppress cytokine production and reduce the inflammation associated with acne (Cordain, 2005). Similarly to HGL diets and dairy products, omega-3 fatty acids have been reported to alter levels of IGF-1 (Bhathena et al., 1991). Although further investigation is clearly needed, the relationship between diet and acne cannot be overlooked. The authors suggest counseling patients on the potential effects of glycemic load and dairy on acne flares. If patients suspect a relationship between their diet and acne, especially in terms of HGL diets, physicians should advise patients to minimize consumption of these foods.

Probiotics

Dermatologists John H. Stokes and Donald M. Pillsbury first proposed a gut–brain–skin unifying theory over 70 years ago. In brief, Stokes and Pillsbury suggested that alterations in the microbial flora of the gastrointestinal tract may lead to local and systemic inflammation. Stokes and Pillsbury even suggested the therapeutic use of "acidophil organisms in cultures like *Bacillus acidophilus*," now referred to as "probiotics" (Stokes & Pillsbury, 1930). More contemporary evidence does support their theory and indicates a role for probiotics in acne as well as mental and gastrointestinal health.

Several in vitro studies have demonstrated the ability of probiotics like lactobacillus to reduce skin inflammation and improve the barrier function of the skin (Gueniche et al., 2010; Philippe et al., 2010). One of these studies also reported that probiotics are able to reduce substance P-mediated skin inflammation (Gueniche et al., 2010), which is important because substance P may be responsible for stress-induced skin inflammation (Lee et al., 2008). In vitro studies have shown antimicrobial effects of probiotics, where certain strains of probiotics were found to inhibit *P. acnes* growth (Al-Ghazzewi & Tester, 2010; Kang et al., 2009). One of the authors (WPB) has demonstrated that a friendly bacterium of the oropharynx known as *Streptococcus salivarius* is capable of producing an inhibitory substance that halts the growth of *P. acnes* in vitro (Bowe et al., 2006).

Probiotics have also been shown to contribute to glucose tolerance (Kleerebezem & Baughan, 2009), while the oral intake of *Bifidobacterium lactis* can improve fasting insulin levels (Burcelin, 2010).

Although there is accumulating basic science evidence supporting the role of probiotics in acne therapy, few studies have directly investigated the use of probiotic supplementation in acne patients. In an Italian study, the addition of 250 mg freeze-dried *L. acidophilus* and *B. bifidum* to standard acne treatment seemed to improve antibiotic compliance and tolerance (Marchetti et al., 1987). One study performed in Russia reported that the addition of probiotics to standard acne therapy decreased time to clinical improvement (Volkova et al., 2001). Another study showed a significant improvement in inflammatory acne lesions with the application of a topical probiotic lotion (Kang et al., 2009). The anti-inflammatory and antimicrobial effects of probiotics as well as their influence on glucose control all suggest a potential role for probiotics in acne therapy. Continued research is required to more accurately understand this role and to determine whether oral or topical administration of probiotics would be a preferable treatment in acne.

Stress and Acne

The notion that stress can exacerbate acne is not a new one, but only recently have researchers begun to better elucidate the nature of this relationship. As discussed in the pathophysiology section of this chapter, a number of neuronal hormones (CRH and melanocortins) and their receptors are present in the skin. Recent basic science research has also suggested the importance of the neuropeptide substance P in the link between stress and acne (Zouboulis & Bohm, 2004). Substance P nerve fibers have been detected in high quantities near the sebaceous glands of acne patients (Toyoda et al., 2002). In another study, substance P was shown to enhance the production of cytokines in cultured sebocytes (Lee et al., 2008).

Although the exact mechanism of stress-induced acne has yet to be determined, several important studies have documented a significant correlation between increased stress levels and acne. A prospective cohort study by Chiu and colleagues (2003) evaluated the effects of examination-induced stress in 22 university students. Results showed that patients had a higher mean grade of acne severity ($p < 0.01$) and a higher mean perceived stress score ($p < 0.01$) during examination periods. Even when adjusting for changes in sleep hours, sleep quality, and diet, results showed that increased acne severity was significantly correlated with increased levels of stress ($p < 0.01$). Similarly, a study by Rizvi and colleagues (2010) reported a significant positive correlation ($p = 0.029$) between pre-examination stress level and acne severity among adolescents in Singapore. Two additional studies documented exacerbations in acne severity during periods of stressful life events (Ghodsi et al., 2009; Yospiovitch et al., 2007).

Given the many reports that stress has been shown to exacerbate acne, the authors believe that activities designed to decrease one's stress level such as meditation, yoga, and massage might prove therapeutic for acne. Although there is limited evidence of these techniques in the literature, the authors did find one early study in which biofeedback relaxation and cognitive imagery were effective in acne therapy (Hughes et al., 1983).

Procedural Therapies

LIGHT AND HEAT

Light and heat therapies are increasingly attractive to patients because they represent "cutting-edge" alternatives to conventional acne treatments (Bowe & Shalita, 2011). The "at-home" and "do-it-yourself" products offer affordability, convenience, ease of use, and privacy (Brown, 2011). Many of these products have been approved by the U.S. Food and Drug Administration (FDA) for use in mild to moderate inflammatory acne and are available without a prescription. The efficacy of light therapy lies in its anti-inflammatory (Shnitkind et al., 2006) and antimicrobial effects. *P. acnes* produces photoactive substances called porphyrins that, when exposed to visible light, produce toxic reactive oxygen species that destroy the bacteria (Lee et al., 1978). Blue light alone has been shown to decrease inflammatory lesions and erythema (Gold et al., 2011; Wheeland & Koreck, 2012). Blue light is the most effective wavelength in acne therapy as it best induces the *P. acnes* photochemical reaction; however, it has limited skin penetration. By combining blue and red light therapy, skin penetration can be enhanced (Goldbert & Russell, 2006). A recent study examined the use of a combined 415-nm blue-light- and 633-nm red-light-emitting device in 21 subjects with inflammatory acne. Subjects alternated between four 20-minute blue-light and four 30-minute red-light self-administered treatments over the course of 4 weeks. Results showed a 69% reduction in lesion counts 2 months after the final treatment (Sadick, 2008). Several "at-home" light devices are available for the treatment of acne vulgaris and range in price from $225 to $400.

In addition to light devices, some of the FDA-approved over-the-counter therapies utilize heat to treat acne. Heat therapy is thought to work by activating *P. acnes* heat-shock proteins that cause the bacteria to self-destruct (Sadick et al., 2010). Devices on the market can reach temperatures as high as 212°F. At such high temperatures, the device is applied for only about 2.5 seconds. Other devices combine the use of heat and light therapy, which is thought to accelerate the *P. acnes* photochemical production of reactive oxygen species (Sadick et al., 2010). A placebo-controlled, double-blind study by Sadick and colleagues (2010) evaluated a combined light and heat energy device in 63 subjects. Results showed a statistically significant improvement in lesion counts and a shorter time to lesion improvement with the combined device compared to placebo. Although there are benefits to these "do-it-yourself" devices, it is important to note that therapies are often significantly weaker than comparable in-office procedures.

Conclusion

Over the past several years there have been numerous advancements in acne therapy, with the successful creation of novel drug combinations, formulations, and innovative drug-delivery systems. Additionally, the use of integrative therapies in acne has been increasing as knowledge of acne pathophysiology grows. Recent research has suggested a role for antioxidants and botanicals in acne therapy. Dermatologists have also begun to recognize the importance of dietary factors, probiotics, and stress on acne progression. Lastly, procedural treatments that utilize light and/or heat serve as adjuncts to traditional acne treatments.

REFERENCES

Adebamowo, C. A., Spiegelman, D., Berkey, C. S., et al. (2006). Milk consumption and acne in adolescent girls. *Dermatology Online Journal, 12*, 1.

Adebamowo, C. A., Spiegelman, D., Berkey, C. S., et al. (2008). Milk consumption and acne in teenaged boys. *Journal of the American Academy of Dermatology, 58*, 787–793.

Adebamowo, C. A., Spiegelman, D., Danby, F. W., et al. (2005). High school dietary dairy intake and teenage acne. *Journal of the American Academy of Dermatology, 52*, 207–214.

Akamatsu, H., Horio, T., & Hattori, K. (2003). Increased hydrogen peroxide generation by neutrophils from patient with acne inflammation. *International Journal of Dermatology, 42*, 366–369.

Arican, O., Kurtus, E. B., & Sasmaz, S. (2005). Oxidative stress in patients with acne vulgaris. *Mediators of Inflammation*, 380–384.

Al-Ghazzewi, F. H., & Tester, R. F. (2010). Effect of konjac glucomannan hydrolysates and probiotics on the growth of the skin bacterium *Propionibacterium acnes* in vitro. *International Journal of Cosmetic Science*, 32, 139–142.

Bassett, I. B., Pannowitz, D. L., & Barnetson, R. S. (1990). A comparative study of tea-tree oil versus benzoyl peroxide in the treatment of acne. *Medical Journal of Australia*, 153, 455–458.

Bellew, S., Thiboutot, D., & Del Rosso, J. Q. (2011). Pathogenesis of acne vulgaris: what's new, what's interesting and what may be clinically relevant. *Journal of Drugs in Dermatology*, 10, 582–585.

Bhathena, S. J., Berlin, E., Judd, J. T., et al. (1991). Effects of omega 3 fatty acids and vitamin E on hormones involved in carboydrate and lipid metabolism in men. *American Journal of Clinical Nutrition*, 54, 684–688.

Bohm, M., Schiller, M., Stander, S., et al. (2002). Evidence of expression of melanocortin-1 receptor in human sebocytes in vitro and in situ. *Journal of Investigative Dermatology*, 118, 533–539.

Bowe, W. P., Filip, J. C., DiRenzo, J. M., et al. (2006). Inhibition of *Propionibacterium acnes* by bacteriocin-like inhibitory substances (BLIS) produced by *Streptococcus salivarius*. *Journal of Drugs in Dermatology*, 5, 868–870.

Bowe, W. P., Joshi, S. S., & Shalita, A. R. (2010). Diet and acne. *Journal of the American Academy of Dermatology*, 63, 124–141.

Bowe, W. P., & Logan, A. C. (2010). Clinical implications of lipid peroxidation in acne vulgaris: old wine in new bottles. *Lipids in Health and Disease*, 9, 141.

Bowe, W. P., & Logan, A. C. (2013). Antioxidants in acne vulgaris and aging: focus on green tea and feverfew. *Journal of Drugs in Dermatology*.

Bowe, W. P., Patel, N., & Logan, A. C. (2012). Acne vulgaris: the role of oxidative stress and the potential therapeutic value of local and systemic antioxidants. *Journal of Drugs in Dermatology*, 11(6), 742–746.

Bowe, W. P., & Shalita, A. R. (2011). Procedural treatments for acne. In: A. R. Shalita, J. Q. D. Rosso, & G. F. Webster (Eds.), *Acne vulgaris* (pp. 208–217). New York and London: Informa Healthcare.

Brown, A. S. (2011). At-home laser and light-based devices. *Current Problems in Dermatology*, 42, 160–165.

Burcelin, R. (2010). Intestinal microflora, inflammation and metabolic disease. Abstract 019, Keystone Symposia on Diabetes, Whistler, British Columbia, Canada.

Chiba, K., Yoshizawa, K., Makino, I., et al. (2001). Changes in the levels of glutathione after cellular and cutaneous damaged induced by squalene monohydroperoxide. *Journal of Biochemical and Molecular Toxicology*, 15, 150–158.

Chiu, A., Chon, Y., & Kimball, A. (2003). The response of skin disease to stress: changes in the severity of acne vulgaris as affected by examination stress. *Archives of Dermatology*, 139, 897–900.

Cordain, L. (2005). Implications for the role of diet in acne. *Seminars in Cutaneous Medicine & Surgery*, 24, 84–91.

Cordain, L., Lindeberg, S., Hurtado, M., et al. (2002). Acne vulgaris: a disease of Western civilization. *Archives of Dermatology, 138,* 1584–1590.

Darling, J. A., Laing, A. H., & Harkness, R. A. (1974). A survey of steroids in cow's milk. *Journal of Endocrinology, 62,* 291–297.

D'Auria, F. D., Laino, L., Strippoli, S., et al. (2001). In vitro activity of tea tree oil against *Candida albicans* mycelial conversion and other pathogenic fungi. *Journal of Chemotherapy, 13,* 377–383.

Docherty, J. J., McEwen, H. A., Sweet, T. J., et al. (2007). Resveratrol inhibition of *Propionibacterium acnes. Journal of Antimicrobial Chemotherapy, 59,* 1182–1184.

Donnelly, L. E., Newton, R., Kennedy, G. E., et al. (2004). Anti-inflammatory effects of resveratrol in lung epithelial cells: molecular mechanisms. *American Journal of Physiology Lung Cellular & Molecular Physiology, 287,* 774–783.

Dreno, B., Foulc, P., Reynaud, A., et al. (2005). Effect of zinc gluconate on *Propionibacterium acnes* resistance to erythromycin in patients with inflammatory acne: in vitro and in vivo study. *European Journal of Dermatology, 15,* 152–155.

Eisenberg, D. M. (1998). Trends in alternative medicine in the United States, 1990–1997, results of a follow-up national survey. *Journal of the American Medical Association, 280,* 1569–1575.

Eisinger, M., Li, W. H., Anthonavage, M., et al. (2011). A melanocortin receptor 1 and 5 antagonist inhibits sebaceous gland differentiation and the production of sebum-specific lipids. *Journal of Dermatology Science, 63,* 23–32.

Elsaie, M. L., Abdelhamid, M. F., Elsaaiee, L. T., et al. (2009). The efficacy of topical 2% green tea lotion in mild-to-moderate acne vulgaris. *Journal of Drugs in Dermatology, 8,* 358–364.

Enshaieh, S., Jooya, A., Hossein, A., et al. (2007). The efficacy of 5% topical tea tree oil gel in mild to moderate acne vulgaris: a randomized, double-blind placebo-controlled study. *Indian Journal of Dermatology, Venereology & Leprology, 73,* 22–25.

Fabbrocini, G., Staibano, S., De Rosa, G., et al. (2011). Resveratrol-containing gel for the treatment of acne vulgaris. *American Journal of Clinical Dermatology, 12,* 133–141.

Gancevicience, R., Graziene, V., Bohm, M., et al. (2007). Increased in situ expression of melanocortin-1 receptor in sebacous glands of lesional skin of patients with acne vulgaris. *Experimental Dermatology, 16,* 547–552.

Ghodsi, S. Z., Orawa, H., & Zouboulis, C. C. (2009). Prevalence, severity and severity risk factors of acne in high school pupils: a community-based study. *Journal of Investigative Dermatology, 129,* 2136–2141.

Gold, M. H., Sending, W., & Biron, J. A. (2011). Clinical efficacy of home-use blue light therapy for mild-to moderate acne. *Journal of Cosmetic Laser Therapy, 12,* 308–314.

Goldberg, D. J., & Russell, B. A. (2006). Combination blue (415 nm) and red (633 nm) LED phototherapy in the treatment of mild to severe acne vulgaris. *Journal of Cosmetic Laser Therapy, 8,* 71–75.

Grange, P. A., Raingeaud, J., Calvez, V., et al. (2009). Nicotinamide inhibits *Propionibacterium acnes*-induced IL-8 production in keratinocytes through NF-kappaB and MAPK pathways. *Journal of Dermatologic Science, 56,* 106–112.

Gueniche, A., Benyacoub, J., Philippe, D., et al. (2010). *Lactobacillus paracasei* CNCM I-2116 (ST11) inhibits substance P-induced skin inflammation and accelerates skin barrier function recovery in vitro. *European Journal of Dermatology*, *20*, 731–737.

Harper, J. C., & Thiboutot, D. M. (2003). Pathogenesis of acne: recent research advances. *Advances in Dermatology*, *19*, 1–10.

Hartmann, S., Lacorn, M., & Steinhart, H. (1998). Natural occurrence of steroid hormones in food. *Food Chemistry*, *62*, 7–20.

Holland, D. B., & Jeremy, A. H. (2005). The role of inflammation in the pathogenesis of acne and acne scarring. *Seminars in Cutaneous Medicine & Surgery*, *24*, 79–83.

Hughes, H., Brown, B. W., Lawlis, G. F., et al. (1983). Treatment of acne vulgaris by biofeedback relaxation and cognitive imagery. *Journal of Psychosomatic Research*, *27*, 185–191.

Hunt, M. J., & Barnetson, R. S. (1992). A comparative study of gluconolactone versus benzoyl peroxide in the treatment of acne. *Australasian Journal of Dermatology*, *33*, 131–134.

Iinuma, K., Noguchi, N., Nakaminami, H., et al. (2011). Susceptibility of *Propionibacterium acnes* isolated from patients with acne vulgaris to zinc ascorbate and antibiotics. *Clinical, Cosmetic, & Investigative Dermatology*, *4*, 161–165.

Ikeno, H., & Nishikawa, T. (2008). An open study comparing efficacy of 5% sodium L-ascorbyl-2-phosphate lotion with 1% clindamycin gel in the treatment of facial acne vulgaris. *Journal of the American Academy of Dermatology*, *58*, Suppl 2, AB2.

Ikeno, H., Tochio, T., Tanaka, H., et al. (2011). Decrease in glutathione may be involved in pathogenesis of acne vulgaris. *Journal of Cosmetic Dermatology*, *10*, 240–244.

Inui, S., Aoshima, H., Nishiyama, A., et al. (2011). Improvement of acne vulgaris by topical fullerene application: unique impact on skin care. *Nanomedicine*, *7*, 238–241.

Jeremy, A. H., Holland, D. B., Roberts, S. G., et al. (2003) Inflammatory events are involved in acne lesion initiation. *Journal of Investigative Dermatology*, *121*, 20–27.

Kang, B. S., Seo, J. G., Lee, G. S., et al. (2009). Antimicrobial activity of enterocins from *Enterococcus faecalis* SL-5 against *Propionibacterium acnes*, the causative agent in acne vulgaris, and its therapeutic effect. *Journal of Microbiology*, *47*, 101–109.

Kleerebezem, M., & Vaughan, E. E. (2009). Probiotic and gut lactobacilli and bifidobacteria: molecular approaches to study diversity and activity. *Annual Record of Microbiology*, *63*, 269–290.

Klock, J., Ikeno, H., Ohmori, K., et al. (2005). Sodium ascorbyl phosphate shows in vitro and in vivo efficacy in the prevention and treatment of acne vulgaris. *International Journal of Cosmetic Science*, *27*, 171–176.

Kono, M., Nagata, H., Umemura, S., et al. (2001). In situ expression of corticotrophin-releasing hormone (CRH) and proopiomelanocortin (POMC) genes in human skin. *FASEB Journal*, *15*, 2297–2299.

Krause, K., Schnitger, A., Fimmel, S., et al. (2007). Corticotrophin-releasing hormone skin signaling is receptor-medicated and is predominant in the sebacous glands. *Hormone & Metabolic Research*, *39*, 166–170.

Kwon, H. H., Yoon, J. Y., Hong, J. S., et al. (2012). Clinical and histological effect of a low glycaemic load diet in treatment of acne vulgaris in Korean patients: a randomized, controlled trial. *Acta Dermato-Venereologica*, *92*, 241–246.

Law, M. P., Chuh, A. A., Molinari, N., et al. (2010). An investigation of the association between diet and occurrence of acne: a rational approach from a traditional Chinese medicine perspective. *Clinical & Experimental Dermatology, 35*, 31–35.

Lee, H. E., Ko, J. Y., Kim, Y. H., et al. (2011). A double-blind randomized controlled comparison of APDDR-0901, a novel cosmeceutical formulation, and. 1% adapalene gel in the treatment of mild-to-moderate acne vulgaris. *European Journal of Dermatology, 21*, 959–965.

Lee, J. H., Shim, J. S, Chung, M. S., et al. (2009). In vitro anti-adhesive activity of green tea extract against pathogen adhesion. *Phytotherapy Research, 23*, 460–466.

Lee, W. J., Jung, H. D., Lee, H. J., et al. (2008). Influence of substance-P on cultured sebocytes. *Archives of Dermatology Research, 300*, 311–316.

Lee, W. L., Shalita, A. R., & Poh-Fitzpatrick, M. B. (1978). Comparative studies of porphyrin production in *Propionibacterium acnes* and *Propionibacterium granulosum*. *Journal of Bacteriology, 133*, 811–815.

Li, Q., Zhao, H., Zhao, M., et al. (2010). Chronic green tea catechins administration prevents oxidative stress-related brain aging in C57BL/6J mice. *Brain Research, 1353*, 28–35.

Liao, S., & Hiipakka, R. A. (1995). Selective inhibition of steroid 5 alpha-reductase isozymes by tea epicatechin-3-gallate and epigallocatechin-3-gallate. *Biochemistry Biophysics Research Communication, 214*, 833–838.

Lorincz, A. L. (1965). Human skin lipids and their relation to skin disease. *AD467008 Armed Services Technical Information Report*, 1–12.

MacLennan, A. H., Wilson, D. H., & Taylor, A. W. (2002). The escalating cost and prevalence of alternative medicine. *Preventive Medicine, 35*, 166–173.

Magin, P. J., Adams, J., Heading, G. S., et al. (2006). Complementary and alternative medicine therapies in acne, psoriasis, atopic eczema: results of a qualitative study of patients' experiences and perceptions. *Journal of Alternative & Complementary Medicine, 12*, 451–457.

Mahmood, T., Akhtar, N., Khan, B. A., et al. (2010). Outcomes of 3% green tea emulsion on skin sebum production in male volunteers. *Bosnian Journal of Basic Medical Science, 10*, 260–264.

Marchetti, F., Capizzi, R., & Tulli, A. (1987). Efficacy of regulators of the intestinal bacterial flora in the therapy of acne vulgaris. *Clinical Therapeutics, 122*, 339–343.

Melnik, B. C. (2010a). Acneigenic stimuli coverage in phosphoinositol-3kinase/Akt/Foxo1 signal tranduction. *Journal of Clinical & Experimental Dermatology, 101*, 1–8.

Melnik, B. C. (2010b). Foxo1: the key for the pathogenesis and therapy of acne? *J Journal der Deutschen Dermatologischen Gesellschaft, 8*, 105–114.

Melnik, B. C. (2010c). The role of transcription factor Foxo1 in the pathogenesis of acne vulgaris and the mode of isotretinoin action. *Giornale Italiano di Dermatologia e Venereologia, 145*, 559–571.

Melnik, B. C., & Schmitz, G. (2009). Role of insulin, insulin-like growth factor-1, hyperglycemic food and mlk consumption in the pathogenesis of acne vulgaris. *Experimental Dermatology, 18*, 833–841.

Morganti, P., Berardesca, E., Guarneri, B., et al. (2011). Topical clindamycin 1% vs. linoleic acid-rich phosphatidylcholine and nicotinamide 4% in the treatment of acne: a multicentre-randomized trial. *International Journal of Cosmetic Science, 33,* 467–476.

Niyomkam, P., Kaewbumrung, S., Kaewnpparat, S., et al. (2009). Antibacterial activity of Thai herbal extracts on acne involved microorganism. *Pharmaceutical Biology, 48,* 375–380.

Ottaviani, M., Alestas, T., Flori, E., et al. (2006). Peroxidated squalene induces the production of inflammatory mediators in HaCat keratinocytes: a possible role in acne vulgaris. *Journal of Investigative Dermatology, 126,* 2430–2437.

Otte, N., Borelli, C., & Korting, H. C. (2005). Nicotinamide: biologic actions of an emerging cosmetic ingredient. *International Journal of Cosmetic Science, 27,* 255–261.

Perricone, N. V. (1993). The photoprotective and anti-inflammatory effects of topical ascorbyl palmitate. *Journal of Geriatric Dermatology, 1,* 5–10.

Philippe, D., Blum, S., & Benyacoub, J. (2010). Oral *Lactobacillus paracasei* improves skin barrier function recovery and reduces local skin inflammation. *European Journal of Dermatology, 21,* 279–278.

Prasad, A. S. (2008). Clinical, immunological, anti-inflammatory and antioxidant roles of zinc. *Experimental Gerontology, 43,* 370–377.

Raman, A., Weir, U., & Bloomfield, S. F. (1995). Antimicrobial effects of tea-tree oil and its major components on *Staphylococcus aureus, Staph. epidermidis* and *Propionibacterium acnes. Letters in Applied Microbiology, 21,* 242–245.

Reuter, J., Merfort, I., & Schempp, C. M. (2010). Botanicals in dermatology: an evidence-based review. *American Journal of Clinical Dermatology, 11,* 247–267.

Rizvi, A. H., Awaiz, M., Ghanghro, Z., et al. (2010). Pre-examination stress in second year medical students in a government college. *Journal of Ayurvedic Medical College of Abbottabad, 22,* 152–155.

Ruamrak, C., Lourith, N., & Natakankitkul, S. (2009). Comparison of clinical efficacies of sodium ascorbyl phosphate, retinol and their combination in acne treatment. *International Journal of Cosmetic Science, 31,* 41–46.

Rutherford, T., Nixon, R., Tam, M., et al. (2007). Allergy to tea tree oil: retrospective review of 41 cases with positive patch tests over 4.5 years. *Australasian Journal of Dermatology, 48,* 83–87.

Sadick, N. S. (2008). Handheld LED array device in the treatment of acne vulgaris. *Journal of Drugs in Dermatology, 7,* 347–350.

Sadick, N. S., Laver, Z., & Laver, L. (2010). Treatment of mild-to-moderate acne vulgaris using a combined light and heat energy device: home-use clinical study. *Journal of Cosmetic Laser Therapy, 12,* 276–383.

Saint-Leger, D., Bague, A., Cohen, E., et al. (1986). A possible role for squalene in the pathogenesis of acne. I. In vitro study of squalene oxidation. *British Journal of Dermatology, 114,* 535–542.

Sardana, K., & Garg, V. K. (2010). An observational study of methionine-bound zinc with antioxidants for mild to moderate acne vulgaris. *Dermatologic Therapy, 23,* 411–418.

Sato, T., Takahashi, A., Kojima, M., et al. (2007). A citrus polymethoxy flavonoid, nobiletin inhibits sebum production and sebocyte proliferation, and augments sebum excretion in hamsters. *Journal of Investigative Dermatology, 127,* 2740–2748.

Shalita, A. R., Smith, J. G., Parish, L. C., et al. (1995). Topical nicotinamide compared with clindamycin gel in the treatment of inflammatory acne vulgaris. *International Journal of Dermatology, 34,* 434–437.

Sharma, M., Schoop, R., Suter, A., et al. (2010). The potential use of Echinacea in acne: control of *Propionibacterium acnes* growth and inflammation. *Phytotherapy Research, 25,* 517–521.

Shnitkind, E., Yaping, E., Geen, S., et al. (2006). Anti-inflammatory properties of narrow-band blue light. *Journal of Drugs in Dermatology, 5,* 605–610.

Slominiski, A., Wortsman, J., Luger, T., et al. (2000). Cortiocotropin releasing hormone: and propiomelanocortin involvement in the cutaneous response to stress. *Physiological Reviews, 80,* 979–1020.

Smith, R. N., Braue, A., Varigos, G. A., et al. (2008). The effect of a low glycemic load diet on acne vulgaris and the fatty acid composition of skin surface triglycerides. *Journal of Dermatologic Science, 50,* 41–52.

Smith, R. N., Mann, N. J., Braue, A., et al. (2007a). A low-glycemic-load diet improves symptoms in acne vulgaris: a randomized controlled diet. *American Journal of Clinical Nutrition, 86,* 107–115.

Smith, R. N., Mann, N. J., Braue, A., et al. (2007b). The effect of of a high-protein, low glycemic load diet versus a conventional, high glycemic-load diet on biochemical parameters associated with acne vulgaris: a randomized, investigator-masked controlled trial. *Journal of the American Academy of Dermatology, 57,* 247–256.

Stokes, J. H., & Pillsbury, D. H. (1930). The effect on the skin of emotional and nervous states: theoretical and practical consideration of a gastrointestinal mechanism. *Archives of Dermatology & Syphilology, 22,* 962–993.

Toyoda, M., Nakamura, M., Makino, T., et al. (2002). Sebacous glands in acne patients express high levels of neutral endopeptidases. *Experimental Dermatology, 11,* 241–247.

Volkova, L. A., Khalif, I. L., & Kabanova, I. N. (2001). Impact of the impaired intestinal microflora on the course of acne vulgaris. *Klinichekaia Meditsina (Moskva), 79,* 39–41.

Wheeland, R. G., & Koreck, A. (2012). Safety and effectiveness of a new blue light device for the self-treatment of mild-to-moderate acne. *Journal of Clinical & Aesthetic Dermatology, 5,* 25–31.

White, G. M. (1998). Recent findings in epidemiologic evidence, classification and subtypes of acne vulgaris. *Journal of the American Academy of Dermatology, 39,* S34–37.

Woolery-Lloyd, H., Baumann, L., & Ikeno, H. (2010). Sodium L-ascorbyl-2-phosphate 5% lotion for the treatment of acne vulgaris: a randomized, double-blind, controlled trial. *Journal of Cosmetic Dermatology, 9,* 22–27.

Xu, Y., Zhang, J. J., Xiong, L., et al. (2010). Green tea polyphenols inhibit cognitive impairment induced by chronic cerebral hypoperfusion via modulating oxidative stress. *Journal of Nutritional Biochemistry, 21,* 741–748.

Yospiovitch, G., Tang, M., Dawn, A. G., et al. (2007). Study of psychological stress, sebum production and acne vulgaris in adolescents. *Acta Dermato-Venereology, 87,* 135–139.

Zhang, L., Li, W. H., Anthonavage, M., et al. (2011). Melanocortin-5 receptor and sebogenesis. *European Journal of Pharmacology, 660*, 202–206.

Zouboulis, C., & Bohm, M. (2004). Neuroendocrine regulation of sebocytes—a pathogenetic link between stress and acne. *Experimental Dermatology, 13*, 31–35.

Zouboulis, C. C., Seltmann, H., Hiroi, N., et al. (2002). Corticotrophin-releasing hormone: an autocrine hormone that promotes lipogenesis in human sebocytes. *Proceedings of the National Academy of Sciences USA, 99*, 7148–7153.

13

Integrative Management of Hair Loss and Hair Care

NICOLE E. ROGERS

Key Concepts

♣ Currently, the only medications approved by the U.S. Food and Drug Administration for hair loss are Rogaine® and Propecia.® However, exciting research into natural botanical ingredients may offer more treatment options.

♣ Some of these include procyanidins derived from apples, grape seeds, and barley, as well as isoflavones, ginseng, gingko, plant-based 5-alpha-reductase inhibitors, essential oils, vitamin C, and amino acids such as taurine and L-carnitine.

♣ In this chapter we discuss these as well as other natural compounds for hair care, hair coloring, and hair protection.

Introduction

For both men and women, hair is a powerful indicator of health and fertility. The most common cause of hair loss is inherited androgenetic alopecia, also known as male or female pattern hair loss (Figs. 13.1 and 13.2). Hair breakage or dullness may signal overprocessing of the hair, especially in developed countries, where there is ready access to chemical relaxers, colorants, and heating devices. The cosmeceutical industry has exploded in recent years as manufacturers have incorporated various plant extracts into products for hair care and hair loss. In this chapter we will focus on active ingredients with scientific data supporting their role in hair protection, hair growth, and hair care.

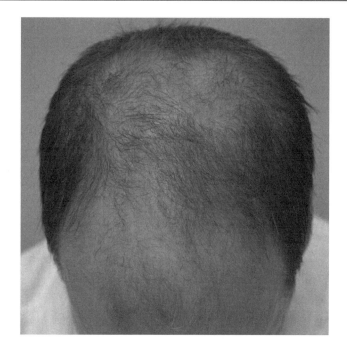

FIGURE 13.1 Male pattern hair loss.

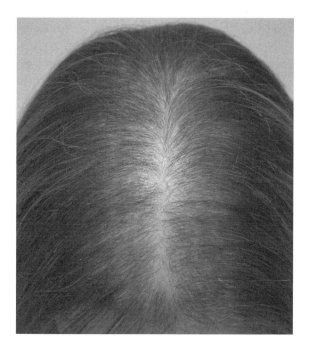

FIGURE 13.2 Female pattern hair loss.

Products for Hair Growth

At present, there are only two medications for hair loss that are approved by the U.S. Food and Drug Administration (FDA) and one medical device that has FDA 510K approval. These include topical minoxidil, sold under the trade name Rogaine® (for men and women), oral finasteride (trade name Propecia®, approved for men only), and the HairMax LaserComb, a hand-held device emitting a 655-nm low-level laser beam (for men and women). However, there has been a surprising amount of research to identify new ingredients that will help grow or improve hair. The data vary from in vitro cell culture to in vivo rat studies to a few human studies. Box 13.1 provides a summary of some of the proposed plant-based mechanisms of action on hair growth.

POLYPHENOLS: GRAPE SEED, APPLE EXTRACT, BARLEY, AND RASPBERRY

Antioxidants such as polyphenols (including flavonoids) have long been used for anti-aging skin care regimens (Wayne, 1996). They are known for their abilities to scavenge free radicals and thus reduce the deleterious effects of oxidative stress from ultraviolet radiation and environmental pollution.

One group of Japanese researchers investigated the role of procyanidins in stimulating hair growth. Their initial research (involving an examination of about 1,000 different kinds of plant extracts) demonstrated the growth-promoting effects of proanthocyanidins from **grape seeds** (Chardonnay variety) (Takahashi et al., 1998). The oligomeric form increased the proliferation of mouse hair follicle cells in vitro to about 230% of levels seen with controls. This was even more effective than minoxidil, which had a proliferative activity of 160% of controls. In vivo, the 3% proanthocyanidin

---

Box 13.1 Proposed Mechanisms for Hair Growth

Inhibition of 5-alpha-reductase
Downregulation of TGF-β
Upregulation of IGF-1
  – Via increased release of CGRP
  – Mediated by phosphatidylinositol 3-kinase
Activation of NF-κB
Inhibition of protein kinase C
Upregulation of Shh and β-catenin
Increased VEGF and increased uptake of cysteine

extract was as effective as 1% minoxidil in converting the hair of C3H mice from telogen to anagen phase. Epicatechin, the monomeric form of proantho-cyanidins, was less effective, showing 160% of controls' growth in vitro and with no effect in vivo.

In further studies, this same group demonstrated that the dimeric and tri-meric forms of these phenolic compounds were consistently more effective at stimulating hair growth than the monomeric forms (Takahashi et al., 1999). Specifically, they found that the procyanidin B-2 (an epicatechin dimer) exhib-ited the greatest in vitro growth-promoting activity for hair epithelial cells. No other flavonoid compounds examined exhibited higher proliferative activities than the procyanidins.

In 2001 the first clinical trial tested the topical application of a 1% procy-anidin B-2 tonic for hair growth in humans (Takahashi et al, 2001). In this double-blind, placebo-controlled study involving 29 male subjects with andro-genetic alopecia (19 treated, 10 placebo), 78.9% of the treatment group showed an increase in mean hair diameter, while only 30% of the placebo group showed any increase. There were significantly more hairs measuring greater than 40 microns in diameter in the treatment versus the placebo groups ($p < 0.02$), and there was a significant increase in the total number of hairs in the designated scalp area of procyanidin B-2 treatment compared with placebo (gain of $3.67 \pm 4.09/0.25$ cm^2 vs. a loss of $2.54 \pm 4.00/0.25$ cm^2 ($p < 0.001$). No adverse effects were reported in either group.

In a second double-blind clinical trial, 0.7% apple (*Malus pumila*) procy-anidin oligomers were applied to the scalps of men with androgenetic alopecia over a 12-month period (Fig. 13.3) (Takahashi et al., 2005). Twenty-one men in the treatment group and 22 men in the placebo group applied a 2-mL dose of topical procyanidins B-1, B-2, and C-1 twice daily for 6 months, and then the study was extended an additional 6 months for the treatment group. The hair density in a designated 0.8-cm^2 area was assessed after 6 and 12 months. After 6 months, the treatment group had an increase of $3.3 \pm 13.0/0.5$ cm,^{2} whereas the placebo group had a decrease of $3.6 \pm 8.1/0.5$cm^2 ($p < 0.001$ in a two-sample t-test). By 12 months, the treatment group had a significant increase in hair count above baseline ($11.5 \pm 16.5/0.5$ cm^2, $p < 0.005$, paired t-test). Hair caliber was not assessed in this study.

These studies raise additional questions about the mechanism of action of various plant procyanidins. A number of growth factors, such as TGF-β, FGF-5, TNF-α, IL-1α, and IL-1β, are known to negatively regulate hair growth (Danilenko et al., 1996; Foitzik et al., 2000). Based on this evidence, Kamimura and Takahashi investigated the ability of procyanidin B-3, isolated from the seed husks of **barley** (*Hordeum vulgare* L. var *distichon* Alefeld), to counter-act the inhibitory effects of TGF-β1 on hair growth (Kamimura et al., 2002b).

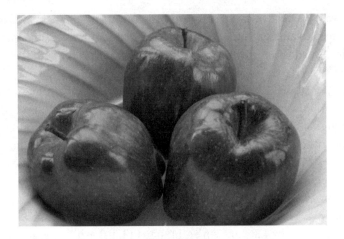

FIGURE 13.3 Apples are an important source of procyanidin extract.

They found that the addition of TGF-β to hair epithelial cell cultures dose-dependently decreased cell growth, and that the addition of procyanidin B-3 neutralized these growth-inhibiting effects. The authors concluded that procyanidin B-3 could directly promote hair cell growth in vitro and could potentially stimulate anagen growth in vivo.

An additional mechanism of action proposed for these procyanidins is the inhibition of the protein kinase C (PKC). PKC is a differentiation signal for epidermal keratinocytes (Chakravathy et al., 1995) and exerts an inhibitory effect on hair growth (Harmon et al., 1995, 1997). The expression of PKC-α, β, and ζ has been demonstrated in the outer root sheath of cultured keratinocytes. In mouse studies, it was found that PKC-α, βI, βII, and η were expressed in the outer root sheaths of both anagen and telogen hair follicles. Researchers found that procyanidin B-2 reduced the expression of all four of these isoenzymes, inhibiting their translocation to the particulate fraction of hair cells and reducing their ability to inhibit hair growth (Kamimura & Takahashi, 2002a).

Commercially available products containing polycyadins include Poly-GRO™ Procyanidin B-2, manufactured by Apple Poly LLC (Morrill NE) and Spectral RS (DS Laboratories).

RASPBERRY

Raspberry may also have a role in treating hair loss (Fig. 13.4). Based on previous work showing that capsaicin could increase facial skin elasticity and promote hair growth, researchers tested raspberry ketone (RK), a structurally similar aromatic compound contained in red raspberries (*Rubus idaeus*), for

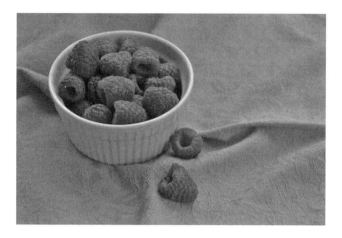

FIGURE 13.4   Raspberry extract may be a source of hair loss treatment.

similar effects. A 0.01% concentration of RK was applied to wild-type mice and was found to increase dermal levels of insulin-like growth factor I (IGF-I) (Harada et al., 2008). This effect appears to be mediated through calcitonin gene-related peptide (CGRP) because it was not seen in CGRP-knockout mice. When applied to the scalps, 0.01% RK promoted hair growth in 50% of humans with alopecia areata (n = 10) after 5 months. The black raspberry (*Rubus occidentalis L.*) may also be interesting for future research given its high phenolic content (Dossett et al., 2010).

ISOFLAVONES AND SOY

Isoflavones are organic compounds that have biologic activities similar to estrogens, hence their other name "phytoestrogens." Similar to capsaicin and raspberry ketone, they stimulate the release of CGRP, which subsequently increases IGF-I expression and hair growth. In one study, dietary isoflavones increased both the number of hair follicles and IGF-I expression within the follicles of wild-type C57BL/6 mice, whereas this effect was not seen in CGRP-knockout mice (Zhao et al., 2011). In another study both isoflavone (75 mg/day) and capsaicin (6 mg/day) were administered to 31 human volunteers. Significantly more hair growth was seen in the treatment group (20/31, 64.5%) than in the placebo group (2/17, 11.8%) (Harada et al., 2007).

Dietary soy was given to C3H/HeJ rats grafted with skin from alopecia areata rats and was found to have a dose-dependent protective effect on the hair follicles, with lower rates of alopecia observed in the 5% and 20% groups versus the 1% soy diet groups. In the same study, some of the mice were injected with genistein three times per week for 10 weeks; they found to have lower rates of alopecia areata development (4/10 vs. 9/10 in the control group) (McElwee et al., 2003).

A soy peptide derivative called soymetide-4 was investigated for its ability to prevent chemotherapy-induced alopecia in rats. Their work showed that oral soymetide-4 did have an alopecia-preventing effect and that it appeared to be mediated through prostaglandin E_2 (PGE_2) (Tsuruki et al., 2005). This effect was blocked by pyrrolidine dithiocarbamate (PDTC), a known inhibitor of NF-κB. These results suggested that PGE_2, which was activated by soymetide-4, could suppress apoptosis of hair follicles by activating NF-κB.

GINSENG, GINGKO, AND RELATIVES

Ginseng has been investigated extensively for its role in potentially treating male and female pattern hair loss. *Panax ginseng*, the Asian ginseng root, exists as red ginseng (which has been heated or steamed) and white ginseng (which has been dried). The plant can be separated into the main root, the fibrous root, and the rhizome. The active ingredients are believed to be saponins, of which 26 have been isolated and identified. These are categorized into panaxadiols, panaxatriols, and oleananes. Within each group, Rb_1, Rg_1, and G-Ro are the most abundant in ginsengs, respectively.

Red ginseng was shown to have superior efficacy over white ginseng in promoting hair growth in cultured mouse vibrissal hair follicles (Matsuda et al., 2003). The active ingredient, Rb_1, showed the most significant promotion of hair growth on cultured mouse vibrissal hair follicles. Red ginseng also was shown to have a protective effect against gentamicin-induced hearing loss in rats, as demonstrated by more hair cells with intact stereocilia in the treatment group (Choung et al., 2011). As above, Rb_1 was shown to be the most effective component in preventing cell apoptosis. Similarly anti-apoptotic and anti-oxidant effects were observed when Korean red ginseng was found to protect against cisplatin-induced ototoxicity in vitro (Im et al., 2010).

In another study, the fruit of the ginseng plant was also found to exert a proliferative effect on C57BL6 mouse hair follicles (Park et al., 2011). There was a significant elongation of the anagen phase as well as enhanced anti-apoptotic (Bcl-2) expression and decreased pro-apoptotic (Bax) expression. An additional mechanism of action was identified when the red ginseng rhizome was found to inhibit the enzyme 5-alpha-reductase (5-AR) in testosterone-treated mice (Murata et al., 2011). So far only one human clinical trial has been published, but it showed that oral consumption of Korean red ginseng extract (3,000 mg/day) for 24 weeks effectively increased hair density and thickness in alopecia patients (Kim et al., 2009).

One older study demonstrated hair regrowth using a 70% ethanolic extract from the leaves of *Ginkgo biloba* in C3H strain mice (Kobayashi et al., 1993). Interestingly, ginkgo has also been shown to have protective effects against gentamicin- and cisplatin-induced ototoxicity, suggesting similarly antioxidant and anti-apoptotic effects as seen with red ginseng (Huang et al., 2007; Yang et al., 2011).

Plant-Derived 5-Alpha-Reductase Inhibitors

A crucial mechanism in the pathogenesis of male (and possibly female) pattern hair loss is the conversion of testosterone to dihydrotestosterone (DHT) by the enzyme 5-AR. DHT is believed to exert a miniaturizing effect on the hair follicle. When DHT levels are reduced by inhibiting 5-AR, ongoing hair loss can be arrested and regrowth can even be observed. At present, finasteride (Propecia®) is the only FDA-approved medication that works by this mechanism. However, there are some side effects related to the use of finasteride, such as breast enlargement or tenderness, a loss of libido, or erectile dysfunction (reported in less than 2% of patients in clinical trials). Therefore a number of plant products have been investigated for 5-AR activity but with fewer side effects. They are listed in Table 13.1.

Saw palmetto (*Serenoa repens*) has been used widely as an alternative to finasteride in treating urinary symptoms of benign prostatic hypertrophy in men. Its active ingredients, liposterolic extract and β-sitosterol, have 5-AR–inhibiting properties. However, the only data we have examining its role in treating hair loss come from a small trial from 1999 in which six of 10 men treated with oral saw palmetto had subjective improvement after oral intake of softgels containing saw palmetto extract for 5 months (Prager et al., 2002). Although it was a randomized, double-blind placebo-controlled trial, no objective measures were used to assess hair follicle diameter or density.

Green tea is consumed widely around the world and is touted for its potential antioxidant and anticancer benefits. It was identified as a 5-AR inhibitor in 1995 (Liao & Hiipakka, 1995), and it was suggested as a treatment for androgenetic alopecia in 2002 (Hiipakka et al., 2002). However, its efficacy is somewhat limited in its native state (epigallocatechin gallate [EGCG]). Researchers observed that its ability to inhibit 5-AR increased when the gallate ester in EGCG was replaced with a long-chain fatty acids, such as lauric (10 carbon chain), myristic (12 chain carbon), and stearic acid (16 carbon chain). The most potent inhibitor of 5-AR was formed with the addition of palmitic acid (14 carbon chain) (Lin et al., 2010).

Another plant investigated for its ability to block 5-AR is *Sophora flavescens*. This plant has been widely used in Chinese medicine for the treatment

Table 13.1. Summary of Plant-Derived 5-Alpha-Reductase Inhibitors

Plant	Latin Name	Active Ingredient(s)	Reference
Saw palmetto, American dwarf palm	Serenoa repens Sabal serrutala	Oleic acid Lauric acid Myristic acid γ-linoleic acid (Liang & Liao, 1992) β-sitosterol	Neiderprum et al. (1994)
Black pepper	Piper nigrum leaf	Active lignin 1* Active lignin 2* Piperine (high in linoleic, oleic, and palmitic acids)	Hirata et al. (2007)
Green tea extract	Epicatechin	With palmitic acid	Lin et al. (2010)
Japanese false nettle	Boehmeria nipononivea	α-linoleic acid Elaidic acid Stearic acid	Shimizu et al. (2000)
Safflower	Carthamus tinctorius L.	Carthamin Carthamidin Isocarthamidin	Kumar et al. (2012)
Lingzhi mushroom	Ganoderma lucidum	Triterpenoids	Fujita et al. (2005)
Red bayberry bark	Murica rubra	Myricanol Myricanone	Matsuda et al. (2001)
White cedar seed	Thuja occidentalis	Unknown	Park et al. (2003)
Japanese climbing fern	Lygodium japonicum	Oleic, linoleic, and palmitic acids	Matsuda et al. (2002)
Puereria flower	Puerariae flos	Soyasaponin I Kaikasaponin III	Murata et al. (2012a)
Rosemary (herb)	Rosmarinus officialis	Unknown	Murata et al. (2012b)
Red ginseng	Ginseng rhizome and Ginsenoside Ro	Triterpine saponins Ginsenoside Rg1	Murata et al. (2012c)
Dried root of plant	Sophora flavescens	unknown	Roh et al. (2002)

*Interestingly, these two lignans also demonstrated stimulation of melanogenesis, which could be applied toward the treatment of gray hair.

of cancers and inflammation. When it was applied to the backs of C57BL/6 mice, the anagen cycle was initiated earlier than in control groups, but it did not affect dermal papillae cells in culture (Roh et al., 2002). It specifically induced mRNA levels of growth factors such as insulin-like growth factor and keratinocyte growth factor and was found to significantly inhibit 5-AR levels in comparison with controls.

ESSENTIAL OILS

Scientists in Korea demonstrated the hair-growth–promoting effects of *Zizyphus jujuba* essential oil. It is a thorny rhamnaceous plant that is already used as an analgesic as well as to prevent pregnancy and diabetes. Researchers applied 0.1%, 1%, and 10% concentrations of the essential oil to the backs of shaved BALB/c mice and observed their growth over 21 days. They found that the mice treated with the 1% and 10% solution had significantly longer hair (9.96 and 10.02 mm) than the control group (8.94 mm) (Yoon et al., 2010).

In India, the seeds of the teak tree (*Tectona grandis*) were used by ancient tribesmen to prevent hair loss. Their hair-growth–promoting activity was recently demonstrated to be equal or better than minoxidil 2% solution. Researchers in India tested 5% and 10% petroleum ether extract on the shaved denuded skin of albino mice. They found that the treated groups had a greater number of follicles entering the anagen phase (64% and 51%) than minoxidil-treated follicles (49%) (Jaybhaye et al., 2010).

VITAMIN C

Vitamin C has long been known for its antioxidant effects, but its use in cosmetics has been made more difficult by its lack of stability. Therefore, researchers investigated the use of a more stable vitamin C derivative, L-ascorbic acid 2-phosphate, to stimulate hair growth. They found that it induced an earlier telogen-to-anagen conversion in C57BL/6 mice compared with the control group (Sung et al., 2006). There was also a greater elongation of hair shafts in cultures treated with L-ascorbic 2-phosphate. This and a subsequent study both found a significant increase in mRNA expression of IGF-1 in treated cell lines, specifically mediated by phosphatidylinositol 3-kinase (PI3K) (Kwack et al., 2009).

AMINO ACIDS AND THEIR DERIVATIVES

Taurine is a naturally occurring β-amino acid produced by methionine and cysteine metabolism. Its production by mammals is limited, so dietary intake is crucial. When human hair follicles were treated with taurine in vitro, there was significantly greater hair elongation in the treated groups versus the control (Collin et al., 2006). When follicles were exposed to TGF-β1, their growth was compromised, but taurine was found to have a protective effect.

L-carnitine is an amino acid necessary for the transport of fatty acids into the mitochondria for subsequent β-oxidation and energy production. It has been shown to increase hair shaft elongation in vitro as well as to prolong anagen by upregulating proliferation and downregulating apoptosis in organ-cultured human scalp hair follicles (Foitzik et al., 2006). In a subsequent study, L-carnitine-L-tartrate was also shown to promote hair growth in a prospective, randomized, placebo-controlled observational study of human volunteers. The treatment group (N = 26) patients with androgenetic alopecia applied 2% carnitine hair tonic to a defined scalp area twice daily for 6 months. The control group (N = 25) applied placebo. After 6 months the treatment group showed a 13.5% increase in the total number of hair follicles ($p < 0.05$) using the Trichoscan technique, with an increase in the number of anagen follicles and a decrease in the number of telogen follicles (Foitzik et al., 2007).

MISCELLANEOUS PLANT ACTIVES

A number of other plants have demonstrated hair growth properties. These include *Polygonum multiflorum* (Chinese "fo-ti"), which appears to upregulate sonic hedgehog (Shh) and β-catenin (Park et al., 2011). *Eclipta alba* ("false daisy") is another plant with hair-growth–promoting activity. Topical studies in C57/BL6 mice demonstrated that the methanolic extract induced anagen in telogen-phase hair follicles at rates comparable to minoxidil (Datta et al., 2009). In another study *E. alba* was combined with extract from *Cuscuta reflexa* (Roxb.) and *Citrullus colocynthis* (Schrad.) and again was found to shorten the time for anagen initiation in rats in comparison with controls (Roy et al., 2007).

The plant *Asiasari radix* was found to promote hair growth in mice as well as human dermal papilla cells. The mechanism was proposed to be through either increased uptake of cysteine or upregulation of vascular endothelial growth factor (VEGF). There was no effect on the 5-AR mechanism. Extract of *Illicium anisatum* was found to stimulate prolonged hair growth in mouse vibrissae follicles through increased IGF-1, keratinocyte growth factor, and VEGF (Sakaguchi et al., 2004). Another plant native to South Korea called *Schisandra nigra* was applied in extract form to the backs of C57BL/6 mice and found to induce anagen progression of the hair shaft (Jabg Hum Kim et al., 2009). Its mechanism was identified as the downregulation of TGF-β.

Products for Hair Coloring

Since the ancient Egyptian days of Cleopatra, women have used various plant extracts and vegetable dyes to darken and color their hair. One of the most common of these is henna, a plant with leaves that render a burgundy-colored compound called lawsone. It is primarily concentrated in the leaves and has an affinity for protein. When the lawsone is dissolved in an acidic liquid such as lemon juice, it can be applied to the hair and will bind to the proteins after several hours of leave-in. The widespread use of henna is somewhat limited by availability and the risk of contact dermatitis. Most modern hair dyes contain manufactured ingredients such as para-phenylene diamine.

Recently, researchers have investigated other plant compounds for possible sources of hair coloring. Typically, the hair coloring process involves the application of dye precursors (usually p-diamines and p-aminophenols) followed by an oxidizing agent (usually H_2O_2). This is done at an alkaline pH because the hair swells, the cuticle lifts, and it becomes easier for dyes to penetrate the hair shaft. However, this alkaline pH can cause damaging side reactions to the hair follicle.

Therefore, different researchers have investigated the use of laccase, an enzyme produced by various fungi, plants, bacteria, and insects, as an alternative oxidizing agent. One group used the laccase enzyme from *Trametes versicolor* (also called the Turkey tail for its resemblance to the tail of a wild turkey) to oxidize natural plant-derived phenolic compounds (Jong-Rok et al., 2010). A second group used laccase from the Japanese mushroom *Flammulina velutipes* (Saito et al., 2012). Both groups had excellent results, achieving optimal coloring and withstanding subsequent shampooing.

Products for Hair Care and Protection

Hair can suffer from a process called "weathering," due to ultraviolet radiation, environmental pollution, and the repeated use of heat and chemicals in hairstyling. A number of natural remedies exist for hair protection as well as correction of dry, damaged, or frizzy hair. They effectively coat the cuticle, protecting it from heat or environmental insult. In this section we discuss various products with scientific data (where available) to support their use (Table 13.2). Products such as olive oil and coconut oil can smooth and protect curly or Afrocentric hair (Fig. 13.5).

PEPTIDES

Afrocentric hair can be extremely difficult to style due to its tight curl. As a result, many people resort to chemical straighteners or repeated application of flatirons or curling irons to smooth the hair and make it more manageable.

Table 13.2. Natural Remedies for Hair Care and Protection

Product	Applications
Aloe vera juice	Mix with wheat germ and coconut oil to increase hair softness. Can reduce dandruff. Risk of allergic contact dermatitis.
Apricot kernel oil	High in oleic and linoleic acid, known to soften hair and skin
Argan oil (Moroccan oil)	High in vitamin E and fatty acids, used to add shine to hair
Avocado oil	Contains monounsaturated fats: best results as a leave-in treatment for dry hair
Camellia oil	High in vitamin E and fatty acids, also known for antioxidant properties
Castor seed oil	Humectant with antifungal properties
Coconut oil	Highest ability to penetrate inside the hair shaft based on low molecular weight and linear structure, thus preventing protein loss (Rele & Mohile, 2003)
Glycerin	Creates layer of oil over hair strand, aiding in the retention of moisture
Hemp oil	Omega fatty acids provide emollient properties to soften hair shaft and prevent moisture loss
Honey	Light humectant with antibacterial properties
Jojoba oil	Wax ester with humectant properties. Multicultural applications (Keenan et al., 2011).
Extra-virgin olive oil	No machines involved in its production. May be used as a pre-shampoo or deep conditioner.
Macadamia nut oil	Antioxidant (Quinn & Tang, 1996)
Shea butter	Emollient
Tea tree oil (Melaleuca oil)	Antiseptic, antibacterial, antifungal properties (Pazyar et al., 2012); Satchell et al. (2002). Soothing to dry scalp. Can cause allergic or irritant contact dermatitis (Rutherford et al., 2007).

However, this can result in a further compromise in the hair strength and leave it even more brittle and prone to breakage. Hair surface tends to be negatively charged and becomes even more negatively charged when it is damaged. Therefore, peptides that have a positive charge are used to coat and repair the cuticle. There is evidence that the location of the positive charge (on the C-terminal end, which is smaller than the N-terminal end) allows for better penetration of the peptide component (Silva et al., 2007).

One group developed a keratin-based peptide that contains 13 amino acids and mimics a fragment of the human keratin type II cuticular protein, encoded by the KRT85 gene. When applied to black relaxed hair, it was found

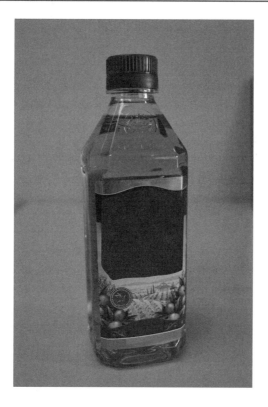

FIGURE 13.5 Extra-virgin olive oil can be used to coat and protect the hair follicle.

to improve both mechanical and thermal properties (Fernandes et al., 2012). This corroborated previous results showing that the same keratin peptide could also restore properties of over-bleached, damaged hair (Fernandes & Cavaco-Paolo, 2012).

CASSIA PLANT

Researchers at Proctor and Gamble demonstrated that extracts from the plant *Cassia tora* and *Cassia obtusifolia* can provide an alternative to the chemical cationic polymers traditionally used in the conditioning process (Staudigel et al., 2007). The endosperm of the *Cassia* plant contains a quaternized galactomannan, which has a positive charge that binds to anionic surfactants to form a water-insoluble complex called coacervate. This complex helps reduce friction from combing of wet hair and thus reduces breakage. Researchers found that the ability to use this plant extract reduced the amount of chemical polymer needed. This is an advantage because the chemical polymer can negatively affect the lather and stability.

HONEYDEW

The cotton honeydew also offers smoothing and protective effects on the hair shaft. The honeydew contains a number of oligosaccharides such as fructose, glucose, inositol, and trehalose, among others (Fig. 13.6). One half-head study showed that patients treated with a 1% honeydew extract had increased smoothness compared with the control side (Oberta et al., 2004). Also, scanning electron microscopy showed that the cuticle scales of treated hair appeared to lie more smoothly and were less prone to chipping. Honeydew is already available in several shampoos and conditioners.

EUCALYPTUS

A group of Japanese researchers conducted a study applying scalp lotions with eucalyptus extract of varying concentrations (0.5% to 3.0%) to a total of 149 individuals (men and women, Japanese and Caucasian backgrounds) (Mamada et al., 2008). The extract was applied to half of the head and placebo lotion was applied to the other half of the head. After a usage period of 2.5 to 3 months, there was found to be a significant increase in hair elasticity and a 10% increase in hair gloss intensity. More than 70% of the participants subjectively felt that the treated hair fibers had improved physical properties. One explanation may be an observed increase in the molar fraction of beta-sheets in the hair cortex, which are believed to lend strength to the hair fiber. On histologic examination, there was no noticeable change in hair caliber between the treated and untreated hair fibers.

Eucalyptus is currently available in commercial "root-awakening" formulas.

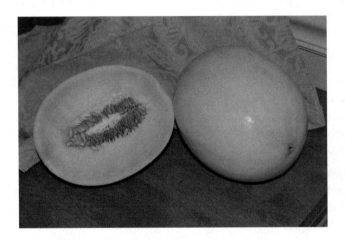

FIGURE 13.6 Honeydew elements may improve hair quality.

Products to Cosmetically Treat Thinning Hair

There are many "camouflage" products that can help to reduce the contrast between hair color and scalp color. Most of these contain synthetic keratin fibers, which electromagnetically cling to the hair shaft and scalp. However, other commercially available products contain wheat or quinoa protein or various root extracts to leave a coating on the hair follicle that increases the feeling of fullness. The major downside of these products is that they last only until the next hair washing.

Conclusion

A surprisingly large number of natural products have applications within hair care and hair loss treatment. This is exciting given that we are relatively limited in the number of FDA-approved treatments available. As more research is conducted, we must continue to evaluate the strength of the data and consider how these new treatments compare in efficacy and safety to existing treatment options.

REFERENCES

Chakravarthy, B. R., Isaacs, R. J., Morley, P., et al. (1995). Stimulation of protein kinase C during Ca+-induced keratinocyte differentiation. *Journal of Biological Chemistry*, *270*, 1362–1368.

Choung, Y. H., Kim, S. W., Tian, C., et al. (2011). Korean red ginseng prevents gentamycin-induced hearing loss in rats. *Laryngoscope, 121*, 1294–1302.

Collin, C., Gautier, B., Gaillard, O., et al. (2006).Protective effects of taurine on human hair follicle grown in vitro. *International Journal of Cosmetic Science, 28*, 289–298.

Danilenko, D. M., Ring, B. D., & Pierce, G. F. (1996). Growth factors and cytokines in hair follicle development and cycling: recent insights from animal models and the potentials for clinical therapy. *Molecular Medicine Today, 2*, 460–467.

Datta, K., Singh, A. T., Mukherjee, A., et al. (2009). *Eclipta alba* extract with potential for hair growth promoting activity. *Journal of Ethnopharmacology, 124*, 450–456.

Dossett, M., Lee, J., & Finn, C. E. (2010). Variation in anthocyanins and total phenolics of black raspberry populations. *Journal of Functional Foods, 2*, 292–297.

Fernandes, M., & Cavaco-Paulo, A. (2012). Protein disulfide isomerase-mediated grafting of cysteine-containing peptides onto over-bleached hair. *Biocatalysts & Biotransformation, 30*, 10–19.

Fernandes, M. M., Lima, C. F., Gomes, A. C., et al. (2012). Keratin-based peptide: biological evaluation and strengthening properties on relaxed hair. *Journal of Cosmetic Science* (Epub ahead of print).

Foitzik, K., Hoting, E., Heinrich, U., et al. (2007). Indications that topical L-carnitine-L-tartrate promotes human hair growth in vivo. *Journal of Dermatologic Science, 48*, 141–144.

Foitzik, K., Hoting, E., Pertile, P., et al. (2006). L-carnitine tartrate promotes human hair growth in vitro. *Journal of Investigative Dermatology, 126*, s27 (P146).

Foitzik, K., Lindner, G., Mueller-Roever, S., et al. (2000). Control of murine hair follicle regression (catagen) by TGF-β in vivo. *FASEB Journal, 14*, 752–760.

Fujita, R., Liu, J., Shimizu, K., et al. (2005). Anti-androgenic activities of *Ganoderma lucidum*. *Journal of Ethnopharmacology, 102*, 107–112.

Harada, N., Okajima, K., Arai, M., et al. (2007). Administration of capsaicin and isoflavone promotes hair growth by increasing insulin-like growth factor-I production in mice and in humans with alopecia. *Growth Hormone & IGF Research, 17*, 408–415.

Harada, N., Okajima, K., Narimatsu, N., et al. (2008). Effect of topical application of raspberry ketone on dermal production of insulin-like growth factor-I in mice and on hair growth and skin elasticity in humans. *Growth Hormone and IGF Research, 18*, 335–344.

Harmon, C. S., Nevins, T. D., & Bollag, W. B. (1995). Protein kinase C inhibits human hair follicle growth and hair fiber production in organ culture. *British Journal of Dermatology, 133*, 686–693.

Harmon, C. S., Nevins, T. D., Ducote, J., et al. (1997). Bisindolymaleimide protein-kinase-C inhibitors delay the decline in DNA synthesis in mouse hair follicle organ cultures. *Skin Pharmacology, 10*, 71–78.

Hiipakka, R. A., Zhang, H. Z., Dai, W., et al. (2002). Structure-activity relationships for inhibition of human 5α-reductases by polyphenols. *Biochemical Pharmacology, 63*, 1165–1176.

Hirata, N., Tokunaga, M., Naruto, S., et al. (2007). Testosterone 5A-reductase inhibitory active constituents of *Piper nigrum* leaf. *Biological & Pharmaceutical Bulletin, 30*, 2402–2405.

Huang, X., Whitworth, C. A., & Rybak, L. P. (2007). *Ginkgo biloba* extract (EGb 761) protects against cisplatin-induced ototoxicity in rats. *Otology & Neurotology, 28*, 828–833.

Im, G. J., Chang, J. W., Choi, J., et al. (2010). Protective effect of Korean red ginseng extract on cisplatin ototoxicity in HEI-OC1 auditory cells. *Phytotherapy Research, 24*, 614–621.

Jabg Hum Kim, S. C., Hyun, J. H., Park, D. B., et al. (2009) Promotion effect of *Schisandra nigra* on the growth of hair. *European Journal of Dermatology, 19*(2), 119–125.

Jaybhaye, D., Varma, S., Gagne, N., et al. (2010). Effect of *Tectona grandis* Linn. seeds on hair growth activity of albino mice. *International Journal of Ayurveda Research, 1*, 211–215.

Jong-Rok, J., Eun-Ju, K., Kumarasamy, M., et al. (2010). Laccase-catalysed polymeric dye synthesis from plant-derived phenols for potential application in hair dyeing: Enzymatic colourations driven by homo- or hetero-polymer synthesis. *Microbial Biotechnology, 3*, 324–335.

Kamimura, A., & Takahashi, T. (2002a). Procyanidin B-2, extracted from apples, promotes hair growth: a laboratory study. *British Journal of Dermatology, 146*, 41–51.

Kamimura, A., & Takahashi, T. (2002b). Procyanidin B-3, isolated from barley and identified as a hair-growth stimulant, has the potential to counteract inhibitory regulation by TGF-β1. *Experimental Dermatology, 11*, 532–541.

Keenan, A. C., Antrim, R. F., & Powell, T. (2011). Characterization of hair styling formulations targeted to specific multicultural needs. *Journal of Cosmetic Science, 62*, 149–160.

Kim, J. H., Yi, S. M., Choi, J. E., et al. (2009). Study of the efficacy of Korean red ginseng in the treatment of androgenetic alopecia. *Journal of Ginseng Research, 33*, 223–228.

Kobayashi, N., Suzuki, R., Koide, C., et al. (1993). Effect of leaves of *Ginkgo biloba* on hair regrowth in C3H strain mice. *Yakagaku Zasshi, 113*, 718–724.

Kumar, N., Rungseevijitprapa, W., Narkkhong, N-A., et al. (2012). 5α-reductase inhibition and hair growth promotion of some Thai plants traditionally used for hair treatment. *Journal of Ethnopharmacology, 139*, 765–771.

Kwack, M. H., Shin, S. H., Kim, S. R., et al. (2009). L-Ascorbic acid 2-phosphate promotes elongation of hair shafts via the secretion of insulin-like growth factor-1 from dermal papilla cells through phosphatidylinositol 3-kinase. *British Journal of Dermatology, 160*, 1157–1162.

Liang, T., & Liao, S. (1992). Inhibition of steroid 5a reductase by specific aliphatic unsaturated fatty acids. *Biochemistry Journal, 285*, 557–562.

Liao, S., & Hiipakka, R. A. (1995). Selective inhibition of steroid 5-alpha-reductase isoenzymes by tea epicatechin-3-gallate and epigallocatechin-3-gallate. *Biochemistry & Biophysics Research Communications, 214*, 833–838.

Lin, S. F., Lin, Y. S., Lin, M., et al. (2010). (2010). Synthesis and structure-activity relationship of 3-0-acylated (-)-epigallocatechins as 5a reductase inhibitors. *European Journal of Medicinal Chemistry, 45*, 6068–6076.

Mamada, A., Ishihama, M., Fukuda, R., et al. (2008). Changes in hair properties by *Eucalyptus* extract. *Journal of Cosmetic Science, 59*, 481–496.

Matsuda, H., Yamazaki, M., Matsuo, K., et al. (2001). Anti-androgenic activity of Myricae cortex—isolation of active constituents of bark of *Myrica rubra*. *Biological & Pharmaceutical Bulletin, 24*, 259–263.

Matsuda, H., Yamazaki, M., Naruto, S., et al. (2002). Anti-androgenic and hair growth promoting activities of *Lygodii spora* (Spore of *Lygodium japonicum*) I. Active constituents inhibiting Testosterone 5α-reductase. *Biological & Pharmaceutical Bulletin, 25*, 622–626.

Matsuda, H., Yamazaki, M., Asanuma, Y., et al. (2003). Promotion of hair growth by Ginseng Radix on cultured mouse vibrissal hair follicles. *Phytotherapy Research*, 797–800.

McElwee, K. J., Niiyama, S., Freyschmidt-Paul, P., et al. (2003). Dietary soy oil content and soy-derived phytoestrogen genistein increase resistance to alopecia areata onset in C3H/HeJ mice. *Experimental Dermatology, 12*, 30–36.

Murata, K., Noguchi, K., Kondo, M., et al. (2012a). Inhibitory activities of *Puerariae flos* against testosterone 5α-reductase and its hair growth promotion activities. *Journal of Natural Medicines, 66*, 158–165.

Murata, K., Noguchi, K., Kondo, M., et al. (2012b). Promotion of hair growth by *Rosmarinus officinalis* leaf extract. *Phytotherapy Research* (Epub ahead of print).

Murata, K., Takeshita, F., Samukawa, K., et al. (2012c). Effects of Ginseng rhizome and Gensenoside Ro on testosterone 5α-reductase and hair re-growth in testosterone-treated mice. *Phytotherapy Research, 26*, 48–53.

Niederprum, H. J., Schweikert, H. U., & Zanker, K. S. (1994). Testosterone 5A reductase inhibition by free fatty acids from *Sabal serrulata* fruits. *Phytomedicine, 1*, 127–133.

Oberta, G., Bauza, E., Berchi, A., et al. (2005). Cotton honeydew (*Gossypium hirutum* L.) extract offers very interesting properties for hair cosmetics and care products. *Drugs Under Experimental & Clinical Research, 31*, 131–140.

Park, H., Zhang, N., & Park, D. K. (2011). Topical application of *Polygonum multiflorum* extract induces hair growth of resting hair follicles through upregulating Shh and β-catenin expression in C57BL/6 mice. *Journal of Ethnopharmacology, 135*, 369–375.

Park, S., Shin, W-S., & Ho, J. (2011). *Fructus panax ginseng* extract promotes hair regeneration in C57BL/6 mice. *Journal of Ethnopharmacology, 138*, 340–344.

Park, W., Lee, C., Lee, B., et al. (2003). The extract of *Thujae occidentalis semen* inhibited 5α-reductase and androchronogenetic alopecia of B6CBAF1/j hybrid mice. *Journal of Dermatologic Science, 31*, 91–98.

Pazyar, N., Yaghoobi, R., Bagherani, N., et al. (2012). A review of applications of tea tree oil in dermatology. *International Journal of Dermatology* (Epub ahead of print).

Prager, N., Bickett, K., French, N., et al. (2002). A randomized, double-blind, placebo-controlled trial to determine the effectiveness of botanically derived inhibitors of 5-α-reductase in the treatment of androgenetic alopecia. *Journal of Alternative & Complementary Medicine, 8*, 143–152.

Quinn, L. A., & Tang, H. H. (1996). Antioxidant properties of phenolic compounds in macadamia nuts. *Journal of the American Oil Chemists' Society, 73*, 1585–1588.

Rele, A. S., & Mohile, R. B. (2003). Effect of mineral oil, sunflower oil, and coconut oil on prevention of hair damage. *Journal of Cosmetic Science, 54*, 175–192.

Roh, S. S., Kim, C. D., Lee, M. H., et al. (2002). The hair growth promoting effect of *Sophora flavescens* extract and its molecular regulation. *Journal of Dermatologic Science, 30*, 43–49.

Roy, R. K., Thakur, M., & Dixit, V. K. (2007). Development and evaluation of polyherbal formulation for hair growth-promoting activity. *Journal of Cosmetic Dermatology, 6*, 108–112.

Rutherford, T., Nixon, R., Tam, M., et al. (2007). Allergy to tea tree oil: retrospective review of 41 cases with positive patch texts over 4.5 years. *Australasian Journal of Dermatology, 48*, 83–87.

Saito, K., Ikeda, R., Endo, K., et al. (2012). Isolation of a novel alkaline-induced laccase from *Flammulina velutipes* and its application for hair color. *Journal of Bioscience and Bioengineering, 113*, 575–579.

Sakaguchi, I., Ishimoto, H., Matsuo, M., et al. (2004). The water-soluble extract of *Illicium anisatum* stimulates mouse vibrissae follicles in organ culture. *Experimental Dermatology, 13*, 499–504.

Satchell, A. C., Saurajen, A., Bell, C., et al. (2002). Treatment of dandruff with 5% tea tree oil shampoo. *Journal of the American Academy of Dermatology,* 852–855.

Shimizu, K., Kondo, R., Sakai, K., et al. (2000). Steroid 5α-reductase inhibitory activity and hair regrowth effects of an extract from *Boehmeria nipononivea. Bioscience Biotechnology Biochemistry, 64,* 875–877.

Silva, C. J., Vasconcelos, A., & Cavaco-Paulo, A. (2007). Peptide structure: Its effect on penetration into human hair. *Journal of Cosmetic Science, 58,* 339–346.

Staudigel, J. A., Bunasky, K., Gamsky, C. J., et al. (2007). Use of quaternized cassia galactomannan for hair conditioning. *Journal of Cosmetic Science, 58,* 637–650.

Sung, Y. K., Hwang, S. Y., Cha, S. Y., et al. (2006). The hair growth promoting effect of ascorbic acid 2-phosphate, a long-acting vitamin C derivative. *Journal of Dermatologic Science, 41,* 150–152.

Takahashi, T., Kamimura, A., Kagoura, M., et al. (2005). Investigation of the topical application of procyanidin oligomers from apples to identify their potential use as a hair-growing agent. *Journal of Cosmetic Dermatology, 4,* 245–249.

Takahashi, T., Kamimura, A., Yokoo, Y., et al. (2001). The first clinical trial for topical application of procyanidin B-2 to investigate its potential as a hair growing agent. *Phytotherapy Research, 15,* 331–336.

Takahashi, T., Kamiya, T., Hasegawa, A., et al. (1999). Procyanidin oligomers selectively and intensively promote proliferation of mouse hair epithelial cells in vitro and activate hair follicle growth in vivo. *Journal of Investigative Dermatology, 112,* 310–316.

Takahashi, T., Kamiya, T., & Yokoo, Y. (1998). Proanthocyanidins from grape seeds promote proliferation of mouse hair follicle cells in vitro and convert hair cycle in vivo. *Acta Dermatol-Venereologica, 78,* 428–432.

Tsuruki, T., Takahata, K., & Yoshikawa, M. (2005). Anti-alopecia mechanisms of soymetide-4, an immunostimulating peptide derived from soy β-conglycinin. *Peptides, 26,* 707–711.

Wayne, Z. (1996). Pycnogenol and skincare. *Drug and Cosmetic Industry, 158,* 44–50.

Yang, T. H., Toung, Y. H., & Liu, S. H. (2011). EGb 761 (*Ginkgo biloba*) protects cochlear hair cells against ototoxicity induced by gentamycin via reducing reactive oxygen species and nitric oxide-related apoptosis. *Journal of Nutritional Biochemistry,* 886–994.

Yoon, J. I., Al-Reza, S. M., & Kang, S. C. (2010). Hair growth promoting effect of *Zizyphus jujuba* essential oil. *Food and Chemical Toxicology, 48,* 1350–1354.

Zhao, J., Harada, N., Kurihara, K., et al. (2011). Dietary isoflavone increases insulin-like growth factor-I production, thereby promoting hair growth in mice. *Journal of Nutritional Biochemistry, 22,* 227–233.

14

Integrative Management of Atopic Dermatitis

KACHIU C. LEE AND PETER A. LIO

Key Concepts

- ♣ Atopic dermatitis (AD) is a chronic skin disease characterized by itch, an impaired epidermal barrier, inflammation, significant bacterial colonization with frequent skin infections, and a clinical course punctuated by flares and remissions.
- ♣ Stress and sleep deprivation can have a negative impact directly on AD, causing delayed healing of the skin barrier and worsening this condition.
- ♣ AD has a worldwide distribution and a prevalence of more than 20% in developed countries and remains a significant problem without an easy cure.
- ♣ Many integrative modalities are used in the treatment of AD, including traditional Chinese medicine, acupuncture, homeopathy, biofeedback, hypnotherapy, natural oils, bathing modifications, probiotics, and dietary restrictions.

Introduction

Atopic dermatitis (AD) is a chronic skin disease characterized by itch, an impaired epidermal barrier, inflammation, significant bacterial colonization with frequent skin infections, and a clinical course punctuated by flares and remissions. Although a number of stimuli may trigger a flare, psychological stress has been shown to play a role in this disease as well (Suarez et al., 2012). While this complex etiopathogenesis signifies a large number of potential targets for treatment, it simultaneously underscores the unsatisfying state of understanding of this disease. With a worldwide distribution and a prevalence of more than 20% in developed countries, AD remains a significant problem without an easy cure. Perhaps then it is not surprising that the majority of patients with AD report using complementary and alternative medicine (CAM) in the treatment of their disease (Jensen, 1990).

Reasons for Using CAM in AD

Several factors drive patients to choose CAM over, or in conjunction with, conventional medications. In a large survey of 227 Norwegians with AD, the primary reason for use of CAM was lack of satisfaction of physician-provided therapy related to poor improvement in disease severity (Jensen, 1990). Part of this dissatisfaction may stem from the diverging views on disease severity between physician and patient. Although both parties are usually in agreement about pretreatment disease severity, the perception of treatment effectiveness quickly diverges. While 91% of physicians rated prescription medications as "moderately" or "very" effective, only 46% of patients gave similarly high ratings. Patients were moderately pleased with their overall AD-related medication care, with 42% stating they were "a lot" or "very satisfied" and 8% stating they were dissatisfied (McAlister et al., 2002). This dichotomy likely serves as a root cause for patients seeking CAM over conventional therapies.

The perceived adverse side effects of conventional medications also play a role in usage of CAM. In a survey of 62 Australians using CAM, preference for natural approaches to skin disease and a perceived lesser potential for adverse effects from CAM were the predominant reasons for choosing CAM over conventional medications (Magin et al., 2006). Poor healthcare access to providers and pharmacies dispensing conventional medications was also associated with higher usage of CAM (Adams et al., 2011). Women residing in rural areas were more likely to consult a CAM practitioner (32%) than those residing in urban areas (28%) (Adams et al., 2011a, 2011b). These findings reinforce those of other studies, where perception of side effects due to CAM and the rural–urban divide played a large role in choosing to use CAM (Box 14.1) (Baron et al., 2005; Ben-Arye et al., 2003, Johnston et al., 2003).

Evidence-Based Review of CAM in AD

TRADITIONAL CHINESE MEDICINE

In Eastern cultures, there is a longstanding history of using traditional Chinese medicine (TCM) as a treatment for AD. TCM, considered separately from

---

Box 14.1 Reasons for Choosing Complementary and Alternative Medicines Over Conventional Therapy

Cultural factors (Lee et al., 2004)

Dissatisfaction with conventional medicine (Baron et al., 2005; Jensen, 1990; Johnston et al., 2003)

Desire for natural therapies (Baron et al., 2005)

Skepticism in regards to conventional medications (Baron et al., 2005; Johnston et al., 2003)

Perception of fewer side effects (Baron et al., 2004; Ben-Arye et al., 2003; Johnston et al., 2003)

Desire to try any possible therapy (Berg & Arnetz, 1998; Jensen, 1990)

Differing perceptions of severity of skin disease compared to physician (McAlister et al., 2002)

Poor accessibility to physicians or conventional medications (Adams et al., 2011a, 2011b)

---

acupuncture, consists of herbal preparations taken by mouth or applied to the skin as well as dietary and lifestyle modifications. Each individual's therapy is personalized to his or her disease, which encompasses a more holistic or constitutional approach and is often combined with acupuncture.

Several double-blind, placebo-controlled studies of TCM for AD have shown significant effects, with decrease in erythema, body surface area involvement, and pruritus (Graham-Brown, 1992; Hon et al., 2007; Sheehan et al., 1992). Sheehan and colleagues (1992) treated 40 adult patients with long-standing, refractory, widespread AD in a placebo-controlled, double-blind, crossover study. At the end of active treatment (two months), subjects receiving TCM compared to placebo had decreased erythema and disease severity. There was also subjective improvement in pruritus and sleep disturbance based on survey responses.

Similarly, children with AD have shown benefit from using TCM. Hon and colleagues (2007) recruited 85 children with AD, randomizing them into a placebo-controlled trial. Experimental subjects were treated with a twice-daily concoction of five herbs traditionally used for AD. Over 12 weeks, these subjects demonstrated improvement on the Scoring of Atopic Dermatitis (SCORAD) severity index and Children's Dermatology Life Quality Index (CDLQI). The total amount of topical corticosteroid and oral antihistamine use also decreased significantly. These effects were still evident in the TCM group four weeks after stopping therapy.

While TCM appears to be a promising treatment for AD, several limitations exist. First, herbal preparations vary between studies and, within the context of TCM, between individual patients with AD, making an evidence-based assessment difficult. Second, preparation of herbal decoctions requires a series of time-consuming steps, with some needing up to 90 minutes for preparation. There may be issues with the safety and purity (Shaw et al., 2012), availability, and consistency of the herbs as well, although there are many modern and more standardized preparations that can allay at least some of these concerns. Side effects of TCM range from mild gastrointestinal upset to severe renal or liver toxicity. In studies of TCM, the most commonly reported side effects were gastrointestinal upset, abdominal distention, loose bowels, and flatulence (Cheng et al., 2008).

Zemaphyte, a TCM mixture of herbs used for treatment of AD, has been examined in several studies (Box 14.2). Immunologically, serum from patients taking Zemaphyte was found to have decreased interleukin-4 (IL-4)-mediated induction of CD23. CD23 normally acts as a low-affinity IgE receptor, and levels have been found to be elevated in AD subjects (Banerjee et al., 1998; Latchman et al., 1994). Skin biopsies of patients treated with Zemaphyte showed similar reductions in CD23 levels (Xu et al., 1997). There was no difference in total serum IgE levels after treatment with Zemaphyte (Latchman et al. 1994). The clinical evidence for the effectiveness of Zemaphyte is mixed, with some studies showing substantial benefit and others showing none when compared to placebo (Chung, 2008; Fung et al., 1999; Ramgolam et al., 2000). In a 2005 Cochrane review of TCM of both English- and Chinese-based literature, Zemaphyte was found to reduce erythema and severity of AD with minimal adverse effects across four clinical trials reviewed. However, larger trials are needed to conclusively determine its efficacy and long-term side effects (Zhang et al., 2005).

Box 14.2 Ingredients of Zemaphyte Herbal Mixture in Traditional Chinese Medicine

Ledebouriella seseloides
Potentilla chinensis
Anebia clematidis
Rehmannia glutinosa
Paeonia lactiflora
Lophatherum gracile
Dictamnus dasycarpus
Tribulus terrestris
Glycyrrhiza uralensis
Schizonepeta tenuifolia

Herbs need daily preparation by simmering in water for 90 minutes.

> **Box 14.3 Other Common Ingredients of Traditional Chinese Medicine Used for AD Treatment**
>
> *Dictamus dasycarpus (Faxinella; Bai Xiab Pi)*
> *Lonicera japonica (Lonicera flower; Jin Yin Hua)*
> *Paeonia suffruticosa (Moutan; Mu Dan Pi)*
> *Polygonum multiflorum (Polygonum stem; Ye Jiao Teng)*
> *Rehmannia glutinosa (Rehmannia raw; Sheng Di Huang)*
> *Sophora angustifolia (Sophora root; Ku Shen)*

TCM in combination with acupuncture can also be effective for AD. In a small study of 20 patients, each received acupuncture twice weekly and personalized combinations of herbals three times daily (Box 14.3). At 12 weeks, all patients experienced improvement of their AD on all measured scales (Salameh et al., 2008). Similarly, another study examined children treated with the following regimen: TCM (drinking *Erka Shizheng* herbal tea twice daily), herbal bath soaks for 20 minutes daily, application of an herbal cream three times daily, and acupuncture for three months. At the end of the study, SCORAD reduction ranged from 60% to 90% in 13 of the 14 subjects treated. DLQI scores also improved by 50% in all subjects, and a reduction in usage of topical corticosteroids and antihistamines was also noted. No renal or hepatic side effects were observed in this pediatric population (Wisniewski et al., 2009). However, the complexity of this study makes it difficult for researchers and individuals to reproduce, and the potential cost and complexity make it impractical for some patients. Regardless, the potential effectiveness of TCM with acupuncture on AD severity is encouraging.

ACUPUNCTURE

Acupuncture, perhaps specifically via modulation of pruritus or inflammation, can be effective in controlling AD. In traditional acupuncture, thin, solid needles are inserted into specific acupuncture points through the skin to varying depths. Electro-acupuncture, in which electrical stimulation is applied to acupuncture needles, is another form of acupuncture that has been practiced since at least the 1950s. Both methods are thought to mediate the sensation of itch through stimulation of Aδ or C fibers, aside from their purported effects on mobilization of *qi* (Carlsson & Wallengren, 2010). Although the exact mechanism of acupuncture on AD is unknown, pilot research points to a role of acupuncture in modulating immune responses.

Several placebo-controlled trials have examined the effect of manual and electro-acupuncture in AD patients. A prospective trial of 10 AD patients found decreased itch intensity in the acupuncture group, with decrease in CD63 basophil activation after acupuncture treatment. Decreased itch was evident at day 0 (day of acupuncture treatment), day 15 (after five acupuncture treatments), and day 33 (after 10 acupuncture treatments) (Pfab et al., 2011). In another study, those receiving acupuncture at the large intestine 11 (LI 11) point experienced a reduced duration and intensity of histamine-induced itch compared to those receiving no acupuncture and acupuncture at placebo points. Similar results have also been reported with electro-acupuncture (Belgrade et al., 1984; Heyer & Hornstein, 1999; Lundeberg et al., 1987).

In a blinded, randomized, placebo-controlled, crossover trial specifically with patients with AD, two-point acupuncture stimulation was applied at the *Quchi* (large intestine 11) and *Xue Hai* (spleen 10) points. Comparison groups included "no acupuncture" and "placebo-point acupuncture" groups. Experimental-group participants were found to have smaller wheal and flare responses to artificially histamine-induced itch after 10 minutes of stimulation. Subjective sensation of itch, as measured by the validated Eppendorf Itch Questionnaire, was significantly lower in the acupuncture group (Pfab et al., 2005, 2010).

Another double-blind, randomized controlled pilot trial in adults with AD examined the effect of self-applied acupressure at LI 11 three times weekly for four weeks. In the acupressure group there was a statistically significant decrease in itch and in lichenification compared to the control group (Lee et al., 2012), further supporting the possibility that stimulation of certain points on the body can lead to improvement in AD symptoms.

Electrical ear acupuncture has also been found to be effective in control of histamine-induced itch in a small-scale study of 32 subjects. In those receiving ear acupuncture, histamine-induced itch was significantly reduced five minutes after acupuncture, and also on assessment four weeks later (Kesting et al., 2006).

These preliminary studies show promise for the use of acupuncture in the treatment of AD. Similar to evidence-based TCM, larger-scale studies of acupuncture and related side effects are still needed. Direct comparison of different acupuncture points and protocols, instead of comparison with placebo-point acupuncture, would also provide useful evidence-based comparisons.

HOMEOPATHY

Homeopathy is a widely used but controversial therapy for AD. Developed in 1796, it uses extremely dilute preparations of substances to treat illness (Fisher, 2011). Although generally considered safe, it may actually delay conventional treatment without much therapeutic benefit and may rarely have life-threatening side effects. Regardless, it has strong supporters and is popular among the public. In a survey of 227 Norwegian adults with AD, homeopathy was one of the most commonly used therapies (Jensen, 1990). Surveys of children with AD have shown that approximately 35% of children have tried homeopathy. While conflicting evidence for homeopathy exists for the treatment of general medical conditions, there are significantly fewer data for the use of homeopathy in patients with AD (Altunc et al., 2007; Ernst, 2002; Linde et al., 1997, 1999; Mathie, 2003; Shang et al., 2005; Wright, 1975).

In a study of 17 Japanese patients with intractable AD, patients were given individualized homeopathy treatments from six months to two-and-a-half years. All patients were allowed to continue conventional dermatological treatments. Using the Glasgow Homeopathic Outcome Scale, over 50% improvement was reported by all patients. Itch, one of the most disturbing symptoms of AD, was decreased in 15 patients. Overall quality of life improved in nine of the 12 patients surveyed (Itamura & Hosoya, 2003). Limitations to this study included the lack of a control group and short follow-up time in the subset of patients treated for only six months. In uncontrolled studies, there always remains a question of the power of the placebo effect, even when patients are aware that they are taking placebo medications (Kaptchuk et al., 2010).

Conversely, a study of 135 children with AD found no difference at six months between the experimental (homeopathy) and control (conventional treatment) groups based on the SCORAD (Witt et al., 2009). The most frequently used homeopathy components were *Calcium carbonicum* (8.2%), *Tuberculinum* (7.2%), and *Medorrhinum* (6.8%) (Witt et al., 2009). Importantly, these preparations are generally diluted to the point that not even a single molecule is given to the patient (Jonas et al., 2003).

Case reports of severe side effects related to homeopathy have been reported. One nine-month-old girl developed bullous pemphigoid while being treated with a homeopathic regimen for AD. Components of her regimen included sulfur, mercury, cantharides, and *Rhus* (*Toxicodendron*) (Kuenzli et al., 2004). Another six-month-old boy developed limb edema and hypoalbuminemia after two months of treatment with homeopathy with nine medications, including iron and arsenic (Goodyear & Harper, 1990). This treatment modality should be approached with caution, as insufficient evidence exists to support the beneficial effects of homeopathy, and severe side effects have been documented.

STRESS- AND BEHAVIOR-MODIFYING METHODS

Stress

Stress itself can have a negative impact directly on AD, causing delayed healing of the skin barrier and worsening this condition. Similarly, psychosocial stress and sleep deprivation can disrupt skin barrier function, even in healthy patients (Muizzuddin et al., 2003; Robles, 2007). Immunologically, stress and sleep deprivation can cause increases in IL-1β, tumor necrosis factor-α, and natural killer cell activity, all of which may play a role in the inflammation of AD (Altemus et al., 2001). In a study of stimulated stressors, patients given a stressful stimulus had delayed skin barrier recovery by 10% at two hours after skin disruption (Robles, 2007).

In contrast, laughter may improve AD through a decrease in IgE production. In a study of 24 patients with eczema, IgE production by B cells was significantly decreased after viewing a humorous film (*Modern Times*, featuring Charlie Chaplin), although the overall severity of AD was not measured or followed up for this study (Kimata, 2009). Viewing a humorous film also improved nighttime awakenings in children with AD, whereas it had no effect on children without AD (Kimata, 2007).

Biofeedback

Biofeedback uses physical instruments to provide information about various physiological functions, with the goal being for the patient to recognize and alter these activities at will. Examples of such processes include muscle tone, skin conductance, breathing, heart rate, and sensory perception. This field evolved from the principle that the mind and body are connected, and that individuals can be trained to use this connection to consciously improve their health and function. The effect of biofeedback on dermatological conditions is preliminary but promising, especially in the areas of hyperhidrosis, Raynaud's disease, and lichen simplex chronicus (Freedman, 1989; Middaugh et al., 2001; Sarti, 1998; Shenefelt, 2002, 2003).

Biofeedback as a treatment for AD has been investigated since the 1970s, and focusing on breaking the itch–scratch cycle can be effective. Using biofeedback, patients can be conditioned to associate the itch sensation with activities other than scratching, thus breaking the itch–scratch cycle (Jordan & Whitlock, 1972). In one study, 12 patients demonstrated mild improvement in itch after biofeedback sessions (Haynes et al., 1979). Large-scale studies of biofeedback in AD are lacking but it remains a promising treatment for AD, especially in cases in which behavioral patterns are playing a significant role in fueling the disease process.

Hypnotherapy

Hypnotherapy combines cognitive and behavioral dimensions to encourage positive change in individuals. In a study of 18 adults and 20 children with severe AD nonresponsive to conventional therapy, all subjects treated with hypnotherapy showed subjective and objective benefit. Adults maintained benefit up to two years afterward, while children maintained benefit up to 18 months afterward. Limitations included the lack of a control group and the lack of blinding among researchers and subjects (Stewart & Thomas, 1995). Systemic reviews on hypnotherapy for AD have found insufficient evidence (Ersser et al., 2007; Hoare et al., 2000). The time and expense of hypnotherapy can also place this therapeutic option out of reach for some patients, but books and online resources can potentially fill this void. Though untested, the book *Skin Deep: A Mind/Body Program for Healthy Skin* by Grossbart and Sherman (2009) can be obtained freely and teaches some of the methods for self-hypnosis.

NATURAL OILS

A disrupted barrier function is a defining characteristic of AD. A mainstay of conventional therapy, applications of various emollients and occlusive agents help to prevent moisture loss. Similarly, natural oil application remains a popular alternative therapeutic approach with the goal of moisturizing the skin and enhancing barrier function.

Sunflower seed oil is a common alternative therapy used for skin disorders, including AD. This oil naturally contains high levels of essential fatty acids, especially linoleic acid in triglyceride form, which is thought to enhance skin barrier properties. Linoleic acid converts to arachidonic acid, which serves as a precursor to prostaglandin E2 and modulates cutaneous inflammation (Goldyne, 1975; Prottey, 1977; Prottey et al., 1975). Alternatively, linoleic acid may directly enhance barrier function independent of prostaglandin metabolism (Elias et al., 1980).

In a study of sunflower oil and AD, both adults (n = 20) and children (n = 227) with AD improved after twice-daily application of a cream containing 2% sunflower oil distillate. Subjects had significant reductions in dryness, flaking, and redness (Piccardi et al., 2001). Sunflower oil has also been shown to be effective at improving both infant's and children's quality of life and severity of AD (Elias et al., 1980; Msika et al., 2008).

Like sunflower oil, evening primrose oil (*Oenothera biennis*) contains high levels of essential fatty acids, in the form of gamma-linoleic acid and omega-6 (Bayles & Usatine, 2009; Morse & Clough, 2006; Senapati et al., 2008). An initial study performed in 1989 demonstrated positive results of using evening primrose oil for subjects with AD, sparking increased research interest in this medication (Morse et al., 1989). In recent years, small-scale studies have found some benefit in AD, although several confounding variables and limitations prevent interpretation of these results (Morse & Clough, 2006; Senapati et al., 2008; Williams & Grindlay, 2008). Additionally, aggregate reviews of studies on evening primrose oil have not shown much benefit for AD, nor have studies of high-dose oral gamma-linoleic acid intake when compared to placebo (Bamford et al., 1985; Berth-Jones & Graham-Brown, 1993; Hoare et al., 2000; Takwale et al., 2003; Williams, 2003).

Coconut oil (*Cocos nucifera*) is used for the treatment of AD directly as an oil or incorporated into creams. It demonstrated promising properties as an emollient and as an antibacterial agent. One study of 26 subjects found that compared to olive oil, coconut oil decreased staphylococcal colonization by 95% when applied twice daily for four weeks. Although larger-scale studies are needed to confirm this finding before evidence-based conclusions can be drawn, this is a promising natural ingredient that may have desirable properties in the treatment of AD (Gong et al., 2006).

At the very least, sunflower and coconut oils appear to have minimal side effects with possible positive benefits for those with AD. The risk of developing an allergy to these oils, which could then lead to food allergies to coconut or sunflower seeds themselves or to cross-reacting allergens, remains a possibility. Additional studies are necessary to determine the rate of sensitization in subjects using these oils regularly, and the long-term benefit for AD.

PROBIOTICS

Probiotics are potentially beneficial bacteria of healthy gut flora, and their use in AD has yielded mixed results. One particular strain, *Lactobacillus rhamnosus* (*Lactobacillus* GG), has been used for the treatment of food allergies and AD. In a study of the perinatal and immediate postnatal period, *Lactobacillus* GG or placebo was given to 132 pregnant mothers for two weeks before delivery, and then to infants from birth to six months. Infants in the experimental group were half as likely as the control group to develop AD at two years, with postulation that gut microflora may be a source of immunomodulators relevant to the develop of AD (Kalliomaki et al. 2001). Results of this study were not reproduced in a similar study of probiotic supplementation in a trial of 105 subjects in which *Lactobacillus* GG was given perinatally (four to six weeks prior to birth), and postnatally for up to six months. There was no difference in the likelihood of developing AD or in the severity of AD in either the placebo or *Lactobacillus* groups (Kopp et al., 2008). The findings of other studies and meta-analysis of probiotic supplementation in children and adults have been equally mixed (Betsi et al., 2008; Brouwer et al., 2006; Gerasimov et al, 2010; Lee et al., 2008; Sistek, 2006; van der Aa et al., 2010). A Cochrane review of the subject is in process, but until there is better understanding about the types of probiotics, the timing of administration, the dosage, and even the subtypes of AD that may particularly benefit from probiotics, this will be difficult to untangle.

VITAMIN SUPPLEMENTATION

Vitamin supplementation is a promising and perhaps effective adjunctive therapy for treatment of AD. Although the mechanism is unclear, several small-scale studies of vitamin D and B12 supplementation have shown some effect on severity of AD.

UVB light has long been used as a treatment for AD, with epidemiological evidence suggesting that latitude may affect AD prevalence (Byremo et al., 2006; Weiland et al., 2004). A small but impressive study of 11 children with mild AD demonstrated significant improvement after oral supplementation with vitamin D during the winter. Improvement was noted in 17% of controls versus 80% of the experimental group (Sidbury et al., 2008). Similar results were reproduced in a study of 45 AD subjects supplemented with 1,600 IU of vitamin D3, with improvement on the SCORAD after 60 days (Javanbakht et al., 2011). Corroborating these results was another study finding a significant inverse correlation between vitamin D levels and eczema severity (Peroni et al., 2011). However, topical vitamin D, while helpful for psoriasis, may actually exacerbate AD due to induction of analogues that trigger Th2 inflammation (Feily & Namazi, 2010).

Vitamin B12 (cobalamin) may also improve AD by inhibiting nitric oxide synthase, a component of the inflammatory pathway that may be related to AD flares. Topical vitamin B12 was effective in a split-body, randomized, placebo-controlled trial of 49 adults and 21 children, with a decrease in AD severity on the side where vitamin B12 cream was applied (Januchowski, 2009; Stucker et al., 2004). Another observational study of 763 maternal–fetal pairs found no correlation between vitamin B12 intake perinatally and risk of development of atopic diseases (Miyake et al., 2011). We remain hopeful that there may be a role for vitamin supplementation, whether orally or topically, in the treatment of AD; at least for now, vitamin D supplementation appears to be becoming less "alternative" and a more mainstream component of care.

FOOD RESTRICTIONS

There is considerable interest in the link between dietary intake and AD, and many patients and families focus on this aspect of the disease. Interestingly, although many are often convinced that foods are driving the AD or at least playing a significant role, in one clever study, after the AD was controlled with topical preparations, there was a dramatic drop in the perception of food reactions of some 80% (Thompson & Hanifin, 2005). Fortunately, this suggests that foods may not be playing as significant a role as once thought.

Several studies have aimed to assess for the benefit of organic versus conventional health foods (Dangour et al., 2010; Kremmydra et al., 2011; Kummeling et al., 2008). While the majority have found no significant relationship, one Dutch birth cohort noted a decreased risk of eczema in children consuming organic dairy products only (Kummeling et al., 2008). However, several confounding factors and limitations to this study prevent us from drawing any definitive conclusions.

A Cochrane review on food allergies reviewed nine randomized controlled studies and found no benefit in choosing a dairy- or egg-free diet for subjects with AD. In contrast, there could be benefit for egg avoidance in infants suspected of having an egg allergy who have positive IgE to eggs on venous blood sampling. There was no benefit in elemental liquid diets (Beth-Hextall et al., 2008).

Other studies funded by Nestlé, a manufacturer of partially hydrolyzed formulas, have found a reduced risk of AD when infants consumed partially hydrolyzed formulas (Alexander & Cabana, 2010; Alexander et al., 2010; Szajewska & Horvath, 2010). These results contradict a previously published Cochrane review that found no benefit of partially hydrolyzed formulas for children with AD (Osborn & Sinn, 2006).

Recently, the gluten-free diet has become increasingly popular for a number of diseases outside of its well-known indication in gluten-sensitive enteropathy (celiac disease), including AD (El-Chammas & Danner, 2011). One provocative study found that 30% of adults with AD had detectable antibodies to gliadin (a part of gluten) compared to only 6.5% of normal controls in the general population (Finn et al., 1985). However, another study looked at this phenomenon from the opposite perspective and found that in 90 children with proven celiac disease, there was no increase in personal or family history of AD or allergies, compared to children without celiac disease (Cataldo et al., 2001). If gluten sensitivity were really associated with AD, we would have expected to see an increase in those patients with proven celiac disease, and this was not borne out. Perhaps most importantly, however, was that the study showed one year of a gluten-free diet did not change the amount of AD or food allergies in those with celiac disease.

Certain foods may contribute to inflammation in the body beyond those that cause obvious allergy, and perhaps there may be foods that do the opposite as well. However, until there are more concrete data, it is difficult to advise such diets.

BATHING

Bathing in dilute bleach baths (sodium hypochlorite) may be useful in reducing staphylococcal colonization on the skin of infants with AD and a history of infection. One randomized, placebo-controlled study of 31 patients noted decreased clinical severity of AD in those receiving dilute bleach baths and mupirocin ointment to the nares (Craig et al., 2010; Huang et al., 2009, 2011). It is unclear whether the baths alone would be sufficient to decrease AD severity or whether the mupirocin component is essential.

Colloidal oatmeal preparations (creams, lotions, bath additives) are another popular treatment preparation for AD (Sompayrac & Ross, 1959). Oatmeal's anti-inflammatory properties are thought to sooth irritated, eczematous skin (Cerio et al., 2010). Randomized placebo-controlled studies are needed to confirm the benefits of oatmeal and AD.

Conclusion

Many CAM modalities show promise for the treatment of AD, although most lack adequate evidence-based studies demonstrating benefit or harm. We eagerly await future investigations on treatment modalities for AD to add to our arsenal of conventional medications.

REFERENCES

Adams, J., Sibbritt, D., & Lui, C. W. (2011a). The urban-rural divide in complementary and alternative medicine use: a longitudinal study of 10,638 women. *BMC Complementary and Alternative Medicine, 11*, 2.

Adams, J., Sibbritt, D., Broom, A., et al. (2011b). A comparison of complementary and alternative medicine users and use across geographical areas: A national survey of 1,427 women. *BMC Complementary and Alternative Medicine, 11*, 85.

Alexander, D. D., & Cabana, M. D. (2010). Partially hydrolyzed 100% whey protein infant formula and reduced risk of atopic dermatitis: a meta-analysis. *Journal of Pediatric Gastroenterology and Nutrition, 50*, 422–430.

Alexander, D. D., Schmitt, D. F., Tran, N. L., et al., (2010). Partially hydrolyzed 100% whey protein infant formula and atopic dermatitis risk reduction: a systematic review of the literature. *Nutrition Reviews, 68*, 232–245.

Altemus, M., Rao, B., Dhabhar, F. S., et al. (2001). Stress-induced changes in skin barrier function in healthy women. *Journal of Investigative Dermatology, 117*, 309–317.

Altunc, U., Pittler, M. H., & Ernst, E. (2007). Homeopathy for childhood and adolescence ailments: systematic review of randomized clinical trials. *Mayo Clinic Proceedings, 82*, 69–75.

Bamford, J. T., Gibson, R. W., & Renier, C.M. (1985). Atopic eczema unresponsive to evening primrose oil (linoleic and gamma-linolenic acids). *Journal of the American Academy of Dermatology, 13*, 959–965.

Banerjee, P., Xu, X. J., Poulter, L. W., et al., (1998). Changes in CD23 expression of blood and skin in atopic eczema after Chinese herbal therapy. *Clinical and Experimental Allergy, 28*, 306–314.

Baron, S. E., Goodwin, R. G., Nicolau, N., et al., (2005). Use of complementary medicine among outpatients with dermatologic conditions within Yorkshire and South Wales, United Kingdom. *Journal of the American Academy of Dermatology, 52,* 589–594.

Bath-Hextall, F., Delamere, F. M., & Williams, H. C. (2008). Dietary exclusions for established atopic eczema. *Cochrane Database of Systematic Reviews.*

Bayles, B., & Usatine, R. (2009). Evening primrose oil. *American Family Physician, 80,* 1405–1408.

Belgrade, M. J., Solomon, L. M., & Lichter, E. A. (1984). Effect of acupuncture on experimentally induced itch. *Acta Dermato-Venereologica, 64,* 129–133.

Ben-Arye, E., Ziv, M., Frenkel, M., et al. (2003). Complementary medicine and psoriasis: linking the patient's outlook with evidence-based medicine. *Dermatology, 207,* 302–307.

Berg, M., & Arnetz, B. (1998). Characteristics of users and nonusers of alternative medicine in dermatologic patients attending a university hospital clinic: a short report. *Journal of Alternative & Complementary Medicine, 4,* 277–279.

Berth-Jones, J., & Graham-Brown, R. A. (1993). Placebo-controlled trial of essential fatty acid supplementation in atopic dermatitis. *Lancet, 341,* 1557–1560.

Betsi, G. I., Papadavid, E., & Falagas, M. E. (2008). Probiotics for the treatment or prevention of atopic dermatitis: a review of the evidence from randomized controlled trials. *American Journal of Clinical Dermatology, 9,* 93–103.

Brouwer, M. L., Wolt-Plompen, S. A., Dubois, A. E., et al. (2006). No effects of probiotics on atopic dermatitis in infancy: a randomized placebo-controlled trial. *Clinical and Experimental Allergy, 36,* 899–906.

Byremo, G., Rod, G., & Carlsen, K. H. (2006). Effect of climatic change in children with atopic eczema. *Allergy, 61,* 1403–1410.

Carlsson, C. P., & Wallengren, J. (2010). Therapeutic and experimental therapeutic studies on acupuncture and itch: review of the literature. *Journal of the European Academy of Dermatology and Venereology, 24,* 1013–1016.

Cataldo, F., Marino,V., Di Stefano, P. (2001). Celiac disease and risk of atopy in childhood. *Pediatric Asthma, Allergy & Immunology, 15,* 77–80.

Cerio, R., Dohil, M., Jeanine, D., et al. (2010). Mechanism of action and clinical benefits of colloidal oatmeal for dermatologic practice. *Journal of Drugs in Dermatology 9,* 1116–1120.

Cheng, C. W., Bian, Z. X., Li, Y. P., et al. (2008). Transparently reporting adverse effects of traditional Chinese medicine interventions in randomized controlled trials. *Journal of Chinese Integrative Medicine, 6,* 881–886.

Chung, L. Y. (2008). Antioxidant profiles of a prepared extract of Chinese herbs for the treatment of atopic eczema. *Phytotherapy Research, 22,* 493–499.

Craig, F. E., Smith, E. V., & Williams, H. C. (2010). Bleach baths to reduce severity of atopic dermatitis colonized by *Staphylococcus. Archives of Dermatology, 146,* 541–543.

Dangour, A. D., Lock, K., Hayter, A., et al. (2010). Nutrition-related health effects of organic foods: a systematic review. *American Journal of Clinical Nutrition, 92,* 203–210.

El-Chammas, K., & Danner, E. (2011). Gluten-free diet in nonceliac disease. *Nutrition in Clinical Practice, 26*, 294–299.

Elias, P. M., Brown, B. E., & Ziboh, V. A. (1980). The permeability barrier in essential fatty acid deficiency: evidence for a direct role for linoleic acid in barrier function. *Journal of Investigative Dermatology, 74*, 230–233.

Ernst, E. (2002). A systematic review of systematic reviews of homeopathy. *British Journal of Clinical Pharmacology, 54*, 577–582.

Ersser, S. J., Latter, S., Sibley, A., et la., (2007). Psychological and educational interventions for atopic eczema in children. *Cochrane Database of Systematic Reviews*.

Feily, A., & Namazi, M. R. (2010). Vitamin A + D ointment is not an appropriate emollient for atopic dermatitis. *Dermatitis, 21*, 174–175.

Finn, R., Harvey, M. M., Johnson, P. M., et al. (1985). Serum IgG antibodies to gliadin and other dietary antigens in adults with atopic eczema. *Clinical and Experimental Dermatology, 10*, 222–228.

Fisher, P. A. (2011). What about the evidence base for homoeopathy? *British Medical Journal, 343*, d6689.

Freedman, R. R. (1989). Quantitative measurements of finger blood flow during behavioral treatments for Raynaud's disease. *Psychophysiology, 26*, 437–441.

Fung, A. Y., Look, P. C., Chong, L. Y., et al. (1999). A controlled trial of traditional Chinese herbal medicine in Chinese patients with recalcitrant atopic dermatitis. *International Journal of Dermatology, 38*, 387–392.

Gerasimov, S. V., Vasjuta, V. V., Myhovych, O. O., et al. (2010). Probiotic supplement reduces atopic dermatitis in preschool children: a randomized, double-blind, placebo-controlled, clinical trial. *American Journal of Clinical Dermatology, 11*, 351–361.

Goldyne, M. E. (1975). Prostaglandins and cutaneous inflammation. *Journal of Investigative Dermatology, 64*, 377–385.

Gong, J. Q., Lin, L., Lin, T., et al. (2006). Skin colonization by *Staphylococcus aureus* in patients with eczema and atopic dermatitis and relevant combined topical therapy: a double-blind multicentre randomized controlled trial. *British Journal of Dermatology, 155*, 680–687.

Goodyear, H. M., & Harper, J. I. (1990). Atopic eczema, hyponatraemia, and hypoalbuminaemia. *Archives of Disease in Childhood, 65*, 231–232.

Graham-Brown, R. (1992). Toxicity of Chinese herbal remedies. *Lancet, 340*, 673–674.

Grossbart, T. A., & Sherman, C. (2009). *Skin Deep: A Mind/Body Program* for Healthy Skin. Albuquerque: Health Press.

Haynes, S. N., Wilson, C. C., Jaffe, P. G., et al. (1979). Biofeedback treatment of atopic dermatitis: controlled case studies of eight cases. *Biofeedback and Self-Regulation, 4*, 195–209.

Heyer, G. R., & Hornstein, O. P. (1999). Recent studies of cutaneous nociception in atopic and non-atopic subjects. *Journal of Dermatology, 26*, 77–86.

Hoare, C., Li Wan Po, A., & Williams H. (2000). Systematic review of treatments for atopic eczema. *Health Technology Assessment, 4*, 1–191.

Hon, K. L., Leung, T. F., Ng, P. C., et al. (2007). Efficacy and tolerability of a Chinese herbal medicine concoction for treatment of atopic dermatitis: a randomized, double-blind, placebo-controlled study. *British Journal of Dermatology, 157,* 357–363.

Huang, J. T., Abrams, M., Tlougan, B., et al. (2009). Treatment of *Staphylococcus aureus* colonization in atopic dermatitis decreases disease severity. *Pediatrics, 123,* e808–814.

Huang, J. T., Rademaker, A., & Paller, A. S. (2011). Dilute bleach baths for *Staphylococcus aureus* colonization in atopic dermatitis to decrease disease severity. *Archives of Dermatology, 147,* 246–247.

Itamura, R., & Hosoya, R. (2003). Homeopathic treatment of Japanese patients with intractable atopic dermatitis. *Homeopathy, 92,* 108–114.

Januchowski, R. (2009). Evaluation of topical vitamin B(12) for the treatment of childhood eczema. *Journal of Alternative & Complementary Medicine, 15,* 387–389.

Javanbakht, M. H., Keshavarz, S. A., Djalali, M., et al. (2011). Randomized controlled trial using vitamins E and D supplementation in atopic dermatitis. *Journal of Dermatological Treatment, 22,* 144–150.

Jensen, P. (1990). Alternative therapy for atopic dermatitis and psoriasis: patient-reported motivation, information source and effect. *Acta Dermato-Venereologica, 70,* 425–428.

Johnston, G. A., Bilbao, R. M., & Graham-Brown, R. A. (2003). The use of complementary medicine in children with atopic dermatitis in secondary care in Leicester. *British Journal of Dermatology, 149,* 566–571.

Jonas, W. B., Kaptchuk, T. J., & Linde, K. (2003). A critical overview of homeopathy. *Annals of Internal Medicine, 138,* 393–399.

Jordan, J. M., & Whitlock, F. A. (1972). Emotions and the skin: the conditioning of scratch responses in cases of atopic dermatitis. *British Journal of Dermatology, 86,* 574–585.

Kalliomaki, M., Salminen, S., Arvilommi, H., et al. (2001). Probiotics in primary prevention of atopic disease: a randomised placebo-controlled trial. *Lancet, 357,* 1076–1079.

Kaptchuk, T. J., Friedlander, E., Kelley, J. M., et al. (2010). Placebos without deception: a randomized controlled trial in irritable bowel syndrome. *PloS One, 5,* e15591.

Kesting, M. R., Thurmuller, P., Holzle, F., et al. (2006). Electrical ear acupuncture reduces histamine-induced itch (alloknesis). *Acta Dermato-Venereologica, 86,* 399–403.

Kimata, H. (2007). Viewing a humorous film improves nighttime wakening in children with atopic dermatitis. *Indian Pediatrics, 44,* 281–285.

Kimata, H. (2009). Viewing a humorous film decreases IgE production by seminal B cells from patients with atopic eczema. *Journal of Psychosomatic Research, 66,* 173–175.

Kopp, M. V., Hennemuth, I., Heinzmann, A., et al. (2008). Randomized, double-blind, placebo-controlled trial of probiotics for primary prevention: no clinical effects of Lactobacillus GG supplementation. *Pediatrics, 121,* e850–856.

Kremmyda, L. S., Vlachava, M., Noakes, P. S., et al. (2011). Atopy risk in infants and children in relation to early exposure to fish, oily fish, or long-chain omega-3 fatty acids: a systematic review. *Clinical Reviews in Allergy & Immunology, 41,* 36–66.

Kuenzli, S., Grimaitre, M., Krischer, J., et al. (2004). Childhood bullous pemphigoid: report of a case with life-threatening course during homeopathy treatment. *Pediatric Dermatology, 21,* 160–163.

Kummeling, I., Thijs, C., Huber, M., et al. (2008). Consumption of organic foods and risk of atopic disease during the first 2 years of life in the Netherlands. *British Journal of Nutrition, 99,* 598–605.

Latchman, Y., Whittle, B., Rustin, M., et al. (1994). The efficacy of traditional Chinese herbal therapy in atopic eczema. *International Archives of Allergy and Immunology, 104,* 222–226.

Lee, G. B., Charn, T. C., Chew, Z. H., et al. (2004). Complementary and alternative medicine use in patients with chronic diseases in primary care is associated with perceived quality of care and cultural beliefs. *Family Practice, 21,* 654–660.

Lee, J., Seto, D., & Bielory, L. (2008). Meta-analysis of clinical trials of probiotics for prevention and treatment of pediatric atopic dermatitis. *Journal of Allergy and Clinical Immunology, 121,* 116–121 e11.

Lee, K. C., Keyes, A., Hensley, J. R., et al. (2012). Effectiveness of acupressure on pruritus and lichenification associated with atopic dermatitis: a pilot trial. *Acupuncture in Medicine, 30,* 8–11.

Linde, K., Clausius, N., Ramirez, G., et al. (1997). Are the clinical effects of homeopathy placebo effects? A meta-analysis of placebo-controlled trials. *Lancet, 350,* 834–843.

Linde, K., Scholz, M., Ramirez, G., et al. (1999). Impact of study quality on outcome in placebo-controlled trials of homeopathy. *Journal of Clinical Epidemiology, 52,* 631–636.

Lundeberg, T., Bondesson, L., & Thomas, M. (1987). Effect of acupuncture on experimentally induced itch. *British Journal of Dermatology, 117,* 771–777.

Magin, P. J., Adams, J., Heading, G. S., et al. (2006). Complementary and alternative medicine therapies in acne, psoriasis, and atopic eczema: results of a qualitative study of patients' experiences and perceptions. *Journal of Alternative & Complementary Medicine, 12,* 451–457.

Mathie, R. T. (2003). The research evidence base for homeopathy: a fresh assessment of the literature. *Homeopathy, 92,* 84–91.

McAlister, R. O., Tofte, S. J., Doyle, J. J., et al. (2002). Patient and physician perspectives vary on atopic dermatitis. *Cutis, 69,* 461–466.

Middaugh, S. J., Haythornthwaite, J. A., Thompson, B., et al. (2001). The Raynaud's Treatment Study: biofeedback protocols and acquisition of temperature biofeedback skills. *Applied Psychophysiology and Biofeedback, 26,* 251–278.

Miyake, Y., Sasaki, S., Tanaka, K., et al. (2011). Maternal B vitamin intake during pregnancy and wheeze and eczema in Japanese infants aged 16–24 months: the Osaka Maternal and Child Health Study. *Pediatric Allergy and Immunology, 22,* 69–74.

Morse, N. L., & Clough, P. M. (2006). A meta-analysis of randomized, placebo-controlled clinical trials of Efamol evening primrose oil in atopic eczema. Where do we go from here in light of more recent discoveries? *Current Pharmaceutical Biotechnology, 7,* 503–524.

Morse, P. F., Horrobin, D. F., Manku, M. S., et al. (1989). Meta-analysis of placebo-controlled studies of the efficacy of Epogam in the treatment of atopic eczema. Relationship between plasma essential fatty acid changes and clinical response. *British Journal of Dermatology, 121*, 75–90.

Msika, P., De Belilovsky, C., Piccardi, N., et al. (2008). New emollient with topical corticosteroid-sparing effect in treatment of childhood atopic dermatitis: SCORAD and quality of life improvement. *Pediatric Dermatology, 25*, 606–612.

Muizzuddin, N., Matsui, M. S., Marenus, K. D., et al. (2003). Impact of stress of marital dissolution on skin barrier recovery: tape stripping and measurement of trans-epidermal water loss (TEWL). *Skin Research & Technology, 9*, 34–38.

Osborn, D. A., & Sinn, J. (2006). Formulas containing hydrolysed protein for prevention of allergy and food intolerance in infants. *Cochrane Database of Systematic Reviews.*

Peroni, D. G., Piacentini, G. L., Cametti, E., et al. (2011). Correlation between serum 25-hydroxyvitamin D levels and severity of atopic dermatitis in children. *British Journal of Dermatology, 164*, 1078–1082.

Pfab, F., Athanasiadis, G. I., Huss-Marp, J., et al. (2011). Effect of acupuncture on allergen-induced basophil activation in patients with atopic eczema:a pilot trial. *Journal of Alternative & Complementary Medicine, 17*, 309–314.

Pfab, F., Hammes, M., Backer, M., et al. (2005). Preventive effect of acupuncture on histamine-induced itch: a blinded, randomized, placebo-controlled, crossover trial. *Journal of Allergy and Clinical Immunology, 116*, 1386–1388.

Pfab, F., Huss-Marp, J., Gatti, A., et al. (2010). Influence of acupuncture on type I hypersensitivity itch and the wheal and flare response in adults with atopic eczema—a blinded, randomized, placebo-controlled, crossover trial. *Allergy, 65*, 903–910.

Piccardi, N., Piccardi, A., Choulot, J. C., Msika, P. (2001). Sunflower oil oleodistillate for atopy treatment: an in vitro and clinical evaluation. *Journal of Investigative Dermatology, 117*, 390–423. [Abstract 169].

Prottey, C. (1977). Investigation of functions of essential fatty acids in the skin. *British Journal of Dermatology, 97*, 29–38.

Prottey, C., Hartop, P. J., & Press, M. (1975). Correction of the cutaneous manifestations of essential fatty acid deficiency in man by application of sunflower-seed oil to the skin. *Journal of Investigative Dermatology, 64*, 228–234.

Ramgolam, V., Ang, S. G., Lai, Y. H., et al. (2000). Traditional Chinese medicines as immunosuppressive agents. *Annals of the Academy of Medicine Singapore, 29*, 11–16.

Robles, T. F. (2007). Stress, social support, and delayed skin barrier recovery. *Psychosomatic Medicine, 69*, 807–815.

Salameh, F., Perla, D., Solomon, M., et al. (2008). The effectiveness of combined Chinese herbal medicine and acupuncture in the treatment of atopic dermatitis. *Journal of Alternative & Complementary Medicine, 14*, 1043–1048.

Sarti, M. G. (1998). Biofeedback in dermatology. *Clinics in Dermatology, 16*, 711–714.

Senapati, S., Banerjee, S., & Gangopadhyay, D. N. (2008). Evening primrose oil is effective in atopic dermatitis: a randomized placebo-controlled trial. *Indian Journal of Dermatology, Venereology and Leprology, 74*, 447–452.

Shang, A., Huwiler-Muntener, K., Nartey, L., et al. (2005). Are the clinical effects of homoeopathy placebo effects? Comparative study of placebo-controlled trials of homoeopathy and allopathy. *Lancet, 366*, 726–732.

Shaw, D., Graeme, L., Pierre, D., et al. (2012). Pharmacovigilance of herbal medicine. *Journal of Ethnopharmacology, 140,* 513–518.

Sheehan, M. P., Rustin, M. H., Atherton, D. J., et al. (1992). Efficacy of traditional Chinese herbal therapy in adult atopic dermatitis. *Lancet, 340,* 13–17.

Shenefelt, P. D. (2002). Complementary psychotherapy in dermatology: hypnosis and biofeedback. *Clinics in Dermatology, 20,* 595–601.

Shenefelt, P. D. (2003). Biofeedback, cognitive-behavioral methods, and hypnosis in dermatology: is it all in your mind? *Dermatologic Therapy, 16,* 114–122.

Sidbury, R., Sullivan, A. F., Thadhani, R. I., et al. (2008). Randomized controlled trial of vitamin D supplementation for winter-related atopic dermatitis in Boston: a pilot study. *British Journal of Dermatology, 159,* 245–247.

Sistek, D., Kelly, R., Wickens, K., et al. (2006). Is the effect of probiotics on atopic dermatitis confined to food sensitized children? *Clinical and Experimental Allergy, 36,* 629–633.

Sompayrac, L. M., & Ross, C. (1959). Colloidal oatmeal in atopic dermatitis of the young. *Journal of the Florida Medical Association, 45,* 1411–1412.

Stewart, A. C., & Thomas, S. E. (1995). Hypnotherapy as a treatment for atopic dermatitis in adults and children. *British Journal of Dermatology, 132,* 778–783.

Stucker, M., Pieck, C., Stoerb, C., et al. (2004). Topical vitamin B12—a new therapeutic approach in atopic dermatitis-evaluation of efficacy and tolerability in a randomized placebo-controlled multicentre clinical trial. *British Journal of Dermatology, 150,* 977–983.

Suarez, A. L., Feramisco, J. D., Koo, J., et al. (2012). Psychoneuroimmunology of psychological stress and atopic dermatitis: pathophysiologic and therapeutic updates. *Acta Dermato-Venereologica, 92,* 7–15.

Szajewska, H., & Horvath, A. (2010). Meta-analysis of the evidence for a partially hydrolyzed 100% whey formula for the prevention of allergic diseases. *Current Medical Research and Opinion, 26,* 423–437.

Takwale, A., Tan, E., Agarwal, S., et al. (2003). Efficacy and tolerability of borage oil in adults and children with atopic eczema: randomised, double blind, placebo controlled, parallel group trial. *British Medical Journal, 327,* 1385.

Thompson, M. M., & Hanifin, J. M. (2005). Effective therapy of childhood atopic dermatitis allays food allergy concerns. *Journal of the American Academy of Dermatology, 53,* S214–219.

van der Aa, L. B., Heymans, H. S., van Aalderen, W. M., et al. (2012). Probiotics and prebiotics in atopic dermatitis: review of the theoretical background and clinical evidence. *Pediatric Allergy and Immunology, 21,* e355–367.

Weiland, S. K., Husing, A., Strachan, D. P., et al. (2004). Climate and the prevalence of symptoms of asthma, allergic rhinitis, and atopic eczema in children. *Occupational and Environmental Medicine, 61,* 609–615.

Williams, H. C. (2003). Evening primrose oil for atopic dermatitis. *British Medical Journal, 327,* 1358–1359.

Williams, H. C., & Grindlay, D. J. (2008). What's new in atopic eczema? An analysis of the clinical significance of systematic reviews on atopic eczema published in 2006 and 2007. *Clinical and Experimental Dermatology, 33,* 685–688.

Wisniewski, J., Nowak-Wegrzyn, A., Steenburgh-Thanik, E. Sampson, H., et al. (2009). Efficacy and safety of traditional Chinese medicine for treatment of atopic dermatitis (AD). American Academy of Asthma, Allergy and Immunology (AAAAI) Annual Meeting: Abstract 131.

Witt, C. M., Brinkhaus, B., Pach, D., et al. (2009). Homoeopathic versus conventional therapy for atopic eczema in children: medical and economic results. *Dermatology*, *219*, 329–340.

Witt, C. M., Ludtke, R., & Willich, S. N. (2009). Homeopathic treatment of children with atopic eczema: a prospective observational study with two years follow-up. *Acta Dermato-Venereologica*, *89*, 182–183.

Wright, J. E. (1975). The role of surgery in the management of orbital tumours. *Modern Problems in Ophthalmology*, *14*, 553–556.

Xu, X. J., Banerjee, P., Rustin, M. H., et al. (1997). Modulation by Chinese herbal therapy of immune mechanisms in the skin of patients with atopic eczema. *British Journal of Dermatology*, *136*, 54–59.

Zhang, W., Leonard, T., Bath-Hextall, F., et al. (2005). Chinese herbal medicine for atopic eczema. *Cochrane Database of Systematic Reviews*.

15

Integrative Management of Cutaneous Infectious Diseases

NIANDRA REID, LESLIE ROBINSON-BOSTOM, AND SHOSHANA LANDOW

Key Concepts

♣ Gram-positive *Staphylococcus aureus*, including the methicillin-resistant variety (MRSA), accounts for many common skin infections such as impetigo, folliculitis, ecthyma, abscesses, and cellulitis. Appropriate antibiotic measures can be supplemented with herbal topical treatments such as tea tree oil, black tea extract, honey, and immunomodulating herbs.

♣ Gram-positive *Streptococcus pyogenes* can also produce impetigo and erysipelas. It has shown sensitivity to several herbs, herb combinations, and immunomodulating natural compounds.

♣ *Corynebacterium* is involved in acne and erythrasma. In addition to conventional antibiotic therapy it can respond to photodynamic therapy, red light therapy, blue light therapy, clove and thyme extracts, tea tree oil, and other herbal extracts.

♣ Gram-negative *Pseudomonas aeruginosa* can cause skin and nail infections. While antibiotics are often effective, alternatives include honey, tea tree oil, green tea extracts, henna extracts, dilute vinegar soaks, and certain Chinese herbs.

♣ Cutaneous fungal infections may affect the scalp, nails, feet, groin, and other skin areas. Oral therapy is usually required for hair and nails, while topical antifungals usually manage other dermatophyte infections. Alternatives include tea tree oil, *S. alata*, ozonized sunflower oil, ajoene, and others.

(continued)

♣ Cutaneous candidiasis often involves moist areas such as groin, inframammary folds, and oral cavity. It usually responds to topical or oral antifungals. Alternatives include gentian violet, tea tree oil, and others.

♣ Seborrheic dermatitis, tinea versicolor, and *Pityrosporum* folliculitis are caused by *Malassezia* organisms. Alternatives include *S. alata*, *S. chrysotrichum*, and others.

♣ Herpes virus infections include cold sores, chickenpox, shingles, and others. Conventional antivirals inhibit viral polymerase activity. Alternatives include a number of herbs, such as *Echinacea* and others.

♣ Wart virus infections produce benign skin tumors and in the case of a few strains of genital wart virus may produce squamous cell cervical cancer. In addition to multiple types of conventional treatments, alternative treatments such as hypnotherapy, garlic extracts, green tea catechins, and others may be beneficial.

♣ Pox viruses can produce skin infections, the most common being molluscum contagiosum. In addition to conventional therapies, alternatives such as garlic extracts, turmeric, and apple cider vinegar may be used.

Introduction

Complementary and alternative medicine is of great interest to patients and providers and is commonly used to supplement or replace more traditional allopathic treatment modalities. The objective of this chapter is to provide readers with an overview of traditional and complementary treatment options for the most common cutaneous bacterial, fungal, and viral skin infections encountered in clinical practice.

Bacterial Cutaneous Infections

Although conventional allopathic therapies usually provide adequate antibiotic therapies for bacterial skin infections, there is an increased need to develop new treatment modalities due to antibiotic resistance. There are a variety of alternative medicines that have been proposed to possess antibacterial properties and have been used as primary treatment or to complement traditional therapy. In this section, we will review the established allopathic treatments and alternative therapies for the most common bacterial cutaneous infections.

GRAM-POSITIVE BACTERIA

Staphylococcal and Streptococcal Skin Infections

Skin infections are a very common complaint in the dermatology clinic. The majority of skin infections in immunocompetent patients are caused by staphylococci, including methicillin-resistant *Staphylococcus aureus* (MRSA) and streptococci (Bolognia et al., 2008; Celestin et al., 2007; Geria & Schwartz, 2010; Iwatsuki et al., 2006; Morgan, 2011; Rajan, 2012).

Impetigo is a superficial infection commonly affecting children and can present either in a nonbullous form (superficial erosions with yellow "honey-colored" crusts) or a bullous form (vesicles and bullae). *S. aureus* and less commonly *Streptococcus pyogenes* are the cause of the infection. Nonbullous impetigo can extend deep into the dermis, causing a "punched-out" ulceration with a purulent or necrotic base (ecthyma), most commonly caused by *S. pyogenes*. In bacterial folliculitis there is infection of the hair follicle, which can progress to a furuncle when the surrounding tissue is affected. Community-acquired MRSA frequently presents as furunculosis. Spreading of infection to multiple follicles can result in a carbuncle. An abscess refers to a walled-off collection of pus anywhere on the body. When infection affects the deep dermis and subcutaneous tissues, cellulitis develops, which classically presents with the four signs of inflammation: *dolor, rubor, tumor*, and *calor* (pain, erythema, swelling, and warmth of the involved extremity). *S. aureus* and *S. pyogenes* are the usual cause of cellulitis, although gram-negative bacteria can be present as well if the cellulitis is associated with a diabetic ulcer. In erysipelas, most commonly caused by *S. pyogenes*, cellulitis involves the lymphatics, resulting in a well-demarcated area of cellulitis commonly on the face or the lower extremities.

More serious infections can occur as a result of staphylococcal and streptococcal infections. In staphylococcal scalded skin syndrome, a disease primarily of young children, superficial bullae form as a result of the epidermolysins secreted by *S. aureus* and MRSA, which eventually exfoliate, leaving behind areas of moist skin. In toxic shock syndrome, due to exotoxin production by *S. aureus,* a severe clinical picture develops that includes high fevers, a diffuse exanthem, erythema of the mucous membranes, and progression to hypotension and multiorgan involvement; it can lead to death.

Established Treatments

Antibiotics with gram-positive coverage, either topical or oral, are the standard therapy for treating staphylococcal and streptococcal skin infections. Local wound care is important in impetigo for removal of crusts. Mupirocin 2% ointment is most commonly used for uncomplicated superficial infections,

Table 15.1. Summary of Treatment Modalities for Staphylococcal
and Streptococcal Skin Infections

Diseases	Established Treatment	Alternative Therapies
Impetigo	• Local wound care, cleansing, wet dressings, topical antibiotics such as mupirocin 2% ointment • Oral antibiotics: penicillin, macrolides, cephalosporins, Bactrim™ (sulfamethoxazole and trimethoprim), clindamycin • Intravenous antibiotics for severe cases: penicillin, cephalosporins, vancomycin	• A variety of medicinal plant extracts for topical use • Essential oils • Herbal treatments to boost the immune system • Honey • Bleach baths
Bacterial folliculitis
Abscesses, furuncles, and carbuncles
Ecthyma
Staphylococcal scalded skin syndrome
Toxic shock syndrome
Erysipelas
Cellulitis
MRSA infections

(Hirschmann, 2007; Morgan, 2011; Rajan, 2012)

followed by beta-lactamase–resistant penicillin or macrolide/cephalosporin and intravenous cephalosporin for more complicated infections. Superficial bacterial folliculitis can be treated with antibacterial washes and lotions/ointments. Warm compresses and incision and drainage are needed for fluctuant lesions. Antibiotic coverage for MRSA should be considered in severe infections since the incidence of community-acquired MRSA is increasing. Staphylococcal scalded skin syndrome if generalized requires intravenous antibiotics and hospitalization, as well as wound care for denuded areas. Toxic shock syndrome treatment involves treatment of hypotension with fluids and vasopressors, removal of any source of infection, and intravenous treatment with beta-lactamase–resistant antibiotics.

S. aureus and MRSA

Alternative Therapies

Herbal Treatments For centuries, traditional medicine has used hundreds of plants in the treatment of bacterial infections. Every region of the world has different systems of medicine that utilize medicinal plants. In some parts of the world, herbal medicine is still the main system of healthcare employed by medicine practitioners. In vitro screenings have been performed for a large number of herbal extracts from different regions of the world, showing various degrees of efficacy against gram-positive bacteria, including MRSA. Very few controlled clinical trials studying the efficacy of herbal medicines with antibacterial activity have been performed.

a) *Tea tree (Melaleuca alternifolia) oil (TTO)*
   The essential oil of the Australian native plant *Melaleuca alternifolia*, TTO is a very popular antimicrobial agent. In vitro, it has been shown to have antibacterial activity against a wide range of bacteria, including *S. aureus* (including MRSA) and streptococci. In vivo, one clinical trial compared the rates of MRSA decolonization in inpatients using a combination of 4% TTO nasal ointment and 5% TTO body wash with a standard 2% mupirocin nasal ointment and triclosan body wash (Caelli et al., 2000). Although more patients in the intervention group cleared the infection, the difference was not statistically significant and the number of patients treated was too small. In an uncontrolled, open-label pilot study of TTO solution used in cleansing of acute and chronic wounds of mixed etiology including MRSA, no conclusion could be drawn due to the small number of participants (Edmondson et al., 2011). In a randomized controlled study of 10% TTO cream versus silver sulfadiazine cream, more wounds (16 out of 34 [46%]) were cleared of MRSA in the TTO group compared with the standard topical regimen (8 out of 24 [31%]) (Dryden et al., 2004). A more recent study used a 5% TTO body wash as part of a MRSA decolonization regimen in nursing home residents with good results (Bowler et al., 2010). More controlled clinical studies are needed to determine the efficacy of TTO in vivo.

b) Black tea (*Thea assamica*, also known as *Camellia sinensis*)
   Extracts of tea have been shown to have antibacterial properties in vitro. In a clinical trial of 104 patients with impetigo contagiosa, tea extracts in aqueous or petrolatum-based lotions were compared with framycetin/gramicidin ointment and oral cephalexin (Sharquie, al-Turfi et al., 2000). The cure rates in the 5% petrolatum extract group were similar to the antibiotic group, although the number of patients in the study was low and the study was not randomized (Sharquie et al., 2000).

c) Essential oils other than TTO
   Essential oils from various species of plants have been used as topical antiseptics in traditional medicine. Several in vitro studies have been published analyzing the antibacterial activity of essential oils. One study examined the fruit oil of *Eucalyptus globulus* (Myrtaceae) and the leaf oils of other eucalyptus plants against multidrug-resistant bacteria and found good activity against MRSA (Mulyaningsih et al., 2011). Another study analyzed antibacterial effects of five Zingiberaceae essential oils—ginger (*Zingiber officinale* Roscoe.), galanga (*Alpinia galanga* Sw.), turmeric (*Curcuma longa* L.), kaempferia (*Boesenbergia pandurata* Holtt.), and bastard cardamom (*Amomum xanthioides* Wall)—and found good activity against gram-positive bacteria, including *S. aureus* (Norajit et al., 2007) Other in

vitro studies analyzed the antibacterial activity of essential oils obtained from fresh bulbs of garlic, *Allium sativum* L., and leek, *Allium porrum* L. (Alliaceae) (Casella et al., 2012). *A. sativum* (garlic) essential oil showed good antimicrobial activity against *S. aureus* (Casella et al., 2012). Other essential oils reported to have good in vitro activity against *S. aureus*, including MRSA, include thyme (Sienkiewicz et al., 2012) oregano (Alexopoulos et al., 2011), coriander (Casetti et al., 2012), *Retama raetam* (Awen et al., 2011), *Hofmeisteria schaffneri* (Perez-Vasquez et al., 2011), peppermint, and spearmint (Imai et al., 2001).

Honey The use of honey for various wounds and burn injuries has been documented for hundreds of years. The bactericidal activity of honey has been studied in a number of in vitro and wound-healing studies using honey from different parts of the world: New Zealand (manuka honey), Malaysia (tualang honey), India, Turkey, Saudi Arabia, Brazil, the United States and other countries (Al-Waili et al., 2011a, 2011b). Honey has consistently showed good antibacterial activity against *Staphylococcus* species, including MRSA (Al-Waili et al., 2011a, 2011b). It is unclear how much of the antibacterial activity is due to its hyperosmolar nature versus an inherent antibacterial property (Al-Waili et al., 2011a, 2011b). Production of H_2O_2, pH, and production of NO metabolites are also believed to play a role (Al-Waili et al., 2011a, 2011b). Honey is also believed to play an immunomodulatory role by inducing cytokine production by its MJP1 protein and to promote wound healing (Majtan et al., 2010).

While there are numerous in vitro studies showing good antimicrobial activity of various types of honey, very few randomized trials have been conducted studying honey compared with standard treatment. In a recent thorough Cochrane review of honey as a topical treatment for wounds, it was found that honey may improve healing times in mild to moderately superficial and partial-thickness burns compared with conventional dressings (Jull et al., 2008). Overall, though, there is insufficient-high quality clinical evidence of the benefits of honey dressings in chronic and acute wounds compared with standard dressings. Further complicating the quality of the evidence is that various types of honey may have different properties based on species of bee, geographical location, and processing conditions.

Immune System-Boosting Treatments Some herbal medicines are believed to play a role in immune modulation by regulating a variety of cytokines. In a review of studies investigating herbal immunomodulators, 49 studies were found showing in vivo or in vitro activity of various botanicals in influencing cytokine production, including interleukin (IL)-1, tumor necrosis factor (TNF)-alpha, interferon (IFN)-gamma, and IL-2, -4, -5,

-6, -8, and -10 (Spelman et al., 2006). Of note, *Astragalus membranaceus*, traditionally used in Chinese medicine, lowers IL-6 production, which is implicated in a number of inflammatory disorders. *A. sativum* (garlic) also lowers IL-6 production in vitro and can reduce the pro-inflammatory cytokines IL-1, TNF, and IL-8 (Spelman et al., 2006). Further in vivo and clinical studies are needed to definitively establish a role of herbal medicines in immunomodulation.

Dilute Bleach Baths Patients with atopic dermatitis have high rates of colonization with *S. aureus,* and the density of colonization increases with clinical severity (Leyden et al., 1974). It is believed that *S. aureus* superantigens activate keratinocytes and promote inflammation, and therefore reducing colonization may improve atopic dermatitis (Cardona et al., 2006). Bleach is a common cleaning antiseptic used in a variety of settings, and it has both in vivo and in vitro activity against *S. aureus,* including MRSA. In a recent randomized placebo-controlled study of patients with moderate to severe atopic dermatitis, patients in the group receiving dilute bleach baths and intranasal mupirocin showed significantly decreased atopic dermatitis severity than the control group (Huang et al., 2009). Additional studies are needed to assess the efficacy of dilute bleach baths in decreasing *S. aureus* colonization and the relationship between decolonization and the severity of atopic dermatitis.

Sunflower Oil In a prospective, randomized, controlled study of preterm infants, daily topical treatment with sunflower oil resulted in a statistically significant reduction in neonatal mortality rates compared with a control group who did not receive emollient therapy (Darmstadt et al., 2008). In another randomized controlled study (Darmstadt et al., 2004), the rate of nosocomial infections in preterm infants was significantly lower after topical therapy with sunflower seed oil three times daily, suggesting that it may provide an alternative to improve skin barrier function and prevent skin infections.

S. pyogenes

Alternative Treatments
Herbal Treatments Similarly to *S. aureus,* hundreds of botanical extracts have been tested in vitro for antibacterial activity against *S. pyogenes*. Some of the botanicals with activity against *S. pyogenes* include *Capsicum* species (Cichewicz & Thorpe 1996) (chili peppers), stem bark extracts of *Phyllanthus* (Brusotti et al., 2011) (Euphorbiaceae), black tea (Sharquie et al., 2000), and various essential oils of aromatic plants (Edris, 2007). Clinical trials are needed to investigate the potential benefits of herbal extracts in *S. pyogenes* skin infections.

Hainosankyuto *Hainosankyuto* is a traditional herbal Japanese medicine (Kampo medicine) composed of six herbs (*Platcodi radix, Glycyrrhizae radix, Aurantii fructus immaturus, Paoniae radix, Zizyphi fructus, Zinzigeris rhizoma*) that has been used for the treatment of various skin infections, including carbuncles, furuncles, palmoplantar pustulosis, and suppurative wounds (Kawahara et al., 2011). In a recent paper, a murine skin infection model was used to investigate the protective effects of oral *hainosankyuto* against *S. pyogenes*. Mice treated with the medicine showed increased survival rates and serum levels of inflammatory cytokines, suggesting a protective effect (Minami et al., 2011). In another paper, infants with perianal abscess were treated with oral *hainosankyuto* as initial treatment with good results (Kawahara et al., 2011). More studies are needed to evaluate the protective effects of this herbal preparation against *S. pyogenes*.

Cordyceps sinensis *C. sinensis*, a member of the Ascomycetes class of fungi, has been used in Chinese herbal medicine as an immune modulator, believed to stimulate host immune responses (Kuo et al., 2005). In a recent study, an air-pouch bacterial inoculation model in mice was used to investigate the protective effects of *C. sinensis* extract against group A streptococcal infection. Mortality in mice fed with *C. sinensis* extract was decreased compared to controls and there was an increase in IL-12 and IFN-gamma mRNA expression in the *C. sinensis* treatment group, suggesting a beneficial immune modulation in the context of group A streptococcal infection (Kuo et al., 2005). More studies are needed to further investigate these findings.

Si-Ni-Tang

Si-Ni-Tang (composed of processed *Zingiber officinale, Glycyrrhiza uralensis,* and *Aconitum carmichaeli*) is an herbal remedy that has been documented in ancient Chinese medicine to be helpful in treating patients with sepsis and septic shock (Chen et al., 2011). A randomized controlled trial was proposed in 2011 to study whether this herbal remedy is beneficial for patients in septic shock (Chen et al., 2011). No other data are available studying this herbal remedy in septic shock.

Table 15.2. Summary of Treatment Modalities for *Corynebacterium* Skin Infections

Diseases	Established Treatments	Alternative Therapies

Erythrasma
Pitted keratolysis
Trichomycosis axillaris
	• Antibacterial soaps
	• Clindamycin/
	  erythromycin lotions
	• Oral erythromycin for
	  resistant cases
		• Photodynamic therapy
		• Red light therapy
		• Thyme oil
		• Golden seal, cleavers,
		  tea tree oil

Corynebacterium Skin Infections

Corynebacterium skin infections include erythrasma, pitted keratolysis, and trichomycosis axillaris (Blaise et al., 2008). Erythrasma is a superficial skin infection of intertriginous sites caused by *Corynebacterium minutissimum*. Pink, well-defined scaly patches that exhibit bright red fluorescence with Wood's lamp are the characteristic clinical presentation. Pitted keratolysis, most commonly caused by *Kytococcus sedentaris*, presents with small crateriform pits on the soles, associated with hyperhidrosis and malodor. Trichomycosis axillaris presents with adherent yellow nodules of the hair shafts of axillary or pubic hair.

Established Therapy Topical therapies for erythrasma include antibacterial soaps and creams (clindamycin, erythromycin), 10% to 20% aluminum chloride and miconazole cream (Blaise et al., 2008). Oral erythromycin can be used in resistant cases. Similarly, pitted keratolysis responds well to topical erythromycin, clindamycin, and miconazole. Feet need to be kept dry. Antibacterial soaps/lotions and shaving are used for trichomycosis axillaris.

Alternative Therapy

Photodynamic Therapy Photodynamic therapy (PDT) involves killing microbes by treatment with a photosensitizer agent, followed by exposure to light. The killing activity is believed to be due to the reactive oxygen species created in the process. In an in vitro study, methylene blue was used as a photosensitizer and polychromatic visible light was used to assess the effects of PDT on organisms of normal skin flora, including *C. minutissimum* (Zeina et al., 2001).

Red Light Therapy In an in vivo study, 13 patients with erythrasma were treated with red light without exogenous photosensitizer. Results showed complete recovery in three patients and various degrees of improvement in the rest (Darras-Vercambre et al., 2006), suggesting that this technique may be used as an alternative therapy.

Clove and Thyme Extracts Essential oils have been used in traditional medicine as antimicrobials. An in vitro study of clove and thyme extracts showed activity against *Corynebacterium* spp. (Nzeako et al., 2006).

Other suggested natural remedies ("Erythrasma," 2010) include golden seal paste (*Hydrastasis canadensis*), cleavers compresses (*Galium aparine*), and TTO, but no published studies were found investigating these treatments specifically against *Corynebacterium* spp.

Other Gram-Positive Bacteria: Propionibacterium acnes

P. acnes is a gram-positive bacterium that is thought to contribute to acne formation by increasing inflammation of the comedones (Eady & Cove, 2000).

Table 15.3. Summary of Treatment Modalities for *Propionibacterium acnes* Skin Infections

Diseases	Established Treatments	Alternative Therapies
Acne	• Antibacterial washes and topical lotions • Oral antibiotics	• Tea tree oil • *Ocimum gratissimum* oil • Thai herbal extracts, *Linum usitatissimum* extracts • Ayurvedic herbal preparations • Dietary changes: Paleolithic diet, South Beach diet, low-carbohydrate diet • Blue light and PDT

This topic is summarized here with respect to *P. acnes* treatment but is more fully explored in the chapter on integrative management of acne (Chapter 12).

Established Therapy

Standard acne therapies include benzoyl peroxide washes and gels, antibiotic topical gels, retinoids, and oral antibiotics of the tetracycline class (Leyden et al., 2009). *P. acnes* can be killed by both topical and oral antibiotics as well as topical benzoyl peroxide.

Alternative Therapy

TTO In a randomized double-blind clinical trial of 60 patients with mild to moderate acne vulgaris, there was significant improvement in the acne severity index in the patients using 5% TTO gel compared to placebo after a course of six weeks (Enshaieh et al., 2007). An older study found that 5% TTO gel was comparable in effect with 5% benzoyl peroxide lotion, although it had a slower onset of action (Bassett et al., 1990). More studies are needed to better establish a role for TTO in acne treatment.

Occimum gratissimum Oil In a recent clinical trial, *O. gratissimum* oil was compared with 10% benzoyl peroxide and placebo in efficacy of treating acne in students. Two of the preparations (2% and 5% *O. gratissimum* oil in alcohol) were more active than benzoyl peroxide, although the 5% preparation was irritating (Martin & Ernst, 2003). Larger studies are needed to evaluate this alternative therapy for acne.

Thai Basil Oils and Linum usitatissimum In an in vitro study of Thai basil oils (*Ocimum basilicum, Ocimum sanctum, Ocimum americanum*) and their micro-emulsions of activity against *P. acnes, O. basilicum* oil had good activity against *P. acnes* (Viyoch et al., 2006). Similarly, in an in vitro study of *L. usitatissimum* extracts, the oil extract had activity against *P. acnes* (Nand et al.,

2011). In vivo studies are needed to assess whether these findings could translate into clinical practice.

Ayurvedic Herbal Extracts Ayurvedic herbal extracts have been used for hundreds of years in traditional Indian medicine to treat acne. In a randomized, double-blind, placebo-controlled trial in 53 patients using oral Ayurvedic preparations with or without Ayurvedic topical preparations it was found that combined treatment with oral and topical formulations showed the best results in improving acne lesions (Lalla et al., 2001).

Paleolithic Diet and Other Insulin-Lowering Diets The Western lifestyle has been suggested to play a role in acne through its insulinotropic activity (Lindeberg, 2012). Populations consuming a Paleolithic diet that excludes dairy, sugar, and grains have low basal insulin levels and do not develop acne (Melnik et al., 2011). It is believed that IGF-1 plays an important role in acne formation by stimulating lipogenesis and androgen receptor signaling (Melnik et al., 2011). Thus, consuming a Paleolithic diet may help improve acne symptoms by decreasing IGF-1 signaling and decreasing insulin levels. Other insulin-lowering diets such as the South Beach diet or Atkins may have similar effects.

Blue Light and PDT P. acnes has been showed to be able to produce porphyrins (Gribbon et al., 1994). In vitro, blue light is able to cause damage to the bacterial membrane, leading to death (Ashkenazi et al., 2003). Red light is known to have anti-inflammatory effects by inducing cytokine release from macrophages (Young et al., 1989). In one study, a combination of blue and red light therapy reduced the number of inflammatory lesions to a greater extent than benzoyl peroxide alone or blue light alone (Kim & Armstrong, 2011). In a study of the efficacy and tolerability of a hand-held blue light device in the treatment of mild to moderate facial acne, it was found that treatment with blue light was significantly associated with a decrease in inflammatory lesions compared to baseline (Wheeland & Dhawan, 2011). Similarly, PDT using aminolevulinic acid followed by red light reduces the number of inflammatory lesions in acne (Kim & Armstrong, 2011).

Azelaic Acid Another treatment option for mild to moderate inflammatory acne is azelaic acid. It provides the effectiveness of other topical agents but without the local irritation of other topical agents and without the systemic side effects of oral antibiotics (Mackrides & Shaughnessy, 1996). In addition, it is considered to be Pregnancy Category B.

Heat Devices A variety of heat devices are available on the market to treat acne (e.g., Zeno Acne Clearing Device). In a randomized, placebo-controlled, double-blind study, patients treated with a hand-held device that emits both light and heat showed significant improvement rates in acne inflammatory lesions compared to the control group (Sadick et al., 2010).

GRAM-NEGATIVE BACTERIA

P. aeruginosa

P. aeruginosa is a common gram-negative bacterium that can be associated with severe hospital-acquired infections and is often antibiotic resistant (Agger & Mardan, 1995; Estahbanati et al., 2002). It causes a number of primary skin and soft tissue infections in immunocompetent individuals (Table 15.4). It is one of the most common pathogens in burn patients and can spread through the burn eschar, producing bacteremia. In green nail syndrome, *P. aeruginosa* can infect the nail, producing a characteristic greenish-blue discoloration. Pseudomonal folliculitis can result from the use of hot tubs, whirlpools, or other nonchlorinated pools. Otitis externa and malignant otitis externa can also develop secondary to pseudomonal infection. In pseudomonal hot-foot syndrome, painful red nodules develop on the soles secondary to swimming in water containing *P. aeruginosa*. In ecthyma gangrenosum, an ulcer with central gray-black eschar develops in patients with *P. aeruginosa* septicemia.

Established Treatments

In green nail syndrome, topical antibiotics (fluoroquinolones) and clipping back the nail are used. Treatment of otitis externa involves antibiotic eardrops and local cleaning of the auditory canal. Topical gentamicin can be used in pseudomonal folliculitis, although the condition is usually self-limiting. Similarly, hot-foot syndrome is self-limiting and does not

Table 15.4. Summary of Treatment Modalities for *Pseudomonas aeruginosa* Skin Infections

Diseases	Established Treatment	Alternative Therapies
Green nail syndrome	• Surgical debridement of eschar, drainage of abscesses • Oral or intravenous antibiotic therapy	• Honey • *Melaleuca alternifolia* (tea tree) oil • Green tea extracts • Henna extracts • Dilute vinegar soaks • Chinese herbal medicine • *Shiunko*
Pseudomonal pyoderma		
Otitis externa and malignant otitis externa		
Pseudomonal folliculitis		
Pseudomonas hot-foot syndrome		
Echthyma gangrenosum		
Burn infections		

require antibiotic treatment. Systemic antibiotics and wound care are used in pseudomonal pyoderma. Intravenous antibiotics (aminoglycosides) are needed once the diagnosis of ecthyma gangrenosum is made, since this is a manifestation of septicemia (Bolognia et al., 2008; Werlinger & Moore, 2004; Wu et al., 2011).

Alternative Therapies

Honey Honey has been used as a microbicidal and wound-healing promoter since ancient times. A number of in vitro studies have looked at the activity of honey against antibiotic-susceptible and resistant strains of *P. aeruginosa*. In one study, 50 strains of *P. aeruginosa* were isolated from different types of wound infections, including burn wounds. All the strains were found to be sensitive to a polyfloral honey (Agmark grade) using an agar dilution method (Shenoy et al., 2012). In another study, manuka honey was found to be effective in killing *P. aeruginosa* bacterial biofilms (Alandejani et al., 2009). A few reports have also shown that honey can be useful in dressing wounds, including burn wounds (Dunford et al., 2000; Molan, 2006) and can increase wound healing by increasing granulation tissue and wound contraction (Khoo et al., 2010).

TTO An in vitro broth microdilution study of TTO and its components' antibacterial activity against 30 isolates of *P. aeruginosa* found that *Pseudomonas* spp. are susceptible to TTO, although less susceptible than other bacteria (Papadopoulos et al., 2006). Clinical studies are needed to further investigate these findings.

Green Tea Extracts Water-soluble green tea extracts were tested in one in vitro study against 43 strains of *P. aeruginosa* collected from clinical specimens at two hospitals in Tehran, Iran (Jazani et al., 2007). About half of the strains were multidrug resistant. The extracts showed good bactericidal action against the resistant strains. In vivo studies are needed to assess whether green tea extracts would show benefit in treated *P. aeruginosa*-infected wounds.

Henna Extracts *Lawsonia inermis* (henna) is another herb used in various parts of the world as an antifungal and antibacterial agent. One study found good in vitro activity of henna extracts against *P. aeruginosa* (Al-Rubiay et al., 2008).

Dilute Vinegar Soaks Dilute vinegar has been used since ancient times as a wound antiseptic (Hansson & Faergemann, 1995; Landis, 2008). As a 0.25% to 0.5% solution, it is bactericidal against many gram-positive and gram-negative organisms, including *P. aeruginosa* (Hansson & Faergemann, 1995). It is believed that vinegar lowers the local pH in wounds, thus reducing the bacterial load. In one study, acetic acid-wetted dressings reduced both the gram-negative and *S. aureus* bacterial load in venous leg ulcers (Hansson & Faergemann, 1995).

Chinese Herbal Medicine   A disc diffusion study of the antibacterial activity of ethanol extracts of 58 Chinese herbal medicines against 89 nosocomial antibiotic-resistant strains of *P. aeruginosa* showed that 26 of the extracts had antibacterial activity, possibly related to the presence of flavonoid compounds in the extracts (Liu et al., 2007).

Shiunko

Shiunko is a two-component topical herbal medicine (*Lithospormi radix* and *Angelica sinensis*) used in China and Japan to treat burns, cuts, and abrasions (Huang et al., 2004). In an in vivo study in rats, wound infections following *P. aeruginosa* inoculation into skin were lower in the *Shiunko*-treated group than the control group and the *Shiunko*-treated group had higher rates of complete epithelialization (Huang et al., 2004).

Fungal Cutaneous Infections

Fungi exist throughout our environment but grow best in places that are cool, dark, and humid. They can be found in air, soil, plants, and animals. Fungal infections of the skin and adnexal structures have the ability to subsist on keratin, a protein found in the hair, nails, and skin of humans. Otherwise healthy individuals can experience cutaneous fungal infections given the right host and environmental conditions; however, persons with compromised immune systems tend to have more frequent and extensive infections.

Cutaneous mycoses involve the epidermis and dermis, hair, and nails; superficial-type mycoses can invade only the outermost layers of the skin and hair (Murray et al., 2005). Deep fungal infections are beyond the scope of this chapter. Cutaneous fungal infections in humans are labeled by body location. Since different organisms can affect the same location, the location alone is not enough to identify the type of fungus. The most common skin infection pathogens are the dermatophytes *Epidermophyton*, *Trichophyton*, and *Microsporum*. Less common are nondermatophyte fungi such as *Malassezia furfur* and *Candida*.

Treatment can be challenging, and many fungal infections will recur. Some types are highly contagious and should be treated promptly. Topical medicines, both allopathic and herbal, are first line for tinea corporis, tinea pedis, tinea cruris, tinea manuum, tinea faciei, tinea versicolor, seborrheic dermatitis, pityriasis folliculitis, and most types of candidiasis. Oral therapy is usually required for tinea capitis, tinea barbae, and onychomycosis.

TINEA CAPITIS, TINEA BARBAE, AND ONYCHOMYCOSIS

Tinea Capitis

This is a fungal infection of the scalp, referred to by laypersons as "ringworm of the scalp," that usually affects children between 3 and 7 years of age. It is characterized by irregular or well-demarcated, often itchy, bald patches and scaling, sometimes with broken-off hairs. At times it may present more subtly and look like common dandruff. Family members should be assessed for treatment because tinea capitis is highly contagious.

Systemic antifungals must be used as the organisms invade hair follicles and cannot be reached with topical therapy. Secondary bacterial infection should be treated with oral antibiotics. In severely inflammatory cases, systemic corticosteroids may also be required to prevent scarring alopecia.

The pathogen dermatophytes are *T. mentagrophytes, T. tonsurans, T. verrucosum, T. equinum, T. violaceum, T. schoenleninii, M. canis,* and *M. audouinii* (Table 15.5).

Tinea Barbae

Tinea barbae is informally known as ringworm of the beard, or barber's itch. It is a local inflammatory reaction in the beard area of men. Often it is seen in people who work with animals, most commonly cattle and dogs, as the transmission is most commonly from animals to humans.

The pathogen dermatophytes are *T. mentagrophytes, T. verrucosum, T. schoenleinii, T. megnini,* and *M. canis* (Table 15.6).

Table 15.5. Summary of Treatment Modalities for Tinea Capitis Infections

Established Treatments	Complementary Treatments
Griseofulvin 20–25 mg/kg/day for 6–12 weeks	*Selenium* Selenium is an essential trace mineral found in soil, water, and some foods. Antifungal shampoos containing selenium sulfide may reduce scaling and contagiousness in patients and close contacts. It has been shown to be an effective adjunctive agent to griseofulvin in the treatment of tinea capitis (Allen et al., 1982).
Fluconazole 6 mg/kg/day for six weeks	
Terbinafine at 62.5 mg/day (less than 20 kg), 125 mg/day (20–40 kg), 250 mg/day (more than 40 kg) for two to six weeks	
Fluconazole at 6 mg/kg/day for six weeks	Prescription-strength shampoos such as Selsun Rx or Exsel contain 2.5% selenium sulfide. It should be massaged into wet hair and remain on the scalp for two to three minutes. Use two or three times weekly for about one month.
Itraconazole at 3–5 mg/kg/day for six weeks	

Table 15.6. Summary of Treatment Modalities for Tinea barbae Infections

Established Treatments	Alternative Treatments
Griseofulvin 330–375 mg daily or twice daily until two to three weeks after clearance	*Shaving and warm compresses*
Terbinafine 250 mg daily for four weeks	*Neem*
Itraconazole 200 mg daily for two weeks	Also known as *Azadirachta indica*, neem is a natural antiseptic extract from the plant's leaves that can be applied to the affected area (Subapriya & Nagini, 2005).
Prednisone for severe inflammation and to prevent scarring. Start with 40 mg daily and taper over two weeks.	

Onychomycosis

Onychomycosis is a fungal infection of the nails. It may cause nail plate discoloration and thickening with subungual debris, roughness, and crumbling, powdery edges. It is often of great cosmetic concern to patients, and it can be painful. These infections are difficult to treat, requiring lengthy courses of medication, and may recur. Risk factors for this infection include aging, diabetes, poorly fitting shoes, working in a humid or moist environment, perspiring heavily, and the presence of tinea pedis (Hainer, 2003).

Patients should never be treated with systemic antifungals without confirming the infection by culture or fungal stain, since nail changes due to traumatic dystrophy and psoriasis can appear identical to those induced by fungal infections. Conservative therapy such as observation or nonprescription topicals is acceptable if a patient has no complicating comorbidities or associated symptoms. Concurrent tinea pedis should be treated with topical medication (see the section above on tinea pedis).

The pathogen dermatophytes are *T. rubrum*, *T. mentagrophytes*, *T. tonsurans*, *T. megninii*, and *E. floccosum*. Nondermatophytes are *S. brevicaulis*, *Scytalidium* spp., *Candida albicans*, *Aspergillis terreus*, *Acremonium* spp., and *Fuscarium* spp (Table 15.7).

TINEA CORPORIS, TINEA PEDIS, TINEA CRURIS, TINEA MANUUM, AND TINEA FACIEI

Tinea corporis, pedis, cruris, manuum, and faciei are closely related in terms of presentation, pathogens, and management. These infections often appear as scaly, red patches with occasional papules and vesicles. Tinea infections that have been empirically treated with topical corticosteroids may present in an atypical way and are labeled tinea incognito.

Tinea cruris affects the genitals, inner upper thighs, and buttocks. It typically spares the penis and scrotum (vs. candidiasis). Tinea corporis affects

Table 15.7. Summary of Treatment Modalities for Onychomycosis

Established Treatments	Alternative Treatments
Topical antifungal treatments such as imidazole, urea, and ciclopirox nail lacquer usually do not work alone but may reduce or stabilize infection and may augment the efficacy of oral antifungals.	*Tea tree oil* Buck and colleagues (1994) compared 100% tea tree oil with 1% clotrimazole solution. After six months the two groups showed comparable results on the basis of mycologic cure (11% for clotrimazole and 18% for tea tree oil), as well as clinical assessment and subjective rating of appearance and symptoms (61% for clotrimazole and 60% for tea tree oil).
Nondermatophyte molds are often resistant to oral antifungals but may respond to topical therapy.	*Ozonized sunflower oil* Menendez and colleagues (2011) found that topical ozonized sunflower oil demonstrated effectiveness in the treatment of onychomycosis superior to that of 2% ketoconazole cream without side effects.
Oral treatment with (1) terbinafine 250 mg daily for 12 weeks, (2) itraconazole 200 mg daily for 12 weeks, or (3) fluconazole 150–200 mg daily for nine months	*Thyme* Wilson (1965) reported successful treatment of onycholysis and paronychia with thyme due to its antifungal properties. *Vinegar soaks* Vinegar soaks daily for 15–20 minutes in a mixture of one part vinegar to two parts warm water may inhibit the growth of fungi (Sulaiman et al., 2005). *Vicks VapoRub™* Derby and colleagues (2011) found that Vicks VapoRub™ demonstrated positive treatment effect in 83% of participants and mycologic and clinical cure at 48 weeks in 27.8% of patients.

the torso and some parts of the extremities. Tinea pedis affects the moist area between the toes and occasionally the foot itself.

Permanent cure of any of these infections may not be possible, but control can be established. Keep the affected areas cool and dry. Old footwear should be discarded as it may be the cause of tinea pedis reinfection.

The pathogen dermatophytes are *T. rubrum, T. mentagrophytes,* and *E. floccosum.* Nondermatophytes are *Scytalidium* spp. and *C. albicans* (Table 15.8).

CUTANEOUS CANDIDIASIS

Presentation varies with the sites involved, the duration of infection, and the patient's immune status and usually includes redness, swelling, and papules or

Table 15.8. Summary of Treatment Modalities for Tinea Corporis, Pedis, Cruris, Manuum, and Faciei Infections

Established Treatments	Alternative Treatments
Small, localized lesions treated topically for one to six weeks, and one week after clinical resolution. Regardless of location on foot, topical antifungals should be applied to web spaces and soles.	*Ozonized sunflower oil* In a study by Menendez and colleagues (2002) a complete clinical and mycologic cure was obtained in 75% and 81% of patients treated with ozonized sunflower oil and ketoconazole respectively.
Treated topically to at least 2 cm outside the border of the lesions	*S. alata* Oladele and colleagues (2010) reported clinical improvement of tinea corporis by use of the ethanolic extracts of *S. alata* leaves.
Topically may use (1) terbinafine 1% cream twice daily, (2) clotrimazole 1% cream twice daily, (3) econazole 1% cream twice daily, (4) oxiconazole 1% cream twice daily, (5) ketoconazole 2% cream twice daily, or (6) miconazole 2% cream twice daily	*Ajoene* In a study by Ledezma and colleagues (1996) of 34 patients treated with 0.4% ajoene cream topically once daily, 79% noted clearing within seven days and the remainder had clearing within 14 days. At a three-month follow-up all participants remained free of fungus. It was further reported that the rapid healing of the lesions as well as the lack of recurrence with the use of 0.4% topical ajoene is similar to published results obtained with 1% terbinafine.
Oral treatment for resistant disease includes (1) itraconazole 100–200 mg once daily for two to four weeks; or pulse therapy with 200 mg twice daily for one week each month for one or two months, (2) terbinafine 250 mg once daily for two to six weeks, (3) griseofulvin ultra-microsize 330–750 mg once daily for four to eight weeks, or (4) fluconazole 150 mg once weekly for two to four weeks	*Tea tree oil* Satchell and colleagues (2002) found that concentrations of tea tree oil (25% and 50%), in solution rather than cream because of immiscibility, resulted in mycologic cure rates of 55% and 64% in the 25% and 50% tea tree oil groups, respectively. However, this was lower than results obtained by clotrimazole (90%) and terbinafine (90%) in similarly designed studies.
Hyperkeratotic variants benefit from keratolytic agents such as salicylic acid or urea creams and lotions.	*Seepwillow* A study by DiSalvo (1974) showed an aqueous extract of *Baccharis glutinosa* or seepwillow/water willow has an inhibitory effect on dermatophytes in vitro.

(*continued*)

Table 15.8 (continued)

Established Treatments	Alternative Treatments
Topical corticosteroids are not indicated but may be used in combination with topical antifungals when pruritus is severe. They are absolutely contraindicated in immunosuppressed patients.	*Solanum chrysotrichum* A study by Herrera-Arellano and colleagues (2003) showed that the therapeutic success rate (clinical and mycologic effectiveness plus tolerability) was 74.51% with *S. chrysotrichum* extract and 69.44% with 2% ketoconazole.
Drying agents include gentian violet, Burow's solution (5% aluminum subacetate) foot soaks twice daily, and 20–25% aluminum chloride hexahydrate powder daily.	*Bitter orange oil* An in vitro study by Ramadan and colleagues (1996) showed that oil of bitter orange exerts fungistatic and fungicidal activity against a variety of pathogenic dermatophyte species, including those responsible for tinea corporis, cruris, and pedis.

pustules. Classic infection differs from dermatophyte infections in appearance in that it has satellite lesions outside the main border of the infection. In addition, it will affect the penis and scrotum in men, unlike dermatophyte infections. Candidal infections are associated with any factor that weakens immune activity, including malignancies, diabetes, and corticosteroid use, as well as prolonged antibiotic use.

In general, affected persons should avoid occlusive clothing, keep skin dry after bathing, and avoid immersing the skin in water. Use drying agents such as Burow's™ solution (aluminum acetate) for oozing lesions and gentian violet for toe web spaces. Powdered formulations are best for moist lesions.

The causative pathogen is *C. albicans* (Table 15.9).

SEBORRHEIC DERMATITIS, TINEA VERSICOLOR, *PITYROSPORUM* FOLLICULITIS

Seborrheic dermatitis, tinea versicolor, and *Pityrosporum* folliculitis are closely related in terms of presentation, pathogens, and management. Since they are caused by species of *Malassezia* that are part of the normal cutaneous microflora, they are not strictly speaking infections but rather overgrowth with inflammatory host reactions.

Seborrheic dermatitis can present as greasy, erythematous scaly patches, petaloid shiny or hyperpigmented plaques, or fine, dry scale on the scalp, face, ears, chest, axillae, and groin. Tinea, or pityriasis, versicolor presents clinically as hypopigmented, hyperpigmented, and/or erythematous lesions

Table 15.9. Summary of Treatment Modalities for Cutaneous Candidiasis

Established Treatments	*Alternative Treatments*
Intertriginous Infection	*Gentian violet*
Topical antifungals such as nystatin 100,000 units/g cream, ointment or powder applied two or three times daily or miconazole 2% cream or powder twice daily. Broad-spectrum agents like econazole and ketoconazole can also be effective. Fluconazole 150 mg once weekly for two to four weeks is indicated for extensive intertriginous candidiasis; topical antifungals may be used at the same time.	A study by Kondo and colleagues (2012) showed that clinical yeast isolates are highly susceptible to gentian violet, and that gentian violet is more effective than povidone–iodine to deter candidiasis.
Candidal Diaper Rash	*Solanum chrysotrichum*
More frequent diaper changes, avoidance of disposable diapers with plastic coverings, and an imidazole cream twice daily. Oral nystatin is an option for infants with coexisting oropharyngeal candidiasis: 1 mL of suspension (100,000 units/mL) is placed in each buccal pouch four times daily.	Herrera-Arellano and colleagues (2007) reported the fungicidal and fungistatic activity of in vitro *S. chrysotrichum* for *Candida* species of medical significance.
Oral Candidiasis	*Tea tree, cinnamon, garlic, probiotic, pomegranate, propolis*
Fluconazole 200 mg on the first day, then 100 mg once daily for two to three weeks	Several therapies have been found to be useful in the treatment of oral candidiasis, including tea tree oral solution (Jandourek et al., 1998), cinnamon lozenges (Quale et al., 1996), garlic paste (Sabitha et al., 2005), probiotics (Hatakka et al. 2007), pomegranate (Endo et al., 2010), and propolis (a natural flavonoid-rich resin made by bees) (Santos et al., 2005). However, propolis should be avoided in children as it is a potent allergen and sensitizing agent (Giusti et al., 2004).
Chronic Mucocutaneous Candidiasis	*Solanum nigrescens*
Long-term oral antifungal treatment with ketoconazole 400 mg once daily or itraconazole 200 mg once daily.	In a study by Giron and colleagues (1988), vaginal suppositories containing 10% extract of *Solanum nigrescens* twice daily for 15 days demonstrated equal efficacy to commercial suppositories containing nystatin used twice daily for 15 days. Ninety percent of the experimental group and 94% of the comparative group were culture negative at the end of treatment.
Candida Folliculitis	*Cleanse diet*
Itraconazole 100 mg twice daily for 14 days	*Candida* cleanse diet is intended to restrict intestinal growth by restricting sugar, white flour, yeast, and cheese. There is no scientific, peer-reviewed evidence of effectiveness.

Table 15.10. Summary of Treatment Modalities for Seborrheic Dermatitis and Tinea Versicolor

Established Treatments	Alternative Treatments
Topical treatment for large areas: (1) selenium sulfide lotion 2.5% (10 minutes daily for one week or 24-hour applications weekly for one month), (2) pyrithione zinc 2% shampoo 10 minutes daily for one week, (3) propylene glycol 50% in water twice daily for two weeks, (4) bifonazole 1% shampoo daily for three weeks, or (5) ketoconazole 2% shampoo daily for three weeks, (6) coal tar combined with salicylic acid 10 minutes daily initially, then as needed	*S. alata* Oladele and colleagues (2010) showed that S. *alata* soap, also known as ringworm bush or candle stick, cleared the lesions on 16 subjects (94.1%), 11 with tinea versicolor and five with tinea corporis.
Topical treatment for limited areas: (1) clotrimazole 1% cream twice daily for two to six weeks, (2) sulconazole 1% cream once daily for two weeks, (3) econazole 1% cream once or twice daily for two weeks, (4) ketoconazole 2% cream once or twice daily for two to four weeks, (5) ciclopirox 0.77% cream or lotion once or twice daily for four weeks, or (7) terbinafine 1% cream or solution once or twice daily for one to two weeks	*Acupuncture* Traditional Chinese Medicine treatment with acupuncture focuses on tonifying and regulating the spleen and stomach *qi*, smoothing the liver *qi*, and dispelling dampness (Ferrari, 2012).
Prevention of recurrence with (1) selenium sulfide 2.5% lotion applied on the first and third day of the month, (2) ketoconazole 2% shampoo lathered on scalp and body for 5–10 minutes once per week, (3) ketoconazole 400 mg once monthly, (4) fluconazole 300 mg once monthly, or (5) itraconazole 400 mg once monthly	*S. chrysotrichum* Herrera-Arellano and colleagues (2004) compared the effectiveness and tolerability of standardized extract of S. *chrysotrichum* (applied every third day for four weeks) against topical 2% ketoconazole. The therapeutic success (clinical and mycologic effectiveness plus tolerability) on the local treatment of seborrheic dermatitis associated with *Malessezia* was 64-71% (no significant difference with ketoconazole).
	Biotin Dietary biotin supplementation has been recommended for treatment of dandruff and related seborrhea (Chhavi & Mohamad, 2012).
	Oil, Shampoo, and Toothbrush Mild cases of cradle cap can be treated with application of white petrolatum or mineral oil for several hours, followed by nonmedicated baby shampoo (McDonald & Smith, 1998). Scrubbing an infant's scalp with a soft toothbrush after applying baby oil or olive oil may be effective for cradle cap (McCollough & Sharieff, 2002).
	Bishop's weed and phototherapy for repigmentation (Cooking, 2012)

with fine scale primarily on the trunk. The affected areas of skin will have an inability to tan that will usually resolve after one to two months of treatment. *Pityrosporum* folliculitis presents as acneiform papules and pustules, primarily on the trunk and upper arms. These infections are not contagious and may or may not relate to poor hygiene; they can range from asymptomatic to severely pruritic.

These conditions tend to appear in infancy (as in "cradle cap") and then disappear until adolescence, when the sebaceous glands become reactivated. They tend to flare with higher temperatures, humidity, heavy sweating, infrequent bathing, and oil-based skin care products. Immunosuppression and systemic corticosteroid use can also cause flares.

The pathogen nondermatophytes are *M. globosa* and *M. furfur* (Table 15.10).

Viral Cutaneous Infections

Many viruses can infect the skin. This section will focus on those seen most commonly in clinical practice: herpes, human papilloma, poxviridae, RNA virus, and hepatitis.

The human herpesviridae family, which can be divided into three groups (alpha, beta, gamma), cause a number of skin diseases (Table 15.11).

Medical treatment for the herpes group of viruses centers on antiviral therapy. The antiviral class of medications called nucleoside analogues work to inhibit herpes simplex virus (HSV) polymerase activity. They include acyclovir, penciclovir, valacyclovir, and famciclovir. Reducing the risk of transmission (e.g., barrier protection to reduce sexual transmission, use of gloves

Table 15.11. Human Herpesviridae Family

Alpha herpesviridae	HSV1 (HHV1)	Herpes labialis, herpes gladiatorum, eczema herpeticum (Kaposi's varicelliform eruption), keratoconjunctivitis, neonatal herpes, genital herpes
	HSV2 (HHV2)	Genital herpes, herpetic whitlow, herpes labialis
	VZV (HHV3)	Chickenpox and herpes zoster
Beta herpesviridae	CMV (HHV 5)	TORCH infection, blueberry muffin rash
	HHV 6	Exanthema subitum/sixth disease/roseola
	HHV 7	Exanthema subitum
Gamma herpesviridae	EBV (HHV4)	Burkitt's lymphoma, mononucleosis, oral hairy leukoplakia, nasopharyngeal carcinoma, Gianotti-Crosti syndrome
	HHV 8	Kaposi's sarcoma

(Bolognia et al., 2008)

by dental workers in the prevention of herpetic whitlow, and taking suppressive therapy to reduce viral shedding) is also important from a public health perspective.

ALTERNATIVE MEDICINE TREATMENTS FOR HERPESVIRIDAE

Some herbals have shown promise in treating HSV infections (Table 15.12). One of the most commonly used herbals has been *Echinacea* root (*Echinacea angustifolia*). In a study by Ghaemi and colleagues (2009), *Echinacea* was shown to be an effective mediator for latency prevention of HSV-1.

Andrographis (*Andrographis paniculata*) is another popular herb used in the treatment of HSV; it is known for its immune-boosting abilities. Studies have demonstrated that *Andrographis* has some viricidal activity against HSV-1 and can have a cumulative effect when used with *Echinacea*, vitamin C, and zinc (Wiart et al., 2005). Another extract that has shown protective activity against HSV infection is *Cynanchum paniculatum* (Bunge) Kitagawa. In animal studies it has been shown to have protective effects against HSV (Li et al., 2012).

Other herbals have also been used for the treatment of herpes virus. Some include olive leaf (*Olea europaea*), passionflower (*Passiflora incarnata*), tronodora (*Tecoma stans*), osha root (*Ligusticum porterii*), lomatium root (*Lomatium dissectum*), chaparral leaf (*Larrea tridentata*), goldenseal root (*Hydrastis canadensis*), St. John's wort (*Hypericum perforatum*), and *Usnea* lichen (*Usnea* spp.).

Olive leaf has been shown to have many applications in medical therapy, including in the treatment of herpes and Epstein-Barr viruses. Calcium elenolate, a compound found in olive leaf extract, has antiviral activity against viruses such as herpes and influenza by preventing these viruses from entering the cells (Renis, 1969).

The root of the *Eleutherococcus senticosus* plant, also called Siberian ginseng or Eleuthero, is used in a number of medical conditions. In addition to being used in the treatment of HSV, it is also used for the treatment of high blood

Table 15.12. Summary of Alternative Treatment Modalities for Herpes Simplex Skin Infections

Evidence in literature	• Herbals: *Echinacea*, *Andrographis* (*Andrographis paniculata*), *Cynanchum paniculatum*, olive leaf, *Eleutherococcus senticosus*, *Opuntia streptacantha*. • Bioflavonoids, ascorbic acid
Lower level of evidence in literature	• Herbals: passionflower (*Passiflora incarnata*), tronodora (*Tecoma stans*), osha root (*Ligusticum porterii*), lomatium root (*Lomatium dissectum*), chaparral leaf (*Larrea tridentata*), goldenseal root (*Hydrastis canadensis*), St. John's wort (*Hypericum perforatum*), and *Usnea* lichen (*Usnea* spp.).

pressure, atherosclerosis, and rheumatic heart disease. In a double-blind study of 93 patients with HSV-2, there was a reduction in the number of outbreaks in patients taking Siberian ginseng (Williams, 1995).

The extract of the cactus plant *Opuntia streptacantha* also demonstrates inhibition of viral replication and inactivation of extracellular RNA and DNA viruses (Ahmad et al., 1996).

Some herbals have also had anecdotal benefits, including kava kava (*Piper methysticum*), valerian root (*Valeriana officinalis*), passionflower, jatamansi (*Nardostachys jatamansi*), and chamomile (*Matricaria recutta*). In terms of creating a soothing effect, alkaline baths with oils of tea tree, manuka, ravensare, and lavender can provide some relief. Immune-boosting herbs that have also been used include goldenseal, astragalus (*Astragalus membranaceus*), and lomatium root.

Bioflavonoids are widely recognized as antioxidants that can be helpful in improving the health of the skin. Bioflavonoids in addition to ascorbic acid have been shown to reduce vesiculation, especially when initiated in the prodromal stage of herpes labialis (Terezhalmy et al., 1978).

Another group of viruses that can have skin manifestations is the group of Papillomaviridae (human papillomavirus [HPV]) (Table 15.13).

Medical treatments of cutaneous warts aim to cause physical destruction, reduce autoinoculation, and boost immune recognition of the virus (Table 15.14). Not all warts need to be treated. The indications for treatment are pain, increased risk of malignancy (as with malignant strains of the virus), interference with daily function (as with some digital warts), decrease in quality of life, or cosmetic embarrassment. Please refer to the chapter on integrative management of warts for a complete discussion (Chapter 28).

Table 15.13. Summary of HPV Types Associated with
Specific Kinds of Viral Warts

Papillomaviradae of the Skin	*HPV Types*
Palmoplantar warts	1, 2, 4
Flat warts	3, 10
Butcher's warts	7
Digital squamous cell carcinoma and Bowen's	16
Epidermodysplasia verruciformis	3, 5, 8
Condyloma accuminata, Buschke-Lowenstein tumor, recurrent respiratory papillomatosis, conjunctival papillomatosis	6, 11
Bowenoid papulosis, erythroplasia of Queyrat, condyloma plana	16
Heck's disease	13, 32

Table 15.14. Integrative Treatments for Warts

Established Treatments	Alternative Treatments
Keratolytics (salicylic acid): inexpensive, available OTC, good evidence	Mind–body therapies: hypnotherapy, acupuncture
Cryotherapy, cantharidin, podophyllin: easy, may be painful, good evidence, may need multiple treatments	Garlic extracts, green tea catechins
CO_2 laser, pulsed dye laser, photodynamic therapy, thermotherapy, curettage: scarring, painful	Adhesiotherapy, exothermic topical patches
Bleomycin, *Candida* antigen: injection, can be painful, expensive, intermediate evidence	Oral zinc supplements
Topical retinoids, imiquimod: local irritation, Pregnancy Category C	Diet: vitamin C, carotenoids, tocopherols, folic acids
Surgical excision: scarring	
Oral cimetidine: low evidence, long-term oral therapy	Glutaraldehyde, formaldehyde, squaric acid, dinitrochlorobenzene: low evidence, increased risk of allergic reaction

(Dall'oglio et al., 2012; Sterling et al., 2001)

INTEGRATIVE THERAPIES FOR HPV

Warts are linked to immunological state, and therefore there are a number of integrative therapies that aim to promote a healthy immunological state. Regulating the diet has been an important alternative tool used in the treatment of the HPV virus. Foods rich in antioxidants like vitamin C, carotenoids, tocopherols, and folic acids and green leafy vegetables, as well as yellow vegetables (papaya, pumpkin, oranges) have been shown to be of some benefit.

Mind–body therapies have also been used to treat warts associated with the HPV virus. There have been many case reports that document the use of hypnosis and other mind–body therapies to help with regression of warts. For example, Spanos and colleagues (1990) showed in a study that patients treated with hypnosis saw greater results in wart regression than patients treated with placebo or topical salicylic acid.

Acupuncture has also been used in the treatment of warts. A single-blind randomized controlled study of 60 patients reported successful treatment of flat warts using auricular acupuncture (Ning et al., 2012).

Both aqueous and lipid extracts of garlic have been shown to have an effect in the treatment of warts. In a study of patients between 5 and 62 years of age (both male and female), garlic extracts were shown to cause complete resolution of warts within one to two weeks of twice-daily application to warts on the hands and feet (Dehghani et al., 2005).

Green tea catechins have been used in the treatment of genital warts because of their antiviral, antioxidant, and immunostimulatory properties (Meltzer et al., 2009). In addition, oral zinc supplements have been shown to be of some benefit in treating cutaneous warts. Sixty-one percent of patients treated with 10 mg/kg of oral zinc had complete remission of their warts after one month of treatment (Al-Gurairi et al., 2002).

Other alternative therapies include adhesiotherapy or the use of occlusive therapies such as duck/duct tape (or electrical tape) for the treatment of cutaneous warts. In some studies the success rate with duct tape has been found to be comparable to cryotherapy and salicyclic acid (Focht et al., 2002).

Exothermic topical patches as well as localized heat therapies for warts have also been documented. A randomized controlled trial of 60 patients with plantar warts showed a response rate of 53% in the treatment group versus 11% in the placebo group after five days of 30 minutes of heat treatments at three months of follow-up (Huo et al., 2010).

Last but not least, lifestyle changes such as decreasing sexual transmission of the virus, diet changes (as above), vaccination against genital warts, and reducing alcohol and cigarette smoking may help reduce propagation of warts.

POXVIRIDAE

There are various poxviruses that manifest in the skin, including molluscum contagiosum, smallpox, vaccinia, monkeypox, cowpox, orf, milker's nodules, and tanapox. This chapter will focus only on molluscum contagiosum, as it is a very common viral infection seen commonly in children and less commonly as a sexually transmitted disease in adults. Treatment options include destructive therapies (curettage, cryotherapy, cantharidin, and keratolytics), immunomodulators (imiquimod, cimetidine, and *Candida* antigen), as well as antivirals (cidofovir).

INTEGRATIVE TREATMENTS FOR MOLLUSCUM

Cantharidin, a derivative of the bodies of blister beetles, is a perfect example of the combination of medical therapy with nontraditional means to achieve resolution of a cutaneous disease (Table 15.15). Randomized controlled trials for the efficacy of cantharidin in the treatment of molluscum are lacking. However, in a survey among pediatric dermatologists, 92% of respondents reported satisfaction with cantharidin's efficacy when used in their patients (Coloe & Morrell, 2009). A large retrospective study showed 90% clearance of molluscum lesions after two treatments with cantharidin (Smolinski & Yan, 2005).

Table 15.15. Summary of Treatment Modalities for Molluscum

Established Treatments	Alternative Treatments
Surgical: curette, cryotherapy, cauterization, pulse dye laser	*Calcarea carbonica*
Topical: cantharidin, cidofovir, benzoyl peroxide, imiquimod, phenol, povidone–iodine + salicylic acid, podophyllotoxin, tretinoin, salicylic acid, silver nitrate	Garlic extracts
Systemic: cimetidine, griseofulvin	Turmeric, apple cider vinegar

Garlic has antiviral and antifungal properties in its active ingredient allicin that can be used to treat molluscum lesions, although data are lacking. Turmeric and apple cider vinegar (oral or topical) are also among the alternative therapies for molluscum.

Calcarea carbonica, a homeopathic remedy, has been shown to be superior to placebo in clinical studies (Manchanda et al., 1997).

RNA VIRUSES

There have been alternative therapies used for the treatment of the virus that causes measles (Table 15.16). Integrative therapies for measles include vitamin A. Treatment of patients with measles with vitamin A has been associated with reductions in morbidity and mortality (AAPCID, 1993).

Herbs such as *Echinacea purpurea* and *Astragalus membranaceus* have been used for their antiviral properties. *Astragalus propinquus* (also known as *Astragalus membranaceus*) has a history of use as a herbal medicine and is used in traditional Chinese medicine. Antiviral activity has been reported with the use of *Astragalus* in laboratory and animal studies (Zheng et al., 2009).

Other integrative therapies used in measles that have historical or theoretical uses include homeopathic aconite (*Aconitum napellus*), alkanna (*Alkanna* sp.), annatto (*Bixa orellana*), bamboo, belladonna (*Atropa belladonna*), black pepper (*Piper nigrum*), bovine colostrum, jewelweed (*Impatiens biflora*, *Impatiens pallida*), kudzu (*Pueraria lobata*), pomegranate (*Punica granatum*), raspberry (*Rubus idaeus*), spirulina, and yarrow (*Achillea millefolium*).

Table 15.16. RNA Viruses Associated with Specific Skin Disorders

Picornaviridae	Enteroviruses (coxsackievirus A and B, echoviruses): hand foot and mouth disease, herpangina
Paramyxovirus	Measles (rubeola), mumps
Togaviridae	Rubella (German measles), *chikungunya* fever

Conclusion

Dermatology invites eclectic practice and experimentation. Indeed, according to survey data, 35% to 69% of patients with skin diseases have used complementary and alternative medicine (Bhuchar et al., 2012), with herbal therapies and diet as the two oldest and most frequently relied upon interventions. While some of the same approaches used in modern evidence-based allopathic medicine, such as psoralens for repigmentation (Paul et al., 1987), have been used for thousands of years, most complementary and alternative treatments have not been scientifically proven but rather relied upon anecdotal experience.

Furthermore, although beyond the scope of this chapter to address, users of complementary and alternative medicine should recognize that those treatments, like any other medical intervention, are associated with risks of unwanted side effects. The U.S. Food and Drug Administration does not require manufacturers to prove efficacy or safety information of herbal remedies, so we recommend careful evaluation of any treatment option with a professional healthcare provider. Many treatments have a long history of effectiveness but more evidence in the traditional placebo-controlled, double-blind studies is needed. At this time, most of the alternative treatments cannot be recommended to the exclusion of conventional therapy with confidence; they are best used as adjunct, or integrative, therapy.

REFERENCES

American Academy of Pediatrics Committee of Infectious Diseases (AAPCID) (1993). Vitamin A treatment of measles. *Pediatrics, 91*(5), 1014–1015.

Agger, W. A., & A. Mardan (1995). *Pseudomonas aeruginosa* infections of intact skin. *Clinical Infectious Diseases, 20*(2), 302–308.

Ahmad, A., Davies, J., et al. (1996). Antiviral properties of extract of *Opuntia streptacantha. Antiviral Research, 30*(2–3), 75–85.

Alandejani, T., Marsan, J., et al. (2009). Effectiveness of honey on *Staphylococcus aureus* and *Pseudomonas aeruginosa* biofilms. *Otolaryngology Head and Neck Surgery, 141*(1), 114–118.

Alexopoulos, A., Kimbaris, A. C., et al. (2011). Antibacterial activities of essential oils from eight Greek aromatic plants against clinical isolates of *Staphylococcus aureus. Anaerobe, 17*(6), 399–402.

Al-Gurairi, F. T., Al-Waiz, M., et al. (2002). Oral zinc sulphate in the treatment of recalcitrant viral warts: randomized placebo-controlled clinical trial. *British Journal of Dermatology, 146*(3), 423–431.

Allen, H. B., Honig, P. J., et al. (1982). Selenium sulfide: adjunctive therapy for tinea capitis. *Pediatrics, 69*(1), 81–83.

Al-Rubiay, K. K., Jaber, N. N., et al. (2008). Antimicrobial efficacy of henna extracts. *Oman Medical Journal*, 23(4), 253–256.

Al-Waili, N. S., Salom, K., et al. (2011). Honey and microbial infections: a review supporting the use of honey for microbial control. *Journal of Medicinal Food*, 14(10), 1079–1096.

Al-Waili, N., Salom, K., et al. (2011). Honey for wound healing, ulcers, and burns; data supporting its use in clinical practice. *Scientific World Journal*, 11, 766–787.

Arndt, K., & Stern, R. (1998). Alternative medicine and dermatology: the unconventional issue. *Archives of Dermatology*, 1344(11), 1472.

Ashkenazi, H., Malik, Z., et al. (2003). Eradication of *Propionibacterium acnes* by its endogenic porphyrins after illumination with high intensity blue light. *FEMS Immunology and Medical Microbiology*, 35(1), 17–24.

Awen, B. Z., Unnithan, C. R., et al. (2011). Essential oils of *Retama raetam* from Libya: chemical composition and antimicrobial activity. *Natural Product Research*, 25(9), 927–933.

Bassett, I. B., Pannowitz, D. L., et al. (1990). A comparative study of tea-tree oil versus benzoyl peroxide in the treatment of acne. *Medical Journal of Australia*, 153(8), 455–458.

Bhuchar, S., Katta, R., & Wolf, J. (2012). Complementary and alternative medicine in dermatology: an overview of selected modalities for the practicing dermatologist. *American Journal of Clinical Dermatology*, 13(5), 311–317.

Blaise, G., Nikkels, A. F., et al. (2008). *Corynebacterium*-associated skin infections. *International Journal of Dermatology*, 47(9), 884–890.

Bolognia, J. L., Jorizzo, J. L., & Rapini, R. P. (2008). *Dermatology*, 2nd ed, St. Louis: Mosby.

Bowler, W. A., Bresnahan, J., et al. (2010). An integrated approach to methicillin-resistant *Staphylococcus aureus* control in a rural, regional-referral healthcare setting. *Infection Control and Hospital Epidemiology*, 31(3), 269–275.

Brusotti, G., Cesari, I., et al. (2011). Antimicrobial properties of stem bark extracts from *Phyllanthus muellerianus* (Kuntze) Excell. *Journal of Ethnopharmacology*, 135(3), 797–800.

Buck, D. S., Nidorf, D. M., et al. (1994). Comparison of two topical preparations for the treatment of onychomycosis: *Melaleuca alternifolia* (tea tree) oil and clotrimazole. *Journal of Family Practice*, 38(6), 601–605.

Caelli, M., Porteous, J., et al. (2000). Tea tree oil as an alternative topical decolonization agent for methicillin-resistant *Staphylococcus aureus*. *Journal of Hospital Infections*, 46(3), 236–237.

Cardona, I. D., Cho, S. H., et al. (2006). Role of bacterial superantigens in atopic dermatitis: implications for future therapeutic strategies. *American Journal of Clinical Dermatology*, 7(5), 273–279.

Casella, S., Leonardi, M., et al. (2012). The role of diallyl sulfides and dipropyl sulfides in the in vitro antimicrobial activity of the essential oil of garlic, *Allium sativum* L., and leek, *Allium porrum* L. *Phytotherapy Eesearch* [E-pub before print].

Casetti, F., Bartelke, S., et al. (2012). Antimicrobial activity against bacteria with dermatological relevance and skin tolerance of the essential oil from *Coriandrum sativum* L. fruits. *Phytotherapy Research*, 26(3), 420–424.

Celestin, R., Brown, J., et al. (2007). Erysipelas: a common potentially dangerous infection. *Acta Dermatovenerologica Alpina, Panonica, et Adriatica, 16*(3), 123–127.

Chen, H. C., Chen, W. C., et al. (2011). Simultaneous use of traditional Chinese medicine (si-ni-tang) to treat septic shock patients: study protocol for a randomized controlled trial. *Trials, 12,* 199.

Chhavi S, S. D., Mohammad A (2012). Potential of herbals as antidandruff agents. *International Journal of Pharmacy.* Available at http://www.irjponline.com/vol-issue3/3.pdf (accessed July 4, 2012).

Cichewicz, R. H., & Thorpe, P. A. (1996). The antimicrobial properties of chile peppers (*Capsicum* species) and their uses in Mayan medicine. *Journal of Ethnopharmacology, 52*(2), 61–70.

Coloe, J., & Morrell, D. S. (2009). Cantharidin use among pediatric dermatologists in the treatment of molluscum contagiosum. *Pediatric Dermatology, 26*(4), 405–408.

Cooking W. (2012). Bishop's weed (*Ammi majus*). Available at http://www.whatsin-yourcart.net/ns/DisplayMonograph.asp?storeID=89421731439A489E8444B228509 165F7&DocID=bishopsweed (accessed July 4, 2012).

Dall'oglio, F., D'Amico, V., et al. (2012). Treatment of cutaneous warts: an evidence-based review. *American Journal of Clinical Dermatology, 13*(2), 73–96.

Darmstadt, G. L., Badrawi, N., et al. (2004). Topically applied sunflower seed oil prevents invasive bacterial infections in preterm infants in Egypt: a randomized, controlled clinical trial. *Pediatric Infectious Disease Journal, 23*(8), 719–725.

Darmstadt, G. L., Saha, S. K., et al. (2008). Effect of skin barrier therapy on neonatal mortality rates in preterm infants in Bangladesh: a randomized, controlled, clinical trial. *Pediatrics, 121*(3), 522–529.

Darras-Vercambre, S., Carpentier, O., et al. (2006). Photodynamic action of red light for treatment of erythrasma: preliminary results. *Photodermatology, Photoimmunology & Photomedicine, 22*(3), 153–156.

Dehghani, F., Merat, A., et al. (2005). Healing effect of garlic extract on warts and corns. *International Journal of Dermatology, 44*(7), 612–615.

Derby, R., Rohal, P., et al. (2011). Novel treatment of onychomycosis using over-the-counter mentholated ointment: a clinical case series. *Journal of the American Board of Family Medicine, 24*(1), 69–74.

DiSalvo, A. F. (1974). Antifungal properties of a plant extract. I. Source and spectrum of antimicrobial activity. *Mycopathologia et Mycologia Applicata, 54*(2), 215–219.

Dryden, M. S., Dailly, S., et al. (2004). A randomized, controlled trial of tea tree topical preparations versus a standard topical regimen for the clearance of MRSA colonization. *Journal of Hospital Infection, 56*(4), 283–286.

Dunford, C., Cooper, R., et al. (2000). The use of honey in wound management. *Nursing Standard, 15*(11), 63–68.

Eady, E. A., & Cove, J. H. (2000). Is acne an infection of blocked pilosebaceous follicles? Implications for antimicrobial treatment. *American Journal of Clinical Dermatology, 1*(4), 201–209.

Edmondson, M., Newall, N., et al. (2011). Uncontrolled, open-label, pilot study of tea tree (*Melaleuca alternifolia*) oil solution in the decolonisation of methicillin-resistant

Staphylococcus aureus-positive wounds and its influence on wound healing. *International Wound Journal, 8*(4), 375–384.

Edris, A. E. (2007). Pharmaceutical and therapeutic potentials of essential oils and their individual volatile constituents: a review. *Phytotherapy Research, 21*(4), 308–323.

Endo, E. H., Cortez, D. A., et al. (2010). Potent antifungal activity of extracts and pure compound isolated from pomegranate peels and synergism with fluconazole against *Candida albicans. Research in Microbiology, 161*(7), 534–540.

Enshaieh, S., Jooya, A., et al. (2007). The efficacy of 5% topical tea tree oil gel in mild to moderate acne vulgaris: a randomized, double-blind placebo-controlled study. *Indian Journal of Dermatology, Venereology and Leprology, 73*(1), 22–25.

Erythrasma—Treatment, Prevention and Natural Remedies for Erythrasma (2010). Available at http://ygoy.com/2010/06/11/erythrasma/ (accessed July 5, 2012).

Estahbanati, H. K., Kashani, P. P., et al. (2002). Frequency of *Pseudomonas aeruginosa* serotypes in burn wound infections and their resistance to antibiotics. *Burns, 28*(4), 340–348.

Ferrari, L. F. (2012). Candidiasis: yeast meets west. Available at: http://myyeastinfectionhomeremedy.net/goto/http://www.csomaonline.org/files/public/v17_n01_Ferrari_Candidiasis.pdf (accessed July 5, 2012).

Focht, D. R., 3rd, Spicer, C., et al. (2002). The efficacy of duct tape vs. cryotherapy in the treatment of verruca vulgaris (the common wart). *Archives of Pediatrics & Adolescent Medicine, 156*(10), 971–974.

Geria, A. N., & Schwartz, R. A. (2010). Impetigo update: new challenges in the era of methicillin resistance. *Cutis, 85*(2), 65–70.

Ghaemi, A., Soleimanjahi, H., et al. (2009). *Echinacea purpurea* polysaccharide reduces the latency rate in herpes simplex virus type-1 infections. *Intervirology, 52*(1), 29–34.

Giron, L. M., Aguilar, G. A., et al. (1988). Anticandidal activity of plants used for the treatment of vaginitis in Guatemala and clinical trial of a *Solanum nigrescens* preparation. *Journal of Ethnopharmacology, 22*(3), 307–313.

Giusti, F., Miglietta, R., et al. (2004). Sensitization to propolis in 1255 children undergoing patch testing. *Contact Dermatitis, 51*(5–6), 255–258.

Gribbon, E. M., Shoesmith, J. G., et al. (1994). The microaerophily and photosensitivity of *Propionibacterium acnes. Journal of Applied Bacteriology, 77*(5), 583–590.

Hainer, B. L. (2003). Dermatophyte infections. *American Family Physician, 67*(1), 101–108.

Hansson, C., & Faergemann, J. (1995). The effect of antiseptic solutions on microorganisms in venous leg ulcers. *Acta Dermato-Venereologica, 75*(1), 31–33.

Hatakka, K., Ahola, A. J., et al. (2007). Probiotics reduce the prevalence of oral candida in the elderly—a randomized controlled trial. *Journal of Dental Research, 86*(2), 125–130.

Herrera-Arellano, A., Rodriguez-Soberanes, A., et al. (2003). Effectiveness and tolerability of a standardized phytodrug derived from *Solanum chrysotrichum* on tinea pedis: a controlled and randomized clinical trial. *Planta Medica, 69*(5), 390–395.

Herrera-Arellano, A., Jimenez-Ferrer, E., et al. (2004). Clinical and mycological evaluation of therapeutic effectiveness of *Solanum chrysotrichum* standardized extract on patients with pityriasis capitis (dandruff). A double-blind and randomized clinical trial controlled with ketoconazole. *Planta Medica, 70*(6), 483–488.

Herrera-Arellano, A., Martinez-Rivera Mde, L., et al. (2007). Mycological and electron microscopic study of *Solanum chrysotrichum* saponin SC-2 antifungal activity on *Candida* species of medical significance. *Planta Medica, 73*(15), 1568–1573.

Hirschmann, J. V. (2007). Antimicrobial therapy for skin infections. *Cutis, 79*(6 Suppl), 26–36.

Huang, J. T., Abrams, M., et al. (2009). Treatment of *Staphylococcus aureus* colonization in atopic dermatitis decreases disease severity. *Pediatrics, 123*(5), e808–814.

Huang, K. F., Hsu, Y. C., et al. (2004). Shiunko promotes epithelization of wounded skin. *American Journal of Chinese Medicine, 32*(3), 389–396.

Huo, W., Gao, X. H., et al. (2010). Local hyperthermia at 44 degrees C for the treatment of plantar warts: a randomized, patient-blinded, placebo-controlled trial. *Journal of Infectious Diseases, 201*(8), 1169–1172.

Imai, H., Osawa, K., et al. (2001). Inhibition by the essential oils of peppermint and spearmint of the growth of pathogenic bacteria. *Microbios, 106*(Suppl 1), 31–39.

Iwatsuki, K., Yamasaki, O., et al. (2006). Staphylococcal cutaneous infections: invasion, evasion and aggression. *Journal of Dermatological Science, 42*(3), 203–214.

Jandourek, A., Vaishampayan, J. K., et al. (1998). Efficacy of melaleuca oral solution for the treatment of fluconazole refractory oral candidiasis in AIDS patients. *AIDS, 12*(9), 1033–1037.

Jazani, N. H., Shahabi, S., et al. (2007). Antibacterial effects of water-soluble green tea extracts on multi-antibiotic resistant isolates of *Pseudomonas aeruginosa. Pakistan Journal of Biological Sciences, 10*(9), 1544–1546.

Jull, A. B., Rodgers, A., et al. (2008). Honey as a topical treatment for wounds. *Cochrane Database of Systematic Reviews (Online)*(4), CD005083.

Kawahara, H., Nakai, H., et al. (2011). Management of perianal abscess with *hainosankyuto* in neonates and young infants. *Pediatrics International, 53*(6), 892–896.

Khoo, Y. T., Halim, A. S., et al. (2010). Wound contraction effects and antibacterial properties of Tualang honey on full-thickness burn wounds in rats in comparison to hydrofibre. *BMC Complementary and Alternative Medicine, 10*, 48.

Kim, R. H., & Armstrong, A. W. (2011). Current state of acne treatment: highlighting lasers, photodynamic therapy, and chemical peels. *Dermatology Online Journal, 17*(3), 2.

Kondo, S., Tabe, Y., et al. (2012). Comparison of antifungal activities of gentian violet and povidone-iodine against clinical isolates of *Candida* species and other yeasts: a framework to establish topical disinfectant activities. *Mycopathologia, 173*(1), 21–25.

Kuo, C. F., Chen, C. C., et al. (2005). *Cordyceps sinensis* mycelium protects mice from group A streptococcal infection. *Journal of Medical Microbiology, 54*(Pt 8), 795–802.

Lalla, J. K., Nandedkar, S. Y., et al. (2001). Clinical trials of ayurvedic formulations in the treatment of acne vulgaris. *Journal of Ethnopharmacology, 78*(1), 99–102.

Landis, S. J. (2008). Chronic wound infection and antimicrobial use. *Advances in Skin & Wound Care, 21*(11), 531–540.

Ledezma, E., Sousa, L. D., Jorquera, A., et al. (1996). Efficacy of ajoene, an organosulphur derived from garlic, in the short-term therapy of tinea pedis. *Mycoses, 39*(9–10), 393–395.

Leyden, J. J., Del Rosso, J. Q., et al. (2009). Clinical considerations in the treatment of acne vulgaris and other inflammatory skin disorders: a status report. *Dermatologic Clinics, 27*(1), 1–15.

Leyden, J. J., Marples, R. R., et al. (1974). *Staphylococcus aureus* in the lesions of atopic dermatitis. *British Journal of Dermatology, 90*(5), 525–530.

Li, X. F., Guo, Y. J., et al. (2012). Protective activity of the ethanol extract of *Cynanchum paniculatum* (Bunge) Kitagawa on treating herpes simplex encephalitis. *International Journal of Immunopathology and Pharmacology, 25*(1), 259–266.

Lindeberg, S. (2012). Paleolithic diets as a model for prevention and treatment of Western disease. *American Journal of Human Biology, 24*(2), 110–115.

Liu, C. S., Cham, T. M., et al. (2007). Antibacterial properties of Chinese herbal medicines against nosocomial antibiotic-resistant strains of *Pseudomonas aeruginosa* in Taiwan. *American Journal of Chinese Medicine, 35*(6), 1047–1060.

Mackrides, P. S., & Shaughnessy, A. F. (1996). Azelaic acid therapy for acne. *American Family Physician, 54*(8), 2457–2459.

Majtan, J., Kumar, P., et al. (2010). Effect of honey and its major royal jelly protein 1 on cytokine and MMP-9 mRNA transcripts in human keratinocytes. *Experimental Dermatology, 19*(8), e73–79.

Manchanda R. K., M. N., Bahl, R., Atey, R. (1997). Double-blind placebo controlled clinical trials of homeopathic medicines in warts and molluscum contagiosum. *CCRH Quarterly Bulletin, 19*, 25–29.

Martin, K. W., & Ernst, E. (2003). Herbal medicines for treatment of bacterial infections: a review of controlled clinical trials. *Journal of Antimicrobial Chemotherapy, 51*(2), 241–246.

McCollough, M., & Sharieff, G. Q. (2002). Common complaints in the first 30 days of life. *Emergency Medicine Clinics of North America, 20*(1), 27–48.

McDonald, L. L., & Smith, M. L. (1998). Diagnostic dilemmas in pediatric/adolescent dermatology: scaly scalp. *Journal of Pediatric Health Care, 12*(2), 80–84.

Melnik, B. C., John, S. M., et al. (2011). Over-stimulation of insulin/IGF-1 signaling by Western diet may promote diseases of civilization: lessons learnt from Laron syndrome. *Nutrition & Metabolism, 8*, 41.

Meltzer, S. M., Monk, B. J., et al. (2009). Green tea catechins for treatment of external genital warts. *American Journal of Obstetrics and Gynecology, 200*(3), e231–237.

Menendez, S., Falcon, L., et al. (2002). Efficacy of ozonized sunflower oil in the treatment of tinea pedis. *Mycoses, 45*(8), 329–332.

Menendez, S., Falcon, L., et al. (2011). Therapeutic efficacy of topical OLEOZON(R) in patients suffering from onychomycosis. *Mycoses, 54*(5), e272–277.

Minami, M., Ichikawa, M., et al. (2011). Protective effect of *hainosankyuto*, a traditional Japanese medicine, on *Streptococcus pyogenes* infection in murine model. *PLoS One, 6*(7), e22188.

Molan, P. C. (2006). The evidence supporting the use of honey as a wound dressing. *International Journal of Lower Extremity Wounds, 5*(1), 40–54.

Morgan, M. (2011). Treatment of MRSA soft tissue infections: an overview. *Injury, 42*(Suppl 5), S11–17.

Mulyaningsih, S., Sporer, F., et al. (2011). Antibacterial activity of essential oils from Eucalyptus and of selected components against multidrug-resistant bacterial pathogens. *Pharmaceutical Biology, 49*(9), 893–899.

Murray, P. R., R. K., Pfaller MA (2005). *Medical microbiology.* Philadelphia: Elsevier Mosby.

Nand, P., Drabu, S., et al. (2011). Antimicrobial investigation of *Linum usitatissimum* for the treatment of acne. *Natural Product Communications, 6*(11), 1701–1704.

Ning, S., Li, F., et al. (2012). The successful treatment of flat warts with auricular acupuncture. *International Journal of Dermatology, 51*(2), 211–215.

Norajit, K., Laohakunjit, N., et al. (2007). Antibacterial effect of five Zingiberaceae essential oils. *Molecules (Basel, Switzerland), 12*(8), 2047–2060.

Nzeako, B. C., Al-Kharousi, Z. S., et al. (2006). Antimicrobial activities of clove and thyme extracts. *Sultan Qaboos University Medical Journal, 6*(1), 33–39.

Oladele AT, D. B., Elujoba AA, Oyelami AO (2010). Management of superficial fungal infections with *Senna alata* (alata) soap: A preliminary report. *African Journal of Pharmacy and Pharmacology, 4*(3), 98–103.

Papadopoulos, C. J., Carson, C. F., et al. (2006). Susceptibility of pseudomonads to *Melaleuca alternifolia* (tea tree) oil and components. *Journal of Antimicrobial Chemotherapy, 58*(2), 449–451.

Paul, B. S., Diette, K. M., et al. (1987). Therapeutic photomedicine. In T. B. Fitzpatrick et al., eds., *Dermatology in general medicine* (3rd ed., p. 1547). New York: McGraw Hill.

Perez-Vasquez, A., Capella, S., et al. (2011). Antimicrobial activity and chemical composition of the essential oil of *Hofmeisteria schaffneri. Journal of Pharmacy and Pharmacology, 63*(4), 579–586.

Quale, J. M., Landman, D., et al. (1996). In vitro activity of *Cinnamomum zeylanicum* against azole resistant and sensitive *Candida* species and a pilot study of cinnamon for oral candidiasis. *American Journal of Chinese Medicine, 24*(2), 103–109.

Rajan, S. (2012). Skin and soft-tissue infections: classifying and treating a spectrum. *Cleveland Clinic Journal of Medicine, 79*(1), 57–66.

Ramadan, W., Mourad, B., et al. (1996). Oil of bitter orange: new topical antifungal agent. *International Journal of Dermatology, 35*(6), 448–449.

Renis, H. E. (1969). In vitro antiviral activity of calcium elenolate. *Antimicrobial Agents and Chemotherapy, 9,* 167–172.

Sabitha, P., Adhikari, P. M., et al. (2005). Efficacy of garlic paste in oral candidiasis. *Tropical Doctor, 35*(2), 99–100.

Sadick, N. S., Laver, Z., et al. (2010). Treatment of mild-to-moderate acne vulgaris using a combined light and heat energy device: home-use clinical study. *Journal of Cosmetic and Laser Therapy, 12*(6), 276–283.

Santos, V. R., Pimenta, F. J., et al. (2005). Oral candidiasis treatment with Brazilian ethanol propolis extract. *Phytotherapy Research, 19*(7), 652–654.

Satchell, A. C., Saurajen, A., et al. (2002). Treatment of interdigital tinea pedis with 25% and 50% tea tree oil solution: a randomized, placebo-controlled, blinded study. *Australasian Journal of Dermatology, 43*(3), 175–178.

Sharquie, K. E., al-Turfi, I. A., et al. (2000). The antibacterial activity of tea in vitro and in vivo (in patients with impetigo contagiosa). *Journal of Dermatology, 27*(11), 706–710.

Shenoy, V. P., Ballal, M., et al. (2012). Honey as an antimicrobial agent against *Pseudomonas aeruginosa* isolated from infected wounds. *Journal of Global Infectious Diseases, 4*(2), 102–105.

Sienkiewicz, M., Lysakowska, M., et al. (2012). The antimicrobial activity of thyme essential oil against multidrug-resistant clinical bacterial strains. *Microbial Drug Resistance (Larchmont, N.Y.), 18*(2), 137–148.

Smolinski, K. N., & Yan, A. C. (2005). How and when to treat molluscum contagiosum and warts in children. *Pediatric Annals, 34*(3), 211–221.

Spanos, N. P., Williams, V., et al. (1990). Effects of hypnotic, placebo, and salicylic acid treatments on wart regression. *Psychosomatic Medicine, 52*(1), 109–114.

Spelman, K., Burns, J., et al. (2006). Modulation of cytokine expression by traditional medicines: a review of herbal immunomodulators. *Alternative Medicine Review, 11*(2), 128–150.

Sterling, J. C., Handfield-Jones, S., et al. (2001). Guidelines for the management of cutaneous warts. *British Journal of Dermatology, 144*(1), 4–11.

Subapriya, R., & Nagini, S. (2005). Medicinal properties of neem leaves: a review. *Current Medicinal Chemistry. Anti-Cancer Agents, 5*(2), 149–146.

Sulaiman O, M. R., Hashim R, Sanchis GC. (2005). The inhibition of microbial growth by bamboo vinegar. *Journal of Bamboo and Rattan, 4*(1), 71–80.

Terezhalmy, G. T., Bottomley, W. K., et al. (1978). The use of water-soluble bioflavonoid-ascorbic acid complex in the treatment of recurrent herpes labialis. *Oral Surgery, Oral Medicine, and Oral Pathology, 45*(1), 56–62.

Werlinger, K. D., & Moore, A. Y. (2004). Therapy of other bacterial infections. *Dermatologic Therapy, 17*(6), 505–512.

Wheeland, R. G., & Dhawan, S. (2011). Evaluation of self-treatment of mild-to-moderate facial acne with a blue light treatment system. *Journal of Drugs in Dermatology, 10*(6), 596–602.

Wiart, C., Kumar, K., et al. (2005). Antiviral properties of ent-labdene diterpenes of *Andrographis paniculata nees,* inhibitors of herpes simplex virus type 1. *Phytotherapy Research, 19*(12), 1069–1070.

Williams, M. (1995). Immuno-protection against herpes simplex type II infection by eleutherococcus root extract. *International Journal of Alternative & Complementary Medicine, 13,* 9–12.

Wilson, J. W. (1965). Paronychia and onycholysis, etiology and therapy. *Archives of Dermatology, 92*(6), 726–730.

Viyoch, J., Pisutthanan, N., et al. (2006). Evaluation of in vitro antimicrobial activity of Thai basil oils and their micro-emulsion formulas against *Propionibacterium acnes. International Journal of Cosmetic Science, 28*(2), 125–133.

Wu, D. C., Chan, W. W., et al. (2011). *Pseudomonas* skin infection: clinical features, epidemiology, and management. *American Journal of Clinical Dermatology, 12*(3), 157–169.

Young, S., Bolton, P., et al. (1989). Macrophage responsiveness to light therapy. *Lasers in Surgery and Medicine, 9*(5), 497–505.

Zeina, B., Greenman, J., et al. (2001). Killing of cutaneous microbial species by photodynamic therapy. *British Journal of Dermatology, 144*(2), 274–278.

Zheng, Y., Gu, R., et al. (2009). Chinese medicinal herbs for measles. *Cochrane Database of Systematic Reviews (Online)*(4), CD005531.

16

Integrative Management of Contact Dermatitis

PHILIP D. SHENEFELT

Key Concepts

- ♣ Irritant contact dermatitis occurs more frequently, tends to be more burning or painful, and heals more rapidly after the irritant is avoided, while allergic contact dermatitis tends to be more itchy and persists for weeks after the allergen is avoided.

- ♣ Allergic contact dermatitis may be superimposed over another skin condition such as atopic dermatitis or stasis dermatitis. When the latter two conditions do not respond as expected to therapy, consider the possibility of an overlying allergic contact dermatitis.

- ♣ Most of the time, patch testing or usage testing is required to confirm allergic contact dermatitis and to identify the specific allergens involved.

- ♣ Desensitization to contact allergens currently is not feasible. Avoidance is the key to improvement of allergic contact dermatitis.

- ♣ Conventional treatments for irritant or allergic contact dermatitis can be supplemented with alternative or complementary treatments to produce an integrated approach to treatment.

- ♣ Some individuals will have their dermatitis persist despite apparent adequate avoidance of the irritant or allergen and despite good treatment.

Introduction

Contact dermatitis results from direct skin contact with an exogenous irritant or allergen. The phase of the dermatitis may be acute, subacute, or chronic. Acute dermatitis consists of usually well-demarcated patches of erythema with or without vesicles. Subacute dermatitis presents with patches of mild erythema with scaling. Chronic dermatitis manifests as dry, often lichenified (thickened) patches or plaques with or without excoriations. The dermatitis occurs within areas of direct contact with the irritant or allergen. Differential diagnosis of contact dermatitis includes atopic dermatitis, dyshidrotic dermatitis, nummular dermatitis, seborrheic dermatitis, stasis dermatitis, psoriasis, patch stage mycosis fungoides (cutaneous T-cell lymphoma), and tinea (fungal infection). The clinical pattern is useful but not always definitive in establishing the diagnosis. Potassium hydroxide wet-mount microscopic examination can often identify fungus if present. A skin biopsy can often help differentiate dermatitis from psoriasis or patch stage mycosis fungoides. A skin biopsy of dermatitis typically has a spongiotic pattern in the epidermis, which is common to several categories of dermatitis and often does not identify the specific type of dermatitis and does not differentiate between irritant and allergic contact dermatitis. Regional location of the dermatitis helps to distinguish the type of dermatitis. Seborrheic dermatitis typically occurs on the scalp, face (especially paranasally), ear canals, central chest, or back, but rarely may be very widespread. Atopic dermatitis typically occurs flexurally in the antecubital fossa and popliteal fossa and sides of the neck but again may be widespread. Dyshidrotic dermatitis occurs on the palms and soles. Stasis dermatitis typically occurs on the lower legs. Irritant or allergic contact dermatitis can be superimposed on any of these other types of dermatitis. Examples would be seborrheic dermatitis with superimposed allergic contact dermatitis, atopic or dyshidrotic hand dermatitis with superimposed irritant or allergic contact dermatitis, or stasis dermatitis with superimposed allergic contact dermatitis. Areas of stasis dermatitis are particularly prone to develop allergic contact dermatitis.

Irritant Contact Dermatitis

Irritant contact dermatitis is quite common, with a prevalence of 2% to 5% in the general population and higher in occupations that have frequent exposure to irritants (Shenefelt, 1996a, 1996b). Age of onset can be wide-ranging, with a peak at 16 to 20 years old. The male-to-female ratio is typically 1 to 3. Clinical manifestations include red, oozing, or dry skin, with or without scales, fissuring, often with a predominance of a burning sensation or soreness more than itching. Diagnosis is made by the clinical pattern and distribution. Differential diagnoses include atopic, allergic contact, dyshidrotic, nummular, seborrheic, or stasis dermatitis, and, on the hands, psoriasis. Pathogenesis occurs from repeated chemical irritant microtrauma to the skin. Typical chemicals include soaps, detergents, water, solvents, oils, plant juices, and many other irritating chemicals. Over 57,000 chemicals are known skin irritants (Belsito, 2005). Frequently, irritant contact dermatitis can be acquired from chemical exposures at work, known as occupational irritant contact dermatitis. Specific occupations typically have specific irritant exposures (Shenefelt, 1995). Individuals with atopic dermatitis are more prone to irritant contact dermatitis due to the defect in their barrier function. Prognosis is that acute or subacute irritant contact dermatitis usually clears in a few days with avoidance of irritant chemicals, although chronic cases may take longer and have less complete clearing.

Allergic Contact Dermatitis

Allergic contact dermatitis is also common, with a prevalence of about 1% in the general population and higher in occupations exposed to allergenic chemicals (Shenefelt, 1996b). Age of onset is any age, with median age of 37 years old. The male-to-female ratio is typically 1 to 2. Clinical manifestations include acute dermatitis with redness with or without blistering, subacute dermatitis with redness and scaling, or chronic dermatitis with or without lichenification and/or excoriations. For allergic contact dermatitis, usually itching predominates over burning sensations. Diagnosis is made from the clinical pattern and distribution and from patch testing. Differential diagnoses include atopic, irritant contact, dyshidrotic, nummular, seborrheic, or stasis dermatitis, and also psoriasis on the hands or scalp. Allergic contact dermatitis may exist alone or may be superimposed on irritant contact dermatitis, atopic dermatitis, dyshidrotic dermatitis, seborrheic dermatitis, stasis dermatitis, psoriasis, or other skin disorder. Pathogenesis is a cell-mediated type IV delayed immunological reaction. Initial sensitization typically takes two to three weeks, but recurrent exposure usually elicits a dermatitis reaction in two to seven days. The prognosis is that acute or subacute allergic contact dermatitis usually takes six to eight weeks to clear because the antigen is fixed to the skin cells of the epidermis and the body continues to react until the skin cells containing the antigen are shed. In chronic cases clearing may take longer and be incomplete (Elfeel et al., 2008). Chromate allergen also fixes to the dermis and clearing can take months. Sensitivity to the specific contact allergen usually persists lifelong. The most common cutaneous locations for allergic contact dermatitis, in descending order of frequency, are the hands (see also section below on hand dermatitis), scattered generalized, face, eyelids, trunk, arm, leg, scalp, foot, lips, anogenital, and neck (Franzway et al., 2013). Common types of allergens include metals (nickel, cobalt, chromate, gold), rubber chemicals, cosmetic and fragrance chemicals, topical antibiotics such as neomycin, preservative and vehicle chemicals, various plants, and many other miscellaneous chemicals. Much more extensive information about specific allergens may be found in *Contact and Occupational Dermatology* (Marks et al., 2002) and in *Fisher's Contact Dermatitis*, 6th edition (Rietschel & Fowler, 2007). Avoidance of the allergen may include protective clothing or gloves. Some allergens will penetrate most gloves. For example, acrylate glues used by dentists and orthopedists easily penetrate gloves. Poison ivy allergen can also penetrate most gloves. Poison ivy allergic contact dermatitis occurs in response to oily urushiols that occur in the leaves and stems of poison ivy, poison oak, poison sumac, India marking nut, Japanese black lacquer, cashew, and a few other plants. Exposure may occur to the moist or dried plant, smoke from burning plants, laundry markings, Japanese black lacquer items, some vegetable-tanned leathers, or animal fur or clothing that has brushed against or otherwise been exposed to the plants.

Patch Testing

Unless the source of the allergen is clear, such as with poison ivy allergic contact dermatitis or nickel sensitivity, patch testing often is indicated to determine the specific allergens involved. Patch testing involves placing a small amount of a pure known allergen in an appropriate dilution in a small chamber (Finn chamber) attached to a hypoallergenic tape backing, proceeding with other allergens until a number of chambers are filled, and then taping the chambers onto the upper back and leaving them in place for two days. The TRUE Test is a ready-made set currently consisting of 36 contact allergens impregnated in squares attached to adhesive backings. It likewise is taped to the upper back and left in place for two days. The tapes are then removed and the reactions are then graded as none, slight (redness with no palpable induration), 1+ (redness with palpable induration), 2+ (redness with some blistering), or 3+ (redness with confluent blistering). Another reading is performed one to five days later. Reactions tend to be slower and often milder in the elderly (Scalf & Shenefelt, 2007). There are over 4,300 known contact allergens (De Groot, 2008) but a smaller number of common contact allergens. This follows the Pareto principle rule of thumb that roughly 20% of the allergens cause 80% of the problems. Common metal salt allergens include nickel, cobalt, chromate, and gold. Fragrance allergens include cinnamates, balsam of Peru, eugenol, oak moss, and a number of others. Topical medicament allergens include neomycin, bacitracin, "-caine" analgesics, quinolones, ethylenediamine dihydrochloride, diphenhydramine, doxepin, various corticosteroids, and others. Preservative allergens include formaldehyde and formaldehyde releasers such as quaternium 15, thiomersol, Cl Me isothiazolinione (Kathon CG), parabens, and others. Vehicle allergens include wool alcohols (lanolin), sorbic acid, and others. Rubber compound delayed contact allergens include thiuram, mercaptobenzothiazole, carbamates, para-phenylenediamines, and others. Latex rubber contact urticaria is a different type I allergic reaction to rubber tree latex proteins and is not tested for with patch testing but can be tested for using RAST or scratch and prick testing for immediate sensitivity. Resin delayed contact allergens include epoxy resin, p-tert-butylphenol formaldehyde resin, colophony, and others (Shenefelt, 1998). Photocontact allergens require sun exposure to activate them. They are tested with photopatch testing, which involves patch testing plus exposure to ultraviolet light at 24 hours. Photo contact allergens include para-amino benzoic acid and benzophenones. The 15 most frequent allergens in 2007–2008 in descending order of frequency were nickel, *Myroxylon pereirae* (balsam of Peru, a fragrance), neomycin, fragrance mix, quaternium 15 (a preservative found in creams, lotions, and shampoos), cobalt, bacitracin, formaldehyde, methyldibromoglutaronitrile/phenoxyethanol (Euxyl K 400, a preservative), para-phenylenediamine (found in black hair dye and black rubber), propolis (a resinous mixture that honeybees collect from tree buds and use to seal small gaps in the hive; commonly used in cosmetics and medicinals), carbamate mix (found in rubber), potassium dichromate (found in leather products and concrete), methylchloroisothiazolinone/ methylisothiazolinone (Kathon CG, a common preservative found in creams, lotions, and shampoos), and thiuram mix (found in rubber) (Franzway et al., 2013). The patch testing differentiates these allergens from phototoxic reactions, for example to certain plants such as lime fruit rind or juice or buttercup plant juice. Differential diagnosis also includes phototoxic or photoallergic drug reactions. Frequently, allergic contact dermatitis can be acquired from chemical exposures at work, known as occupational allergic contact dermatitis (Shenefelt, 1994). Specific occupations typically have specific allergen exposures (Shenefelt, 1995).

Usage Testing

Usage testing can be done with suspected substances provided that they are nonirritating. The material is rubbed onto the antecubital fossa twice daily for four days. A positive reaction will usually occur within a week. Since the substance such as a cream or lotion or cosmetic or other material is a mixture of chemicals, the usage test does not identify what specific chemical is the allergen but does clarify whether the substance is safe for the patient to use.

Conventional Treatment of Irritant Dermatitis

Conventional treatment consists of avoidance of irritants, use of emollient creams, and if necessary use of corticosteroid creams or ointments. The type of vehicle used is important, and the old adage that "if it is wet, dry it, and if it is dry, wet it" still holds. For a wet oozing irritant contact dermatitis, astringents can be useful. Aluminum subacetate solution is a protein precipitant that helps to stop oozing. Inflammation can be reduced using corticosteroid creams of appropriate strength for the body area involved, generally weaker for face and body-fold areas and stronger for other body areas (Tadicherla et al., 2009). The type of vehicle that contains the corticosteroid is equally important. For wet oozing areas, a gel or lotion is often more suitable, while for dry scaly areas, an emollient cream or ointment often performs better.

Integrative Treatment of Irritant Dermatitis

Tannins from tea or oak bark or other vegetable sources containing tannic acid are also astringent and can help to stop oozing. Cool tea compresses or neem oil (*Azadirachta indica*) or aloe vera extract (Kapoor & Saraf, 2010) can be used as mild anti-inflammatories with some antimicrobial activity also. As a cautionary note, neem oil itself has some mild contact allergenic potential (Reutemann & Ehrlich, 2008). Many other ethnobotanical preparations have been used, often depending on local availability, but many do not have empirical scientific evidence to support their use, and some may also be irritant or allergenic themselves. Dry areas can be treated with a topical moisturizing cream or mineral oil or petrolatum. Alternatively, olive oil, cocoa butter, coconut oil, almond oil, or other nonirritating and nonallergenic vegetable oil may be used. Animal fats such as bear grease have been used in the past. Other alternative approaches for treating dermatitis, including traditional Chinese medicine, topical teas, and other modalities, may be found in the chapter on integrative therapies for atopic dermatitis (Chapter 14). Instruction in avoidance of the irritants is key to permitting healing to occur. In occupations that involve wet work this may be difficult, and protective barrier creams or vinyl gloves worn outside of thin cotton gloves may be needed.

Conventional Treatment of Allergic Contact Dermatitis

Immediate washing with soap and water within five minutes may help to prevent reactions. Protective barrier creams have offered partial protection, and many of the above-described treatment strategies for irritant dermatitis can be tried. For severe cases, if not contraindicated, a tapering dose of oral corticosteroid may be used, such as prednisone 40 mg/day for five days, 30 mg/day for five days, 20 mg/day for five days, 10 mg/day for five days, and 5 mg/day for five days. Another systemic option would be triamcinolone acetonide 40 mg intramuscularly, which also provides a slow-release tapering dosage over about a month. In cases resistant to other treatments, phototherapy in the form of narrow-band ultraviolet B or psoralen plus ultraviolet A may be beneficial.

Integrative Treatment of Allergic Contact Dermatitis

The folk remedy of rubbing jewelweed on the area has had mixed reports and recently has been reported to be more efficacious than nothing but less efficacious than washing with soap and water (Abrams Motz et al., 2012). For those with a strong nickel sensitivity, a nickel avoidance diet may be of benefit. This includes avoiding eating canned foods and foods from crops grown in nickel-rich soil.

There have been several interesting experiments on the effect of the mind on contact dermatitis. The effect of hypnotic suggestion on delayed cellular immune responses was significant for erythema size ($p < 0.02$) and palpable induration ($p < 0.01$) in one study (Zachariae et al., 1989) but not in others (Locke et al., 1987, 1994), However, under experimental conditions even simple suggestion has been shown to induce contact dermatitis in an area not touched by Japanese lacquer tree allergen but believed by sensitized individuals to have been so touched; the same individuals did not react when actually touched by lacquer tree allergen but believed that they had not been so touched ($p < 0.01$) (Ikemi & Nakagawa, 1962). Similarly, using hypnosis, volunteers in a double-masked protocol who were told to increase their sensitization to one of two experimental allergens, dinitrochlorobenzene and diphenylcyclopropenone, while decreasing it to the other showed a significant difference in reactions between allergens they were told under hypnosis to enhance and those they were told to diminish ($p < 0.01$) (Zachariae & Bjerring, 1993). As David Spiegel (2011) has said, "it is not all mind over matter, but mind matters." The possible mechanisms of action are becoming somewhat clearer since it has been discovered that nerve endings in the skin can release calcitonin gene-related peptide (CGRP) and other peptides that inhibit Langerhans cell function in the epidermis by modulating activation of NF-κB (Ding et al., 2007). The Langerhans cells are intimately involved in presenting allergens to start the allergic contact dermatitis sequence. Using the hypnotic state to control the release of peptides including CGRP from cutaneous nerve endings, which inhibit the Langerhans cells from presenting the antigen to T lymphocytes, can prevent the occurrence of an episode of allergic contact dermatitis.

Hand Dermatitis

Hand dermatitis can be especially problematic both with respect to diagnosis and with respect to treatment (Menne & Maibach, 2000). Some hand dermatitis is endogenous (coming from within). Common examples include dyshidrosis and atopic hand dermatitis. However, most hand dermatitis is exogenous (coming from the outside). Irritant contact hand dermatitis is the most common, but allergic contact hand dermatitis is often the most troublesome. The differential diagnosis includes irritant contact dermatitis, allergic contact dermatitis, atopic dermatitis, dyshidrotic dermatitis, psoriasis, and tinea (fungal infection). The hands are key to many human activities, so hand dermatitis can cause significant impairment and disability. Impairment is a medical assessment while disability is a quasi-judicial rating. Not uncommonly two or more disease processes may coexist, for example atopic hand dermatitis complicated by irritant contact dermatitis, or irritant contact dermatitis with superimposed allergic contact dermatitis. Scraping the skin for potassium hydroxide wet mount can be performed to check for fungal hyphae. History may help to suggest atopic dermatitis. Patch testing may be needed to determine whether a contact allergy is involved. Biopsy may help to distinguish between dermatitis and psoriasis.

Conventional treatment consists of minimizing handwashing, avoidance of known allergens, use of heavy emollient creams, and use of corticosteroid creams or ointments. If the person is allergic to topical corticosteroids, a noncorticosteroid anti-inflammatory such as tacrolimus or pimecrolimus can be used instead. In some instances overnight occlusion with vinyl gloves with the fingertips cut off may enhance the treatment response. For a discussion of other conventional and integrative treatment strategies, please refer to the sections above on irritant and allergic contact dermatitis.

REFERENCES

Abrams Motz, V., Bowers, C. P., Mull Young, L., et al. (2012). The effectiveness of jewelweed, *Impatiens capensis*, the related cultivar *I. balsamina* and the component lawsone in preventing post poison ivy exposure contact dermatitis. *Journal of Ethnopharmacology, 143*(1):314–318.

Belsito, D. V. (2005). Occupational contact dermatitis: etiology, prevalence, and resultant impairment/disability. *Journal of the American Academy of Dermatology, 53*, 303–313.

De Groot, A. C. (2008). *Patch testing, test concentrations and vehicles for 4350 chemicals* (3rd ed.). Wapserveen, Netherlands: A. C. Degroot Publishing.

Ding, W., Wagner, J. A., & Granstein, R. D. (2007). CGRP, PACAP, and VIP modulate Langerhans cell function by inhibiting NF-kappaB activation. *Journal of Investigative Dermatology, 127*, 2357–2367.

Elfeel, K. A., Shenefelt, P. D., Farghaly, H., et al. (2008). A correlation of allergic contact dermatitis with allergen type and patient categorical variables. *Cutaneous and Ocular Toxicology, 27*(4), 249–270.

Franzway, A. F., Zug, K. A., Belsito, D. V., et al. (2013). North American contact dermatitis group patch-test results for 2007–2008. *Dermatitis, 24*(1), 10–21.

Ikemi, Y., & Nakagawa, S. (1962). A psychosomatic study of contagious dermatitis. *Kyushu Journal of Medical Science, 13*, 335–350.

Kapoor, S., & Saraf, S. (2010). Assessment of viscoelasticity and hydration effect of herbal moisturizers using bioengineering techniques. *Pharmacognosy Magazine, 6*(24), 298–304.

Locke, S. E., Ransil, B. J., Covino, N. A., et al. (1987). Failure of hypnotic suggestion to alter immune response to delayed-type hypersensitivity antigens. *Annals of the New York Academy of Science, 496*, 745–749.

Locke, S. E., Ransil, B. J., Zachariae, R., et al. (1994). Effect of hypnotic suggestion on the delayed type hypersensitivity response. *Journal of the American Medical Association, 272*, 47–52.

Marks, J. G., Elsner, P., & DeLeo, V. A. (2002). *Contact and occupational dermatology* (3rd ed.). St. Louis, MO:, Mosby.

Menne, T., & Maibach, H. I. (Eds.) (2000). *Hand eczema* (2nd ed.). Boca Raton, FL: CRC Press.

Reutemann, P., & Ehrlich, A. (2008). Neem oil: an herbal therapy for alopecia causes dermatitis. *Dermatitis, 19*(3), E12–15.

Rietschel, R. L, & Fowler, J. F. (2007). *Fisher's contact dermatitis* (6th ed.). Hamilton, Ontario: B. C. Decker.

Scalf, L. A., & Shenefelt, P. D. (2007). Contact dermatitis: diagnosing and treating skin conditions in the elderly. *Geriatrics, 62*(6), 14–19.

Shenefelt, P. D. (1994). Clinical aspects of occupational allergic contact dermatitis. In D. J. Hogan (ed.), *Occupational skin disorders* (pp. 1–12). New York: Igaku-Shoin.

Shenefelt, P. D. (1995). Two-way tables listing irritant or allergen versus occupation. *American Journal of Contact Dermatitis, 6*(2), 105–109.

Shenefelt, P. D. (1996a). Epidemiology of irritant contact dermatitis. In P. G. M. Van der Valk & H. I. Maibach (eds.), *The irritant contact dermatitis syndrome* (pp. 17–22). Boca Raton, FL: CRC Press.

Shenefelt, P. D. (1996b). Descriptive epidemiology of contact dermatitis in a university student population. *American Journal of Contact Dermatitis, 7*(2), 88–93.

Shenefelt, P. D. (1998). Limits of ICD-9-CM code usefulness in epidemiologic studies of contact and other types of dermatitis. *American Journal of Contact Dermatitis, 9*(3), 176–178.

Spiegel, D. (2011). Mind matters in cancer survival. *Journal of the American Medical Association, 305*(5), 502–503.

Tadicherla, S., Ross, K., Shenefelt, P. D., et al. (2009). Topical corticosteroids in dermatology. *Journal of Drugs in Dermatology, 8*(12), 1093–1105.

Zachariae, R., & Bjerring, P. (1993). Increase and decrease of delayed cutaneous reactions obtained by hypnotic suggestions during sensitization. *Allergy, 48*, 6–11.

Zachariae, R., Bjerring, P., & Arendt-Nielsen, L. (1989). Modulation of type I immediate and type IV delayed immunoreactivity using suggestion and guided imagery during hypnosis. *Allergy, 44*, 537–542.

17

Integrative Management of Hyperhidrosis

REENA N. RUPANI, MD AND MARY TEEPLE, MD

Key Concepts

- ♣ Hyperhidrosis is defined as perspiration in excess of what is needed for physiologic thermoregulation.
- ♣ Conventional therapies include topical and oral anticholinergics, onabotulinum toxin A injections, iontophoresis and microwave technology, and surgical approaches.
- ♣ An integrative approach would also take into account dietary factors, botanical supplements, mind–body interventions including biofeedback, acupuncture, and hypnosis, and psychotherapy.

Introduction

Hyperhidrosis is defined as perspiration in excess of what is needed for physiologic thermoregulation. Primary focal hyperhidrosis, the most common type, is excessive regional sweating that is idiopathic in nature (i.e., not related to medications or medical comorbidities such as hyperthyroidism), and with localization following the distribution of eccrine sweat glands, which are most densely concentrated in the face, axillae, palms, and soles. These glands are innervated by the sympathetic nervous system and respond to the neurotransmitter acetylcholine. While thermoregulatory sweating is coordinated by the preoptic region near the rostral hypothalamus, primary hyperhidrosis falls more under the category of emotional sweating, which is regulated by the limbic system (Schlereth et al., 2009).

Theoretical etiologies for hyperhidrosis would include dysfunction of the cerebral cortex, the sweat gland, or any sympathetic ganglia or fibers in the enjoining pathway. In primary hyperhidrosis, the cause is not thought to be due to the gland or duct itself (which is typically histologically and functionally intact) but instead is an abnormal or exaggerated central response to normal emotional stress. Although a psychiatric explanation is often attempted, and many individuals with hyperhidrosis describe subjective feelings of anxiety, depression, or social isolation, studies have shown that the majority of patients with essential hyperhidrosis lack overt psychopathology and these symptoms are more likely a result, rather than a primary etiology, of excessive sweating (Ruchinskas et al., 2002).

Unlike primary hyperhidrosis, secondary hyperhidrosis is excessive sweating due to an underlying condition rather than a primary dysfunction of the sweating mechanism itself. There are a multitude of such secondary etiologies, and the treatment essentially lies in removal of the underlying condition (Freedberg et al., 2003). As such, treatment and integrative therapy of primary, rather than secondary, hyperhidrosis will be reviewed here.

Conventional Therapy

Conventional treatment of hyperhidrosis offers many options, ranging from topical therapy to invasive surgery. Because hyperhidrosis is a difficult disease process that is not entirely understood, it is important to explore patients' expectations and counsel them about the limitations and complications associated with therapy.

Topical Therapy

Over-the-counter antiperspirants may provide adequate therapy for treating very mild symptoms. These generally contain aluminum or zirconium salts and exert their effect by creating a mechanical obstruction at the opening of eccrine sweat gland ducts. Prescription-strength antiperspirants may be useful in treating mild to moderate palmar, plantar, and axillary hyperhidrosis. Various formulations include 20% aluminum chloride in ethanol or 6.25% aluminum tetrachloride. In addition to forming a physical obstruction, these antiperspirants cause atrophy of the secretory cells. Skin irritation may limit therapy with prescription-strength products and may be alleviated by applying the antiperspirant to dry skin, adding cornstarch or baking powder, or using adjunctive low-dose corticosteroid cream. The anticholinergic medication glycopyrrolate, compounded to 0.5% to 2% in solution and applied topically with cotton balls nightly, is also effective in some cases (Kim et al., 2008).

Systemic Therapies

Systemic therapies may be attempted in severe or recalcitrant cases of primary focal hyperhidrosis. Oral anticholinergics are effective at decreasing sweating (glycopyrrolate, oxybutynin, propanthelene), but dosing is complicated by side effects such as dry mouth and urinary retention (Paller et al., 2012). Beta-blockers, alpha-agonists, and calcium-channel blockers (such as propranolol, clonidine, and diltiazem) may also be tried; there is mixed efficacy and a relatively low incidence of side effects in young and healthy patients (Walling, 2012).

In addition to medications, iontophoresis is another potential therapy. Also known as electromotive drug therapy, this noninvasive procedure introduces ionized substances to the body by applying a current or electromotive force through water. Although the exact mechanism of action in its treatment of hyperhidrosis is unknown, it is thought that the process temporarily blocks sweat glands via accumulation of H^+ anion within the acrosyringium (Kreyden, 2004). Iontophoresis may be performed with tap water at home, and anticholinergics may be added to the solution for increased effect. While side effects are minimal and mainly involve dry hands, treatment is limited due to the time required to complete the process (typically 20 to 30 minutes daily).

Noninvasive microwave-based technology (MiraDry™) was approved by the U.S. Food and Drug Administration (FDA) in 2011 for the treatment of axillary hyperhidrosis. Microwave energy penetrates to the dermis and generates heat, resulting in thermolysis of eccrine glands with minimal collateral damage via use of a concurrent hydroceramic cooling system (Lupin et al., 2011). So far results are promising, although accessibility and cost are limiting factors for patients.

Onabotulinum Toxin A

Onabotulinum toxin A is a neurotoxin that blocks the release of acetylcholine from the presynaptic junction of cholinergic autonomic neurons. By decreasing stimulation of cholinergic receptors, sweat production may be temporarily reduced (typical dosing is 50 units of reconstituted product per axillary vault, duration three to four months). Although the FDA currently approves its use only for the treatment of axillary hyperhidrosis, several studies have shown onabotulinum toxin's effectiveness in palmar hyperhidrosis as well (Saadia et al., 2001). Adverse effects include pain with injection, temporary weakness of thenar eminence musculature, and reduction of the pincer grip. Cryoanalgesia with ice packs or refrigerant sprays as well as topical anesthetics and nerve blocks may be used to decrease pain. Drug penetration with improper placement can be limited by the thick stratum corneum of the palms and soles.

Surgery

If symptoms of hyperhidrosis are refractory to all of the aforementioned therapies, surgery is a last-resort option. Skin excision has historically been used to remove axillary eccrine sweat glands and treat hyperhidrosis (Lawrence & Lonsdale Eccles, 2006). However, ineffectiveness as well as permanent scarring has limited its use. Another surgical technique is endoscopic transthoracic sympathectomy. This procedure entails permanent interruption of the upper thoracic sympathetic chain in order to inhibit the sympathetic drive for perspiration (Herbst et al., 1994). While this therapy is effective, it also has significant adverse effects, such as compensatory sweating, that limit its desirability and use. As a result, an alternative and temporary approach is thoracic sympathetic clipping, in which the sympathetic chain is not severed but rather temporarily interrupted. Finally, there are newer surgical techniques such as minimally invasive suction curettage (liposuction) that remove axillary sweat glands with a greater success rate and with fewer side effects; drawbacks are common relapse and expense (Lillis & Coleman, 1990).

An Integrative Approach

Conventional treatment for primary focal hyperhidrosis is often limited by adverse effects or its invasive component—therefore, an integrative approach can play a fundamental role in the treatment of hyperhidrosis. There are several modalities through which relief may be obtained, and application of these may be tailored to the specific complaints and goals of the individual. Depending on the severity of disease as well as patient expectations, a stepwise approach may be implemented.

Diet

First, dietary modifications to avoid potentially exacerbating elements can be employed. This would include foods/beverages that increase basal metabolic rate or are vasodilatory or stimulants. As such, the following foods should be avoided.

Onions have been traditionally consumed to prevent cardiovascular disease due to their proven vasodilatory effect. It has been demonstrated that raw onion extracts decrease vascular tone in both endothelium-dependent and endothelium-independent manners. Low doses of raw onion extract produce endothelium-released nitric oxide, resulting in vasodilatation, whereas high doses of raw onion extracts have been shown to produce endothelium-independent vasorelaxation. Such vasodilating effects will exacerbate sweating (Chen et al., 1999).

Caffeine has long been known to be a stimulant of the central nervous system. Its lipophilic properties permit penetration of the blood–brain barrier, where it acts as an adenosine receptor antagonist and causes a disinhibitory effect on neural activity. It is additionally a phosphodiesterase inhibitor, resulting in elevated cyclic AMP and thereby affecting multiple cell processes, most notably including heart rate control and metabolic function (Davis, 2003). Caffeine metabolites such as theobromine and theophylline additionally produce vasodilatory and positive chronotropic and inotropic effects, respectively. Thus caffeine functions through multiple mechanisms of action, and its stimulatory nature increases basal metabolic rate, heart rate, and ultimately thermal regulation.

Alcohol affects many physiological processes. Most noteworthy here, it may directly exacerbate hyperhidrosis and cause excessive sweating. While studies have shown variable thermoregulatory responses to alcohol in humans, it has traditionally been thought that alcohol induces peripheral vasodilatation and thereby results in perspiration. As such, avoiding alcohol is recommended in those with hyperhidrosis (Desruelle et al., 1996).

Spicy foods have long been known to require extensive digestive effort, resulting in elevated basal metabolic rate, thermogenesis, and sweat production or exacerbation. Furthermore, one active component of spicy foods, capsaicin, is a member of the vanilloid family and stimulates a receptor called the vanilloid receptor subtype 1 (Terumasa et al., 2002). Stimulation of this receptor induces a similar sensation to that of excessive heat. The result of such stimulation may be a burning sensation or even perspiration.

Garlic is a component of many foods and contains sulfuric compounds. Although it does not directly induce sweating or exacerbate hyperhidrosis, the sulfuric compounds in garlic produce strong odors that may be appreciated through sweat. Therefore, avoidance of garlic may decrease the unpleasant aroma of perspiration and avoid further emotional distress (Ellis, 2012).

By the opposite logic, any food that eases digestive effort, lowers core body temperature, or has astringent activity may theoretically aid in decreasing sweat burden (Ellis, 2012). Drinking water or eating food products with high water content may also lower core body temperature, yielding a cooling effect that minimizes any thermal impetus for perspiration. Furthermore, eating food products with astringent activity favors vasoconstriction, which decreases the sweat burden (Ellis, 2012). With the above concepts in mind, the following dietary recommendations are made to decrease excessive perspiration: water, apple cider vinegar, fruit, whole grains, olive oil, foods high in B vitamins (such as fish, eggs, red meat, nuts, avocados, carrots, and peas), calcium, and magnesium (Ellis, 2012).

Botanical Supplements

Supplementing with botanical products may provide additional sweat relief. Particularly, botanicals with astringent and stress- or anxiety-relieving properties may help decrease sweat burden. As primary focal hyperhidrosis is considered an aberrant response to normal emotional stressors, the idea is that reducing the impact of these as much as possible could confer healing benefit. The following botanicals are anecdotally recommended for hyperhidrosis.

Sage is an herb that has an extensive history of medicinal use. Currently, the primary proposed uses include hyperhidrosis, sore throat, and dyspepsia, and Germany's Commission E has approved sage for the treatment of excessive sweating. Although there have been no double-blind, placebo-controlled studies to confirm this effect, there has been such a study indicating that sage leaf may play a role as an antianxiety agent. Thus, while more studies are needed, introducing sage into the diet may alleviate sweating. The recommended dose is 1 to 3 grams of dried sage taken up to three times daily, and the sage may be consumed as a tea, gargle, tincture, or extract (Consumer Labs, 2012). Of cautionary note, however, some species of sage (particularly *Salvia officinalis,* common garden sage) contain a chemical compound called thujone, which can trigger hypoglycemia, hypertension, miscarriage, and seizures. Thujone additionally can interact with diabetic medications, anticonvulsants, and sedatives.

Schisandra is an East Asian herb that has a history of medicinal use in Russian and Chinese cultures. While there have not been controlled trials demonstrating effectiveness in treatment of hyperhidrosis, schisandra is thought to have antioxidant, expectorant, and, most notably, astringent activity. As such, it is thought to be particularly effective for perspiration. Schisandra is available in several forms, including tincture, powder, tablets, capsules, and extracts, and the recommended dosage is 1.5 to 6 grams daily (Consumer Labs, 2012). Possible side effects can include increased intracranial pressure, seizures, gastroesophageal reflux, and uterine contractions. Schisandra may interact with medications metabolized by CYP3A4, 2C9, with warfarin, and with tacrolimus.

Lemon balm is native to southern Europe and is often referred to by its Latin binomial, *Melissa officinalis*. It has traditionally been used for the treatment of wounds and is most commonly used in modern medicine for the treatment of oral and genital herpes. However, there is evidence that lemon balm has a sedative effect via inhibition of GABA transaminase by its constituent rosmarinic acid, and is therefore used to treat insomnia and anxiety. Lemon balm may also be combined with other herbs such as valerian, and in this form it is particularly effective at reducing anxiety. By acting as an anxiolytic, lemon balm may mitigate the emotional source of sweating. When consuming lemon balm for its sedative effect, the recommended dose is 1.5 to 4.5 grams of dried herb daily. When using the lemon balm in extract or tincture form, follow label instructions (Consumer Labs, 2012). Caution should be used when administering lemon balm to patients who take sedative medications, due to potential additive effects.

Kava kava has a long history of being a ceremonial drink for Pacific Islanders and is a member of the pepper family. Active ingredients called kavalactones have been isolated and discovered to have sedative, analgesic, and relaxing effects. There have been several placebo-controlled studies of kava and its effect on anxiety, with the majority of them concluding that kava is an effective anxiolytic (Pittler & Ernst, 2000). Another double-blind study compared kava to standard antianxiety medication and found both therapies to be equally effective (Boerner et al., 2003). By effectively reducing anxiety, kava may reduce the emotional drive to sweat. However, recent data have indicated that hepatotoxicity is a potential adverse effect to taking kava, and regulatory agencies have banned or restricted its sale in several countries. Therefore, while kava may be effective, physician approval is recommended before consuming it regularly.

St. John's wort is from the species *Hypericum perforatum* and has long been used as therapy for emotional disorders. Several double-blind studies have compared the efficacy of St. John's wort to both placebo and antidepressant medications (Linde et al., 1996). While results are somewhat mixed, evidence as a whole indicates that it is likely more effective than placebo and as effective as antidepressant medications in the treatment of depression, with many fewer adverse effects than standard antidepressant medications. Again, through its calming and antidepressant effect, St. John's wort is proposed to be effective in the treatment of hyperhidrosis. Like many other medications, it is metabolized through the cytochrome P450 system and therefore may affect the metabolism of other drugs. Dosage is generally 300 mg taken three times per day. The effect of the herb may not be appreciated for four weeks (Consumer Labs, 2012). There are, however, may potential concerning side effects with this herb, including photosensitivity, inability to conceive, perioperative cardiac complications, and exacerbation of mania, attention-deficit/hyperactivity disorder, and psychosis.

White peony root, a traditional Chinese remedy, is a dried root that may be chopped or powdered. It is often used to treat menstrual irregularities as well as hot flashes associated with menopause and has been found anecdotally to be effective in decreasing sweat burden. The root may be consumed in teas, tinctures, or encapsulations (Caelia, 2012).

Mind–Body Medicine

If implementing dietary modifications and botanical supplementation has not provided sufficient relief, various stress management techniques such as massage, yoga, and biofeedback may provide additional benefit. Several studies have provided substantial evidence that massage and yoga aid those who suffer from a wide range of conditions. Massage therapy has been proven to decrease levels of stress hormones, increase endogenous levels of serotonin, ease anxiety and depression, and create an overall sense of relaxation (Field et al., 2005). Furthermore, several controlled studies demonstrate the effectiveness of yoga on many health conditions and have specifically concluded that there is a positive effect of yoga on perceived stress and associated psychological outcomes (Michalsen et al., 2005). By incorporating massage and yoga into one's daily or weekly routine, the perceived stress burden may be reduced, thereby perhaps decreasing the emotional stimulus for sweating.

Biofeedback can also help to regulate sweating. This technique trains patients to control bodily processes that are normally involuntary, including heart rate, muscle tension, and skin temperature or moisture level. There are various mechanisms to monitor biofeedback, including electromyography to measure muscle tension, electroencephalography to measure brain wave activity, and galvanic skin response to measure electrical skin conductance. During a biofeedback session, a patient undergoes behavioral and emotional stimuli while being monitored by one of the aforementioned mechanisms, thereby illuminating physical responses. The eventual goal is learning to control these responses without monitoring. Many controlled studies have demonstrated the beneficial effects of biofeedback on bodily processes, and some have specifically demonstrated its successful therapeutic use in treating hyperhidrosis. One such study demonstrated that six weeks after completing biofeedback therapy, clinical improvement was achieved in 11 out of 14 adults with chronic hyperhidrosis (Duller & Gentry, 1980).

Acupuncture is another therapeutic modality that can be integrated into the treatment armamentarium. Stimulation of certain anatomic sites via insertion of fine needles can decrease overexcitation of nerve endings and therefore regulate sweat production. Studies have indicated that sensory stimulation accomplished through acupuncture may modulate both sympathetic and parasympathetic autonomic activity, depending on the site of stimulation (Haker et al., 2000), and one study found that acupuncture used at specific *Huatuojiaji* points had a total effectiveness rate of 96.7% when treating spontaneous hyperhidrosis (Wang & Zhao, 2008).

Hypnosis is another valuable technique. Its efficacy in different dermatologic conditions has been long established, with even more substantial results in those conditions with a psychosomatic component (Shenefelt, 2000). Although the exact pathophysiological mechanism has yet to be established, it is known that many of the effects of hypnosis are exerted through regulation of autonomic functions such as blood flow and neurohormonal modulation (Shenefelt, 2003). Hypnosis essentially produces a state of relaxation and ultimately may be used as a treatment strategy to diminish situational stress, improve healthful behaviors, and reduce disease-related symptoms such as excessive sweating. While hypnosis may be used as an independent modality to treat hyperhidrosis, one study also found it to be extremely effective at eliminating the pain associated with onabotulinum toxin A administration (Maillard et al., 2007). Thus, hypnosis may play multiple roles in treating a patient with hyperhidrosis.

If all of the aforementioned treatment strategies do not provide adequate relief, psychotherapy may be attempted. However, such a strategy must be approached with caution, as it will not be effective in all patients. As previously described, while it is believed that primary hyperhidrosis is an exaggerated central response to an emotional stimulus, the presence of hyperhidrosis alone is not indicative of an underlying psychopathology (Lerer & Jacobowitz, 1981). As such, it is appropriate to consider psychotherapy in a patient with emotionally situational hyperhidrosis. In one case study, a 23-year-old man was treated with psychotherapy that was specifically tailored to his particular social anxieties. Although he was not completely cured of his hyperhidrosis, he nonetheless achieved significant improvement and was more functional in social settings (Kraft & Kraft, 2007). Therefore, as emotional stressors and hyperhidrosis can create something of a vicious cycle, psychotherapy may be a useful adjunctive treatment.

Conclusion

Several integrative treatment modalities may be implemented to decrease excessive sweating associated with primary hyperhidrosis, and given the lack of definitive/curative conventional therapies, a combination approach may yield more satisfying results.

REFERENCES

Boerner, R. J., et al. (2003). Kava-kava extract LI 150 is as effective as opipramol and buspirone in generalised anxiety disorder: an 8-week randomized, double-blind multi-centre clinical trial in 129 out-patients. *Phytomedicine, 10*, 38–49.

Caelia, A. (2012). Natural herbs for sweaty hands. Available at http://www.ehow.com/about_5270410_natural-herbs-sweaty-hands.html (accessed March 7, 2012).

Chen, J. H., et al. (1999). Welsh onion (*Allium fistulosum* L.) extracts alter vascular responses in rat aortae. *Journal of Cardiovascular Pharmacology, 33*(4), 515–520.

Consumer Lab (2012). Available at http://www.consumerlab.com (accessed April 20, 2012).

Davis, J. M. (2003). Central nervous system effects of caffeine and adenosine on fatigue. *American Journal of Physiology, 284*(2), R399–R404.

Desruelle, A. V., et al. (1006). Alcohol and its variable effect on human thermoregulatory response to exercise in a warm environment. *European Journal of Applied Physiology and Occupational Physiology, 74*(6), 572–574.

Duller, P., & Gentry, W. D. (1980). Use of biofeedback in treating chronic hyperhidrosis: a preliminary report. *British Journal of Dermatology, 103*(2), 143–146.

Ellis, J. (2012). Hyperhidrosis: diet tips to stop excessive sweating. Available at http://www.prlog.org/10224407-hyperhidrosis-diet-tips-to-stop-excessive-sweating.html. (accessed March 7, 2012).

Field, T., et al. (2005). Cortisol decreases and serotonin and dopamine increase following massage therapy. *International Journal of Neuroscience, 115*(10), 1397–1413.

Freedberg, I., et al. (2003). *Fitzpatrick's dermatology in general medicine* (6th ed.). New York: McGraw-Hill.

Haker, E., et al. (2000). Effect of sensory stimulation (acupuncture) on sympathetic and parasympathetic activities in healthy subjects. *Journal of the Autonomic Nervous System, 79*(1), 52–59.

Herbst, F., et al. (1991). Endoscopic thoracic sympathectomy for primary hyperhidrosis of the upper limbs. A critical analysis and long-term results of 480 operations. *Annals of Surgery, 220*(1), 86.

Kim, W. O., Kil, H. K., Yoon, K. B., et al. (2008). Topical glycopyrrolate for patients with facial hyperhidrosis. *British Journal of Dermatology, 158*(5), 1094–1097.

Kraft, T., & Kraft, D. (20077). An integrative approach to the treatment of hyperhidrosis: a case study. *London Psychotherapy, 24*(1), 38–45.

Kreyden, O. P. (2004). Iontophoresis for palmoplantar hyperhidrosis. *Journal of Cosmetic Dermatology, 3*(4), 211–214.

Lawrence, C. M., & Lonsdale Eccles, A. A. (2006). Selective sweat gland removal with minimal skin excision in the treatment of axillary hyperhidrosis: a retrospective clinical and histological review of 15 patients. *British Journal of Dermatology, 155*(1), 115–118.

Lerer, B., & Jacobowitz, J. (1981). Treatment of essential hyperhidrosis by psychotherapy. *Psychosomatics, 22*(6), 536–538.

Lillis, P. J., & Coleman, W. P. 3rd. (1990). Liposuction for treatment of axillary hyperhidrosis. *Dermatologic Clinics, 8*(3), 479.

Linde, K., et al. (1996). St John's wort for depression—an overview and meta-analysis of randomised clinical trials. *British Medical Journal, 313*(7052), 253–258.

Lupin, M. L., Hong, C. H., & O'Shaughnessy, K. F. (2011). A multi-center evaluation of the MiraDry System to treat subjects with axillary hyperhidrosis. The 31st Annual Conference of the American Society for Laser Medicine and Surgery. Grapevine, TX.

Maillard, H., et al. (2007). Efficacy of hypnosis in the treatment of palmar hyperhidrosis with botulinum toxin type A. *Annals of Dermatology & Venereology, 134*(8–9), 653–654.

Michalsen, A., et al. (2005). Rapid stress reduction and anxiolysis among distressed women as a consequence of a three-month intensive yoga program. *Medical Science Monitor, 11*(12), CR555–561.

Paller, A. S., Shah, P. R., Silverio, A. M., et al. (2012). Oral glycopyrrolate as second-line treatment for primary pediatric hyperhidrosis. *Journal of the American Academy of Dermatology, 67*(5), 918–923.

Pittler, M. H., & Ernst, E. (2000). Efficacy of kava extract for treating anxiety: systematic review and meta-analysis. *Journal of Clinical Psychopharmacology, 20*(1), 84–89.

Ruchinskas, R. A., et al. (2002). The relationship of psychopathology and hyperhidrosis. *British Journal of Dermatology, 147*(4), 733–735.

Saadia, D., et al. (2001). Botulinum toxin type A in primary palmar hyperhidrosis: Randomized, single-blind, two-dose study. *Neurology, 57*(11), 2095–2099.

Schlereth, T., et al. (2009). Hyperhidrosis—causes and treatment of enhanced sweating. *Deutsches Ärzteblatt International, 106*(3), 32–37.

Shenefelt, P. (2000). Hypnosis in dermatology. *Archives of Dermatology, 136*, 393–399.

Shenefelt, P. D. (2003). Biofeedback, cognitive-behavioral methods, and hypnosis in dermatology: Is it all in your mind? *Dermatologic Therapy, 16*(2), 114–122.

Terumasa, N., et al. (2002). Activation of central terminal vanilloid receptor-1 receptors and methylene-ATP-sensitive P2X receptors reveals a converged synaptic activity onto the deep dorsal horn neurons of the spinal cord. *Journal of Neuroscience, 22*(4), 1228–1237.

Walling, H. W. (2012). Systemic therapy for primary hyperhidrosis: a retrospective study of 59 patients treated with glycopyrrolate or clonidine. *Journal of the American Academy of Dermatology, 66*(3), 387–392.

Wang, W. Z., & Zhao, L. (2008). Acupuncture treatment for spontaneous polyhidrosis. *Journal of Traditional Chinese Medicine, 28*(4), 262–263.

18

Integrative Management of Lichen Planus

REENA N. RUPANI, MD AND MARY TEEPLE, MD

Key Concepts

♣ Lichen planus is a challenging disease entity to treat.

♣ Conventional therapy yields clinical improvement, but it is limited by adverse effects and disease recurrence, with much of its benefit being palliative in nature.

♣ By integrating additional therapeutic modalities such as dietary modification and vitamin and herbal supplementation, one may improve the overall health state of the body and therefore prevent recurrence.

♣ Nonprescription topical agents such as aloe vera gel are also effective at improving clinical disease and symptomology, and relaxation techniques such as hypnosis and biofeedback can provide substantial healing benefit.

♣ Treatment plans should be patient-specific, with appropriate modality implementation being determined by each patient's needs.

Introduction

Lichen planus is an inflammatory disorder affecting 1% to 2% of the population that typically involves flexural skin, oral and genital mucous membranes, and nails, but it can be diffuse in distribution and can also affect the scalp. The classic cutaneous lesion of lichen planus is an erythematous to violaceous, flat-topped, polygonal papule (purple, pruritic, polygonal, planar papules), but it can also include erosive, atrophic, or bullous subtypes (Lavanya et al., 2011). Whitish puncta or reticulated networks often develop on the surface of papules and are termed Wickham striae, which are distinguished from "scale"

(Sachdeva et al., 2011). Oral lichen planus is often characterized by bilateral white striations, papules, or plaques that may become erythematous or erosive and are located on the buccal mucosa, tongue, or gingiva. Overall lesions may be asymptomatic but are most often pruritic, and even considerably painful on mucosal skin.

While typically described as self-limiting, the lesions of lichen planus can persist for months to sometimes years and can significantly affect the patient's quality of life through clinical appearance, associated symptoms, subsequent scarring (scalp and nails), and cutaneous postinflammatory hyperpigmentation.

Pathogenesis

The precise etiology of lichen planus is unknown, but an immunological mechanism involving CD8[+] T-cell–mediated destruction of basal keratinocytes has been proposed. Lichen planus may coexist with other diseases of altered immune reactivity, such as primary biliary cirrhosis, ulcerative colitis, alopecia areata, vitiligo, and lichen sclerosus.

The inflammatory process is thought to be initiated by an unknown antigenic stimulus, which may arise from either an exogenous or endogenous source. Potential exogenous stimuli include allergens, infectious agents, proteins, or drugs, whereas a potential endogenous stimulus would likely be an autoreactive peptide. Antigen-specific mechanisms of disease would include antigen presentation by basal keratinocytes and subsequent keratinocyte apoptosis mediated by CD8[+] cytotoxic T cells. Nonspecific mechanisms could include mast cell degranulation and matrix metalloproteinase (MMP) activation. One study concluded, with respect particularly to oral lichen planus, that these mechanisms may combine to cause T-cell accumulation in the superficial lamina propria, basement membrane disruption, intraepithelial T-cell migration, and keratinocyte apoptosis (Sugerman et al., 2002). The authors went on to propose that chronicity of disease (again, particularly with respect to oral lichen planus) may be due, in part, to deficient antigen-specific TGF-β1–mediated immunosuppression (Sugerman et al., 2002).

Hypothesized associations with lichen planus include emotional stress, tobacco use, and oral or gastrointestinal candidiasis. The question of association with hepatitis C has been studied with mixed results, but a systematic review from 2010 found that lichen planus patients have a significantly higher risk than controls of being hepatitis C virus (HCV) seropositive, and a similar odds ratio of having lichen planus was found among HCV patients (Lodi et al., 2010). However, subgroup analysis revealed that the strength of this association varied geographically. Certainly a lichen planus patient with positive risk factors for HCV should undergo serologic testing.

Conventional Therapy

Disease management can be difficult due to the chronicity of lichen planus and associated symptoms. Many treatments are effective only partially (and temporarily, at best). Additionally, adverse effects can limit traditional therapy.

High-potency topical steroids are first-line treatment for both mucosal and cutaneous lichen planus (Usatine & Tinitigan, 2011). In oral lichen planus, steroids compounded in Orabase™, an occlusive material that provides membranous protection from extensive glucocorticoid contact and prevents salivary removal of medication, are particularly useful. Prophylactic measures to prevent the development of oral candidiasis include the use of chlorhexidine gluconate mouthwashes and topical anticandidal medication such as miconazole ointment. Topical anesthetic gels or compounded mouthwashes ("Magic" mouthwash) are useful prior to meals. Nonsteroidal topical immunomodulators such as tacrolimus and pimecrolimus may also confer benefit in cutaneous disease.

Systemic steroid therapy in doses ranging from 0.5 to 1 mg/kg/day, tapered slowly over six to eight weeks, can be used in cases of severe erosive mucocutaneous disease. Unfortunately, disease relapse with steroid taper is common (Usatine & Tinitigan, 2011), and the longer time course of treatment increases the myriad risks of steroid side effects. Systemic retinoids (acitretin) can be used as monotherapy or in conjunction with steroids, as can other immunosuppressive agents, including cyclosporine, azathioprine, or mycophenolate mofetil. Methotrexate is another immunomodulating treatment that may provide benefit (Ganesan & Shekar, 2011). These medications introduce the need for frequent laboratory monitoring, and potential fetal toxicity is important for women of childbearing years.

Phototherapy (narrow-band UVB) can be useful in some forms of cutaneous lichen planus (Habib, 2005) but may confer an increased risk of postinflammatory pigmentary alteration.

An Integrative Approach

Although conventional therapy provides benefit for some, and to varying degrees, such treatment is often merely palliative in nature and is limited by adverse effects; cessation frequently leads to disease recurrence. Therefore, in addition to conventional therapy, an individual may experience immense long-term benefit by integrating supplemental treatment modalities that influence the overall health of the body. The goal of such treatment is to minimize pain, resolve current lesions, prevent future lesions, and decrease the risk of oral cancer. Integration may begin with lifestyle modifications such as hygiene improvement and dietary change and then progress to more extensive therapy such as topical regimens and hypnosis. Outlined below is a recommended approach to the integrative management of lichen planus.

Hygiene

The first step in establishing care for lichen planus from an integrative approach is ensuring adequate general and dental hygiene. For cutaneous lichen planus, caution must be taken when using shower or bath products. Wash affected skin with plain water and nonsoap cleansers, and avoid all contact with irritating shampoo or soap products (particularly chemicals like sodium lauryl sulfate, preservatives, fragrances, and dyes). For oral lichen planus, dental hygiene maintenance is essential, despite oral pain. To minimize irritation while brushing teeth, fluoride-free toothpaste, alcohol-free mouthwash, and soft-bristle toothbrushes are recommended (Ganesan & Shekar, 2011). Dental restorations or prostheses that are composed of potentially irritating material such as gold, mercury, and palladium salts should also be addressed (Ganesan & Shekar, 2011).

Dietary Modification

Dietary modification has particular significance for individuals with oral lichen planus. When oral lesions are present, avoiding hard/sharp-edged foods, spicy, and acidic foods will provide substantial pain relief. While spicy foods are easy to recognize and thus easy to avoid, acidic foods may be less obvious. The following is a list of some common acidic food products to avoid (Rail, 2012):

- Fruits: glazed fruits, canned fruits, blueberries, cranberries, currants
- Vegetables: corn, squash, lentils, olives
- Dairy products: processed dairy products, cheese, milk, butter
- Animal protein: processed meats, bacon, sausage, ham, pork, organ meats, red meats, corned beef, salmon, tuna
- Grains: processed grains, flour, white rice, white bread, pasta, pastries

- Nuts, fats, and oils: peanuts, cashews, pecans, walnuts, pistachios, avocado oil, corn oil, canola oil, sunflower oil
- Beverages: alcohol, caffeine, sweeteners, fruit juices
- Miscellaneous: ketchup, mustard, vinegar, pepper

Altering the diet may also play a role in lowering the risk of cancer development in individuals with lichen planus. Although the exact risk is unknown, individuals with oral lichen planus are considered to have a slightly increased chance of developing oral squamous cell carcinoma relative to the general population. As such, decreasing alcohol consumption and smoking cessation in tobacco users are imperative to reduce this risk (Maserejian et al., 2006). Furthermore, despite some vegetables and fruits having a high acid content, as previously discussed, several case–control studies have demonstrated an inverse relationship between oral cancer and fruit and vegetable consumption. However, one prospective cohort study that investigated such a relationship found that fruit consumption decreased the risk of oral premalignant lesions, while vegetable consumption had no consistent association. Synthesizing all of this information to initiate a diet plan therefore must be specific to the patient. Avoiding particularly acidic fruits and vegetables may be helpful in a patient with painful oral lesions, but increased consumption of less-acidic fruits and perhaps vegetables in a person with fewer lesions or minimal pain may decrease the risk of developing oral cancer (Maserejian et al., 2006).

Supplements

Vitamin and botanical supplements may also provide benefit in the treatment and prevention of recurrence of lichen planus. Lichen planus is associated with decreased antioxidant defense and increased oxidative damage, so vitamins and herbs with antioxidant activity are thought to be particularly effective. Vitamin A, vitamin C, vitamin E, omega-3 fatty acid, beta-carotene, zinc, and cod liver oil supplements are all recommended as part of the therapeutic regimen. A comparative cross-sectional study conducted in New Delhi, India, investigated salivary levels of vitamins E and C in individuals with oral lichen planus. Results indicated that these vitamin levels were statistically significantly lower than those in controls, and it was concluded that these known antioxidants may be utilized to counteract free radical-mediated cell disturbances (Rai et al., 2008). In another study, individuals with lichen planus pigmentosus were treated with several 15-day courses of a vitamin A regimen, and many of them obtained clinical improvement (Gaby, 2011). Vitamin supplementation is therefore a useful modality in therapy of lichen planus.

Botanical supplements may also ameliorate disease. Purslane (*Portulaca oleracea*) is an antioxidant-rich herbal medicine that was recently studied in a randomized, double-blind, placebo-controlled trial. The trial was conducted on individuals with documented oral lichen planus and results were determined using the Visual Analog Scale (VAS) as well as clinical improvement measured by lesion type and size (Agha-Hosseini et al., 2010). Results indicated that patients in the purslane group experienced significantly more benefit than those treated with placebo, and all purslane-treated individuals had either a partial or complete response based on VAS scoring. This trial, in addition to several other studies, concluded that purslane is both a safe and efficacious treatment for oral lichen planus. Recommended dosage is 235 mg per day.

In addition to purslane, curcuminoids have been found to be efficacious in the treatment of lichen planus. A randomized, double-blind, placebo-controlled clinical trial was recently conducted in which individuals with oral lichen planus were treated with 6,000 mg per day of curcuminoid product in three divided doses (Chainani-Wu et al., 2012). Symptoms were qualified using the Numerical Rating Scale and signs were determined using the Modified Oral Mucositis Index. After the year-long trial, it was determined that curcuminoids at this dose have an acceptable safety profile, with few adverse effects, and provide benefit in improving the signs and symptoms of oral lichen planus.

While purslane and curcuminoids have been shown to treat clinical signs and symptoms of lichen planus, several other herbal supplements may also be effective. Thunder god vine root bark (*Tripterygium wilfordii*) is an immunosuppressive agent that may provide therapeutic benefit, and astringent agents such as tormentil (*Potentilla erecta*) with a high tannin content coat ulcerative lesions, preventing salivary and nutritional irritation. The following is a list of additional herbal therapies that may provide benefit in treating lichen planus: licorice root, marshmallow leaf or root, hollyhock leaf or root, comfrey leaf, ginger, meadowsweet flowering top, yarrow flowering top, calendula flower, hops strobili, creosote bush herb, bigleaf sagebrush leaf, hawthorn leaf, blackberry and raspberry leaf and root, blueberry and bilberry leaf and fruit, bayberry bark, bistort leaf, black tea, and agrimony herb (Yarnell et al., 2010).

Aloe Vera

A randomized, double-blind, placebo-controlled trial was conducted in which the efficacy of aloe vera gel and placebo were compared in the treatment of 54 patients with oral lichen planus. Results indicated that therapy with aloe vera gel was statistically significantly more effective than placebo at improving the clinical state of the disease and decreasing symptomology. Two patients treated with aloe vera experienced complete clinical remission (Choonhakarn et al., 2008). Aloe vera may be obtained directly from the plant or purchased at any local drugstore; it is applied topically.

Mind–Body Approaches

Hypnosis and biofeedback are additional valuable therapeutic techniques. The precise pathophysiological mechanism of hypnosis is unknown; however, many of its effects are thought to be derived through autonomic regulation (Shenefelt, 2000). Hypnosis is particularly effective at decreasing inflammation and associated inflammatory discomfort and is therefore specifically applicable to inflammatory skin disorders such as lichen planus (Shenefelt, 2008). Additional benefits are relaxation, diminishing social stress, and improving an individual's attitude about the disease state.

Biofeedback is a technique that trains patients to voluntarily control normally involuntary processes. Patients undergo mental exercises, while being physically monitored by various mechanisms, to observe the direct effect of the mind on bodily function. Patients may thereby learn to regulate and control autonomic function, as well as symptomatic sensations such as itch or pain. Although no direct evidence has demonstrated biofeedback's effect on individuals with lichen planus, its widespread application in other dermatologic diseases makes it nonetheless a promising modality. Furthermore, some studies have shown that biofeedback and hypnosis work synergistically (Shenefelt, 2003).

Finally, there are some miscellaneous modalities that one may utilize to enhance the above therapeutic regimens, such as ice pack application to decrease inflammation and pain and aromatherapy, yoga, meditation, and massage for stress relief. By incorporating these adjuncts patients may maximize treatment benefit, decrease pain, and develop a positive outlook about their treatment, expectations, and goals.

REFERENCES

Agha-Hosseini, F., et al. (2010). Efficacy of purslane in the treatment of oral lichen planus. *Phytotherapy Research, 24*(2), 240–244.
Chainani-Wu, N., et al. (2012). High-dose curcuminoids are efficacious in the reduction in symptoms and signs of oral lichen planus. *Journal of the American Academy of Dermatology, 66*(5), 752–760.

Choonhakarn, C., et al. (2008). The efficacy of aloe vera gel in the treatment of oral lichen planus: a randomized controlled trial. *British Journal of Dermatology, 158*(3), 573–577.

Gaby, A. R. (2011). *Nutritional medicine.* Concord, NH: Fritz Perlberg Publishing.

Ganesan, S., & Shekar, C. (2011). Oral lichen planus. *Journal of Dental Sciences & Research, 2*(1), 62–87.

Lavanya, N., Jayanthi, P., Rao, U. K., et al. (2011). Oral lichen planus: An update on pathogenesis and treatment. *Journal of Oral & Maxillofacial Pathology, 15*(2), 127–132.

Lodi, G., Pellicano, R., & Carrozzo, M. (2010). Hepatitis C virus infection and lichen planus: a systematic review with meta-analysis. *Oral Disease, 16*(7), 601–612.

Maserejian, N. N., et al. (2006). Prospective study of fruits and vegetables and risk of oral premalignant lesions in men. *American Journal of Epidemiology, 164*(6), 556–566.

Rai, B., et al. (2008). Salivary vitamin E and C in lichen planus. *Gomal Journal of Medical Sciences, 6*(2), 91–92.

Rail, K. (2012). High acidic foods list. Available at http://www.livestrong.com/article/2 3346-high-acidic-foods-list/ (accessed on April 20, 2012).

Sachdeva, S., Sachdeva, S., & Kapoor, P. (2011). Wickham striae: etiopathogenesis and clinical significance. *Indian Journal of Dermatology, 56*(4), 442–443.

Shenefelt, P. (2000). Hypnosis in dermatology. *Archives of Dermatology, 136*, 393–399.

Shenefelt, P. D. (2003). Biofeedback, cognitive-behavioral methods, and hypnosis in dermatology: is it all in your mind? *Dermatologic Therapy, 16*(2), 114–122.

Shenefelt, P. D. (2008). Relaxation, meditation, and hypnosis for skin disorders and procedures. In B. N. De Luca (Ed.), *Mind-Body and relaxation research focus* (pp. 45–63). Hauppauge, NY: Nova Science Publishers.

Sugerman, P. B., Savage, N. W., Walsh, L. J., et al. (2002). The pathogenesis of oral lichen planus. *Critical Reviews in Oral Biology & Medicine, 13*(4), 350–365.

Usatine, R., & Tinitigan, M. (2011). Diagnosis and treatment of lichen planus. *American Family Physician, 84*(1), 53–60.

Yarnell, E., & Abascal, K. (2010). Herbal treatment for lichen planus. *Alternative and Complementary Therapies, 16*(4), 217–222.

19

Integrative Management of Neurodermatitis

REENA N. RUPANI, MD AND DANIEL C. BUTLER, BS

Key Concepts

- ♣ Neurodermatitis refers to chronic scratching due to cutaneous, neuropathic, or psychogenic disease, which leads to lichenification and an endless itch/scratch cycle.
- ♣ Neuropathic pruritus may be due to nerve impingement or underlying medical disease.
- ♣ Psychogenic pruritus may stem from underlying psychiatric illness or comorbid depression.
- ♣ Aside from treatment of any underlying etiologic factors, pharmacologic management of neurodermatitis remains inconsistently effective.
- ♣ Bringing a psychiatrist on board can be very beneficial.
- ♣ Topical capsaicin, hypnosis, and acupuncture have some evidence of therapeutic benefit.

Introduction

Neurodermatitis, also known as lichen simplex chronicus, is a disorder characterized by excessive, vigorous scratching to relieve an itch that can be cutaneous, neuropathic, or psychogenic in origin. The chronicity of the itch/scratch cycle is the hallmark of the disease. Lichenification is the characteristic skin change, and the lesional patterns of the condition can clue an astute clinician to the diagnosis. Although not always easy to diagnose, neurodermatitis typically occurs on body parts that are within reach. The cycle is self-propagating,

as scratching leads to increased release of pruritogenic inflammatory mediators. This chapter will focus on neuropathic and psychogenic sources of neurodermatitis, as cutaneous pruritus has been discussed separately.

Neuropathic Neurodermatitis

Neuropathic itch can result from pathology located at any point along the afferent pathway of the nervous system. Damage to the peripheral nervous system
(such as in postherpetic neuropathy, brachioradial pruritus, or notalgia paresthetica) or the central nervous system (tumors and demyelinating diseases
such as multiple sclerosis) can lead to chronic pruritus (Yosipovitch & Samuel,
2008). Some of the proposed mechanisms include local nerve damage, deficient
afferent nervous signaling (causing central itch neurons to fire excessively), and
central hypersensitivity of nerve fibers (Yosipovitch & Samuel, 2008).

Brachioradial pruritus is a radiculopathy associated with chronic, severe
itch over the dorsal forearm and proximally up to the neck. Studies have
shown diminished nerve endings in the dermis and epidermis (similar to
changes that occur during phototherapy), and while it is considered a primary
neuropathy, the exact mechanism of the sensation is debated (Wallengren &
Sundler, 2005). It is aggravated in many cases with sun exposure, and for some
patients it is also associated with nerve root compression in the C5–C8 distribution (Yosipovitch & Samuel, 2008).

Meralgia and cheiralgia paresthetica refer to severe pruritus of the lateral
thigh and radial aspect of the forearm, respectively. The cause of nerve irritation can be variable but is most commonly entrapment. While the disease can
present as any type of regional paresthesia, including pain, itching is a common complaint.

Notalgia paresthetica, another localized pruritus syndrome, is commonly
associated with degenerative thoracic vertebral changes on imagery (Savk &
Savk, 2005). The hallmark sign is unilateral pruritus of the mid- to upper back,
in the T1–T6 dermatomes, and the clinical appearance is of a hyperpigmented
patch or thin plaque due to release of macular amyloid from chronic scratching.

Postherpetic neuralgia, experienced most frequently as pain after an episode of the neurotropic herpes zoster virus, can also manifest as itch that falls
under neurodermatitis.

Trigeminal trophic syndrome results in chronic itching and pain of the
face secondary to damage to the trigeminal nerve, typically leading to severe
excoriations and ulcerations of the nasal ala, cheek, temple, or frontal scalp
(Yosipovitch & Samuel, 2008). Without a proper history, this can be sometimes be confused with psychogenic neurodermatitis.

Psychogenic Neurodermatitis

Psychogenic itch refers to pruritus believed to derive from psychiatric origins, such as neurotic excoriations and delusions of parasitosis. These patients make up 2% of visits to dermatology clinics (Arnold et al., 2001). Without a syndromal pattern or underlying inflammatory disease, patients can be thus categorized only by exclusion, although a careful history and global examination can provide important clues.

Studies show that psychiatric illness is common in patients with chronic itch, and there is a significant correlation between emotional stress and itching (Dalgard et al., 2007; Laihinen, 1991). While there are several psychiatric conditions that are commonly diagnosed along with psychogenic neurodermatitis (including obsessive-compulsive disorder, anxiety, and psychosis), depression is the primary associated disease in these patients (Dalgard et al., 2007).

Psychogenic pruritus often leads to mechanically harmful behavior, including hair pulling, compulsive picking, and skin-breaking excoriation. The face is the most commonly involved/affected site for patients with psychogenic itch (Gupta et al., 2005). Clinical diagnostic clues include secondary skin changes such as erosions, thickened ulcers, hyperpigmented nodules, and hypopigmented atrophic scars.

Conventional Treatment of Neuropathic and Psychogenic Neurodermatitis

If any medical conditions (such as nerve entrapment, spinal tumors, or demyelinating disease) are discovered, treatment of these is paramount for symptom relief. Other pharmacology aimed particularly at the nerves includes gabapentin, pregabalin, antiepileptics (carbamazepine and phenytoin), topical capsaicin, topical anesthetics, and regional nerve blocks. Onabotulinum toxin A is also used by some to ameliorate neurogenic itching (Yosipovitch & Samuel, 2008). The literature also supports a positive response to transcutaneous electrical nerve stimulation. The proposed mechanism of action is by inhibiting C-fiber nociception transmission through electric impulse stimulation (Yüksek et al., 2011). Physical therapy may also benefit patients with neuropathic itch.

If treatable psychiatric disease such as depression is present in psychogenic pruritus, first-line treatment should be aimed at relieving this. In patients with psychosis, such as delusions of parasitosis, antipsychotics and pimozide have shown therapeutic benefit (van Vloten, 2003) by altering neurotransmitter concentrations and blocking overactive dopamine pathways. One review found close to 70% efficacy when patients were compliant with antipsychotics (Lee, 2008); however, pimozide use can be limited by extrapyramidal side effects and potential cardiac toxicity. Additionally, patients with psychogenic pruritus are often in strong denial of their condition and firmly believe their problem to be primarily dermatologic, making the discussion of psychopharmacotherapy (or even psychiatric referral) rather delicate.

Integrative Treatment of Neuropathic and Psychogenic Neurodermatitis

Psychotherapy is an important component of therapy not only for those with a clear psychiatric basis for their itch but also for any patient with neurodermatitis. Counseling and education on coping strategies for handling the subsequent psychological distress of feeling chronically itchy, as well as stress management, can have universal benefit. Helping patients gain insight into their pathology, as well as ways to avoid skin-damaging behaviors of picking and scratching, can help break the vicious cycle. One study indicated that therapy focused on positive reinforcement, stress reduction, and progressive muscle relaxation could diminish the cutaneous pruritus of atopic dermatitis by decreasing anxiety levels (Bae et al., 2012), and practitioners may try extrapolating this clinical benefit to patients with neurodermatitis.

Topical Remedies

Ice packs can be helpful both by acting as an anesthetic to numb the skin and also by stimulating temperature-sensing nerve fibers and perhaps "distracting" the itch fibers. There is some concern, however, that frequent use of ice packs may cause thermal injury that ultimately worsens symptoms of brachioradial pruritus (Bernhard & Bordeaux, 2005).

Capsaicin, available in cream and a newer 8% patch form, is the active ingredient in chili peppers and is helpful in treating neuropathic neurodermatitis (Gooding et al., 2010). It interferes with the retrograde transport of nerve growth factor to the cell bodies of sensory nerves, which leads to decreased synthesis of substance P, and overall a decreased perception of itch (Burks et al., 1985). Newer theories, however, purport that depleted substance P is a mere correlate of capsaicin treatment, and that actual pain/itch relief comes from a process described as "defunctionalization" of nociceptor fibers, including temporary loss of membrane potential, inability to transport neurotrophic factors leading to altered phenotype, and reversible retraction of epidermal and dermal nerve fiber terminals (Anand & Bley, 2011).

Hypnotherapy

Several cases have been reported in which long-term resolution of neuro-dermatitis symptoms occurred with hypnosis (Iglesias, 2005; Lehman, 1978). Several cases of successful treatment of acne excoriée (a form of psychogenic neurodermatitis) with hypnosis were reported by Hollander (1959) and then by Shenefelt (2004).

Acupuncture

Acupuncture continues to be used and studied as a remedy for recalcitrant pruritus. Iliev (1998) has reviewed applications in various dermatologic ill-nesses, including neurodermatitis, and the *Journal of Traditional Chinese Medicine* has published several reports of multiple cases of neurodermatitis treated with acupuncture (Liu, 1987; Yang, 1997).

Homeopathy, Supplements, and Nutrition

Studies on other integrative options are limited for the specific treatment of neurodermatitis, but there is anecdotal evidence for St. John's wort (*Hypericum perforatum*) and witch hazel (*Hamamelis virginiana*). The anesthetic, anti-inflammatory, and mood-improving properties of these remedies, along with their positive safety profiles, lend benefit to neurodermatitis (Deutsches Grünes Kreuz, 2005).

One published homeopathic approach to neurodermatitis advocated the use of hydrocotyle, thuja, graphites, kali bich, and sulphur. Partial relief of itch-ing was seen when these homeopathic medications were used to treat lichen simplex chronicus (Gupta et al., 2006).

Maintaining adequate nutrition may be critical to preserving intact cell-mediated immunity and suppressing varicella zoster virus and subsequent postherpetic neuralgia (Chen et al., 2012). Administration of intravenous vita-min C immediately relieved postherpetic neuralgia in one reported case (Byun & Jeon, 2011). This result has been confirmed in a multicenter prospective cohort study (Schencking et al., 2012), demonstrating a real potential role for ascorbic acid in the treatment of zoster and postherpetic neuralgia.

REFERENCES

Anand, P., & Bley, K. (2011). Topical capsaicin for pain management: therapeutic potential and mechanisms of action of the new high-concentration capsaicin 8% patch. *British Journal of Anaesthesia, 107*(4), 490–502.

Arnold, L. M., Auchenbach, M.B., & McElroy, S. L. (2001). Psychogenic excoriation. Clinical features, proposed diagnostic criteria, epidemiology and approaches to treatment. *CNS Drugs,15*(5), 351–359.

Bae, B. G., Oh, S. H., Park, C. O., et al. (2012). Progressive muscle relaxation therapy for atopic dermatitis: objective assessment of efficacy. *Acta Dermato-Venereologica, 92*(1), 57–61.

Bernhard, J. D., & Bordeaux, J. S. (2005). Medical pearl: the ice-pack sign in brachioradial pruritus. *Journal of the American Academy of Dermatology, 52*(6), 1073.

Burks, T. F., Buck, S. H., & Miller, M. S. (1985). Mechanisms of depletion of substance P by capsaicin. *Federation Proceedings, 44*(9), 2531–2534.

Byun, S. H., & Jeon, Y. (2011). Administration of vitamin C in a patient with herpes zoster—a case report. *Korean Journal of Pain, 24*(2), 108–111.

Chen, J. Y., Chang, C. Y., Lin, Y. S., et al. (2012). Nutritional factors in herpes zoster, postherpetic neuralgia, and zoster vaccination. *Population Health Management, 15*(6), 391–397.

Dalgard, F., Lien, L., & Dalen, I. (2007). Itch in the community: associations with psychosocial factors among adults. *Journal of the European Academy of Dermatology & Venereology, 21*(9), 1215–1219.

Deutsches Grünes Kreuz, e. V. (2005). St. John's wort treatment relieves skin inflammation and pruritus in neurodermatitis. *Kinderkrankenschwester, 24*(11), 479.

Gooding, S. M., Canter, P. H., Coelho, H. F., et al. (2010). Systematic review of topical capsaicin in the treatment of pruritus. *International Journal of Dermatology, 49*(8), 858–865.

Gupta, M. A., Gupta, A. K., Ellis, C. N., et al. (2005). Psychiatric evaluation of the dermatology patient. *Dermatology Clinics, 23*(4), 591–599.

Gupta, R., Manchanda, R. K., & Arya, B. S. (2006). Homoeopathy for the treatment of lichen simplex chronicus: a case series. *Homeopathy, 95*(4), 245–247.

Hollander, M. B. (1959). Excoriated acne controlled by post-hypnotic suggestion. *American Journal of Clinical Hypnosis, 1,* 122–123.

Iglesias, A. (2005). Three failures of direct suggestion in psychogenic dermatitis followed by successful intervention. *American Journal of Clinical Hypnosis, 47*(3), 191–198.

Iliev, E. (1998). Acupuncture in dermatology. *Clinics in Dermatology, 16,* 659–688

Laihinen, A. (1991). Assessment of psychiatric and psychosocial factors disposing to chronic outcome of dermatoses. *Acta Dermato-Venereologica Suppl (Stockh), 156,* 46–48.

Lee, C. S. (2008). Delusions of parasitosis. *Dermatologic Therapy, 21*(1), 2–7.

Lehman, R. E. (1978). Brief hypnotherapy of neurodermatitis: a case with four-year follow-up. *American Journal of Clinical Hypnosis, 21*(1), 48–51.

Liu, J. X. (1987). Treatment of 86 cases of local neurodermatitis by electro-acupuncture (with needles inserted around diseased areas). *Journal of Traditional Chinese Medicine, 7*(1), 67.

Oaklander, A. L. (2011). Neuropathic itch. *Seminars in Cutaneous Medicine & Surgery, 30*(2), 87–92.

Savk, O., & Savk, E. (2005). Investigation of spinal pathology in notalgia paresthetica. *Journal of the American Academy of Dermatology, 52*(6), 1085–1087.

Schencking, M., Vollbracht, C., Weiss, G., et al. (2012). Intravenous vitamin C in the treatment of shingles: results of a multicenter prospective cohort study. *Medical Science Monitor, 18*(4), CR215–224.

Shenefelt, P. D. (2004). Using hypnosis to facilitate resolution of psychogenic excoriations in acne excoriée. *American Journal of Clinical Hypnosis, 46*(3), 239–245.

van Vloten, W. A. (2003). Pimozide: use in dermatology. *Dermatology Online Journal, 9*(2), 3.

Wallengren, J., & Sundler, F. (2005). Brachioradial pruritus is associated with a reduction in cutaneous innervation that normalizes during the symptom-free remissions. *Journal of the American Academy of Dermatology, 52*(1), 142–145.

Yang, Q. (1997). Acupuncture treatment of 139 cases of neurodermatitis. *Journal of Traditional Chinese Medicine, 17*(1), 57–58.

Yosipovitch, G., & Samuel, S. (2008). Neuropathic and psychogenic itch. *Dermatologic Therapy, 21*, 32–41.

Yüksek, J., Sezer, E., Aksu, M., et al. (2011). Transcutaneous electrical nerve stimulation for reduction of pruritus in macular amyloidosis and lichen simplex. *Journal of Dermatology, 38*(6), 546–552.

20

Integrative Management of Postherpetic Neuralgia

ROBERT A. NORMAN, JOSEPH SALHAB, AND SABA ALAQILI

Key Concepts

- ♣ Postherpetic neuralgia (PHN) is a debilitating consequence of herpes zoster ("shingles"), which is a blistering skin condition caused by the virus varicella zoster.
- ♣ The virus is identical to the one that causes chickenpox in the pediatric population; once a patient is infected with chickenpox, the virus lies dormant in the sensory dorsal root ganglia.
- ♣ If the virus is reactivated, it returns as shingles, characterized by the classic vesicular dermatomal rash that produces a sharp, burning pain in the area of distribution.
- ♣ Herpes zoster and PHN predominately affect patients over the age of 60.
- ♣ Topical capsaicin, oral and topical steroids, antivirals, anticonvulsants, and antidepressants are used for the treatment of PHN.
- ♣ Integrative approaches toward the treatment of neuropathic pain are becoming more popular and include acupuncture, meditation, relaxation techniques, and Chinese herbs.

Introduction

Postherpetic neuralgia (PHN) is a debilitating consequence of herpes zoster (Fig. 20.1), which is a blistering skin condition caused by the virus varicella zoster. The virus is identical to the one that causes chickenpox. Once a patient

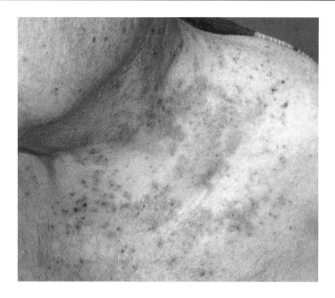

FIGURE 20.1 Herpes zoster

is infected with chickenpox, the virus lies dormant in the sensory dorsal root ganglia. If reactivated, it returns as herpes zoster or shingles, characterized by the classic vesicular dermatomal rash that produces a sharp, burning pain in the area of distribution (Gilden et al., 2011).

Most cases of shingles, however, remit within weeks to months after onset. When the pain persists for longer periods (greater than three months), especially after the rash has faded, the syndrome is now classified as PHN. PHN is characterized as an unrelenting gnawing and burning pain confined to the area on the body that was initially affected. Often the pain is so severe that it hinders basic living functions and often causes insomnia, depression, and anorexia (due to loss of appetite) (Gupta, 2012).

During the primary infection phase, the DNA virus gains access to the dorsal root ganglia and enters a latency period. Although the mechanism of the cause of the neuropathic pain is unclear, one postulated theory is that the virus alters the genetic expression of certain dorsal root sensory neurons, along with inducing physical injury to the neurons themselves. The inflammatory reaction of the body in combating the virus likely adds to the nerve damage. Subsequent nerve damage and physiological destruction to both afferent and central neurons leads to the impairment of inhibitory neurons, hyperexcitability of sodium channels, and upregulation of NMDA glutamate receptors, all of which contribute to the neuropathic nature of PHN (Gupta, 2012).

Epidemiology: Causes, Incidence, and Risk Factors

Herpes zoster and PHN predominately affect patients over the age of 60. In fact, the development of herpes zoster has been observed to approximately double in incidence each decade after the age of 50. Although the most significant risk factor is advanced age, other risk factors include impaired immunity secondary to infection with human immunodeficiency virus (HIV), chronic corticosteroid use, malignancies and consequent chemotherapy, and radiation therapy. Other established risk factors that increase the likelihood of developing neuralgia later include the development ophthalmic zoster and prodromal pain prior to visualization of epidermal lesions. Impaired healing of the inflamed nerve after the viral infection has subsided tends to occur with aging and with other factors that impair healing, contributing to the persistent pain. Vaccination with Zostavax at age 60 is recommended to reduce the likelihood of developing zoster by half and to limit the severity of the zoster if it does occur.

Estimates reveal that approximately one million patients a year contract herpes zoster, and of those, roughly 20% progress to PHN. Although the prevalence of PHN is increased in individuals over the age of 60, recent studies have shown that race plays an important role in determining an individual's susceptibility to this disease process: African Americans have a 25% greater chance of developing this condition than Caucasians.

Reemergence of dormant varicella zoster virus in the dorsal root ganglion is believed to most likely be due to the progressive decline in cell-mediated immunity as a consequence of aging.

Statistically, HIV-positive patients have approximately a 15 times higher incidence of herpes zoster than HIV-negative patients. Moreover, it is estimated that about 1 in 4 patients with Hodgkin's lymphoma will progress to reactivation of the varicella zoster virus and subsequent herpes zoster.

Clinical Presentation

Once the herpes zoster infection resolves, pain that remains in that area of distribution for more than three consecutive months is defined as PHN (Gupta, 2012). There is often a characteristic sharp and burning pain on the area of the body where the shingles outbreak transpired. Typically in both a dermatomal and unilateral distribution, the most common area for PHN to develop is on the face, trunk, and arms. The pain can last from as little as month to as long as several years following the shingles infection (Mustafa et al., 2009).

Although the most common symptom is pain, the intensity and description of the pain can vary from individual to individual. The pain can be mild or severe and can also wax and wane, causing intermissions of pain-free intervals. Most patients would describe the pain as aching, burning, or lancinating; others often describe it as an "electric shock." The area affected is also sensitive to extraneous stimuli, such as temperature changes, physical palpation, and tight clothing. Rarely, there have been patients who have expressed muscular symptoms, such as general weakness, paralysis, numbness, and tremors. Although the mechanism is unclear, it may be attributed to the dissemination of the virus through nerves that control muscular movement.

Although theoretically any dermatome may be affected by the virus, T5 and T6 are the most frequently involved vertebral dermatomes. The dermatomal distribution for these nerves extends into the fifth intercostal spaces, covering both the nipples and part of the xiphoid process. If located on the face, the most commonly involved nerve is the trigeminal nerve, more specifically its ophthalmic division. This nerve delivers only sensory information and innervates the eyelids, eyebrow, and part of the forehead and a share of the nose. If the ophthalmic division is affected, potential complications can include anterior uveitis, episcleritis, and keratitis. If the oculomotor, trochlear, and abducens nerves are affected, this may cause paralysis of ocular motility and thus "double vision" (Stankus et al., 2000).

From a psychiatric perspective, those with unresolved pain may have fluctuations in mood, depression and social withdrawal, bouts of insomnia, and unintentional weight loss.

Approaches to Treatment

TOPICAL TREATMENTS

Capsaicin cream, also called Zostrix, is the only drug approved by the U.S. Food and Drug Administration for PHN treatment. This cream contains ingredients from hot chili peppers normally found in the wild. The mechanism of action includes the depletion of substance P from nerve skin fibers, causing analgesia in the area of pain. Substance P is a neuropeptide that regulates pain activity, and its increased concentration is associated with amplified pain signals. The cream is applied three to five times daily on the affected area (Backonja et al., 2012; Stankus et al., 2000).

Xylocaine patches are small bandages that contain the local anesthetic lidocaine. Once applied directly to the area of pain, the bandage causes analgesia and pain relief from four to 12 hours (Davies et al., 2004; Stankus et al., 2000).

SYSTEMIC TREATMENTS

Co-codamol is a combination of paracetamol (acetaminophen, a nonopioid) and codeine phosphate, a weaker opioid. This over-the-counter drug has been used with varied success. If it is not efficacious, an individual can try prescription opioids, which include higher amounts of codeine, morphine, and tramadol. Tramadol is a nonnarcotic and has sedating effects that are beneficial for sleep. Although first-line drugs may include acetaminophen and other nonsteroidal anti-inflammatories (NSAIDs), studies have not demonstrated their effectiveness in controlling PHN (Nurmiko et al., 2010; Stankus et al., 2000).

Antidepressants are often used in PHN treatment because of the way they interfere with pain pathways by affecting various levels of brain chemicals. Although they do not eliminate the source of the pain itself, their effect mentally allows the patient to endure and tolerate it until symptoms resolve. Typically, clinicians will prescribe antidepressants for PHN at lower dosages than for a case of clinical depression. (Nurmiko et al., 2010; Stankus et al., 2000).

Tricyclic antidepressants such as amitriptyline and nortriptyline have had the best results for neuropathic pain in their class. Most of the side effects of the tricyclics are due to their antimuscarinic properties; they include dry mouth, blurry vision, constipation, arrhythmias, urinary retention, and liver toxicity. Although most tricyclics across the board share these side effects, nortriptyline is better tolerated because it is associated with less anticholinergic properties. Tricyclic antidepressants should be used with caution in the elderly due to the severity of some of these side effects. Studies have also shown that nortriptyline is as effective as amitriptyline. Due to the tricyclics' slow mechanism of action, a trial of at least three months is necessary before efficacy is judged. For amitriptyline (Elavil), the recommended starting dosage is 10 to 25 mg orally, best taken before bedtime. If response is inadequate, raise the dose by 25 mg every two to four weeks until effective. Maximum dose is 150 mg per day (Stankus et al., 2000). For nortriptyline (Pamelor), the recommended starting dosage is 10 to 25 mg orally, best taken before bedtime. If response is inadequate, raise the dose by 25 mg every two to four weeks until effective. Maximum dose is 125 mg per day (Stankus et al., 2000).

Selective serotonin reuptake inhibitors (SSRIs) such as venlafaxine and duloxetine aren't as efficacious but are better tolerated and often have fewer side effects than tricyclics in general. These may be considered if there are any contraindications for the use of tricyclics or if the patient cannot tolerate them (Nurmiko et al., 2010; Stankus et al., 2000).

Anticonvulsants have also been used with some success to regulate and reduce the pain associated with PHN. These medications regulate neuropathic pain both centrally and peripherally by correcting the imbalance in electrical activity caused when nerves are injured and irritated. The most commonly prescribed anticonvulsants for this purpose are gabapentin (Neurontin) and lamotrigine (Lamictal). These drugs are often better tolerated than other drugs in the class. Clinical trials have demonstrated that most of these anticonvulsants seem to be equally effective, so drug selection depends on side effects and tolerance. Failure of one anticonvulsant to work does not mean that other drugs in the same class will also fail. As with antidepressants, clinicians often prescribe lower doses than if they were treating, for example, epilepsy. Side effects can be moderate and severe and can include liver toxicity, thrombocytopenia, drowsiness, and peripheral edema. Gabapentin, especially, may increase the risk of suicide (Mustafa et al., 2009; Stankus et al., 2000).

For gabapentin (Neurontin), the recommended starting dosage is 100 to 300 mg orally, best taken before bedtime. If response is inadequate, raise the dose by 100 to 300 mg every three days until effective. Maximum dose is 900 mg three times daily (Stankus et al., 2000). For lamotrigine (Lamictal), the recommended starting dosage is 25 mg orally, best taken before bedtime. If response is inadequate, raise the dose by 50 mg every two weeks until a maintenance dosage of 225 to 375 mg per day is achieved (Stankus et al., 2000).

There are conflicting studies on whether prednisone therapy is efficacious in both preventing and reducing the pain associated with PHN. Prednisone usually works best when given early in the course of zoster along with antiviral therapy. By decreasing inflammation, prednisone may reduce nerve damage. Some studies show benefit for six to 12 months, while others show no benefit over placebo. In either case, it can be used as adjunctive treatment if there are no absolute contraindications to its use. Because of the harsh side effect profile of steroids, however, it may be wise to use it only as preventive adjunctive therapy in patients over the age of 50, due to the increased risk of developing PHN with age (Chen et al., 2010; Stankus et al., 2000). The recommended starting dosage for prednisone is 30 mg twice daily for the first week. Decrease the dosage to 15 mg twice daily for the second week. Decrease the dosage again to 7.5 mg twice daily for the third week. Reevaluate at that time (Stankus et al., 2000).

INTEGRATIVE APPROACH

Although conventional medicine may cover a vast array of treatments for PHN, integrative approaches toward the treatment of neuropathic pain are becoming more popular. Many patients, especially older ones, do not want to start on drugs that have severe side effects, especially if they are more difficult to deal with than the actual pain itself. Moreover, there is a growing trend for clinicians to use integrative treatments as adjunctive therapy on top of other drugs to increase their efficacy. In fact, Hui and colleagues (1999) demonstrated in 56 patients with PHN that combination treatment with alternative and integrative therapy along with conventional medicines decreased the intensity of pain by an average of 72%, which is both a promising and drastic inference. The clinical trial was also repeated with some variations in 2012 (Hui et al., 2012), using a three-week interval of complementary and alternative medicine along with procaine 1%. The authors concluded that in just three weeks pain was significantly reduced; in some patients, pain relief lasted for at least two years. Some of the alternative treatments used in this study are listed and outlined below.

Acupuncture originated in ancient China and has been used to treat muscle pain, back pain, headaches, and carpel tunnel syndrome. By manipulating the skin using thin needles, it is hypothesized to work by stimulating the release of endorphins and monoamines from the central nervous system, which can block pain receptors at peripheral sites. In addition, acupuncture encourages cell repair, cell membrane regeneration, and healing of the affected skin (Han, 2004).

Wang and colleagues (2007), at the Yale School of Medicine, studied the effects of acupuncture on the treatment of PHN and produced some promising results. They demonstrated that 10 acupuncture treatments, administered over a two-month interval, produced a significant decrease in pain and its side effects, such as nausea and impaired appetite.

In the cupping technique, cups are placed on the skin to increase blood circulation and the delivery of homeostatic proteins to the affected region. Growth factors such as PDGF are delivered to the affected area, promoting cell proliferation and regeneration when injury has occurred. Cupping has been used both in Western and Eastern civilizations to treat a variety of conditions, including acute myelitis, hemophilia, arthritis, bronchopneumonia, and eczema (Albedah et al., 2011).

Meditation and relaxation techniques are useful because they lead to a decrease in stress hormones. This has been shown to decrease the incidence of chronic pain, depression, and anxiety. Meditation, which provokes a deep, relaxing state of mind, helps both stabilize the autonomic nervous system and limit anxiety states. Stress, along with these other factors, can prolong and exacerbate neuropathic pain. Other relaxation-based techniques that may be used along with meditation include breathing and visualization exercises (Walloch et al., 1998). Hypnosis has been shown to alleviate the pain of PHN through its action at the anterior cingulate cortex.

Willow bark tea contains certain compounds that may offer pain relief. When made into a tea, the phenolic glycoside esters within the plant become ingestible. Once they enter the body, these compounds are oxidized into other compounds, one being salicylic acid, which is found in pain-relieving drugs such as aspirin. One study showed that willow bark tea has moderate effectiveness for relieving other causes of pain, such as lower back pain (Vlachojannis et al., 2009).

Hui and colleagues (2012) used Chinese herbs along with acupuncture, cupping, and neural therapy. Chinese herbs that have been used in the past to treat PHN include Radix Bupleuri, Poria, and Rhizoma Atractylodis Macrocephalae. Many of these herbs were used in combination with one another and were given to patients in pill form.

Lavender, eucalyptus, and peppermint oils are essential oils that can be applied topically to the skin to produce local analgesic effects. Passionflower may have sedative effects, and it may allow for sleep in those who have insomnia due to the intense pain of PHN (Dunning et al., 2006; Ngan et al., 2011).

Other forms of alternative treatment may include the use of heat and cold packs on the affected area. It is not known whether this form of treatment is as efficacious as other forms of combination treatment.

Prevention of PHN

Although PHN is a devastating complication of shingles, there are steps that can be taken to decrease the incidence of PHN once shingles takes its course.

Acyclovir and famciclovir are antiviral agents that are typically given to a patient with a shingles outbreak. These drugs work by inhibiting DNA polymerase, affecting viral replication by causing premature chain termination. Studies have shown that if started within 72 hours of the outbreak, they can drastically reduce the duration or even eliminate the complication of subsequent neuropathic pain. However, other studies provide conflicting reports, finding that acyclovir produced no improvement in PHN, even if started within 72 hours after the outbreak. Therefore, the results regarding the initiation of antivirals are variable, so the clinician must decide under what circumstances to start these drugs (Carrasco et al., 2000; Stankus et al., 2000).

Of these agents, the archetypal nucleoside analogue is acyclovir (Zovirax). This agent can be given orally or intravenously. The benefit of using the intravenous route is that it has a higher bioavailability than the oral route. Valacyclovir is characterized as a pro-drug version of acyclovir; compared with acyclovir, it has higher bioavailability, is given at shorter intervals, and may be overall more efficacious at decreasing the pain and duration of PHN. Side effects of these antivirals are generally well tolerated and can include nausea, drowsiness, constipation, and headache (Stankus et al., 2000).

For acyclovir (Zovirax), the recommended starting dosage is 800 mg five times a day orally for seven to 10 days (Stankus et al., 2000). For valacyclovir

(Valtrex), the recommended starting dosage is 1,000 mg three times a day orally for seven days (Stankus et al., 2000).

A herpes zoster vaccine is now available to the general public and is typically indicated for adults over the age of 50. In fact, it is now recommended that all adults over the age of 50, in absence of any contraindications, should receive the zoster vaccine as part of their regular medical care. The zoster vaccine (Zostavax) is a single subcutaneous injection. Because it reduces the risk of shingles outbreaks, it also prevents the occurrence of PHN by default. Contraindications to Zostavax include immunocompromise, pregnancy, and hypersensitivity to gelatin or neomycin. (Gilden et al., 2011).

REFERENCES

Albedah, A., Khalil, M., Elolemy, A., et al. (2011). Hijama (cupping): a review of the evidence. *Focus on Alternative and Complementary Therapies, 16*, 12–16.

Backonja, M. M. (2010). High-concentration capsaicin for the treatment of post-herpetic neuralgia and other types of peripheral neuropathic pain. *European Journal of Pain Supplements, 4*, 170–174.

Breuer, J. (2009). Varicella zoster. In A. J. Zuckerman, J. E. Banatvala, B. D. Schoub, et al. (Eds.), *Principles and practice of clinical virology* (6th ed.). Chichester, UK: John Wiley & Sons, Ltd.

Carrasco, D. A., Straten, M. V., & Tyring, S. K. (2000). Treatment of varicella-zoster virus and postherpetic neuralgia. *Dermatologic Therapy, 13*, 258–268.

Chen, N., Yang, M., He, L., et al. (2010). Corticosteroids for preventing postherpetic neuralgia. *Cochrane Database of Systematic Reviews*, Issue 12.

Davies, P. S., & Galer, B. S. (2004). Review of lidocaine patch 5% studies in the treatment of postherpetic neuralgia. *Drugs, 64*(9), 937–947.

Dunning, T., & Chaitow, L. (2006). Complementary approaches to managing pain. In T. Dunning (Ed.), *Complementary therapies and the management of diabetes and vascular disease: a matter of balance*. Chichester, UK: John Wiley & Sons, Ltd.

Gilden, D., Mahalingam, R., Nagel, M. A., et al. (2011). Review: The neurobiology of varicella zoster virus infection. *Neuropathology and Applied Neurobiology, 37*, 441–463.

Goh, L., & Khoo, L. (1997). A retrospective study of the clinical presentation and outcome of herpes zoster in a tertiary dermatology outpatient referral clinic. *International Journal of Dermatology, 36*, 667–672.

Gupta, R. (2012). Post-herpetic neuralgia. *Continuing Education in Anaesthesia Critical Care Pain, 12*(4), 181–185.

Han, J. (2004). Acupuncture and endorphins. *Neuroscience Letters, 361*, 258–261.

Hui, F., Boyle, E., Vayda, E., et al. (2012). A randomized controlled trial of a multifaceted integrated complementary-alternative therapy for chronic herpes zoster-related pain. *Alternative Medicine Review, 17*(1), 57–68.

Hui, F., Cheng, A., Chiu, M., et al. (1999). Integrative approach to the treatment of postherpetic neuralgia: a case series. *Alternative Medicine Review 4*(6), 429–435.

Mustafa, M. B., Arduino, P. G., & Porter, S. R. (2009). Varicella zoster virus: review of its management. *Journal of Oral Pathology & Medicine, 38*, 673–688.

Ngan, A., & Conduit, R. (2011). A double-blind, placebo-controlled investigation of the effects of *Passiflora incarnata* (passionflower) herbal tea on subjective sleep quality. *Phytotherapy Research, 25*, 1153–1159.

Nurmikko, T. J. (2010). Postherpetic neuralgia. In C. F. Stannard, E. Kalso, & J. Ballantyne (Eds.), *Evidence-based chronic pain management*. Oxford, UK: Wiley-Blackwell.

Stankus, J., Dlugopolski, M., & Packer, D. (2000). Management of herpes zoster (shingles) and postherpetic neuralgia. *American Family Physician, 61*(8), 2437–2444.

Sterling, J. C. (2008). Virus infections. In T. Burns, S. Breathnach, N. Cox, et al. (Eds.), *Rook's textbook of dermatology* (7th ed.). Malden, MA: Blackwell Publishing.

Walloch, C. L. (1998). Neuro-occupation and the management of chronic pain through mindfulness meditation. *Occupational Therapy International, 5*, 238–248.

Wang, S. M. (2007). An integrative approach for treating postherpetic neuralgia—a case report. *Pain Practice, 7*(3), 274–278.

21

Integrative Management of Pruritus

REENA N. RUPANI, MD AND DANIEL C. BUTLER, BS

Key Concepts

- ♣ Pruritus is a common complaint, both as a primary disease entity and also secondary to cutaneous inflammation. A thorough workup may be necessary to elucidate the cause.
- ♣ Conventional treatment options for primary cutaneous pruritus include topical and oral antihistamines, topical and oral steroids or other anti-inflammatory drugs, GABA-agonists, cooling agents such as menthol and phenol, and newer applications of neurokinin-1 receptor antagonists.
- ♣ Integrative management includes various herbal remedies such as milky oats, chamomile, tannins, St. John's wort, licorice extract, and others.
- ♣ Nutrition may play a role in management of some forms of pruritus.

Introduction

Pruritus is a common symptom that can have significant morbidity. The inciting stimulus for cutaneous pruritus can be central, metabolic, or within peripheral nerve endings in the skin, and careful evaluation is required to highlight primary dermatologic or systemic causes.

An initial workup for pruritus of unknown origin should include a thorough history of timing and inciting factors, associated symptoms, medical comorbidities, medications, allergies, current skin care practices, a full review of systems, and perhaps a travel history. A physical examination by a primary care provider, in combination with a full skin examination, should follow. Based on any information thus generated, targeted laboratory testing (complete blood count with differential, blood urea nitrogen/creatinine, liver function enzymes and bilirubin, thyroid function tests and thyroid antibodies, urinalysis, PPD, hepatitis serologies, HIV testing), chest radiography, and skin biopsy if indicated can help reveal the etiology. Finally, a thorough workup should include an assessment of the patient's mental state and any associated symptoms of anxiety or depression.

As the differential diagnosis is broad and treatment of secondary pruritus (related to metabolic, infectious, or neoplastic processes) depends on addressing the underlying causative factor, this chapter will focus on traditional and integrative treatment strategies for primary cutaneous pruritus related to skin disease.

Pathophysiology

Histamine is the classically known mediator of pruritus, but apart from this, several other mediators and receptors, including the neurotrophins nerve growth factor (NGF), brain-derived neurotrophic factor, neurokinins/neuropeptides such as substance P, gastrin-releasing peptide, cytokines such as interleukin-31, autotaxin, and the histamine H4 receptor, have been identified as playing a role in the pathophysiology of itch (Raap et al., 2011). Mast cells, eosinophils, lymphocytes, and even keratinocytes interact with neuronal cells via cytokines, neurotrophins, and neuropeptides, adding novel regulatory pathways for the modulation of itch.

Traditional Therapies

ORAL MEDICATIONS

Current treatments for pruritus are limited and often suboptimal. Systemic antihistamines are generally used first line, although the efficacy of antihistamines in pruritic diseases other than urticaria is often unreliable. When released from circulating mast cells and basophils, histamine binds to one of its four receptors and produces the itch sensation, among other symptoms (Metz & Ständer, 2010). Antihistamines function by competing for binding sites with the active molecule. The H1 sedating class is the first generation of antihistamines and has peripheral as well as central effects (Cevikbas et al., 2011). The CNS penetration and associated sedation differentiates the first generation from the second and third generation of H1 agents. H2 blockers are also used, but less frequently. Additional medications with antihistaminic properties include the antidepressant doxepin.

Steroids are another common first-line pharmaceutical approach to pruritus. The principal mechanism of action is immune suppression through the inhibition of nuclear factor kappa-light-chain-enhancer of activated B cells (NF-kB), a transcription factor that is essential for the synthesis of several inflammatory cytokines and proteins. Additionally, cellular immunity is suppressed via inhibition of the genes encoding interleukins 1, 2, 3, 4, 5, and 8, which are generally responsible for T-cell response and proliferation. This therapeutic approach is particularly useful (yet still not universally effective) in illnesses such as atopic dermatitis or psoriasis that are immunologic in nature. Other systemic agents for pruritus include cyclosporine, tacrolimus, and azathioprine; they have different mechanisms of action, but all function to suppress the immune system. Adverse effects, the need for frequent monitoring, and potential toxicities make these agents second- or third-line choices.

Gabapentin and pregabalin are medications used for neurogenic pruritus. Both are agonists of the GABA receptor (neurotransmitter gamma-aminobutyric acid) responsible for nerve signaling. By binding to GABA receptors, these molecules are able to prevent release of active molecules such as glutamate, noradrenaline, substance P, and calcitonin gene-related peptide. The effect of the medications on the nervous system allows for treatment of pruritus initiated primarily by nerve irritation.

Aprepitant is a newer addition to the therapeutic armamentarium for pruritus. An antiemetic, it functions via blockade of the neurokinin 1 receptor and is in the class of substance P antagonists. Some researchers have found efficacy in treatment of severe pruritus related to antiepidermal growth factor receptor therapy in cancer patients (Santini et al., 2012), and another study examined its use in brachioradial pruritus (Ally et al., 2013). It has also been studied in combination with Korean red ginseng (*Panax ginseng*) for the treatment of atopic dermatitis and associated pruritus (Lee & Cho, 2011).

TOPICAL MEDICATIONS

Topical medications, many available over the counter, offer acute relief but require frequent application. Menthol ointment or cream is known for its pleasant smell and soothing qualities. It acts on the noxious cold stimuli thermoreceptors and results in blunting of the pruritic response (Peier et al., 2002). This is an inexpensive, safe, easily accessible option for low-grade persistent pruritus, but there is little evidence of its efficacy in severe cases (Riser et al., 2003).

Phenol is another soothing agent similar to menthol that can be used in combination or as monotherapy for itch relief. Phenol is the active ingredient in calamine lotion (Millikan, 2003). Owing to its variety of effects, including antiseptic and analgesic, it is a chemical precursor to a variety of medications, including aspirin. It is the analgesic effect that is thought to confer efficacy against pruritus, despite the known separation of itch and pain fibers. One important detail, however, is that phenol has potentially toxic renal and cardiac effects. Its penetration of normal skin is of minimal concern (such as in the treatment of pruritus related to varicella), but in cases of significant epidermal compromise (such as severe atopic dermatitis), the concern is heightened (Millikan, 2003).

Coal tar has a long history of use not only for its antipruritic properties but also for its antibacterial and anti-inflammatory effects. There are over 200 active substances in tar, one of which is the aforementioned phenol. Used primarily as second-line therapy due to its undesirable staining properties, it is available in several formulations, allowing for customizable use. The carcinogenic potential of coal tar has been questioned, but a study of over 13,000 patients showed no increase in skin and non-skin cancers with its use (Roelofzen et al., 2010).

Finally, topical steroids/immunosuppressants and topical antihistamines (mechanisms of action previously discussed under oral therapies above) are also available both by prescription and over the counter, with variable efficacy. The greatest utility is in the treatment of pruritus with a clear disease-based etiology (such as contact dermatitis, atopic dermatitis, psoriasis, or lichen planus), with lower efficacy in neurocutaneous causes of itch or difficult-to-characterize disease entities such as pruritus ani, prurigo nodularis, or lichen simplex chronicus.

Integrative Therapies

Traditional approaches to pruritus management are beneficial, yet often suboptimal or incomplete. The purpose of an integrative approach is to maximize treatment efficacy by combining the benefits of all available therapeutic options. While rigorous trials are still mostly lacking, many herbal/botanical, nutritional, and mind–body approaches have been described anecdotally and in small studies.

HERBAL REMEDIES

Practitioners and healers worldwide have historically used (and continue to use) herbal remedies for pruritus. Through the process of purification, preparations can be made that isolate the active substances within the herb. Both individual herbs and combinations of herbs have been studied.

Oatmeal/wild milky oats (*Avena sativa*) is well known for its high colloid protein content and has long been used to ease itch stemming from pruritic papulosquamous disorders and contact dermatitis (Millikan, 2003). An article by Rino and colleagues (2010) highlighted a substance called avenanthramide within colloidal oatmeal that decreased the transcription of pro-inflammatory factors due to direct inhibition of NF-kB. A stark inverse relationship between the avenanthramide content and NF-kB activity was found. Baths containing oatmeal are easily added to topical or systemic therapeutic regimens for pro-phylaxis or acute management of pruritus. Other plants with similar protein makeup have the potential to function equally as well in pruritus manage-ment. These include flax, fenugreek, English plantain, hearts ease, marshmal-low, mulberry, mullein, and slippery elm (Bedi & Shenefelt, 2002).

Tannins are also useful in treating pruritus. The exact mechanism of action is unclear but may be due to coagulation of proteins at the skin's surface. Witch hazel (*Hamamelis virginiana*) is a tannin-rich herb used for its antipruritic properties. Others include oak bark, English walnut leaf, goldenrod, Labrador tea, lady's mantle, lavender, and St. John's wort. Anecdotal evidence has long been available suggesting the use of witch hazel in pruritic disease, but one study demonstrated the efficacy of witch hazel in treating patients with atopic dermatitis (Brown & Dattner, 1998). Teas, wines, fruits, and spices are other common sources.

St. John's wort (*Hypericum perforatum*) also contains tannins. It is best known for its use in depression, but in the treatment of pruritus, topical oint-ments and creams have demonstrated positive results. A study examining both the anti-inflammatory and antibiotic properties of St. John's wort found that its topical use was superior to placebo in decreasing the severity of skin lesions and decreasing skin colonization by pathogenic organisms (Schempp et al., 2003).

Arnica (*Arnica montana*) is a flowering herb that, when used topically, may help alleviate pruritus by reducing associated inflammation and providing analgesia. Studies have shown benefits in a wide variety of pruritic disease, such as acne, insect bites, and psoriasis (Millikan, 2003). It has been shown to decrease transcription of interleukins, including IL-1, IL-2, IL-6, IL-8, and TNF-alpha (Lass, 2008). However, given that arnica contains sesquiterpene lactones, there is a risk of allergic contact dermatitis among those sensitive to the Compositae family. Additionally, there are severe risks of toxicity if taken orally, or even if applied over large surface areas for long periods of time or to a compromised skin barrier. Caution is also advised during pregnancy.

German chamomile (*Matricaria chamomilla*) essential oil contains the ter-pene bisabolol, as well as chamazulene, and flavonoids (Millikan, 2003). It is consumed primarily as a tea but can also be used as a topical agent, and the antipruritic properties are found to be partially due to its anti-inflammatory effects. It has been studied and compared to topical hydrocortisone (Albring, 1983), with one study showing superior efficacy against 1% hydrocortisone ointment in healing periostomy skin lesions (Charousaei et al., 2011). Additionally, antihistamine effects have been documented highlighting the multifactorial nature of chamomile's efficacy (Kobayashi, 2005)). As a member of the Asteraceae family, however, chamomile also carries a risk of allergic contact dermatitis, and there have even been reports of anaphylaxis after tea ingestion (Andres et al., 2009).

Licorice (*Glycyrrhiza glabra*) has been shown to treat atopic dermatitis and associated pruritus (Eichenfield et al., 2007; Saeedi et al., 2003). Tested as a gel and commonly used in herbal combination therapies, it possesses an active molecule called glycyrrhizin, a triterpene saponin (Brown & Dattner, 1998). Its derivative glycyrrhetinic acid has been found to inhibit cortisol metabolism (Whorwood et al., 1993). Specifically, it inhibits the action of 11-beta hydroxysteroid dehydrogenase (11β-HSD), which results in an inhibition of the conversion of hydrocortisone to the inactive cortisone. Licorice also has the added benefit of helping with postpruritic/postinflammatory hyperpigmentation (Eichenfield et al., 2007). Compresses can be prepared by adding 3 g (1 tsp) of the 10% extract to 150 mL water (Graf, 2000). Caution must be exercised in oral administration with hypertensive patients, and systemic licorice should be avoided in those with known cardiac or renal disease. Elevations in blood pressure have been reported.

Aloe vera (*Aloe barbadensis*) is well known for its role in wound healing and the treatment of burns. Combined with traditional pharmaceuticals such as hydrocortisone, aloe can also provide augmented therapeutic effect for inflammatory skin disorders. One study examined aloe as a biologically active vehicle for hydrocortisone 21-acetate, both systemically and topically (Davis et al., 1991). Results were that aloe, when used systemically with steroids, showed enhanced anti-inflammatory effects such as an 88.1% decrease in edema and a 91% decrease in polymorphonuclear leukocytic activation (topical inhibition of edema was 97%). Another study revealed aloe vera's efficacy in diminishing pruritus related to psoriasis, where a dramatic 83.3% response rate was noted versus 6.6% with the placebo hydrophilic cream (Syed et al., 1996). Another nice feature of aloe is that it is relatively "inert" in that allergic reactions and contact dermatitis are rare (for oral consumption, patients must take care to choose "aloin-free" supplements to avoid untoward gastrointestinal effects). Overall safe and effective, aloe is likely underused.

Medicinal mushrooms (*Ganoderma lucidum*) are turning out to be nature's "panacea"; unsurprisingly, they may also play a role in pruritus management.

One study examined their efficacy in treating mosquito saliva-related pruritus (mimicking a bite) and found *Ganoderma* to be beneficial (Andoh et al., 2010). However, the exact mechanism of action and targeted molecules continue to be studied (Zhang et al., 2010).

Nutrition

The role of nutrition in skin disease is increasingly under study, and with respect to pruritus, the anti-inflammatory diet has strong potential impact. This approach to food (see Chapter 3) emphasizes low-glycemic choices, as well as a more balanced omega-3 to omega-6 fatty acid ratio, thus theoretically leading to decreased downstream systemic inflammation, disease burden, and associated pruritus. In atopic dermatitis and psoriasis, disease states that are found to have upregulated inflammatory mediators and cytokines, the overall philosophy of the anti-inflammatory diet may have practical applications.

There is much debate about the specific role of food choices and allergens with respect to atopic dermatitis. Yeast-free diets, fatty acid-rich diets, and egg/milk-free diets have not shown a generalized benefit, but there are individual cases of success—logically, these are in patients who have proven allergies to the withheld food item (Bath-Hextall et al., 2008).

Weight loss in itself is therapeutic for psoriasis. Additionally, the antioxidant properties of fish and fish oils (via modification of polyunsaturated fatty acid metabolism and eicosanoid profiles) have been shown to diminish disease severity in several uncontrolled trials (Wolters, 2005).

Finally, the gluten-free diet for treating dermatitis herpetiformis, an often intensely pruritic skin disease associated with gluten-sensitive enteropathy, is the hallmark of dietary approaches to skin disease and associated pruritus. Patients can experience substantial symptom relief by strict adherence to this diet, even without pharmacological therapy. Increasingly, individual application of gluten-free diets (on a case-by-case basis) is also playing a role in the management of other cutaneous diseases, psoriasis being one example.

REFERENCES

Albring, M., Albrecht, H., Alcorn, G., Lüker, P. W. (1983). The measuring of the anti-inflammatory effect of a compound on the skin of volunteers. *Meth Find Exp Clin Pharmacol*, 5, 75-77.

Ally, M. S., Gamba, C. S., Peng, D. H., et al. (2013). The use of aprepitant in brachioradial pruritus. *JAMA Dermatology*, 149(5), 627–628.

Andoh, T., Zhang, Q., Yamamoto, T., et al. (2010). Inhibitory effects of the methanol extract of *Ganoderma lucidum* on mosquito allergy-induced itch-associated responses in mice. *Journal of Pharmacologic Science*, *114*(3), 292–297.

Andres, C., Chen, W. C., Ollert, M., et al. (2009). Anaphylactic reaction to chamomile tea. *Allergology International*, *58*(1), 135–136.

Bath-Hextall, F., Delamere, F. M., & Williams, H. C. (2008). Dietary exclusions for established atopic eczema. *Cochrane Database of Systematic Reviews*, (1), CD005203.

Bedi, M. K., & Shenefelt, P. D. (2002). Herbal therapy in dermatology. *Archives of Dermatology*, *138*, 232–242.

Brown, D., & Dattner, A. (1998). Phytic therapeutic approaches to common dermatologic conditions. *Archives of Dermatology*, *134*, 1401–1404.

Cevikbas, F., Steinhoff, M., & Ikoma, A. (2011). Role of spinal neurotransmitter receptors in itch: new insights into therapies and drug development. *CNS Neuroscience & Therapeutics*, *17*, 742–749.

Charousaei, F., Dabirian, A., & Mojab, F. Using chamomile solution or a 1% topical hydrocortisone ointment in the management of peristomal skin lesions in colostomy patients: results of a controlled clinical study. *Ostomy Wound Management*, *57*(5), 28–36.

Davis, R. H., Parker, W. L., & Murdoch, D. P. (1991). Aloe vera as a biologically active vehicle for hydrocortisone acetate. *Journal of the American Podiatric Medicine Association*, *81*, 1–9.

Eichenfield, L. F., Fowler, J. F. Jr., Rigel, D. S., et al. (2007). Natural advances in eczema care. *Cutis*, *80*(6 Suppl), 2–16.

Graf, J. (2000). Herbal anti-inflammatory agents for skin disease. *Skin Therapy Letters*,

Kobayashi, Y., Takahashi, R., Ogino, F. (2005) Antipruritic effect of the single oral administration of German chamomile flower extract and its combined effect with antiallergic agents in ddY mice. *Journal of Ethnopharmacology*, *101*(1–3), 308–312.

Lass, C., Vocanson, M., Wagner, S., Schempp, C. M., Nicolas, J. F., Merfort, I., Martin, S. F. (2008). Anti-inflammatory and immune-regulatory mechanisms prevent contact hypersensitivity to Arnica montana L. *Experimental Dermatology*, *10*, 849–857.

Lee, J. H., & Cho, S. H. (2011). Korean red ginseng extract ameliorates skin lesions in NC/Nga mice: an atopic dermatitis model. *Journal of Ethnopharmacology*, *133*(2), 810–817.

Lipton, R. A. (1958). Comparison of jewelweed and steroid in the treatment of poison ivy contact dermatitis. *American Allergy*, *16*, 526–556.

Metz, M., & Ständer, S. (2010). Chronic pruritus—pathogenesis, clinical aspects and treatment. *Journal of the European Academy of Dermatology & Venereology*, *24*, 1249.

Millikan, L. E. (2003), Alternative therapy in pruritus. *Dermatologic Therapy*, *16*, 175–180.

Peier, A. M., Moqrich, A., Hergarden, A. C., et al. (2002). A TRP channel that senses cold stimuli and menthol. *Cell*, *108*, 705–715.

Raap, U., Ständer, S., & Metz, M. (2011). Pathophysiology of itch and new treatments. *Current Opinion Allergy & Clinical Immunology*, *11*(5), 420–427.

Rino Cerio MD, Magdalene Dohil MD, Jeanine Downie MD FAAD, Sofia Magina MD, Emmanuel Mahé MD, Alexander J. Stratigos MD. (2010). Mechanism of Action and

Clinical Benefits of Colloidal Oatmeal for Dermatologic Practice. *Journal of Drugs in Dermatology, 9*(9),1116–1120.

Riser, R. L., Kowcz, A., Schoelermann, A., et al. (2003). Tolerance profile and efficacy of a menthol-containing itch relief spray in children and atopics. *Pediatric Dermatology, 194*(Suppl 64), S83.

Roelofzen, J. H., Aben, K. K., Oldenhof, U. T., et al. (2010). No increased risk of cancer after coal tar treatment in patients with psoriasis or eczema. *Journal of Investigative Dermatology, 130*, 953–961.

Saeedi, M., Morteza-Semnani, K., & Ghoreishi, M. R. (2003). The treatment of atopic dermatitis with licorice gel. *Journal of Dermatologic Treatment, 14*(3), 153–157.

Santini, D., Vincenzi, B., Guida, F. M., et al. (2012). Aprepitant for management of severe pruritus related to biological cancer treatments: a pilot study. *Lancet Oncology, 13*(10), 1020–1024.

Schempp, C. M., Hezel, S., & Simon, J. C. (2003). Topical treatment of atopic dermatitis with Hypericum cream: A randomised, placebo-controlled, double-blind halfside comparison study. *Hautarzt, 54*, 248–253.

Syed, T. A., Attmad, S. A., Holf, A. H., et al. (1996). Management of psoriasis with aloe vera tract in a hydrophilic cream: a placebo double-blind study. *Tropical Medicine & International Health, 1*, 505–509.

Whorwood, C. B., Sheppard, M. C., & Stewart, P. M. (1993). Licorice inhibits 11β-hydroxysteroid dehydrogenase messenger ribonucleic acid levels and potentiates glucocorticoid hormone action. *Endocrinology, 132*, 2287–2292.

Wolters, M. (2005). Diet and psoriasis: experimental data and clinical evidence. *British Journal of Dermatology, 153*, 706–714.

Zhang, Q., Andoh, T., Konno, M., et al. (2010). Inhibitory effect of methanol extract of *Ganoderma lucidum* on acute itch-associated responses in mice. *Biological & Pharmaceutical Bulletin, 33*(5), 909–911.

22

Integrative Management of Psoriasis

KRISTOPHER DENBY, NANA DUFFY, ROBERT A. NORMAN, PAUL BLACKCLOUD, AND FRANCISCO TAUSK

Key Concepts

♣ Psoriasis is an inflammatory disorder in which the T lymphocyte becomes overactive and initiates a series of biochemical events leading to inflammation.

♣ Psoriasis, which affects 1% to 3% of the population worldwide, is transmitted in a genetically dominant mode with variable penetrance.

♣ In the last 10 years, many studies have reported a link between psoriasis and an increased risk of heart attack.

♣ Patients with psoriasis should seek integrative treatment methods such as diets, herbal therapy, dietary supplements, and meditation to deal with their conditions, using them with standard treatments to achieve the most favorable outcome.

Introduction

Psoriasis is a relatively common cutaneous inflammatory disease that, for many years, has been known to be associated with a specific form of arthritis (psoriatic arthritis) (Fig. 22.1). More recently, a plethora of data has emerged to suggest that psoriasis should in fact be considered a systemic inflammatory disease (Reich, 2012). Specifically, patients with severe psoriasis have been shown to have a higher risk of coronary artery disease (CAD), stroke, metabolic syndrome, cardiovascular mortality, and depression (Kimball et al., 2008). Treatments for psoriasis range from topical therapies for patients with

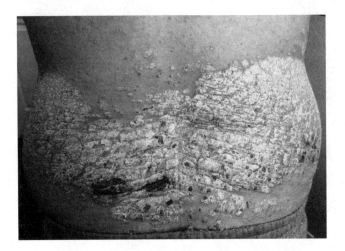

FIGURE 22.1 Psoriasis

mild disease to systemic therapies for patients with moderate to severe skin disease and/or arthritis. For the purposes of this chapter we will discuss "integrative therapy" for psoriasis from two different perspectives. We will first approach integrating complementary and alternative medicine (CAM) with traditional therapies for psoriasis; then we will discuss integrating lifestyle changes with traditional therapy for psoriasis. The latter is becoming increasingly more important as we gain more knowledge about the systemic comorbidities associated with psoriasis.

Complementary and Alternative Medicine

The definition of CAM differs depending on the cultural environment. For example, contrary to what we find in the United States, homeopathic medicine or aromatherapy would not be considered "unconventional" in England or Germany. The definition of CAM will also change as we gain more evidence of efficacy from traditional randomized controlled trials (RCT). Indeed, it is the paucity of evidence of efficacy that defines these modalities as "unconventional."

CAM use is common among patients with skin disease (Fuhrmann et al., 2010), reaching a prevalence ranging from 43% to 69% in subjects with psoriasis (Smith et al., 2009). Many patients with skin diseases use these modalities in a complementary or "integrative" way and are not seeking to replace the mainstream therapies prescribed by their health providers. Patients tend not to disclose spontaneously their usage unless specifically asked (Fuhrmann et al., 2010). This highlights the importance of maintaining an open, nonjudgmental line of communication with our patients regarding this issue in order to prevent possible drug interactions as well as untoward side effects.

CAM use varies in different countries. For example, in the Korean population, the most commonly used treatments for psoriasis were "oriental medicines," balneotherapy, and health supplements (Kim et al., 2012). In the United States, herbal therapies and vitamin/mineral supplements are the most common modalities used among patients with skin diseases (Fuhrmann et al., 2010). In the following section we will describe the CAM modalities used for psoriasis that have the largest and best body of evidence. For the most part the information presented below resulted from RCTs; anecdotal and case reports will not be discussed.

Fish Oil and Omega-3 Fatty Acids

Fish oil supplements and cold-water fish such as mackerel, sardine, trout, salmon, pilchard, kipper, and herring are rich in omega-3 fatty acids, specifically eicosapentaenoic acid (EPA) and docosahexaenoic acid (DHA). Alpha lipoic acid (ALA), another omega-3 fatty acid, is derived from plants (flaxseed, walnuts, leafy green vegetables, soybean, hemp). Because the body must convert ALA into EPA and DHA, it is metabolically more efficient to consume fish oil rather than plant oils. EPA and DHA compete with arachidonic acid (AA) as substrates for cyclooxygenase and lipoxygenase, which thereby produces inflammatory mediators in the odd-numbered classes (leukotriene B5, prostaglandin E3). These products are less inflammatory than the eicosanoids that would have been created from AA; therefore, ingesting fish oil would theoretically result in the reduction of inflammation in patients with psoriasis.

Another potential mechanism of action is related to the discovery of E-series and D-series "resolvins" synthesized from EPA and DHA respectively (De Caterina, 2011; Im, 2012; Miles & Calder, 2012). Resolvins are a relatively recently discovered class of lipids that are synthesized during the resolution of inflammation (Im, 2012). Human data on resolvins are sparse, but a wealth of animal model and in vitro data reveal that they have significant anti-inflammatory effects. Animal models have demonstrated their ability to limit inflammation in a variety of disease states, including sepsis, allergic asthma, acute lung injury, colitis, diabetes, peritonitis, pneumonia, retinopathy, reperfusion injuries following ischemic insults, and periodontitis (Uddin & Levy, 2011). Specific anti-inflammatory mechanisms observed include (1) inhibition of neutrophil recruitment, (2) stimulation of monocytes to clear apoptotic neutrophils, and (3) inhibition of pro-inflammatory cytokine release and transcription (Uddin & Levy, 2011).

Fish oil has been studied in patients with psoriasis in topical, oral, and intravenous forms. Most of the RCTs investigating fish oil for the treatment of psoriasis had positive outcomes (Smith et al., 2009). The studies that showed the greatest improvements in Psoriasis Area and Severity Index (PASI) scores were those in which fish oil was used as integrative or concomitant therapy (with phototherapy or retinoids) or administered intravenously rather than orally (Smith et al., 2009). The range of improvement with fish oil supplements is approximately 40% to 75% reduction in PASI scores, and the dosages of fish oil used in studies were highly variable. If taken as monotherapy, fish oil needs to be taken at high doses (between 3.6 and 14 g daily) and for long periods of time (six weeks to six months) to be effective.

An interesting use for fish oil is seen in patients with both psoriasis and concomitant hypertriglyceridemia. In this case, the fish oil has the potential to improve skin health and modify risk for CAD. The treatment of hypertriglyceridemia with fish oil is well established in terms of efficacy, and the American Heart Association (AHA) recommends that patients with severe hypertriglyceridemia take between 2 and 4 g fish oil daily (EPA and DHA) (Saravanan et al., 2010). One option for a fish oil supplement is a prescription-grade omega-3-acid ethyl ester that has U.S. Food and Drug Administration approval for hypertriglyceridemia. Because the primary side effect of a retinoid like acetretin is hypertriglyceridemia and fish oil has been shown to be more effective in combination with retinoids, one may consider recommending a fish oil supplement to a patient taking acetretin for psoriasis.

In all patients, regardless of a history of CAD, the AHA recommends eating fish high in omega-3 fatty acids twice weekly. In patients with a history of CAD, supplementation with 1 g fish oil daily (containing EPA and DHA) is recommended, as studies have shown that people who take fish oil after a myocardial infarction (MI) have a lower mortality than those who do not (Saravanan et al., 2010). This is probably related to a reduction in fatal post-MI arrhythmias. Therefore, a fish oil supplement should be recommend to any psoriasis patient with a history of MI.

Common side effects of fish oil are dyspepsia, taste disturbances, and, most bothersome, a fishy halitosis. The latter side effect can be deceased by refrigerating the capsules, and many companies add flavoring that aims to disguise the odor. Doses larger than 4 g daily have antiplatelet effects and should be used cautiously in conjunction with other anticoagulants (Saravanan et al., 2010). Lipid profiles should be monitored throughout therapy with fish oil supplements, and caution should be taken with patients who have hepatic impairment.

Mercury contamination of fish has been a concern for the public in general, especially for children and pregnant women. The risk of mercury contamination in fish oil supplements is very low for two reasons: first, the fish that contain the highest amounts of omega-3 fatty acids are not the same ones that contain high amounts of mercury (shark, swordfish, tilefish, king mackerel); second, heavy metals bind with proteins in the flesh of fish, not the oil. If one is still concerned about mercury, prescription omega-3-acid ethyl esters can be a good option. Alternatively, one could take a fish oil supplement that is tested by a third party for heavy metals (this should be stated on the label).

Vitamins/Herbal Therapies

This section will be a brief summary of the RCT data for vitamins and herbal therapies, since most of the studies evaluated these interventions as monotherapy for psoriasis and not necessarily as integrative therapy.

There is no evidence that supplementing oral vitamin D in patients with psoriasis is effective; however, topical vitamin D analogues are commonly used and considered standard of care (Smith et al., 2009).

- Vitamin B12 (in a cream containing avocado oil) applied topically showed no difference compared to control (Smith et al., 2009).
- Among psoriasis patients taking lithium and inositol supplementation (6 g/day) showed a statistically significant (albeit modest) improvement compared to placebo (Smith et al., 2009).
- Zinc supplementation has not shown any efficacy (Smith et al., 2009).
- The only study showing evidence for selenium supplementation was a study combining coenzyme Q10, vitamin E, and selenium (Kharaeva et al., 2009). There is some evidence for the effectiveness of topical neem (Choonhakarn et al., 2010; Smith et al., 2009).
- Results of the use of topical aloe vera have been conflicting, with aloe vera cream (Choonhakarn et al., 2010) but not aloe vera gel (Paulsen et al., 2005) showing efficacy.
- A cream containing 10% *Mahonia aquiolium* (barberry or Oregon grape) showed a decrease in PASI compared to placebo (Bernstein et al., 2006).
- A trial using topical oleum horwatheinsis (a mixture of herbs) dissolved in soft paraffin failed to show any efficacy (Smith et al., 2009).
- An extract of sweet whey has been shown in two studies to improve psoriasis (Poulin et al., 2007).
- A pilot study investigating curcuminoids (the active components in turmeric) for the treatment of psoriasis was not encouraging (Kurd et al., 2008).
- In a very recent large RCT, ginger supplementation (0.5 to 1 g daily) was shown to significantly reduce chemotherapy-induced nausea (Ryan et al.,

2011). This could be of assistance in decreasing methotrexate-associated nausea among patients with psoriasis (Kurd et al., 2008).

Climatotherapy

Traditional climatotherapy for psoriasis involves spending about one month at the Dead Sea in Israel or Jordan, bathing in the sea and lying in the sun. This is a form of CAM that is very difficult to replicate in RCTs. That being said, there are a plethora of studies showing that both artificial (bathing in Dead Sea minerals in a bathtub and then undergoing phototherapy) and natural climatotherapy are very effective for psoriasis (Kazandjieva et al., 2008; Klein et al., 2011). Dead Sea climatotherapy may be even more effective for early-onset psoriasis (onset before 40 years of age) (Harari et al., 2011). Dead Sea climatotherapy is not considered "unconventional" by some healthcare systems; in fact it is subsidized by the German healthcare system for patients who fail to respond to other forms of psoriasis treatment, and patients often achieve remissions approaching a year. The effectiveness of Dead Sea climatotherapy appears to be the result of the following synergistic elements: (1) stress reduction, (2) Dead Sea minerals, and (3) unique ultraviolet (UV) characteristics. Patients who undergo climatotherapy are away from work and other stressful situations and are taking one month to focus on their health and wellness. They also have ample time to meet with other patients with psoriasis, so they can empathize with each other and share life experiences. The Dead Sea has the highest salt content of any natural body of water, which prohibits the existence of much marine life. It is rich in magnesium, calcium, sodium, and potassium salts as well as bromine. Studies have suggested that cutaneous absorption of these salts decreases the mitotic rate of keratinocytes; salt water is also keratolytic and hydrating. The particular UV conditions at the Dead Sea are such that most of the rays reaching bathers are UVA and longer-wavelength UVB rays. Due to the very low altitude and evaporation of the salt water into the overlying air, most of the shorter UVB rays that promote erythema are filtered and do not reach the surface (Kudish et al., 2011). Longer-wavelength UVB rays (those responsible for the therapeutic effect in psoriasis patients) are also filtered, but to a lesser degree. Therefore, compared to other places on Earth, there is a greater proportion of therapeutic UVB and longer-wave UVA rays, allowing the sea bathers with psoriasis to spend long periods of time outside without suffering sunburns due to the filtering of lower-wavelength UVB rays (Kudish et al., 2011).

This type of climatotherapy is not feasible for most patients and should be recommended with caution in patients with a history of skin cancer. It would be safer than many systemic agents in pregnancy and children (Ben-Amitai & David, 2009). Artificial Dead Sea climatotherapy would also not be feasible for most private practices or academic institutions but would be easily performed at home if a patient has a home phototherapy booth.

Other areas where climatotherapy has been shown to be effective are at the Canary Islands and the Black Sea (Table 22.1). In a specific type of climatotherapy called balneotherapy, one bathes in hot springs or thermal water. Two specific areas of interest are the Blue Lagoon in Iceland and the Kangal hot springs in Turkey. The Blue Lagoon contains superheated geothermal seawater and the blue-green algae *Lyngbya estuaria* var. *thermalis*. It has been demonstrated that the mud from the Blue Lagoon helps to repair the barrier properties of the epidermis and regulates epidermal differentiation. Blue Lagoon balneotherapy is usually performed in combination with classic phototherapy. The Kangal hot springs offer a very specific type of balneotherapy where very small predatory fish present in the springs actually feed on psoriatic scales—this has been termed "ichthyotherapy" and has led to significant improvement of the disease. In Croatia, the practice of bathing in naphtalan (a black-green tarlike substance), termed naphtalic therapy, is used in the treatment of psoriasis.

Again, most of the studies related to climatotherapy or balneotherapy are not RCTs because of the challenge in replicating these natural conditions in the context of a clinical trial. A summary of locations for climatotherapy and balneotherapy that have been helpful to patients with skin disease, including psoriasis, is presented in Table 22.1 (Kazandjieva et al., 2008).

Mind–Body

The psychological effects of suffering from psoriasis cannot be overstated. The mechanisms by which stress alters the immune system, in psoriasis in particular, have been well described and reviewed (Moynihan et al., 2010). In addition to quality-of-life deficits, patients with psoriasis have higher rates of depression, anxiety, and suicidality (Kurd et al., 2010). Psoriasis patients often observe that their disease worsens with stress, and some identify a stressful event as the initial cause of their disease. Psychiatric comorbidities are common, in particular depression (Rieder & Tausk, 2012).

There are also potential cardiovascular benefits to reducing stress in the psoriasis patient. Psychological stress can both contribute to the development of CAD and precipitate acute cardiac events (Ho et al., 2010). Activation of the sympathetic nervous system increases the adherence of natural killer cells to the endothelium via ICAM-1 and CD11a. Increased recruitment of T cells

Table 22.1. Summary of Climatotherapy Options

Location	Properties
Dead Sea (Israel)	Unique UVA, UVB properties; Dead Sea salts
Black Sea (Bulgaria)	Sunlight, seawater, allergen-free air
Blue Lagoon (Iceland)	Blue-green algae
Kangal hot springs (Turkey)	Doctor fish
La Roche Posay (France)	Selenium
Comano, Montecatini Terme (Italy)	Sulfur
Italy (Levico, Vetriolo)	Arsenic ferruginous*
Dolomite (Italy)	Calcium, magnesium, sulfates
Spain (Panticosta, Fuente Amarga, Segura, Cuntis)	Sulfur
Spain (Archena, Mar Menor)	Peloid treatments (mud)
Poland (Busko-Zdrój, Ladek-Zdrój)	Sulfur, selenium, iodine; radon*, sulfur
Bulgaria (Jagoda, Kjustendil, Marikostinovo)	Sulfur, peloid
Croatia (Ivanić Grad)	Naphtalic therapy
Argentina (Copahue Thermal Basin Complex)	Volcanic water and mud or algae from sulphurous lagoons
New York (Saratoga Springs)	Lithium, magnesium, calcium
West Virginia (White Sulphur Springs)	Sulfur

and platelets is also observed. Activation of recruited T cells results in further amplification of a pro-inflammatory signal, which in turn facilitates the formation of atherosclerotic plaques (Ho et al., 2010). Lastly, chronic stress contributes to coronary events by increasing platelet activation and elevating fibrinogen levels, which increases platelet aggregation.

While several observational studies have shown benefit, most of the RCTs assessing psychological interventions for psoriasis have not had positive results (Smith et al., 2009). This area of CAM is also very difficult to study via RCTs, as appropriate control groups for psychosocial interventions are not easily designed. Until now, the best-documented intervention has been meditation. An RCT comparing patients assigned to meditation with control patients did show a statistically significant decrease in psoriasis severity ratings, and another study using mindfulness-based stress reduction tapes during phototherapy showed that the intervention group cleared their psoriasis more quickly (Smith et al., 2009; Kabat-Zinn et al., 1998). Hypnosis has been reported to significantly improve the skin disease in highly hypnotizable subjects (Tausk & Whitmore, 1999).

Lifestyle Modifications

ALCOHOL

Patient with psoriasis should be counseled to drink at most in moderation, for several reasons. First, alcohol has been implicated in the actual development of psoriasis. A recently published prospective study of 116,430 women confirmed an increased risk of incident psoriasis among those who drank five or more non-light beers per week (Qureshi et al., 2010). The study findings were robust even when the results were adjusted for important potential confounders such as smoking duration, smoking intensity, age, BMI, folate intake, and physical activity. Interestingly, no effect was seen for individuals consuming light beer, wine, or liquor. There is some evidence that patients with psoriasis have a higher prevalence of anti-gliadin antibodies found in those with gluten sensitivity (Michaelsson et al., 1993); this may explain why no effect was seen with these beverages. Similar data exist for alcohol leading to incident psoriasis in men (Poikolainen et al., 1990). Drinking excessively can put psoriasis patients at a higher risk for medication-induced liver toxicity (especially if methotrexate is being used) and treatment resistance (Ricketts et al., 2010) and can be associated with more severe and extensive disease. In a study with patients hospitalized with moderate to severe psoriasis, alcohol consumption was associated with increased mortality (Ricketts et al., 2010).

It is important to counsel patients with psoriasis to drink in moderation—up to one drink per day for women and up to two drinks per day for men (a "drink" is defined as 12 ounces of beer, 5 ounces of wine, or 1.5 ounces of liquor). A patient with psoriasis would best be advised to drink only moderately, and light beer or red wine might be the best options.

OBESITY AND DIET

As chronic inflammation is a characteristic of both psoriasis and obesity, it is not surprising that they are linked (Herron et al., 2005; Love et al., 2011; Puig, 2011). Psoriasis patients are also at an increased risk of developing other aspects of the metabolic syndrome (Kimball et al., 2008), which is defined by the following criteria:

- Waist circumference $\geq$40 inches in men or $\geq$35 inches in women
- Triglycerides >150 mg/dL
- HDL $\leq$40 mg/dL in men or $\leq$50 mg/dL in women
- Blood pressure $\geq$130/85 mmHg
- Fasting glucose $\geq$100 mg/dL

Weight loss in psoriasis patients with metabolic syndrome would theoretically reduce their risk for CAD; however, this has not been explored via RCTs. Regardless, obesity affects how patients respond to therapies and augments their risk for certain side effects.

Interestingly, with the exceptions of ustekinumab, adalimumab, and infliximab, dosing of biologics in psoriasis is generally independent of the patient's weight. As anticipated, there is a trend toward decreased efficacy of fixed-dose biologics in obese psoriasis patients (Puig, 2011). Recently weight reduction has been shown to increase the efficacy of biologics in patients with psoriasis (Bardazzi et al., 2010). Obese patients with psoriasis have experienced marked improvement in their psoriasis following weight loss secondary to gastric bypass surgery (Hossler et al., 2011; Porres, 1977). There is also evidence from an RCT that combining a low-calorie diet with cyclosporine treatment resulted in better outcomes than in the group treated with cyclosporine only (Gisondi et al., 2008).

Psoriasis patients should follow a heart-healthy diet. The AHA recommends the following:

- At least 4.5 cups of fruits and vegetables daily
- At least two 3.5-ounce servings of oily fish daily
- At least three 1-ounce servings of fiber-rich whole grains daily
- Less than 1,500 mg of sodium daily
- No more than 450 calories of sugar-sweetened beverages *per week*
- At least four servings of nuts, legumes, and seeds per week
- No more than two servings of processed meats per week
- Limit saturated fats (animal meat, lard, cream, whole milk, palm oil) and trans fats (commercial baked goods, fried foods, snack foods, vegetable shortening or stick margarine).
- Use monounsaturated (canola oil, olive oil, peanut oil, sunflower oil, avocados) or polyunsaturated (soybean oil, corn oil, safflower oil, oily fish) fats instead.

Finally, there is some evidence that the Mediterranean diet may be better for modifying cardiac risk factors than low-fat diets (Nordmann et al., 2011). This would be especially important among patients with psoriasis who also have severe disease or other risk factors for heart disease such as hypertension, low HDL, family history of premature heart disease, or increased age or those who smoke. Mediterranean diets are characterized by a higher intake of monounsaturated fats (olive oil mostly), plant proteins, and whole grains and fish; moderate alcohol intake; and low consumption of red meat, refined grains, and sweets. The Mediterranean diet generally contains more fat than the traditional diet recommended by the AHA, so this should be recommended with caution to obese patients with psoriasis.

SMOKING

The association between smoking and psoriasis has long been recognized. As gender appears to alter the effects of smoking on other diseases (Bell et al., 1991; Mucha et al., 2006), it is unsurprising that some authors have found gender-specific effects of smoking on psoriasis (Mucha et al., 2006). Research indicates that female smokers have an increased incidence of psoriasis, while male psoriatic patients who smoke experience more severe disease (Behnam et al., 2005; Bell et al., 1991; Braathen et al., 1989). Recent studies have proposed a number of possibly interrelated mechanisms to explain the relationship between smoking and psoriasis (Attwa & Swelam, 2011; Torii et al., 2011). Exposure to tobacco products correlates with higher levels of circulating T_H17 cells, the T-cell population implicated in the development of psoriasis (Torii et al., 2011). Similarly, it has been shown that smoking increases levels of reactive oxygen species and decreases levels of intrinsic antioxidant mechanisms in both smokers (with or without psoriasis) and patients with psoriasis compared to nonsmoking controls (Attwa & Swelam, 2011). Furthermore, in psoriatic patients, the degree of perturbation correlated both with the PASI score and pack-years of smoking (Attwa & Swelam, 2011). Additionally, for both male and female psoriasis patients, smoking is associated with a decreased response to therapy (Behnam et al., 2005).

Of similar import is the manner in which smoking modifies the risk of developing psoriatic arthritis. There are conflicting data on how smoking modifies the risk of developing psoriatic arthritis in patients with preexisting psoriasis. Even studies looking at particular IL-13 gene polymorphisms do not agree on how smoking affects the development of psoriatic arthritis (Duffin et al., 2009; Eder et al., 2011). In psoriasis patients in Utah, Duffin and colleagues (2009) found that the IL-13 polymorphism rs1800925*T (the minor allele) was associated with a decreased risk of developing psoriatic arthritis but that smoking negated this benefit. Surprisingly, they also found that smoking tended to delay the onset of psoriatic arthritis, following the initial diagnosis of psoriasis, regardless of genotype. In Toronto, Eder and colleagues (2011) concluded that rs1800925*C (the major allele) increased the risk of developing psoriatic arthritis in nonsmokers. One explanation for this discrepancy would be co-segregation of this IL-13 polymorphism with another key gene that alters psoriasis risk. As the populations under study were in Utah and Toronto, it seems likely that there may be a significant difference in genetic background, possibly due to a founder effect.

The cytochrome P450 enzymes have been implicated in modulating the effect of smoking on the development of psoriasis and psoriatic arthritis (Richter-Hintz et al., 2003). The question remains of what other genetic differences between these populations modify the effects of smoking on the development of psoriatic arthritis. In light of the other health benefits accrued through smoking cessation, particularly cardiovascular ones (Pipe et al., 2010), and prior studies demonstrating the benefits of smoking cessation on psoriasis disease severity, it remains prudent to counsel patients with psoriasis against smoking. As patients with severe psoriasis have an increased incidence of CAD, it is even more important to address modifiable risk factors such as smoking in this population.

GLUTEN

Gluten is found primarily in wheat, barley, and rye and products made from these ingredients. There is some evidence that psoriasis patients with elevated anti-gliadin antibodies benefit from a gluten-free diet (Michaelsson et al., 2000). If these antibodies are not elevated, a gluten-free diet is not likely to be helpful. Furthermore, there is no evidence to suggest widespread screening of psoriasis for these antibodies. However, inasmuch as a gluten-free diet may be a stepping stone to weight loss, obese patients with psoriasis should not be discouraged from trying a gluten-free diet if desired.

Conclusion

There are a wide variety of possible therapies for psoriasis that fall into the large category of CAM. A number of these therapies have significant evidence of efficacy, while others have either minimal or no evidence. Similarly, lifestyle modifications that represent a nontoxic means of augmenting a standard therapeutic regimen also have varying degrees of evidence for their use.

Fish oil acts to reduce inflammation such as that found in psoriasis both by inhibiting the production of inflammatory mediators and via their role in the synthesis of pro-resolution molecules. Fish oil is most effective when used in conjunction with traditional therapies such as phototherapy or retinoids. Additionally, high-dose fish oil is effective in treating hypertriglyceridemia, a common side effect of retinoid therapy. Prescribing fish oil for psoriasis patients taking retinoids should be part of their treatment regimen. There is no evidence to recommend supplementation with vitamin D, vitamin B12, zinc, curcuminoids, or topical oleum horwatheinsis. Similarly, there is limited evidence of efficacy for selenium, inositol, topical neem, topical aloe vera, and topical *Mahonia aquiolium*. Despite the absence of evidence, the low toxicity of these options does not merit discouraging their use in patients who express an interest in augmenting medical therapy.

Climatotherapy, particularly at the Dead Sea, has also been shown to be effective in treating severe psoriasis. However, for the vast majority of patients, this is not financially feasible. Artificial Dead Sea climatotherapy, utilizing commercial Dead Sea salt products, can be considered if patients own a home phototherapy unit. Interventions directed at reducing stress may be an important adjunct treatment for any patient with psoriasis whose disease is exacerbated by daily stressors. Another mind–body intervention, hypnosis, can be considered as a nontoxic adjunct to traditional therapy, although it is most effective in highly hypnotizable subjects.

Similarly, addressing modifiable lifestyle risk factors can make a significant different in the quality of life of patients with psoriasis. Excessive alcohol intake, particularly of non-light beer, has been shown to increase the incidence of psoriasis. Further, after the onset of psoriasis excessive alcohol intake can worsen the patient's psoriasis, decrease the efficacy of medications, and increase the risk of medication-associated hepatotoxicity. This highlights the value of counseling our patients to drink in moderation.

In light of the pro-inflammatory nature of obesity, it is similarly important to counsel obese patients with psoriasis on weight loss. That biologics are more effective following weight loss underscores the importance of patients with psoriasis achieving a healthy BMI. While gluten intolerance is rare in psoriasis, for patients with anti-gliadin antibodies, gluten avoidance can be helpful. The importance of smoking cessation cannot be overstated, as tobacco usage is implicated in incident psoriasis, increased disease severity, and decreased efficacy of therapeutic interventions. While the relationship between smoking and incident psoriatic arthritis remains unclear, the other health benefits favor smoking cessation.

Physicians familiar with integrative approaches to disease management recognize the value of augmenting traditional psoriasis therapy with a carefully considered selection of the integrative therapies mentioned above. Indeed, roughly half of patients with psoriasis already use CAM alongside their mainstream therapies, but few will voluntarily disclose this to their health provider. Initiating this discussion in a nonjudgmental manner serves three purposes: (1) it improves the therapeutic relationship with patients already using CAM, (2) it allows us to monitor for drug–drug unwanted side effects such as bleeding in patients taking both fish oil and antiplatelet agents, and (3) it provides the opportunity for us to steer our patients toward CAM treatments with the best evidence, such as fish oil, climatotherapy, and stress reduction.

REFERENCES

American Heart Association. (2012). AHA Nutrition Center: Healthy Diet Goals. Retrieved June 24, 2012, from http://www.heart.org/HEARTORG/GettingHealthy/Nutrition Center/HealthyDietGoals/Healthy-Diet- Goals_UCM_310436_SubHomePage.jsp.

Attwa, E., & Swelam, E. (2011). Relationship between smoking-induced oxidative stress and the clinical severity of psoriasis. *Journal of the European Academy of Dermatology and Venereology*, 25(7), 782–787.

Bardazzi, F., Balestri, R., et al. (2010). Correlation between BMI and PASI in patients affected by moderate to severe psoriasis undergoing biological therapy. *Dermatologic Therapy*, 23(Suppl. 1), S14–19.

Behnam, S. M., Behnam, S. E., et al. (2005). Smoking and psoriasis. *Skinmed*, 4(3), 174–176.

Bell, L. M., Sedlack, R., et al. (1991). Incidence of psoriasis in Rochester, Minn, 1980–1983. *Archives of Dermatology*,127(8), 1184–1187.

Ben-Amitai, D., & David, M. (2009). Climatotherapy at the Dead Sea for pediatric-onset psoriasis vulgaris. *Pediatric Dermatology*, 26(1), 103–104.

Bernstein, S., Donsky, H., et al. (2006). Treatment of mild to moderate psoriasis with Relieva, a *Mahonia aquifolium* extract—a double-blind, placebo-controlled study. *American Journal of Therapeutics*, 13(2), 121–126.

Braathen, L. R., Botten, G., et al. (1989). Psoriatics in Norway. A questionnaire study on health status, contact with paramedical professions, and alcohol and tobacco consumption. *Acta Dermato-Venereologica Supplementum*, 142, 9–12.

Choonhakarn, C., Busaracome, P., et al. (2010). A prospective, randomized clinical trial comparing topical aloe vera with 0.1% triamcinolone acetonide in mild to moderate plaque psoriasis. *Journal of the European Academy of Dermatology and Venereology*, 24(2), 168–172.

De Caterina, R. (2011). Omega-3 fatty acids in cardiovascular disease. *New England Journal of Medicine*, 364(25), 2439–2450.

Duffin, K. C., Freeny, I. C., et al. (2009). Association between IL13 polymorphisms and psoriatic arthritis is modified by smoking. *Journal of Investigative Dermatology*, 129(12), 2777–2783.

Eder, L., Chandran, V., et al. (2011). IL13 gene polymorphism is a marker for psoriatic arthritis among psoriasis patients. *Annals of Rheumatic Disease*, 70(9), 1594–1598.

Fuhrmann, T., Smith, N., et al. (2010). Use of complementary and alternative medicine among adults with skin disease: updated results from a national survey. *Journal of the American Academy of Dermatology*, 63(6), 1000–1005.

Gisondi, P., Del Giglio, M., et al. (2008). Weight loss improves the response of obese patients with moderate-to-severe chronic plaque psoriasis to low-dose cyclosporine therapy: a randomized, controlled, investigator-blinded clinical trial. *American Journal of Clinical Nutrition*, 88(5), 1242–1247.

Harari, M., Czarnowicki, T., et al. (2011). Patients with early-onset psoriasis achieve better results following Dead Sea climatotherapy. *Journal of the European Academy of Dermatology and Venereology* May 17 [E-pub before print].

Herron, M. D., Hinckley, M., et al. (2005). Impact of obesity and smoking on psoriasis presentation and management. *Archives of Dermatology, 141*(12), 1527–1534.

Ho, R. C., Neo, L. F., et al. (2010). Research on psychoneuroimmunology: does stress influence immunity and cause coronary artery disease? *Annals of the Academy of Medicine of Singapore, 39*(3), 191–196.

Hossler, E. W., Maroon, M. S., et al. (2011). Gastric bypass surgery improves psoriasis. *Journal of the American Academy of Dermatology, 65*(1), 198–200.

Im, D. S. (2012). Omega-3 fatty acids in anti-inflammation (pro-resolution) and GPCRs. *Progress in Lipid Research, 51*(3), 232–237.

Kabat-Zinn, J., Wheeler, E., et al. (1998). Influence of a mindfulness meditation-based stress reduction intervention on rates of skin clearing in patients with moderate to severe psoriasis undergoing phototherapy (UVB) and photochemotherapy (PUVA). *Psychosomatic Medicine, 60*(5), 625–632.

Kazandjieva, J., Grozdev, I., et al. (2008). Climatotherapy of psoriasis. *Clinics in Dermatology, 26*(5), 477–485.

Kharaeva, Z., Gostova, E., et al. (2009). Clinical and biochemical effects of coenzyme Q(10), vitamin E, and selenium supplementation to psoriasis patients. *Nutrition, 25*(3), 295–302.

Kim, G. W., Park, J. M., et al. (2012). Comparative analysis of the use of complementary and alternative medicine by Korean patients with androgenetic alopecia, atopic dermatitis and psoriasis. *Journal of the European Academy of Dermatology and Venereology* May 23 [E-pub before print].

Kimball, A. B., Gladman, D., et al. (2008). National Psoriasis Foundation clinical consensus on psoriasis comorbidities and recommendations for screening. *Journal of the American Academy of Dermatology, 58*(6), 1031–1042.

Klein, A., Schiffner, R., et al. (2011). A randomized clinical trial in psoriasis: synchronous balneophototherapy with bathing in Dead Sea salt solution plus narrowband UVB vs. narrowband UVB alone (TOMESA-study group). *Journal of the European Academy of Dermatology and Venereology, 25*(5), 570–578.

Kudish, A. I., Harari, M., et al. (2011). The measurement and analysis of normal incidence solar UVB radiation and its application to the photoclimatherapy protocol for psoriasis at the Dead Sea, Israel. *Photochemistry and Photobiology, 87*(1), 215–222.

Kurd, S. K., Smith, N., et al. (2008). Oral curcumin in the treatment of moderate to severe psoriasis vulgaris: A prospective clinical trial. *Journal of the American Academy of Dermatology, 58*(4), 625–631.

Kurd, S. K., Troxel, A. B., et al. (2010). The risk of depression, anxiety, and suicidality in patients with psoriasis: a population-based cohort study. *Archives of Dermatology, 146*(8), 891–895.

Love, T. J., Qureshi, A. A., et al. (2011). Prevalence of the metabolic syndrome in psoriasis: results from the National Health and Nutrition Examination Survey, 2003–2006. *Archives of Dermatology, 147*(4), 419–424.

Michaelsson, G., Gerden, B., et al. (1993). Patients with psoriasis often have increased serum levels of IgA antibodies to gliadin. *British Journal of Dermatology, 129*(6), 667–673.

Michaelsson, G., Gerden, B., et al. (2000). Psoriasis patients with antibodies to gliadin can be improved by a gluten-free diet. *British Journal of Dermatology, 142*(1), 44–51.

Miles, E. A., & Calder, P. C. (2012). Influence of marine omega-3 polyunsaturated fatty acids on immune function and a systematic review of their effects on clinical outcomes in rheumatoid arthritis. *British Journal of Nutrition, 107*(Suppl 2), S171–184.

Moynihan, J., Rieder, E., et al. (2010). Psychoneuroimmunology: the example of psoriasis. *Giornale Italiano di Dermatologia e Venereologia, 145*(2), 221–228.

Mucha, L., Stephenson, J., et al. (2006). Meta-analysis of disease risk associated with smoking, by gender and intensity of smoking. *Gender Medicine, 3*(4), 279–291.

National Center for Complementary and Alternative Medicine (2011).What is complementary and alternative medicine (CAM)? Retrieved August 28, 2011, 2011, from http://nccam.nih.gov/health/whatiscam/.

Nordmann, A. J., Suter-Zimmermann, K., et al. (2011). Meta-analysis comparing Mediterranean to low-fat diets for modification of cardiovascular risk factors. *American Journal of Medicine, 124*(9), 841–851 e842.

Paulsen, E., Korsholm, L., et al. (2005). A double-blind, placebo-controlled study of a commercial Aloe vera gel in the treatment of slight to moderate psoriasis vulgaris. *Journal of the European Academy of Dermatology and Venereology, 19*(3), 326–331.

Pipe, A. L., Papadakis, S., et al. (2010). The role of smoking cessation in the prevention of coronary artery disease. *Current Atherosclerosis Reports, 12*(2), 145–150.

Poikolainen, K., Reunala, T., et al. (1990). Alcohol intake: a risk factor for psoriasis in young and middle aged men? *British Medical Journal, 300*(6727), 780–783.

Porres, J. M. (1977). Jejunoileal bypass and psoriasis. *Archives of Dermatology, 113*(7), 983.

Poulin, Y., Bissonnette, R., et al. (2007). XP-828L in the treatment of mild to moderate psoriasis: randomized, double-blind, placebo-controlled study. *Alternative Medicine Review, 12*(4), 352–359.

Puig, L. (2011). Obesity and psoriasis: body weight and body mass index influence the response to biological treatment. *Journal of the European Academy of Dermatology and Venereology, 25*(9), 1007–1011.

Qureshi, A. A., Dominguez, P. L., et al. (2010). Alcohol intake and risk of incident psoriasis in US women: a prospective study. *Archives of Dermatology, 146*(12), 1364–1369.

Reich, K. (2012). The concept of psoriasis as a systemic inflammation: implications for disease management. *Journal of the European Academy of Dermatology and Venereology, 26*(Suppl 2), 3–11.

Richter-Hintz, D., Their, R., et al. (2003). Allelic variants of drug metabolizing enzymes as risk factors in psoriasis. *Journal of Investigative Dermatology, 120*(5), 765–770.

Ricketts, J. R., Rothe, M. J., et al. (2010). Nutrition and psoriasis. *Clinics in Dermatology, 28*(6), 615–626.

Rieder, E., & Tausk, F. (2012). Psoriasis, a model of dermatologic psychosomatic disease: psychiatric implications and treatments. *International Journal of Dermatology, 51*(1), 12–26.

Ryan, J. L., Heckler, C. E., et al. (2011). Ginger (*Zingiber officinale*) reduces acute chemotherapy-induced nausea: a URCC CCOP study of 576 patients. *Supportive Care in Cancer* August 5 [E-pub before print].

Saravanan, P., Davidson, N. C., et al. (2010). Cardiovascular effects of marine omega-3 fatty acids. *Lancet*, *376*(9740), 540–550.

Smith, N., Weymann, A., et al. (2009). Complementary and alternative medicine for psoriasis: a qualitative review of the clinical trial literature. *Journal of the American Academy of Dermatology*, *61*(5), 841–856.

Tausk, F., & Whitmore, S. E. (1999). A pilot study of hypnosis in the treatment of patients with psoriasis. *Psychotherapy and Psychosomatics*, *68*(4), 221–225.

Torii, K., Saito, C., et al. (2011). Tobacco smoke is related to Th17 generation with clinical implications for psoriasis patients. *Experimental Dermatology*, *20*(4), 371–373.

Uddin, M., & Levy, B. D. (2011). Resolvins: natural agonists for resolution of pulmonary inflammation. *Progress in Lipid Research*, *50*(1), 75–88.

23

Integrative Management of Rosacea

HILARY BALDWIN

Key Concepts

♣ Rosacea is a chronic inflammatory disorder without a cure.

♣ Traditional treatment approaches include benzoyl peroxide, topical and oral antibiotics, sun protection, alpha-blockers, isotretinoin, and trigger avoidance.

♣ Integrative management can include additional topical and oral agents such as green tea, CoffeeBerry, colloidal oatmeal, licorice, niacinamide, feverfew, antioxidants such as pomegranate, and many vitamins such as C, E, and A.

Introduction

Rosacea is a common disorder affecting 16 million people in the United States alone (National Rosacea Society, 2010). Despite earlier beliefs that rosacea was primarily a disease of light-skinned Caucasian women, we now know that it affects all races. Erythema may be more difficult to appreciate in patients with Fitzpatrick skin types IV and V, but papules, pustules, and granulomatous lesions are commonly seen. Although women may have a higher incidence of rosacea than men, men are more likely to develop phymas (Berg & Liden, 1989; Powell, 2005). The diagnosis is most often made in patients in their thirties through fifties (Sobye, 1950).

To truly understand the impact of rosacea on the 16 million sufferers, the psychosocial impact cannot be overlooked. For many of our patients, the stigma of a "rum blossom" or "drinker's nose" and the social and professional isolation that results from low self-esteem and prejudice are far more significant than the clinical reality.

The past decade has seen a much better understanding of the pathophysiology of rosacea, but many pieces of the puzzle remain elusive. It is likely that rosacea is a multifactorial disease with marked individual disparity that results in the great deal of interpatient variation that we observe clinically.

The absence of a one-size-fits-all therapeutic modality is therefore not surprising. In part resulting from our poor understanding of the pathogenesis of this condition, we do not truly treat rosacea, but rather manage it. We cannot offer patients cures, but can mitigate symptoms and transiently improve or even normalize appearance. As with all incurable conditions, frustrations with inadequate therapy and chronicity of therapy plague rosacea treatment plans. Benefits from a combination of medical, complementary, behavioral, and psychological approaches cannot be overemphasized. The overall goal is the improvement of the quality of life of the patient. No two patients will be alike in their needs in this regard.

Due to the unpredictability of response to standard therapy as well as a desire to use products that are more natural, patients are turning more frequently to integrative medicine for the treatment of rosacea. However, data behind the use of nontraditional products in rosacea are imprecise at best. Clinical trials are rare; when performed, they are almost uniformly underpowered, open-label, and unblinded. Still, the absence of conclusive clinical data does not necessarily equate with ineffectiveness, and one must keep an open mind. With many of the modalities mentioned in this paper, promising in vitro data and a good scientific rationale will be the sum total of our evidence base. Looking for a good scientific rationale for rosacea treatments involves an understanding of the pathophysiology of the disease and ultimately includes several broad categories of treatments: barrier repair products, redness reducers, antioxidants, anti-inflammatories, products that improve dermal structure and function, and photoprotectants.

Pathophysiology

Long believed to have an infectious basis, as does acne, recent investigation has demonstrated that rosacea is a chronic inflammatory disorder with neurovascular dysregulation (Del Rosso et al., 2012). Researchers have found aberrations in the natural immune response of the skin producing chronic inflammation. The upregulation of cathelicidins, antimicrobial peptides important in the innate immune system, results in recruitment of immune cells and angiogenesis (Bevins & Liu, 2007; Yamasaki & Gallo, 2009b;

Yamasaki et al., 2007). Increased matrix metalloproteinases (MMPs) and nitric oxide and reactive oxygen species result in chronic ongoing dermal degradation (Wise, 2007).

These observations have helped us to understand that many of our commonly used medications modulate the inflammatory process in rosacea. The tetracycline class of antibiotics downregulate pro-inflammatory cytokines, decrease the production of MMPs and indirectly reduce nitric oxide and reactive oxygen species (Baldwin, 2006; Weinberg, 2005). Both azelaic acid and metronidazole have been shown to reduce neutrophil production of reactive oxygen species and azelaic acid to downregulate the aberrant production of cathelicidins seen in rosacea (McClellan & Noble, 2000; Passi, 1992; Yamasaki & Gallo, 2009a).

Antibiotic resistance is a growing problem worldwide. A review of the literature shows that the prevalence of tetracycline resistance has risen dramatically over the last three decades on a global scale (Ayer et al., 2007; Del Rosso & Leyden, 2007). This has prompted the director of the Centers for Disease Control and Prevention (CDC) to call antibiotic resistance "one of the world's most pressing public health problems" (CDC, 2011). The CDC estimates that half of antibiotic prescriptions written each year are unnecessary (100 million total prescriptions). They recommend prescribing antibiotics only when the diagnosis of bacterial infection is confirmed and they are likely to be of benefit to the patient. Since a bacterial pathogenesis for rosacea has not been demonstrated, guidelines for treatment from the American Acne and Rosacea Society are based on the use of therapy that targets the inflammatory nature of rosacea (Del Rosso et al., 2008). This includes using as first-line treatment the topical and oral agents that are approved by the U.S. Food and Drug Administration (FDA) for the treatment of rosacea: azelaic acid, metronidazole, and oral anti-inflammatory doses of doxycycline. Sodium sulfacetamide, often used for rosacea, was grandfathered in for the treatment of rosacea by a monograph despite the absence of official pivotal trials.

Treatment paradigms have shifted over the last decade as our knowledge of the mechanism of action of traditionally used medications vis-à-vis the pathophysiology of rosacea has crystallized. The enormity of the problem of antibiotic resistance has led us to reconsider or limit the use of antibiotics in rosacea where no bacterial entity has been shown to exist (Del Rosso et al., 2008; Fleisher, 2011). In 2013 we endeavor to improve the health of our patients while minimizing ecologic mischief; the time to be cavalier has passed.

This is all the more reason why nonantibiotic, natural, complementary products are so sensible in the treatment of rosacea, if not as first-line therapies then certainly as integrative adjuncts. This is particularly true for erythema-totelangiectatic rosacea (ETR), for which there is no clear pharmacological therapy.

Classification

Rosacea is a condition characterized by a constellation of findings that can include central facial erythema and telangiectasias, papules and pustules, granulomatous nodules, phyma formation, and ocular changes. The disorder is capricious, with flares and remissions that appear to have no rationale.

For the purpose of discussing therapy, rosacea is best viewed as a collection of several conditions with a common name. Although many patients have polymorphic disease, most have one feature that predominates. Successful treatment of the different predominant features requires quite different approaches.

Historically, rosacea was described as occurring in four stages, from pre-rosacea (flushing and blushing) through severe inflammatory lesions, persistent erythema, and phyma formation. (Cohen & Tiemstra, 2002; Plewig & Kligman, 1993; Wilkin, 1994; Zuber, 2000). This classification system implied gradual progression from pre-rosacea to advanced disease, a clinical course that is uncommonly seen. Clinical trials were hampered by a lack of standardized criteria and data were hard to analyze.

A more useful classification system based on predominant lesion morphology was developed by a committee of the National Rosacea Society and published in 2002 (Wilkin et al., 2002). In this system, patients are classified as having one of four types—erythematotelangiectatic, papulopustular, phymatous or ocular—with a variant form referred to as granulomatous. Individual patients may straddle one or more subtypes, but this system allows us to evaluate therapy based on similar lesion types. Therapeutic options for the various types are easily categorized, and there are few medications or therapies that are significantly effective in more than one category.

Conventional Prescription Medications

Products that have been FDA approved for the treatment of rosacea (azelaic acid 15% gel, metronidazole 0.75% and 1% gel, and anti-inflammatory dose doxycycline) are effective primarily for papulopustular rosacea (PPR). Although some patients may see a modicum of improvement in erythema with the above, by in large ETR has, as yet, no effective pharmacological treatment. Alpha-adrenergic agonists are in development that may offer temporary but highly effective erythema reduction by vasoconstriction (Fowler et al., 2012). Other topical products (benzoyl peroxide/clindamycin combination, calcineurin inhibitors, clindamycin, erythromycin, permethrin, and retinoids) have scant evidence behind them and have met with variable clinical success (Pelle et al., 2004). Oral metronidazole has been used extensively in Europe for PPR (Builhou et al., 1978; Pelle et al., 2004; Pye & Burton, 1976; Stieger, 1979). Isotretinoin can result in dramatic improvement in severe, recalcitrant, or recurring rosacea but unfortunately does not generally offer long-term resolution (Erdogan et al., 1996, 1998; Gajardo, 1994; Hoting et al., 1986; Marsden et al., 1984; Nikolowski & Plewig, 1981; Pelle et al., 2004; Plewig et al., 1982; Rebora, 2002; Schmidt et al., 1984).

Integrative Treatment

As mentioned earlier, there are several broad categories in which complementary therapy could be expected to aid patients with rosacea (Box 23.1). They include barrier repair, redness reduction, antioxidants, anti-inflammatories, products with in vitro evidence to suggest that they might generally improve dermal structural components, and photoprotection. Virtually all of the treatments discussed below have numerous functions. They will be covered in detail in the section in which they have the greatest putative advantage in rosacea.

Barrier Repair

Many studies have demonstrated that barrier dysfunction is present in all forms of rosacea, particularly ETR. Patients complain of burning and stinging and comment that "everything" irritates their skin, even water.

In a National Rosacea Society survey of 1,066 patients, 41% said that their skin care products cause irritation and 27% said cosmetics cause a flare of their

> **Box 23.1 Categories of Activity Potentially Helpful in Rosacea**
>
> Barrier repair and enhancement
> Redness reduction
> Antioxidants
> Anti-inflammatory
> Products that increase dermal structural components
> Photoprotection

rosacea (Rosacea.org, 2013). Unfortunately, this often includes agents that would otherwise improve their rosacea, such as topical medications and sunscreens, and cosmetics that could provide instant concealment.

Why sensitivity is seen is not known. Proposed mechanisms include a defective stratum corneum that may permit exposure to irritating substances, a thinned stratum corneum, increased blood flow to the skin, and direct neuronal influences (Issachaar et al., 1997; Lammintausta & Maibach, 1988). The stinging in rosacea is not necessarily accompanied by erythema, so it cannot be assessed visually (Basketter & Griffiths, 1993). Why patients experience stinging without visible signs of irritation is unknown. It does not appear to be due to contact irritation or allergy as it occurs without positive patch tests (Wilkin, 1994). Lactic acid stinger tests, considered the gold standard for irritancy measurement, are more likely to be positive in rosacea patients who flush (Lonne-Bahm et al., 1999).

Repairing and perhaps enhancing the barrier function of the skin may help to reduce the symptoms and allow for the use of effective therapy and cosmetic camouflage. The goal of topical medications and complementary products, therefore, is to deliver effective treatment without irritating the skin still further (Draelos, 2005a).

Treatments that reduce irritation and increase hydration/barrier repair include oatmeal, niacinamide, and vitamin E (Box 23.2).

OATMEAL

Colloidal oatmeal is a powder derived from the grinding and processing of whole oat grain. The starch-protein fraction is combined with emollients to form a gelatinous hydrocolloid. This forms a protective barrier that hydrates the skin and prevents transepidermal water loss (Kurtz & Wallo, 2007). Additionally, oatmeal contains multiple components that soothe and protect pruritic and irritated skin. Such components include saponins for cleansing and normalizing skin pH, antioxidants such as vitamins A, B, and E, which also act as minor sunscreens, and polysaccharides, which help to maintain barrier integrity (Baumann et al., 2009). Oatmeal also contains phenolic compounds

Box 23.2 Barrier Protection

Niacinamide
Vitamin E
Colloidal oatmeal

such as avenanthramides, which have been shown to be anti-inflammatory because of their ability to reduce pro-inflammatory cytokine production, reduce neutrophil chemotaxis, and inhibit prostaglandin synthesis (Guo et al., 2010; Lee-Manion et al., 2009; Sur et al., 2008).

The anti-inflammatory ability of these phenolic compounds has been shown to be in the realm of 1% hydrocortisone (Fowler et al., 2010). Oatmeal has not been studied in rosacea per se but has the potential to offer reduction in irritation by providing immediate soothing and ultimate barrier repair and enhancement.

NIACINAMIDE

Niacinamide (also known as nicotinamide) has been shown to be effective in the treatment of numerous cutaneous conditions in both oral and topical formulations. Niacinamide is the amide of niacin (nicotinic acid or vitamin B3) and lacks the side effects of flushing and burning seen with niacin (Gehring, 2004).

In rosacea, niacinamide is perhaps most useful in its ability to act as an anti-inflammatory, as an inhibitor of vasoactive amines, and as a barrier repair agent. Its anti-inflammatory ability has been demonstrated in blistering disorders, rosacea, acne, and nitrogen mustard-induced irritation (Gehring, 2004; Iraji & Banan, 2010).

The use of a moisturizer containing niacinamide and glycerin showed an improvement in the integrity of the stratum corneum by corneometry and transepidermal water loss (Christman et al., 2012). Niacinamide-containing cream has also been shown to increase protein synthesis and to stimulate ceramide synthesis (Christman et al., 2012).

In a randomized, investigator-blinded study of 50 patients with rosacea, test moisturizer was applied to the face and one forearm twice daily for four weeks with the other forearm left untreated as control (Draelos et al., 2005). There was improved stratum corneum barrier function and hydration. Additionally, both investigator and patients found improvement in signs and symptoms of rosacea.

In an open-label, unblinded study of 198 patients with acne and/or rosacea, a formulation of oral nicotinamide (750 mg), zinc (25 mg), copper (1.5 mg), and folic acid (500 ug) was given twice daily for eight weeks either as a solo agent or as an add-on to oral antibiotics (Niren & Torok, 2006). Patients reported improvement in global appearance and reduction in inflammatory lesions. Patient satisfaction with the nicotinamide combination alone was comparable to antibiotics plus the nicotinamide combination. There was no difference in the clinical response between the 24% who were taking antibiotic and nicotinamide compared to the 74% taking nicotinamide alone.

Reduction in Erythema

See Box 23.3.

Box 23.3 Redness Reduction

Vitamin C
Licorice
Niacinamide
Xanthine
Golden chamomile
Polypodium leucotomas

FEVERFEW

Feverfew (*Tanacetum parthenium, Chrysanthemum parthenium*) is a ubiqui-tous perennial herb. Its first documentation as an anti-inflammatory dates back before 100 A.D. (Jeffrey, 2013). Since then we have learned that it is an antioxidant and anti-irritant as well. Early physicians used feverfew to treat fever, headache, arthritis, and gastrointestinal disorders. Until more recently, its topical use was limited due to the parthenolides in the plant, which are potent skin sensitizers. A parthenolide-free extract of feverfew (PFE) has been developed that maintains its beneficial aspects without the risk of sensitization.

Anti-irritant, anti-inflammatory, and antioxidant properties of fever-few have been demonstrated in in vitro studies. It has been shown to inhibit pro-inflammatory mediators such as 5-lipoxygenase, to decrease tumor necro-sis factor-alpha, interleukins 2 and 4, and interferon gamma from activated lymphocytes, to reduce neutrophil chemotaxis, and to inhibit NF-kB–depen-dent gene transcription (Martin et al., 2005; Wu, 2008).

In vivo studies have been few and small. However, feverfew has been shown to reduce erythema in several studies. In one, erythema that had been artifi-cially produced by methyl nicotinate and tape stripping was reduced after the application of feverfew (Southall et al., 2004).

In another study on volunteers with Fitzpatrick skin types I and II, the pre-application of feverfew-PFE reduced UV-induced erythema on the back when compared to placebo. This observation was corroborated by chromometry and diffuse reflectance spectrophotometry (Tierney et al., 2005).

Finally, a moisturizer with feverfew-PFE was used by 31 women with self-reported sensitive skin. The investigators reported a significant reduction at weeks 1, 2, and 3 in facial redness, roughness, and irritation. The patients reported less redness, dryness, and tightness and improved texture at week 1 (Nebus et al., 2005).

LICORICE

Licorice extracts (*Glycyrrhiza glabra, G. inflata*) are produced by boiling and condensing the root of the plant. Licochalcone A, the extract from *G. inflata*, is the most commonly used in topical preparations. It has been shown to reduce pro-inflammatory cytokines and inhibit superoxide anion production and cyclooxygenase activity. This presumably accounts for the anti-irritant and anti-inflammatory properties of licorice (Yokota et al., 1998).

Several in vivo studies have demonstrated the ability of licochalcone A extract to reduce redness. When used in atopic patients, preparations containing 1% to 2% licochalcone A extract significantly reduced erythema and itching after two weeks of use (Saeedi et al., 2003).

In a study of 62 patients with mild to moderate redness, a formulation of licochalcone and SPF-15 produced a significant decrease in redness at four and eight weeks that was comparable to that achieved with metronidazole gel and azelaic acid. This was accompanied by an improved quality of life after eight weeks and verification by cross-polarized photography (Weber et al., 2006).

Lastly, in a small placebo-controlled study, UV- and shaving-induced erythema was significantly reduced after twice-daily application of licochalcone A extract for three days (Kolbe et al., 2006).

Antioxidants and Anti-aging Agents

ETR bears a strong resemblance clinically to chronic sun-damaged skin with clinical evidence of standing erythema and telangiectasia. Histologically there are similarities as well with evidence of chronic dermal matrix degradation. Much of this is thought to be due to oxidative damage. There is a scientific rationale, then, for the use of topical antioxidants in the treatment of rosacea. Many of the agents listed here as antioxidants also have strong anti-inflammatory capabilities and may improve rosacea through more than one pathway (Box 23.4).

GREEN TEA

All teas—white, green, oolong, and black—derive from the same species: *Camellia sinensis*. All are excellent sources of the polyphenol catechins that are known to have good antioxidant and anti-inflammatory potential, but

---

Box 23.4 Antioxidant Activity

Vitamins A, C, E
Tea
CoffeeBerry
Chamomile
Soy
Pycnogenol
Colloidal oatmeal
Pomegranate

---

green tea appears to be the most potent (Berson, 2008; Camouse et al., 2005; Chiu et al., 2005).

In vitro studies show several findings that may be germane to rosacea. Anti-inflammatory actions include the inhibition of neutrophil and macrophage chemotaxis with downstream reduction in pro-inflammatory cytokines (Emer et al., 2011). Antioxidant activity includes the inhibition of lipoxygenase, cyclooxygenase, nitric oxide synthetase, and lipid peroxidase (Emer et al., 2011). Additionally, topical green tea extract has been shown to decrease UV-induced erythema. One percent to 10% green tea extract 30 minutes prior to irradiation reduced the erythema response to solar-stimulated light, and black tea reduced UVB-induced erythema when applied to human or mouse skin *after* irradiation (Elmets et al., 2001; Zhao et al., 1999). This may be particularly useful in rosacea patients in whom sun exposure is a trigger and for a natural alternative or adjunct for sun protection (Elmets et al., 2001; Katiyar et al., 2007; Yusuf et al., 2007). Lastly, green tea has been shown to improve skin barrier function (Chiu et al., 2005).

COFFEEBERRY

Extracts taken from berries of the coffee plant (*Coffea arabica*) before they ripen have potent antioxidant activity (Farris, 2007). The polyphenols present in the extracts are good antioxidants and have been shown to protect against both UVA and UVB radiation (Iwai et al., 2004; Scalbert et al., 2005). At least one study has shown that the antioxidant capability (measured by the Oxygen Radical Absorbance Capacity [ORAC] score) of CoffeeBerry is 10 to 15 times the capacity of vitamins C and E, green tea, and pomegranate (Baumann, 2007b; Jancin, 2007). However, it remains unclear if the ORAC score, developed by the U.S. Department of Agriculture for food substances, is relevant to topical products (Ditre et al., 2008). It is not clear if caffeine itself, extracted from the leaves of the plant, is an active ingredient in its own right (Hexsel et al., 2003).

CoffeeBerry extract has been shown to upregulate collagen production and connective tissue growth factor and to downregulate fibronectin and MMPs, all of which might improve the ongoing dermal matrix degradation seen in rosacea (Farris, 2007).

In a six-week split-face study on 10 patients, CoffeeBerry extract was shown to result in global improvement of skin appearance (Baumann, 2007a; Facino et al., 1995). It is interesting that Coffeeberry appears to improve the appearance of rosacea while coffee itself is an often-mentioned trigger for rosacea flares.

POMEGRANATE

Pomegranate (*Punica granatum*) has become extremely popular in recent years, with oral ingestion boasting antioxidative properties similar to green tea and red wine (Baumann et al., 2009). Ingestion of pomegranate tablets has been shown to increase the SPF of topical sunscreens, presumably by modulating UVA-mediated damage in keratinocytes (Syed et al., 2006).

Pomegranate contains ellagic acid, a phenolic compound. It is a potent antioxidant. In vitro studies with extracts from pomegranate seed oil showed a stimulation of keratinocyte proliferation, and peel extracts stimulated type I procollagen synthesis and inhibited MMP-1 from dermal fibroblasts (Aslam et al., 2006). This would suggest the possibility of beneficial dermal structural effects from topical pomegranate extracts in rosacea.

TOPICAL VITAMINS

Vitamins A, C, and E, along with ubiquinones, uric acid, and glutathione, are part of the endogenous antioxidant protection of the skin. However, sun exposure causes oxidative stress to occur faster than the skin can manage. The antioxidants themselves are depleted easily by sun and ozone. Minimal exposure of 1.6 times the minimum erythemal dose was shown to decrease vitamin C by 70% (Katiyar et al., 1995).

Assuming the absence of profound vitamin deficiency, oral administration of vitamins does not supply antioxidant benefit to the skin. Gastrointestinal absorption is the rate-limiting step in skin delivery and the transport mechanisms to the skin are inadequate. Ingestion of large quantities of water-soluble vitamins results in rapid excretion, and lipid-soluble vitamins can be toxic at higher doses.

So the question becomes: Can topical application of vitamins increase the antioxidative abilities of the stratum corneum? As with all topically applied treatments, absorption is hampered by the stratum corneum; without absorption there is no activity. Unlike other products intended for activity in the superficial dermis, however, antioxidants are able to perform their tasks within the epidermis, a slightly smaller hurdle.

VITAMIN E

Vitamin E is the umbrella term for eight different fat-soluble compounds, four tocopherols and four tocotrienols that are identified by the prefixes alpha, beta, gamma, and delta. Synthetic vitamin E contains eight stereoisomers that are generally esterified for increased stability. They must be hydrolyzed to become biologically active. This occurs readily in the stomach, but slowly if at all in the skin when topically applied (Burke, 2004). The once-common practice, then, of opening a capsule of vitamin E and applying the contents to the skin was likely effective as an emollient only.

Vitamin E is a potent antioxidant that prevents, in concert with vitamin C, the propagation of free radicals in tissues. Since it is fat-soluble, vitamin E prevents the hydrophobic cell membranes from oxidative damage. The most widely studied is alpha tocopherol, which is a crucial, perhaps the most important, antioxidant in the glutathione peroxidase pathway (Thiele et al., 2005; Traber & Atkinson, 2007). It scavenges free radical intermediates, becoming oxidized in the process. The oxidized form is subsequently recycled back into use through reduction by other antioxidants such as vitamin C, retinol, or ubiquinol (Wang & Quinn, 1999).

Vitamin E has been shown to be effective topically in several ways that might prove useful for rosacea patients: as an antioxidant, skin protectant, and photoprotectant (Baumann & Spencer, 1999; Thiele et al., 2005). In a vehicle-controlled trial of 13 patients, it was shown that it is possible to deposit alpha tocopherol in the stratum corneum after a 0.15% rinse-off preparation and that such application decreased photo-oxidative stress after UVA irradiation (Ekanayake-Mudiyanselage et al., 2005). It has been shown to reduce UV-induced erythema and edema and histologically to normalize dermal collagen and elastin altered by UV exposure (Burke, 2004; Thiele et al., 2005).

Thus, in rosacea, it is possible that vitamin E could act as an antioxidant, barrier repair cream, and photoprotectant, but clinical proof of this statement is lacking.

VITAMIN C

Vitamin C, a water-soluble vitamin (also known as L-ascorbic acid and ascorbate), is an inclusive term for several compounds that have vitamin C activity, including its acid, salts, and the oxidized form, dehydroascorbic acid. Ascorbate and ascorbic acid interconvert in the body according to pH.

Small amounts of vitamin C are present within the epidermis, but it is highly susceptible to UV exposure and ozone. Topically applied, vitamin C is finicky. Exposed to air, L-ascorbic acid oxidizes and must be esterified to remain stable (Farris, 2005). Additionally, absorption is maximized when the pH is highly acidic—3.5 being optimal for absorption, although not for the integrity of the epidermis (Burke, 2004). If these formulation difficulties are overcome, topical application is a more effective method for skin delivery than is oral (Burgess, 2008).

The scientific rationale for vitamin C use in rosacea is sound. It is a good anti-inflammatory and antioxidant that also promotes collagen synthesis and inhibits degradation (Farris, 2005). As mentioned before, vitamin C aids vitamin E in its efforts as an antioxidant by reducing vitamin E back to its effective state.

In clinical studies, vitamin C 5% topical application to photoaged skin has been shown to increase elastic repair histologically (Humbert et al., 2003). In vivo, it has been shown to stimulate fibroblasts, increase the rate of neocollagenesis, decrease melanin formation, and exhibit anti-inflammatory activity (Reszko et al., 2009). The combination of vitamin C and vitamin E has been shown to have photoprotectant abilities greater when combined than when either agent is used alone (Lin et al., 2003, 2005). The addition of ferulic acid doubles the photoprotective effect, presumably because it improves the stability of both vitamin C and E (Lin et al., 2005; Pinnell et al., 2005).

Vitamin C could be expected therefore to be useful in rosacea, especially in combination with vitamin E for reduction of erythema, ongoing dermal matrix degradation, and photodamage or photo-induced rosacea flare (Farris, 2005).

PYCNOGENOL

Pycnogenol is the extract of pine bark (*Pinus pinaster*). It is rich in proanthocyanidins and oral administration has been reported to have antioxidant, chemoprotective, and photoprotective effects (Blazso et al., 2004; Sime & Reeve, 2004). It may be a useful complement to sunscreens as it has been shown to produce dose-dependent reductions in inflammatory sunburn reaction (Sime & Reeve, 2004).

Anti-inflammatory Agents

See Box 23.5.

Box 23.5 Anti-inflammatory Agents

Vitamin C
Soy
Niacinamide
Feverfew
Licorice
Tea
Chamomile
Aloe vera
Colloidal oatmeal
Witch hazel

ALOE VERA

Aloe vera is another ancient herbal medicine, with early reports dating back to the 16th century B.C. Over the centuries, it has been bestowed with nearly magical powers to rejuvenate, heal, and soothe; unfortunately these claims do not always stand up to rigorous scrutiny (Ernst, 2000; Marshall, 2000).

Aloe vera gel contains numerous potential active ingredients, including salicylic acid, magnesium lactate, and gel polysaccharides. These components may result in anti-inflammatory activities via thromboxane and prostaglandin pathway inhibition, antipruritic capabilities and anti-inflammatory capabilities via immunomodulation respectively (Wu, 2008).

There are conflicting data for the efficacy of aloe in the treatment of wounds. Some studies show that it promotes the rates of healing (Davis et al., 1989; Heggers et al., 1997), others that it causes slower wound healing compared to conventional therapy (Kaufman et al., 1988; Schmidt & Greenspoon, 1991).

Most of the human clinical data for aloe come from its use as an anti-inflammatory and antipruritic for patients with atopic dermatitis and psoriasis. Results in psoriasis were conflicting. One study of 30 patients showed significant improvement in Psoriasis Area and Severity Index (PASI) scores with aloe compared to placebo (Syed et al., 1996), whereas another showed placebo to be superior (Paulsen et al., 2005).

Because of its analgesic, antipruritic, and anti-inflammatory properties, aloe could potentially improve the symptomatology of rosacea in some patients (Bedi & Shenefelt, 2002; Feily & Namazi, 2009). Additionally, in a study on rats with burn wounds, application of aloe produced significant reduction in vasodilatation, suggesting the possibility of reducing erythema in rosacea (Somboonwong et al., 2000).

CHAMOMILE

Chamomile (*Matricaria recutita* and *Chamaemelum nobile*) has been used historically for its soothing effects. Paradoxically, it can be a potent skin sensitizer as it is a member of the ragweed family; therefore, it must be recommended with caution. Chamomile contains terpenoids and flavonoids that have been shown to inhibit cyclooxygenase and lipoxygenase as well as histamine release, therefore suggesting antioxidant, anti-inflammatory, and antipruritic effects (Lee et al., 2010; Merfort et al., 1994). Studies in skin irritation and atopic dermatitis have shown efficacy, with one study showing its anti-inflammatory effect to be nearly 60% that of hydrocortisone 0.25% (Albring et al., 1983).

A cream containing a 1% extract of golden chamomile (*Chrysanthellum indicum*) was studied in 246 patients with moderate rosacea (Rigopoulos et al., 2005). In this randomized, placebo-controlled trial, patients applied the cream twice daily for 12 weeks. Erythema and overall rosacea severity were assessed by the investigator and patients every four weeks. Erythema and overall rosacea severity were significantly reduced ($p < 0.05$) in the treatment group compared to baseline and placebo. Adverse reactions were mild and similar to placebo.

SOY

Soy (*Glycine max*) has anti-inflammatory, antioxidant, moisturizing, and cleansing properties that may be helpful for patients with rosacea, particularly due to its known tolerability for patients with sensitive skin. There are numerous actives in soy that might be beneficial in rosacea. Soybeans are high in protein (38% to 45% by weight) and oils (20% by weight), of which many are fatty acids and phytosterols. Active ingredients include unsaturated fatty acids, soy lipids, lecithin, and phytosterols, which act as moisturizers and provide barrier protection (Baumann et al., 2009). Vitamins A and E act as antioxidants. Large soy proteins have been shown to soften the skin and saponins are gentle cleansers (Liu et al., 2001).

WITCH HAZEL

Witch hazel contains tannins as its primary active ingredient. It has anti-inflammatory activity and may reduce UV-induced erythema. It has not been studied in rosacea (Brown & Dattner, 1998).

Agents That May Improve Dermal Structural Components

Several substances have shown the ability in both in vitro and in vivo studies to alter collagen, elastin, and ground substance in the skin (Box 23.6).

Box 23.6 Promotion of Dermal Health

Pomegranate (increases collagen and decreases MMP-1)
Vitamin C (increased collagen and elastin)
Retinoids (fibroblast proliferation, increased collagen, decreased MMP)
Soy (collagen synthesis)
CoffeeBerry (upregulates collagen production, decreases MMPs)

Considering that rosacea is an inflammatory disorder that results in chronic, ongoing dermal matrix degradation, it stands to reason (although studies are thin) that improving dermal health might improve rosacea signs and symptoms. Vitamin C has been shown to increase collagen and elastin, and soy to increase collagen synthesis. Pomegranate has been shown to stimulate fibroblasts, increase collagen, and decrease MMP-1. CoffeeBerry has been shown to upregulate collagen production and decrease MMPs. It is the retinoids, however, that have the most promise in this regard.

VITAMIN A

Vitamin A is a general term for several compounds, including retinol, retinal, and the carotenoids, including beta-carotene. Retinoids are natural and synthetic derivatives of vitamin A that are lipid-soluble and able to penetrate the epidermis (Sorg et al., 2005). Prescription retinoids include retinoic acid and the synthetic naphthalene derivatives adapalene and tazarotene. Cosmeceutical retinoids include retinyl esters, retinol, retinaldehyde, and the oxoretinoids.

Within the skin, retinol is oxidized into retinaldehyde, which in turn is oxidized into retinoic acid, the biologically active form of vitamin A (Draelos, 2005b; Sorg et al., 2006). It is believed that the efficacy of both retinol and retinaldehyde is related to the conversion into retinoid acid. It appears that the percutaneous absorption profile, however, is as important as its metabolism. Once again, without penetration through the stratum corneum, topical agents are unable to live up to their potential.

Retinoids have an impressive array of activities within the skin. They are potent antioxidants by virtue of their ability to scavenge free radicals (Rittie et al., 2006; Sorg et al., 2005). However, it is in their protean ways of altering the structural components of the dermis that they have their most intriguing potential effects in anti-aging and rosacea. Topical application of retinoic acid has been shown to increase fibroblast and keratinocyte proliferation, increase collagen and extracellular matrix production, and modulate cellular differentiation (Rittie et al., 2006; Sorg et al., 2005; Varani et al., 1998). An increase in MMPs has been demonstrated in rosacea, and retinoids have been shown to decrease MMP-mediated extracellular matrix degradation (Kanada et al., 2012; Rittie et al., 2006; Sorg et al., 2005).

Although prescription retinoids have been shown to have potential efficacy in ETR and PPR, retinoic acid is often too irritating, especially in the patients with ETR who often complain of "sensitive skin" (Chang et al., 2012). Retinol and retinaldehyde are gentler yet still potentially effective alternatives.

There are no in vivo data for the use of topical retinoids in rosacea, but ETR in particular bears a striking histological resemblance to aging skin, for which retinoid data abound (Del Rosso, 2002; Kafi et al., 2007). In combination with hydroquinone 4%, retinol 0.3% was found to be as efficacious as prescription tretinoin 0.05% cream in 41 women with mild to moderate photodamaged skin (Del Rosso, 2002). In a placebo-controlled study of 87 elderly patients, application of retinol 0.4% lotion to the forearm resulted in improvement in fine wrinkle scores (Kafi et al., 2007). Histology of the treated skin showed an increase in glycosaminoglycan and procollagen I. In another randomized, double-blind, controlled study comparing a tri-retinol 1.1% cream to prescription 0.025% tretinoin cream on the face of 34 women with mild to moderate photodamage, both products were equally effective with minimal side effects (Ho et al., 2012).

Photoprotectants

Heightened sensitivity to sunlight is one of the most common triggers reported by rosacea patients. Additionally, biopsies of rosacea, particularly ETR, bear a striking resemblance to chronically sun-damaged skin. This sometimes poses a clinical dilemma as well. Sun protection, then, is an important part of rosacea therapy. The easily irritated skin of rosacea patients is often intolerant of commercial sunscreens, so complementary alternatives are attractive alternatives (Box 23.7). Many of the active agents mentioned in this chapter have

Box 23.7 Photoprotection

Vitamin C
Vitamins E, C, ferulic acid
Soy
Pycnogenol
CoffeeBerry
Tea
Polypodium leucotomas
Pomegranate

potential efficacy in photoprotection. As mentioned in detail in the text above, Vitamins C and E, soy, pycnogenol, CoffeeBerry, green tea, pomegranate, and *Polypodium leucotomas*have all been shown to have in vitro or in vivo data supporting their efficacy either as stand-alone photoprotectants or in combination with each other or chemical and physical sunblocks. At the present time, however, the sun protection factor offered by these products is insufficient to recommend them as routine sun protectants.

POLYPODIUM LEUCOTOMAS

Polypodium leucotomas is a species of fern found in Central America. There are numerous phenolic compounds contained within the plant that have antioxidant and photoprotective properties.(Gombau et al., 2006; Middelkamp-Hup et al., 2004) In a small study of nine patients with Fitzpatrick skin types I and II, ingestion of 7.5 mg/kg of *P. leucotomas* extract resulted in a significant reduction in UV-induced erythema (Middelkamp-Hup et al., 2004). Biopsy of the UV-exposed skin showed fewer sunburn cells, less vasodilation, and a reduction in other signs of UV-induced injury. It is untested in rosacea per se, but based on the in vitro findings, it may have merit in photoprotection and erythema reduction.

Basic Skin Care

Regardless of which products are used, prescription or not, no rosacea visit is complete without a complete discussion of skin care products. Patients must avoid products that may exacerbate their condition or irritate their sensitive skin. This includes the ubiquitous alpha and beta hydroxyacids, retinoids, toners and astringents, detergent soaps, and most notably topical steroids often recommended by pharmacists.

Choice of a barrier repair product is recommended as it will improve the symptoms of irritated skin and also allow the more consistent use of medications, sunscreens, or complementary products. Bathing instructions should include recommendations for mild, synthetic detergent soaps that are fragrance-free and avoidance of hot water, washcloths, and physical and chemical exfoliants. Physical sunblocks are often less irritating than chemical sunscreens, or patients may find the application of a barrier repair cream prior to sunscreen use to be helpful.

Many patients chose to apply concealers to improve their appearance. Often these products are similarly too irritating for consistent use. Several studies have shown that the use of camouflage techniques improves confidence, the sense of well-being, and the quality of life of patients (Baldwin, 2010; Cotterill & Cunliffe, 1997; Nicholson et al., 2007; Seite et al., 2012). General recommendations for camouflage products include the avoidance of heavy cosmetics that will require scrubbing to remove, the use of green-tinted concealers to neutralize redness, and the use of matte-finish cosmetics, which tend to cause less irritation than those with shine and shimmer.

Conclusion

Patients with rosacea have a chronic, life-affecting condition, the extent of which we are only beginning to define. Like many patients with visible deformities, they face daily problems with self-esteem, public reaction, and professional disability.

As our understanding of the pathophysiology of rosacea has crystallized, we have come to recognize that inflammation, neurovascular regulation, barrier dysfunction, and oxidative damage play important roles. This has led to a better understanding of the mechanism of action of many of the medications that we have used for years—because we had found that they worked, not because we understood why. Similarly, we are learning that many botanicals and other complementary agents have roles in reducing inflammation, hypersensitivity, oxidative damage, barrier dysfunction, and neurovascular dysregulation.

As adjuncts or as monotherapy, rosacea patients are asking for additional remedies for their condition. This may be due to disappointment with efficacy (primarily in ETR), or dismay and fear regarding the long-term use of medications that this chronic condition requires. Others just prefer a more natural approach.

Clearly, vigorous evidence-based literature supporting the use of natural products in rosacea is lacking, and we look forward to more rigorous trials in the future. In the meantime, many products have sound scientific rationales and good in vitro data that warrant their use while we await more conclusive data.

REFERENCES

Albring, M., et al. (1983). The measuring of the anti-inflammatory effect of a compound on the skin of volunteers. *Methods & Findings of Experimental & Clinical Pharmacology, 5,* 575–577.

Aslam, M., Lansky, E., & Varani, J. (2006). Pomegranate as a cosmeceutical source: pomegranate fractions promote proliferation and procollagen synthesis and inhibit matrix metalloproteinase-1 production in human skin cells. *Journal of Ethnopharmacology, 103*(3), 311–318.

Ayer, V., Tewodros, W., Manoharan, A., et al. (2007).Tetracycline resistance in group A streptococci: emergence on a global scale and influence on multiple-drug resistance. *Antimicrobial Agents & Chemotherapy, 51*, 1865–1868.

Baldwin, H. (2006). Oral therapy for rosacea. *Journal of Drugs in Dermatology, 5*, 16–21.

Baldwin, H. (2010). A community-based study of the effectiveness of doxycycline 40 mg (30-mg immediate-release and 10-mg delayed-release beads) on quality of life and satisfaction with treatment in participants with rosacea. *Cutis, 86*(5 Suppl), 26–36.

Basketter, D., & Griffiths, H. (1993). A study of the relationship between susceptibility to skin stinging and skin irritation. *Contact Dermatitis, 29*(4), 185–188.

Baumann, L. (2007a). Less-known botanical cosmeceuticals. *Dermatologic Therapy, 20*, 330–342.

Baumann, L. (2007b). Organic skin care. *Skin & Allergy News, 38*, 25.

Baumann, L., & Spencer, J. (1999). The effects of topical vitamin E on the cosmetic appearance of scars. *Dermatologic Surgery, 25*, 311–315.

Baumann, L., Wollery-Lloyd, H., & Friedman, A. (2009). "Natural" ingredients in cosmetic dermatology. *Journal of Drugs in Dermatology, 8*, s5–s9.

Bedi, M., & Shenefelt, P. (2002). Herbal therapy in dermatology. *Archives of Dermatology, 138*, 232–242.

Berg, M., & Liden, S. (1989). An epidemiological study of rosacea. *Acta Dermatologica Venereologica, 69*(5), 419–423.

Berson, D. (2008). Natural antioxidants. *Journal of Drugs in Dermatology, 7*, s7–s12.

Bevins, C., & Liu, F. (2007). Rosacea: skin innate immunity gone awry? *Nature Medicine, 13*, 904–906.

Blazso, G., et al. (2004). Pycnogenol accelerates wound healing and reduces scar formation. *Phytotherapy Research, 18*, 579–581.

Brown, D., & Dattner, A. (1998). Phytotherapeutic approaches to common dermatologic conditions. *Archives of Dermatology, 134*(11), 1401–1404.

Burgess, C. (2008). Topical vitamins. *Journal of Drugs in Dermatology, 7*(7), s2–6.

Burke, K. (2004). Photodamage of the skin: protection and reversal with topical antioxidants. *Journal of Cosmetic Dermatology, 3*, 149–155

Camouse, M., et al. (2005). Protective effects of tea pholyphenols and caffeine. *Expert Reviews Anticancer Therapy, 5*, 1061–1068.

Centers for Disease Control & Prevention (2011). Preserving antibiotics for the future. Available at http://www.cdc.gov/getsmart/healthcare/learn-from-others/factsheets/preserve-future.html. Updated November 4, 2011. Accessed January 2013.

Chang, A., et al. (2012). A randomized, double-blind, placebo-controlled, pilot study to assess the efficacy and safety of clindamycin 1.2% and tretinoin 0.025% combination gel for the treatment of acne rosacea over 12 weeks. *Journal of Drugs in Dermatology, 11*(3), 333–339.

Chiu, A., et al. (2005). Double-blinded, placebo-controlled trial of green tea extracts in the clinical and histologic appearance of photoaging skin. *Dermatologic Surgery, 31*, 855–860.

Christman, J., Fix, D., Lucus, S., et al. (2012). Two randomized, controlled, comparative studies of the stratum corneum integrity benefits of two cosmetic niacinamide/glycerin body moisturizers vs conventional body moisturizers. *Journal of Drugs in Dermatology*, *11*(1), 22–29.

Cohen, A., & Tiemstra, J. (2002). Diagnosis and treatment of rosacea. *Journal of the American Board of Family Practice*, *46*, 584–587.

Cotterill, J., & Cunliffe, W. (1997). Suicide in dermatological patients. *British Journal of Dermatology*, *137*, 246–250.

Davis, R., Leitner, M., Russo, J., et al. (1989). Wound healing. Oral and topical activity of Aloe vera. *Journal of the American Podiatric Medicine Association*, *79*(11), 559–562.

Del Rosso, J. (2002). Feature: topical retinoid therapy. *Skin Aging*, *10*, 50–62.

Del Rosso, J., Baldwin, H., Webster, G. (2008). American Acne and Rosacea Society rosacea medical management guidelines. *Journal of Drugs in Dermatology*, *7*, 531–533.

Del Rosso, J., Gallo, R. L., et al. (2012). Why is rosacea considered to be an inflammatory disorder? The primary role, clinical relevance and therapeutic correlations of abnormal innate immune response in rosacea-prone skin. *Journal of Drugs in Dermatology*, *11*(6), 694–700.

Del Rosso, J., & Leyden, J. (2007). Status report on antibiotic resistance: implications for the dermatologist. *Dermatologic Clinics*, *25*, 127–132.

Del Rosso, J., Leyden, J., Thiboutot, D., et al. (2008). Antibiotic use in acne vulgaris and rosacea: clinical considerations and resistance issues of significance to dermatologists. *Cutis*, *82*(2, suppl 2), 5–12.

Ditre, C., et al. (2008). Innovations in natural antioxidants and their role in dermatology. *Cutis*, *82*(6 Suppl), 2–16.

Draelos, Z. (2005a). Assessment of skin barrier function in rosacea patients with a novel 1% metronidazole gel. *Journal of Drugs in Dermatology*, *4*, 557–562.

Draelos, Z. (2005b). Retinoids and cosmetics. *Journal of Cosmetic Dermatology*, *19*(suppl), s3–s5.

Draelos, Z., Ertel, K., & Berge, C. (2005). Niacinamide-containing facial moisturizer improves skin barrier and benefits subjects with rosacea. *Cutis*, *76*, 135–141.

Ekanayake-Mudiyanselage, S., et al. (2005). Vitamin E delivery to human skin by a rinse-off product: penetration of alpha-tocopherol versus wash-out effects of skin surface lipids. *Skin Pharmacology & Physiology*, *18*, 20–26.

Elmets, C., et al. (2001). Cutaneous photoprotection from ultraviolet injury by green tea polyphenols. *Journal of the American Academy of Dermatology*, *44*, 425–432.

Emer, J., Waldorf, H., & Berson, D. (2011). Botanicals and anti-inflammatories: Natural ingredients for rosacea. *Seminars in Cutaneous Medicine & Surgery*, *30*, 148–155.

Erdogan, F., et al. (1996). Efficacy of low-dose isotretinoin in patients with treatment-resistant rosacea. *Archives of Dermatology*, *34*, 1022–1029.

Erdogan, F., et al. (1998). Efficacy of low-dose isotretinoin in patients with treatment-resistant rosacea. *Archives of Dermatology*, *134*, 884–885.

Ernst, E. (2000). Adverse effects of herbal drugs in dermatology. *British Journal of Dermatologu*, *143*, 923–929.

Facino, R., et al. (1995). Echinacoside and caffeoyl conjugates protect collagen from free radical-induced degradations: A potential use of Echinacea extracts in the prevention of skin photodamage. *Planta Medica, 61,* 510–514.

Farris, P. (2005). Topical vitamin C: a useful agent for treating photoaging and other dermatologic conditions. *Dermatologic Surgery, 31,* 814–818.

Farris, P. (2007). Idebenone, green tea and Coffeeberry extract: New and innovative antioxidants. *Dermatologic Therapy, 20,* 322–329.

Feily, A., & Namazi, M. (2009). Aloe vera in dermatology: a brief review. *Giornale Italiano di Dermatologia e Venereologia, 144,* 85–91.

Fleisher, A. (2011). Inflammation in rosacea and acne: implications for patient care. *Journal of Drugs in Dermatology, 10,* 614–620.

Fowler, J., et al. (2010). Innovations in natural ingredients and their use in skin care. *Journal of Drugs in Dermatology, 9*(6), s72–s81.

Fowler, J., et al. (2012). Once-daily topical brimonidine tartrate gel 0.5% is a novel treatment for moderate to severe facial erythema of rosacea: results of two multicenter, randomized and vehicle-controlled studies. *British Journal of Dermatology, 166*(3), 633–641.

Gajardo, J. (1994). Severe rosacea treated with oral isotretinoin. *Revista Médica de Chile, 122*(2), 177–179.

Gehring, W. (2004). Nicotinic acid/niacinaminde and the skin. *Journal of Cosmetic Dermatology, 3*(2), 88–93.

Gombau, L., et al. (2006). *Polypodium leucotomos* extract: antioxidant activity and disposition. *Toxicology In Vitro, 20,* 464–471.

Guilhou, J., Meynadier, J., Guilhou, E., et al. (1978). Treatment of rosacea with metronidazole [in French]. *Nouvelle Presse Medicale, 7,* 1960–1961.

Guo, W., Nie, L., Wu, D., et al. (2010). Avenanthramides inhibit proliferation of human colon cancer cell lines in vitro. *Nutrition & Cancer, 62,* 1007–1016.

Heggers, J., Elzaim, H., Garfield, R., et al. (1997). Effect of the combination of Aloe vera, nitroglycerin and L-NAME on wound healing in the rat excisional model. *Journal of Alternative & Complementary Medicine, 3*(2), 149–153.

Hexsel, D., Orlandi, C., & Zechmeister do Prado, D. (2003). Botanical extracts used in the treatment of cellulite. *Dermatologic Surgery, 31,* 866–872.

Ho, E., et al. (2012). A randomized, double-blind, controlled comparative trial of the anti-aging properties on non-prescription tri-retinol 1.1% vs. prescription tretinoin 0.025%. *Journal of Drugs in Dermatology, 11*(1), 64–69.

Hoting, E., Paul, E., & Plewig, G. (1986). Treatment of rosacea with isotretinoin. *International Journal of Dermatology, 25,* 660–663.

Humbert, P., et al. (2003). Topical ascorbic acid on photoaged skin. Clinical, topographical and ultrastructural evaluation: double-blind study vs. placebo. *Experimental Dermatology, 12,* 237–244.

Iraji, F., & Banan, L. (2010). The efficacy of nicotinamide el 4% as an adjuvant therapy in the treatment of cutaneous erosions of pemphigus vulgaris. *Dermatologic Therapy, 23*(3), 308–311.

Issachaar, N., et al. (1997). pH measurements during lactic acid stinging test in normal and sensitive skin. *Contact Dermatitis, 36,* 152–155.

Iwai, K., et al. (2004). In vitro antioxidative effects and tyrosinase inhibitory activities of seven hydroycinnamoyl derivatives in green coffee beans. *Journal of Agricultural Food Chemistry, 52*, 4893–4898.

Jancin, B. (2007). Less skin care with daily sunscreen use. *Skin & Allergy News, 38*(7), 1.

Jeffrey, C. (2013). *Tanacetum parthenium*. Mansfield's World Database of Agricultural and Horticultural Crops. Available at http://mansfield.ipk-gatersleben.de/pls/hymldb. Accessed January 29, 2013.

Kafi, R., et al. (2007). Improvement of naturally aged skin with vitamin A (retinol). *Archives of Dermatology, 143*, 606–612.

Kanada, K., Nakatsuji, T., & Gallo, R. (2012). Doxycycline indirectly inhibits proteolytic activation of tryptic kallikrein-related peptidases and activation of cathelicidin. *Journal of Investigative Dermatology, 132*(5), 1435–1442.

Katiyar, S., et al. (1995). Protection against ultraviolet-B radiation-induced local and systemic suppression of contact hypersensitivity and edema responses in C3H/HeN mice by green tea polyphenols. *Photochemistry Photobiology, 62*, 855–861.

Katiyar, S., Elmets, C., & Katiyar, S. (2007). Green tea and skin cancer: photoimmunology, angiogenesis and DNA repair. *Journal of Nutrition Biochemistry, 18*, 287–296.

Kaufman, T., et al. (1988). Aloe vera gel hindered wound healing of experimental second-degree burns: a quantitative controlled study. *Burn Care & Rehabilitation, 9*(2), 156–159.

Kolbe, L., et al. (2006). Anti-inflammatory efficacy of Licochalcone A: Correlation of clinical potency and in vitro effects. *Archives of Dermatologic Research, 298*, 23–30.

Kurtz, E., & Wallo, W. (2007). Colloidal oatmeal: history, chemistry and clinical properties. *Journal of Drugs in Dermatology, 6*, 167–170.

Lammintausta, K., & Maibach, H. (1988). Exogenous and endogenous factors in skin irritation. *International Journal of Dermatology, 27*, 213–222.

Lee, S., Heo, Y., & Kim, Y. (2010). Effect of German chamomile oil application on alleviating atopic dermatitis-like immune alterations in mice. *Journal of Veterinary Science, 11*, 35–41.

Lee-Manion, A., Price, R., Strain, J., et al. (2009). In vitro antioxidant activity and antigenotoxic effects of avenanthramides and related compounds. *Journal of Agricultural Food Chemistry, 57*, 10619–10624.

Lin, F-H., et al. (2005). Ferulic acid stabilizes a solution of vitamins C and E and doubles its photoprotection of the skin. *Journal of Investigative Dermatology, 125*, 826–832.

Lin, J-Y., et al. (2003).UV photoprotection by combination topical antioxidants vitamin C and vitamin E. *Journal of the American Academy of Dermatology, 48*, 866–874.

Liu, J-C., et al. (2001). Poster presented at 59th Annual Meeting of the American Academy of Dermatology, March 2–7, 2001, Washington DC.

Lonne-Bahm, S., Fischer, T., & Berg, M. (1999). Stinging and rosacea. *Acta Dermatologica Venereologica, 79*, 460–461.

Marsden, J., Shuster, S., & Neugebauer, M. (1984). Response of rosacea to isotretinoin. *Clinical & Experimental Dermatology, 9*, 484–488.

Marshall, J. (2000). Aloe vera gel: what is the evidence? *Pharmacy Journal, 244*, 360–362.

Martin, K., et al. (2005). Poster presented at 63rd Annual Meeting of the American Academy of Dermatology, February 18–22, 2005, New Orleans, La.

McClellan, K., & Noble, S. (2000). Topical metronidazole. A review of its use in rosacea. *American Journal of Clinical Dermatology, 1*, 191–199.

Merfort, I., et al. (1994). In vivo skin penetration studies of chamomile flavones. *Pharmazie, 49*, 509–511.

Middelkamp-Hup, M. A., et al. (2004).Oral *Polypodium leucotomos* extract decreases ultraviolet-induced damage of human skin. *Journal of the American Academy of Dermatology, 51*, 910–918.

National Rosacea Society. (2010). Rosacea riddle now threatens more than 16 million Americans. Available at http://www.rosacea.org/press/archive/2010030.1.phb

Nebus J., et al. (2005). Poster presented at 63rd Annual Meeting of the American Academy of Dermatology, February 18–22, 2005, New Orleans, La.

Nicholson, K., et al. (2007). A pilot quality-of-life instrument for acne rosacea. *Journal of the American Academy of Dermatology, 57*, 213–221.

Nikolowski, J., & Plewig, G. (1981). Behandlung der Rosacea mit 13-cis-Retinsaure. *Hautarzt, 32*, 575–584.

Niren, N., & Torok, H. (2006). The nicomide improvement in clinical outcomes study (NICOS), results of an 8-week trial. *Cutis, 77*(1 Suppl), 17–28.

Passi, S. (1993). Pharmacology and pharmacokinetics of azelaic acids. *Review of Contemporary Pharmacotherapy, 4*, 7.

Paulsen, E., Korsholm, L., & Brandrup, F. (2005). A double-blind, placebo-controlled study of a commercial Aloe vera gel in the treatment of slight to moderate psoriasis vulgaris. *Journal of the European Academy of Dermatology & Venereology, 19*, 326–331.

Pelle, M., Crawford, G., & James, W. (2004). Rosacea: II. Therapy. *Journal of the American Academy of Dermatology, 51*(4), 499–512.

Pinnell, S., et al. (2005). *Journal of the American Academy of Dermatology, 52*(3), P158. Abstract P2503.

Plewig, G., & Kligman, A. (1993). *Acne and rosacea* (pp. 433–475). Berlin: Springer-Verlag.

Plewig, G., Nikolowski, J., & Wolff, H. (1982). Action of isotretinoin in acne rosacea and gram-negative folliculitis. *Journal of the American Academy of Dermatology, 6*, 766–785.

Powell, F. (2005). Clinical practice. Rosacea. *New England Journal of Medicine, 352*(8), 793–803.

Pye, R., & Burton, J. (1976). Treatment of rosacea by metronidazole. *Lancet, 1*, 1211–1212.

Rebora, A. (2002). The management of rosacea. *Journal of Clinical Dermatology, 3*, 489–496,

Reszko, A., et al. (2009). Cosmeceuticals: practical applications. *Dermatologic Clinics, 27*, 401–416.

Rigopoulos, D., et al. (2005). Randomized placebo-controlled trial of a flavonoid-rich plant extract-based cream in the treatment of rosacea. *Journal of the European Academy of Dermatology & Venereology, 19*(5), 564–568.

Rittie, L., et al. (2006). Retinoid-induced epidermal hyperplasia is mediated by epidermal growth factor receptor activation via specific induction of its ligands heparin-blinding EGF and amphireulin in human skin in vivo. *Journal of Investigative Dermatology, 126,* 732–739.

Rosacea.org/patients/skincare/index.php (accessed Jan. 30, 2013).

Saeedi, M., Morteza-Semnani, K., & Ghoreishi, M. (2003). The treatment of atopic dermatitis with licorice gel. *Journal of Dermatologic Treatment, 14,* 153–157.

Scalbert, A., Johnson, I., & Saltmarsh, M. (2005). Pholyphenols: antioxidants and beyond. *American Journal of Clinical Nutrition, 81,* 215s–217s.

Schmidt, J., et al. (1984). 13-cis-Retinoid acid in rosacea. Clinical and laboratory findings. *Acta Dermato-Venereologica, 64,* 15–21.

Schmidt, J., & Greenspoon, J. (1991). Aloe vera dermal wound gel is associated with a delay in wound healing. *Obstetrics & Gynecology, 78*(1), 115–117.

Seite, S., et al. (2012). Interest of corrective makeup in the management of patients in dermatology. *Clinical & Cosmetic Investigative Dermatology, 5,* 123–128.

Sime, S., & Reeve, V. (2004). Protection from inflammation, immunosuppression and carcinogenesis induced by UV radiation in mice by topical pycnogenol. *Photochemistry & Photobiology, 79,* 193–198.

Sobye, P. (1950). Aetiology and pathogenesis of rosacea. *Acta Dermato-Venereologica, 30*(2), 137–158.

Somboonwong, J., et al. (2000).Therapeutic effects of Aloe vera on cutaneous microcirculation and wound healing in second degree burn model in rats. *Journal of the Medical Association of Thailand, 83,* 417–425.

Sorg, O., et al. (2005). Proposed mechanisms of action for retinoid derivatives in the treatment of skin aging. *Journal of Cosmetic Dermatology, 4,* 237–244.

Sorg, O., et al. (2006). Retinoids in cosmeceuticals. *Dermatologic Therapy, 19,* 289–296.

Southall, M., et al. (2004). Poster presented at 13th Congress of European Academy of Dermatology and Venereology, November 17–21, 2004, Florence, Italy.

Stieger, M. (1979). Metronidazole (Flagyl) as a therapy variant in "rosacea" and in "perioral dermatitis" (preliminary report) [in German]. *Zeitschrift für Hautkrankheiten, 39,* 403–405.

Sur, R., Nigam, A., Grote, D., et al. (2008). Avenanthramides, polyphenols from oats, exhibit anti-inflammatory and anti-itch activity. *Archives of Dermatologic Research, 300,* 569–574.

Syed, D., et al. (2006). Photochemopreventive effect of pomegranate fruit extract on UVA-mediated activation of cellular pathways in normal human epidermal keratinocytes. *Photochemistry & Photobiology, 82*(20), 398–405.

Syed, T., et al. (1996). Management of psoriasis with Aloe vera extract in a hydrophilic cream: A placebo-controlled, double-blind study. *Tropical Medicine & International Health, 1,* 505–509.

Thiele, J., Hsieh, S., & Ekanayake-Mudiyanselage, S. (2005). Vitamin E: critical review of its current use in sociometic and clinical dermatology. *Dermatologic Surgery, 31,* 805–813.

Tierney, N., et al. (2005). Poster presented at 63rd Annual Meeting of the American Academy of Dermatology, February 18–22, 2005, New Orleans, La.

Traber, M. G., & Atkinson, J. (2007). Vitamin E, antioxidant and nothing more. *Free Radicals in Biology & Medicine, 43*(1), 4–15.

Varani, J., et al. (1998). Molecular mechanisms of intrinsic skin aging and retinoid-induced repair and reversal. *Journal of Investigative Dermatology Symposium Proceedings, 3*, 57–60.

Wang, X., & Quinn, P. J. (1999). Vitamin E and its function in membranes. *Progress in Lipids Research, 38*(4), 309–336.

Weber, T., Ceilley, R., Buerger, A., et al. (20).Skin tolerance, efficacy, and quality of life of patients with red facial skin using a skin care regimen containing Licochalcone A. *Journal of Cosmetic Dermatology, 5*(3), 227–232.

Weinberg, J. (2005). The anti-inflammatory effects of tetracyclines. *Cutis, 75* (suppl 4), 6–11.

Wilkin, J. (1994). Rosacea: pathophysiology and treatment. *Archives of Dermatology, 130*, 359–362.

Wilkin, J., Dahl, M., Detmar, M., et al. (2002).Standard classification of rosacea: report of the National Rosacea Society Expert Committee on the classification and staging of rosacea. *Journal of the American Academy of Dermatology, 46*, 584–587.

Wise, R. (2007). Submicrobial doxycycline and rosacea. *Comprehensive Therapy, 33*, 78–81.

Wu, J. (2008). Anti-inflammatory ingredients. *Journal of Drugs in Dermatology, 7*(7), s13–s17.

Yamasaki, K., Di Nardo, A., Bardan, A., et al. (2007).Increased serine protease activity and cathelicidin promotes skin inflammation in rosacea. *Nature Medicine, 13*, 975–980.

Yamasaki, K., & Gallo, R. (2009a). Azelaic acid (AzA) gel 15% decreases kallekrein 5 in epidermal keratinocytes: critical elements in production of cathelicidin and the pathogenesis of rosacea. Paper presented at Fall Clinical Dermatology Conference, October 15–18, 2009, Las Vegas, NV.

Yamasaki, K., & Gallo, R. (2009b). The molecular pathology of rosacea. *Journal of Dermatologic Science, 55*, 77–81.

Yokota, T., et al. (1998). The inhibitory effect of glabridin from licorice extracts on melanogenesis and inflammation. *Pigment Cell Research, 11*, 355–361.

Yusuf, N., et al. (2007). Photoprotective effects of green tea polyphenols. *Photodermatology, Photoimmulology, Photomedicine, 23*, 48–56.

Zhao, J., et al. (1999). Photoprotective effect of black tea extracts against UVB-induced phototoxicity in skin. *Photochemistry & Photobiology, 70*(4), 637–644.

Zuber, T. (2000). Rosacea. *Primary Care, 27*, 309–318.

24

Integrative Management of Seborrheic Dermatitis

REBECCA F. JACOBSON, KACHIU C. LEE, AND PETER A. LIO

Key Concepts

- ♣ Seborrheic dermatitis is an inflammatory papulosquamous condition, predominately found in the sebaceous regions of the body, and affecting some 3% to 5% of the population.
- ♣ While *Malassezia* (*Pityrosporum*) yeasts are thought to be important players in the pathophysiology of seborrheic dermatitis, other associated factors include genetics, stress, diet, and other microbes.
- ♣ Traditional treatments for dandruff include topical antifungals such as ketoconazole, selenium sulfide, and bifonazole, as well as topical corticosteroids and tar preparations.
- ♣ Many complementary and alternative treatments for seborrheic dermatitis have been used, such as oils, plant and animal products, vitamins, homeopathy, and combinations of natural compounds. These continue to undergo research and efficacy studies.

Introduction

Seborrheic dermatitis is an inflammatory papulosquamous condition, predominately found in the sebaceous regions of the body (Morelli et al., 2010). It is common, affecting some 3% to 5% of the population, and presents with red, well-demarcated plaques with greasy scales that can affect the medial eyebrow, glabella, nasolabial folds, and scalp (Pazyar et al., 2012). Common dandruff represents a mild form of seborrheic dermatitis, with flaking or yellow scaling and erythema that occurs on the scalp (Naldi, 2010).

While *Malassezia* (*Pityrosporum*) yeasts are thought to be important players in the pathophysiology of seborrheic dermatitis, other associated factors include genetics, stress, diet, and other microbes (Morelli & Naldi, 2010). Traditional treatments for dandruff include topical antifungals such as ketoconazole, selenium sulfide, and bifonazole, as well as topical corticosteroids and tar preparations (Naldi, 2010).

Reasons for Using Complementary and Alternative Medicine in Seborrheic Dermatitis

There is increasing demand for natural therapies for dermatologic conditions (Buchness, 1998; Satchell et al., 2002). Approximately 35% to 69% of patients with skin diseases have sought out complementary and alternative medicine (CAM; Bhuchar et al., 2012). Given that antifungal medications, including ketoconazole and ciclopirox, are the mainstays of treatment for seborrheic dermatitis, a chronic and incurable condition, there are also an increasing number of cases of antifungal drug resistance and concern over the safety of topical corticosteroid use, especially in the long term. Consequently, alternative treatment modalities are needed (Emtestam et al., 2012).

Evidence-Based Review of CAM in Seborrheic Dermatitis

NATURAL OILS

Tea Tree Oil

Tea tree oil is known to have antibacterial and antifungal qualities. The oil is distilled from the leaves of the Australian *Melaleuca alternifolia* tree and has been tested as a treatment for dandruff (Payzar et al., 2010; Satchell et al., 2002). It is a mixture of almost 100 substances and its antimicrobial action has been linked to the terpinen-4-ol molecule (Satchell et al., 2002). Several studies have specifically demonstrated antifungal action against the *Malassezia* species (Pazyar et al., 2012).

Satchell and colleagues' (2002) randomized, single-blinded, four-week, parallel-group study of 126 patients showed a 41% improvement with daily use of 5% tea tree oil shampoo compared to 11% of the placebo group ($p < 0.001$). Patients also reported improvement in the total area involved, total severity, itchiness, and greasiness of the skin. There were no reported adverse events and the treatment was well tolerated. Ongoing treatment was suggested beyond the four weeks given the high rate of recurrence (Satchell et al., 2002).

Borage Seed Oil

Borage oil is pressed from the seeds of the *Borago officinalis* plant that is found throughout the Middle East and Mediterranean. It contains a high concentration of gamma-linolenic acid (GLA). It is often used, however, without sufficient evidence, for its anti-inflammatory effects (Borage Seed Oil, 2012).

Tollesson and colleagues (1993) proposed that a deficiency in essential fatty acid metabolism, including the production of GLA, is involved in the pathogenesis of infantile seborrheic dermatitis. This was attributed to a malfunction of the enzyme delta-6-desaturase that desaturates linoleic acid to GLA. In a pilot study of 48 children with seborrheic dermatitis, every child's seborrheic dermatitis resolved within 10 to 12 days of daily use of 0.5 mL borage oil therapy in the diaper region (Tollesson et al., 1993). In a follow-up open study, 21 infants with seborrheic dermatitis were also treated in the diaper region with 0.5 mL borage oil that contained 25% GLA; however, this time there was no change in the growth of *Malassezia furfur* compared to healthy individuals (Tollesson et al., 1997). The role of borage oil in the treatment of infantile seborrheic dermatitis remains unclear.

ANIMAL- AND PLANT-BASED PRODUCTS

Aloe Vera

The composition of extract from the aloe vera plant varies depending on the climate and environment where each species grows. Aloe vera extract contains glucose, uric acid, salicylic acid, creatinine, alkaline phosphatase, cholesterol, triglycerides, lactate, calcium, magnesium, zinc, sodium, potassium, and chloride. It has antifungal properties and an inhibitory effect on the growth of fungi such as *Trichophyton mentagrophytes*. It has also been used as a treatment for wounds, burns, frostbite, and ulcers, but there have been limited studies regarding its use as a treatment for seborrheic dermatitis (Klein & Pennesys, 1988). Zawahry and colleagues' (1973) case study of three patients with dandruff and alopecia showed a decrease in scalp oiliness within one week and an improvement of hair loss within a month; however, it was noted that aloe vera had a drying effect on the skin.

Honey

Honey has been used for wound healing, burns, and infected wounds. Its composition differs depending on the type of bees and plants pollinated. The carbohydrate component contributes to its antimicrobial properties. It also contains four phenol compounds that provide its antimicrobial and antioxidant properties. In a randomized study of 30 subjects, all patients who applied a daily 90% honey mixture on the affected areas had complete resolution of symptoms of their seborrheic dermatitis; however, 75% of subjects in the placebo group experienced recurrence of their symptoms (Cherniack, 2010). Outside of a study situation, the properties of honey in a natural form make patient compliance very unlikely, especially when hair-bearing areas such as the scalp are involved.

Homeopathy

Homeopathy remains controversial despite occasionally vigorous debate (Homeopathy Debate Follow-up, 2012). From a scientific standpoint, it is agreed that there is not a single molecule of active ingredient in homeopathic remedies beyond a certain dilution, and, as a positive consequence, no reports of adverse side effects from these medications. Most importantly, there have been inconsistent results in terms of its effectiveness, with skeptics claiming that the placebo effect and publication bias can explain those studies that show an effect. However, homeopathy remains an extremely popular form of CAM that patients use for their skin conditions (Bhuchar et al., 2012).

Smith and colleagues (2002) tested the therapeutic role of a low-dose homeopathic remedy consisting of oral potassium bromide, sodium bromide, nickel sulfate, and sodium chloride in the treatment of seborrheic dermatitis. The mechanism of action of nickel and bromide remains unclear; however, bromide has been shown to be effective in treating psoriasis and appears to have antipruritic effects (Smith et al., 2002).

In a placebo-controlled, randomized, double-blind parallel-group study of 41 patients, the treatment group experienced an approximately 38.5% mean percent change in the Seborrhea Area and Severity Index (SASI) compared to a minus 10.82% mean percent change in the placebo group ($p = 0.02$). The most common adverse outcomes were stomach upset, stomach pain, and nausea, which occurred in 10.4% of the treatment arm compared to 17.7% of placebo patients (Smith et al., 2002).

VITAMINS

Biotin

Biotin is a coenzyme in the pathway that metabolizes carbohydrates, fats, and inorganic molecules. It can be found in foods such as yeast, liver, and egg yolk or produced by intestinal bacteria (Messaritakis 1975).

Messaritakis and colleagues (1975) conducted a 25-patient study where three different groups of infants with seborrheic dermatitis received (1) 5 mg biotin plus vitamin B complex intravenously (IV) over 24 hours; (2) 5 mg biotin IV over two to three hours; or (3) 5 mg biotin IV over one to two minutes. A fourth group received biotin IV plus antibiotics due to a concomitant infection. In 22 out of 25 patients, seborrheic dermatitis improved over five to eight days without any recurrence between 4 and 27 months. The improvement in all groups points to the efficacy of biotin, which was given IV to all subjects in the study (Messaritakis et al., 1975). The lack of a non–biotin-supplemented control group makes these results very difficult to interpret, however.

In addition, Nissen (1972) anecdotally reported that feeding liver and egg yolk, both rich in biotin, to infants during their first few months of life improved their seborrheic dermatitis. Nissen associated this improvement with biotin's role in long-chain fatty acid synthesis and an impairment of fatty acid synthesis in seborrheic dermatitis.

The use of biotin for seborrheic dermatitis, however, has been controversial. The use of biotin was spurred after Gyorgy's studies on rats with biotin deficiency and Nissenson's work with infants with Leiner's disease that improved on biotin. However, others suggest that studies need to first establish the presence of biotin deficiency prior to supplementing biotin in infants (Barness, 1972). Furthermore, a double-blind placebo-controlled study of 16 infants with seborrheic dermatitis found no benefit to daily supplementation with 5 mg of oral biotin over a two-week period: both the treatment group and the placebo group had a similar duration of illness. This suggests that biotin, at least when given orally, does not affect the course of the illness (Erlichman et al., 1981).

Pyridoxine

Pyridoxine is a water-soluble vitamin that is often found in poultry, fish, white potatoes, starchy vegetables, and non-citrus fruits. The recommended daily dosage is 5 ng/mL. It is used for amino acid, carbohydrate, and lipid metabolism ("Pyridoxine," DynaMed, 2012).

A prospective cohort study from 1952 followed four groups of patients who were treated with oral pyridoxine, parental pyridoxine, pyridoxine ointment, or a combination of modalities. In the first group, 11 patients were treated with 300 mg of daily, oral pyridoxine for four weeks without improvement. In the second group, six patients were treated with 600 to 100 mg of daily parenteral pyridoxine for three weeks followed by 10 mg/g of pyridoxine ointment, which resulted in complete clearance over five to 21 days. In the third group, six patients received pyridoxine ointment alone, which cleared their lesions; however, recurrence occurred three to nine weeks later that was treated unsuccessfully with 100 mg parenteral pyridoxine every four hours for four weeks.

In the fourth group of 13 treatment-resistant patients, three patients failed to respond to 50 mg/g of pyridoxine ointment. Overall, topical pyridoxine ointment appears to be more effective in treating seborrheic dermatitis than parenteral pyridoxine. However, this study did not record the amount of topical medication applied to affected areas (Schreiner et al., 1952).

In subsequent Italian and German studies in the 1970s and 1980s, pyridoxine was used to treat seborrheic dermatitis. Since that time, there have not been any English-based articles regarding this topic (Morelli et al., 2010). Consequently, the role and efficacy of pyridoxine as a treatment for seborrheic dermatitis remain unclear.

Other Molecules

CINNAMIC ACID

Cinnamaldehyde and cinnamic alcohol are two chemicals that are commonly used as part of the European Standard "Fragrance Mix." They are also potent contact sensitizers, including the derivative cinnamic acid (Cheung et al., 2003).

Baroni and colleagues (2000) performed an in vitro study on mycotic growth using cultivated *Malassezia* yeast in a cinnamic acid- or cinnamaldehyde-containing suspension. There was a greater than 50% decline in mycotic growth using 0.005 g/dL of cinnamic acid and cinnamaldeyde compared to controls. At a greater concentration of 0.5 g/dL there was no mycotic growth after 30 minutes. Lower concentrations, including 0.01 g/dL, were shown to have a similar reducing effect (80% reduction) as a higher 0.05-g/dL concentration over 40 minutes. Despite these results, cinnamic acid is more likely to be used than cinnamaldehyde in anti-dandruff cosmetic products because it has fewer allergenic properties (Baroni et al., 2000).

In addition, this group found that reducing the pH and increasing the ionic strength of the environment can lead to growth inhibition; buffered acidic shampoos and lotions were thought to be an alternative antimycotic treatment (Baroni et al., 2000). However, further testing is needed to substantiate and update these relatively dated studies.

UREA, LACTIC ACID, AND PROPYLENE GLYCOL (K301)

K301 is a topical mixture of urea, lactic acid, and propylene glycol with small amounts of glycerol and water that has been used for seborrheic dermatitis. Propylene glycol, lactic acid, and urea have been proven to inhibit bacterial and fungal growth. In addition, urea has keratolytic and possible antipruritic properties. Lactic acid is used for its hydrating characteristics and propylene glycol is a keratolytic that may be effective in treating seborrheic dermatitis. In addition, the combination K301, unlike medicated antifungals, is less likely to induce resistance to treatment (Emtestam et al., 2012).

Emtestam and colleagues (2012) conducted a two-part randomized, double-blind, placebo-controlled multicenter study to test the efficacy of K301 in treating seborrheic dermatitis. In the first treatment group (Study 1), 83 patients received once-daily K301 for four weeks followed by four weeks of maintenance therapy three times per week. In the second treatment arm (Study 2), 195 patients received once-daily K301 for four weeks. Compared to placebo, both studies showed an improvement in mean desquamation scores at four weeks (Study 1, 1.9 placebo vs. 1.3 K301; Study 2, 1.7 placebo vs. 1.3 K301; $p < 0.05$) The most common adverse side effects included a burning sensation, pruritus, or erythema. These adverse events were more common in Study 1 (22–25% K301 vs. 23% placebo) than in Study 2 (16% K301 vs. 9% placebo) (Emtestam et al., 2012). Given that this is the only study to date on K301, further studies are needed to confirm these results.

PETROLATUM, SODIUM CHLORIDE, AND PHENOL

A liquid combination of petrolatum, sodium chloride, and phenol (<1%) was reported in a 1950s case series as an alternative topical therapy for seborrheic dermatitis, psoriasis, and atopic dermatitis. A total of 86 patients, nine of whom had seborrheic dermatitis, applied the mixture to the scalp daily for six to 20 weeks. Five of the six patients had a 75% to 100% subjective improvement, and the remainder of the patients showed no improvement or were lost to follow-up. Patients with seborrheic dermatitis did not report any side effects; however, nine psoriatic and atopic patients reported excess oiliness, pruritus, or burning. Relapses were also common once the liquid was discontinued (Sulzberger & Obadia, 1956). Given the limited scope, lack of follow-up, and isolated nature of this study, further research is needed on this combination.

Conclusion

There are many potential CAM treatments for seborrheic dermatitis, such as oils, plant and animal products, homeopathy, and combinations of natural compounds. However, given that many of these studies are anecdotal or singular in nature, further research is needed to evaluate the effectiveness of these treatments.

REFERENCES

Barness, L. A. (1972). Reply to the editor: Treatment of seborrheic dermatitis with biotin and vitamin B complex. *Journal of Pediatrics, 81*(3), 631.

Baroni, A., De Rosa, R., De Rosa, A., et al. (2000). New strategies in dandruff treatment: growth control of *Malassezia ovalis. Dermatology, 201*, 332–336.

Bhuchar, S., Katta, R., & Wolf, J. (2012). Complementary and alternative medicine in dermatology: an overview of selected modalities for the practicing dermatologist. *American Journal of Clinical Dermatology, 13*(5), 311–317.

Borage Seed Oil. In: *Natural Standard.* Available at http://www.naturalstandard.com. ezproxy.umassmed.edu/databases/sports/all/borageseedoil.asp (accessed 12/30/12).

Buchness, M. R. (1998). Alternative medicine and dermatology. *Seminars in Cutaneous Medicine & Surgery, 17*(4), 284–290.

Cherniack, E. P. (2010). Bugs as drugs, Part 1: Insects. The "new" alternative medicine for the 21st century? *Alternative Medicine Review, 15*(2), 124–135.

Cheung, C., Hotchkiss, S. A., & Smith Please, C. K. (2003). Cinnamic compound metabolism in human skin and the role metabolism may play in determining relative sensitization potency. *Journal of Dermatologic Science, 31*(1), 9–19.

Emtestam, L., Svensson, A., & Rensfeldt, K. (2012). Treatment of seborrhoeic dermatitis of the scalp with a topical solution of urea, lactic acid, and propylene glycol (K301): results of two double-blind, randomized, placebo-controlled studies. *Mycoses, 55*, 393–403.

Erlichman, M., Goldstein, R., Levi, E., et al. (1981). Infantile flexural seborrhoeic dermatitis. Neither biotin nor essential fatty acid deficiency. *Archives of Diseases of Childhood, 56*, 560–562.

Homeopathy Debate Follow-up: Andre Saine & Joe Schwarcz (2012). In McGill Blogs, Office of Science and Society. Available at http://blogs.mcgill.ca/oss/2012/12/20/homeopathy-debate-follow-up-andre-saine-joe-schwarcz/ (accessed January 5, 2013).

Klein, A. D., & Pennesys, N. S. (1988). Aloe vera. *Journal of the American Academy of Dermatology, 18*, 714–720.

Messaritakis, J., Kattamis, C., Karabula, C., et al. (1975). Generalized seborrhoeic dermatitis: clinical and therapeutic data of 25 patients. *Archives of Disease in Childhood, 50*, 871–874.

Morelli, V., Calmet, E., & Jhingade Varalakshmi. Alternative therapies for common dermatologic disorders, Part 1. *Primary Care Clinical Office Practice, 37.* 269–283.

Naldi, L. (2010). Seborrheic dermatitis. *Clinical Evidence (Online),* 1713.

Nissen, A. (1972). Treatment of seborrheic dermatitis with biotin and vitamin B complex. *Journal of Pediatrics, 81*(3), 630–631.

Pazyar, N., Yaghoobi, R., Bagherani, N., et al. (2012). A review of the applications of tea tree oil in dermatology. *International Journal of Dermatology (Online),* 1–7.

Pyridoxine (2012). *DynaMed.* Available at http://search.ebscohost.com/login.aspx?direct=true&site=DynaMed&id=113862

Satchell, A. C., Saurajen, A., Bell, C., et al. (2002). Treatment of dandruff with 5% tea tree oil shampoo. *Journal of the American Academy of Dermatology, 47*(6), 852–855.

Schreiner, A. W., Rockwell, E., & Vilter, R. W. (1952). A local defect in the metabolism of pyridoxine in the skin of persons with seborrheic dermatitis of the "Sicca" type. *Journal of Investigative Dermatology, 19*(2), 95–96.

Smith, S. A., Baker, A. E., & Williams, Jr. J. H. (2002). Effective treatment of seborrheic dermatitis using a low dose, oral homeopathic medication consisting of potassium bromide, sodium bromide, nickel sulfate, and sodium chloride in a double-blind, placebo-controlled study. *Alternative Medicine Review, 7*(1), 59–67.

Sulzberger, M. B., & Obadia, J. (1956). A modified liquid petrolatum preparation: Its use in the management of certain common dermatoses of the scalp. *AMA Archives of Dermatology, 73*(4), 373–375.

Tollesson, A., Frithz, A., & Stenlund, K. (1997). *Malassezia furfur* in infantile seborrheic dermatitis. *Pediatric Dermatology, 14*(6), 423–425.

Tollesson, A., & Frithz, A. (1993). Borage oil, an effective new treatment for infantile seborrheoic dermatitis. *British Journal of Dermatology, 129*(1), 95.

Zawahry, M. E., Hegazy, M. R., & Helal, M. (1973). Use of aloe in treating leg ulcers and dermatoses. *International Journal of Dermatology, 12*(1), 68–73.

25

Integrative Management of Skin Cancer

ROBERT A. NORMAN

Key Concepts

♣ The most common type of cancer in the United States is skin cancer, and the incidence of skin cancer is steadily rising.

♣ The indoor tanning industry continues to be one of the fastest-growing businesses in America; major studies show that tanning increases the risk of melanoma and non-melanoma skin cancer such as squamous cell carcinoma and basal cell carcinoma.

♣ Various studies have been conducted on the use of tea polyphenols in the treatment and prevention of many types of cancer, including cancer of the skin.

♣ Substances found in plants that may help protect the skin from sun-related damage include apigenin, curcumin, resveratrol, and quercetin.

♣ Foods such as fish, beans, carrots, chard, pumpkin, cabbage, broccoli, and vegetables containing beta-carotene and vitamin C may also help protect skin.

Introduction

The importance of skin cancer research, prevention, and treatment is underscored by the fact that the most common type of cancer in the United States is skin cancer (National Cancer Institute, n.d.). While the mortality due to cancer in the United States is declining, the incidence of skin cancer is steadily rising (Snowden, 2010). This is not surprising given that many years ago the oncological potential of the sun was not well known nor was protection, such as sunscreen,

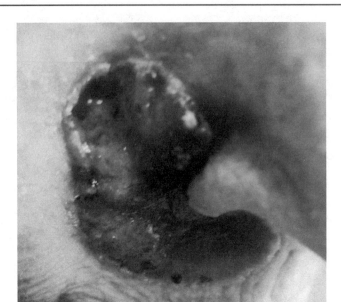

FIGURE 25.1 Basal cell carcinoma

widely promoted. Also, of all of the organs in the human body, the skin is the largest and due to its exterior protection it is more susceptible to environmental exposures (Marieb & Hoehn, 2009). Skin has many types of cells, including squamous, basal, and melanocytes. The three types of skin cancers, squamous cell carcinoma (SCC), basal cell carcinoma (BCC) (Fig. 25.1), and melanoma, are named after the cutaneous cell type that is affected: squamous cells, basal cells, and melanocytes, respectively. In the United States, melanoma is the least common but most fatal type of skin cancer (National Cancer Institute, n.d.).

Skin Cancer Facts

- Skin cancer is the most common form of cancer in the United States. More than 3.5 million cases in two million people are diagnosed annually.
- Each year there are more new cases of skin cancer than the combined incidence of cancers of the breast, prostate, lung, and colon.
- One in five Americans will develop skin cancer in the course of a lifetime.
- BCC is the most common form of skin cancer; an estimated 2.8 million BCCs are diagnosed annually in the United States.

- BCCs are rarely fatal but can be highly disfiguring if allowed to grow.
- SCC is the second most common form of skin cancer. An estimated 700,000 cases are diagnosed each year in the United States, resulting in approximately 2,500 deaths.
- BCC and SCC are the two major forms of non-melanoma skin cancer. Between 40% and 50% of Americans who live to age 65 will have either skin cancer at least once.
- Most BCCs and SCCs occur in chronically sun-exposed areas such as the face, neck, and arms. Melanomas tend to occur more frequently on intermittently sun-exposed areas, such as the back and calves.
- In 2004, the total direct cost associated with the treatment for non-melanoma skin cancers was more than $1 billion.
- About 90% of non-melanoma skin cancers are associated with exposure to ultraviolet (UV) radiation from the sun.
- Up to 90% of the visible changes commonly attributed to aging are caused by the sun.
- Contrary to popular belief, 80% of a person's lifetime sun exposure is not acquired before age 18; only about 23% of lifetime exposure occurs by age 18 (Box 25.1).

Skin Cancer Prevention

From a healthcare perspective, prevention is preferable to cure. This is because when an individual takes steps to prevent a disease, he or she does not have to experience the symptoms of the disease nor have to face the challenge of recovering from the disease, if recovery is even possible. Of course, an individual cannot prevent every disease, but steps can and should be taken to prevent diseases, especially when an individual is at high risk for a disease. The steps of prevention

Box 25.1 Lifetime UV Exposure in the United States*

Ages	Average Accumulated Exposure
1–18	22.73%
19–40	46.53%
41–59	73.7%
60–78	100%

*Based on a 78-year lifespan. Statistics provided by the Skin Cancer Foundation.

do not necessarily guarantee the individual will not get the disease but will reduce the risk of getting it. Due to the various known and undiscovered risk factors for cancer, it should be stressed that prevention only reduces a person's chance of getting cancer and correspondingly lowers the incidence of cancer. Thus, cancer prevention will, it is hoped, also reduce the mortality rate of cancer.

Skin cancer prevention can be approached from two directions: reducing the risk factors associated with skin cancer or increasing the protective factors associated with skin cancer. Certain skin cancer risk factors, such as hereditary traits, are unavoidable, whereas others, such as sun exposure, are avoidable. Even avoidable risk factors are often impossible to avoid all the time, however. For this reason, discovering and promoting protective factors for the development of skin cancer, which may also be beneficial for individuals with unavoidable risk factors, may be a better research approach in the long run. Sunscreen with a Sun Protection Factor (SPF) of at least 15 and protection against both ultraviolet A (UVA) that comes through windows and ultraviolet B (UVB) that is blocked by windows should be applied liberally every two hours during sun exposure and prior to sun exposure. Sunscreens that act as physical blockers, such as titanium or zinc, are effective immediately. Those with darker skin tones can use lower-SPF sunscreens, while fair-skinned individuals and redheads should use at least SPF 35 and in subtropical areas at least SPF 50. Sun-protective clothing is better than sunscreen. Hats with full brims at least three to four inches wide are also recommended.

The National Cancer Institute (n.d.) discusses the risk factors and protective factors associated with skin cancer. They note that risk factors common to all types of skin cancer include male gender, light skin type, smoking, sedentary lifestyle, UV radiation, immunosuppression, increased age, and a high body mass index (BMI). Protective factors include smoking cessation, regular exercise, normal BMI, healthy diet, and antioxidants like polyphenols. The National Cancer Institute (n.d.) notes that some risk factors vary among the different types of skin cancer. The risk factors unique to melanoma, which don't apply to BCC and SCC, are Caucasian race, moles, history of UV burns, and a personal and/or family history of atypical nevi, congenital melanocytic nevi, and melanoma. Researchers have determined the main contributing factor to skin cancer development is UV radiation (LeBlanc et al., 2008), specifically when it causes cutaneous burns. Moreover, Brandon and colleagues (2009) confirm that obesity, defined as a BMI greater than 30 kg/m², increases the size of melanomas.

From a historical perspective, it is essential to look at when melanoma was discovered and/or first diagnosed to see how recent a phenomenon it is and how it has changed with environmental and population changes. Poole and Guerry (2005) note that the first incidence of melanoma was documented in the late 18th century by Dr. John Hunter, a Scottish surgeon. Dr. Hunter preserved the affected tissue, and in the late 1960s, it was confirmed as melanoma. Almost two decades after Dr. Hunter's discovery Dr. René Laennec, a French doctor, categorized melanoma as a skin cancer (Poole & Guerry, 2005). This illustrates the fact that melanoma has been noted in patients for hundreds of years. Recently there has been more awareness of melanomas, with more being diagnosed in earlier and more likely curable stages.

In the United States, the risk of being diagnosed with melanoma over one's lifetime in 1965 was 1 out of 600 people. The risk grew steadily and reached 1 out of 150 people just 20 years later. This distressing risk keeps increasing, and by the end of 2010, the estimated risk is 1 out of 50 people (Curiel-Lewandrowski, 2010). Comparing these risks clearly shows the increasing number of diagnosed melanoma cases since 1965, a disturbing trend that may continue to increase to alarming numbers without increased prevention efforts. Shanklin (2010) discusses the fact that the majority of the UV radiation reaching humans is blocked by the ozone layer. Additionally, the protective effects of the ozone layer against UV radiation have diminished as the ozone hole has grown to an alarming size (Shanklin, 2010). The effects of this environmental catastrophe, which are not yet fully realized, are going to bolster an already alarming trend in primary cutaneous melanoma development.

The National Cancer Institute (n.d.) gives an estimate of 68,130 for the number of newly diagnosed cases of melanoma in the United States in 2010, with a much higher incidence among the Caucasian male population. They also note that the incidence of melanoma is tenfold more common in Caucasians than in African Americans. MacKie, Hauschild, and Eggermont (2009) discuss an odd statistic that they found: a higher prevalence of melanoma among the wealthy. Additionally, melanoma is not specific to any age group and even occurs in young individuals, but its incidence does increase with age (American Cancer Society, 2010). The American Cancer Society (2010) notes that melanoma accounts for only about 5% of skin cancer cases, but a majority of all skin-cancer related deaths are due to melanoma. The 2010 estimation for the number of deaths from melanoma in the United States is 8,700 (National Cancer Institute, n.d.).

It is also valuable to examine the trends of melanoma to evaluate the need for research on this topic and possible risk factors. The recent trend in the United States has shown an increasing incidence of melanoma, which has recently been more prominent in young Caucasian women and older Caucasian men (American Cancer Society, 2010). At first appearance, the trend in the melanoma fatality rate is deceiving, but that is because the trend needs to be viewed as deaths in the population younger or older than age 50 years. The American Cancer Society (2010) discusses that among the population younger than 50 years old there is a decreasing death rate from melanoma, whereas in the population older than 50 years old the rate has possibly increased.

The indoor tanning industry continues to be one of the fastest-growing businesses in America. Why do so many people subject their skin to artificial rays to get a tan? With so many research studies linking UV radiation with skin cancer risks, it might be a good time to close the doors on the "Fake 'n' Bake." According to studies from the American Academy of Dermatology and the U.S. Department of Health & Human Services, tanning increases the risk of melanoma and non-melanoma skin cancer such as SCC and BCC. Tanning increases your rate of skin cancer by 75%—tanning beds are a carcinogen like cigarettes. The excessive exposure to UV radiation during indoor tanning leads to skin aging, immune suppression, and eye damage, including cataracts and ocular melanoma. Yet more than one million people tan in tanning salons on an average day, nearly 70% of them girls and women aged 16 to 29. Almost two million of these patrons are considered "tanning junkies," with almost 100 tanning parlor visits per year.

Research Questions

The number of clinical trials aimed at preventing melanoma is insufficient, especially when taking into account the mortality rate associated with this deadly cancer. According to the National Cancer Institute (n.d.), there are only two clinical trials researching melanoma prevention at this time. The first clinical trial is evaluating a new intervention for melanoma prevention. The trial is examining the role of an anti-inflammatory compound derived from the bark of plants in the prevention of melanoma. The intervention is aimed at treating dysplastic nevi, which are melanoma precursors. The other clinical trial is examining a new tool, a computer program, in physician education on what to look for and how to counsel patients about skin cancer. The National Cancer Institute (n.d.) also shows that there are 308 trials examining the diagnosis and treatment of melanoma. This implies there is 154 times more diagnosis and treatment trials as there are prevention trials. This underscores the need for encouraging more clinical trials for melanoma prevention. One of the goals of research would be to determine the possible efficacy of the use of polyphenols in cutaneous melanoma prevention.

Significance of the Research

The modern version of the Hippocratic Oath, revised by Dr. Louis Lasagna, asserts that it is better to prevent a disease rather than treat it (Association of American Physicians and Surgeons, n.d.). This underlines the importance of determining preventive measures in order to educate patients on the steps that can be taken to avoid an unfortunate path, especially when patients are at higher risk than the general population for developing a disease. This research will be beneficial for everyone since it is almost impossible to prevent sun exposure, but it will be most useful for individuals with genetic predispositions for developing precancerous lesions or melanoma. Others who will greatly benefit from this research are those who have to work outdoors, such as postal workers and farmers, or for those who partake in outdoor hobbies, such as surfing, sailing, or golfing. With the progression of easy global and local transport, the average amount of sun exposure throughout an individual's lifetime will most likely increase. This will increase the likelihood of injuring cutaneous tissue and possibly increase the incidence of melanoma. It is for this reason and many others that there needs to be a push for more activity in the arena of primary cutaneous melanoma prevention. More prevention methods will, we hope, be engendered by research efforts such as this, which will eventually have the potential to reduce the incidence and mortality rate of melanoma.

According to the Skin Cancer Foundation, men have nearly double the rates of SCC and BCC that women have. With melanoma, the deadliest type of skin cancer, men have the highest chances of dying of the disease.

Why men? Men get more UV exposure because of their jobs, use sunscreen less, have higher rates of sunburn, and get later detection of skin cancer. Certain animal studies suggest that male skin may offer less innate protection from SCC because of an apparent inability to retain adequate amounts of antioxidants. Although the researchers caution that more research is needed to validate the findings, such research could lead to gender-specific sunscreen. Men who work indoors during the week and take their shirts off and wear shorts on the weekend get strong intermittent sun exposure. They are at higher risk than outdoor workers to develop melanoma.

Various studies have been conducted on the use of tea polyphenols in the treatment and prevention of many types of cancer, including cancer of the skin, esophagus, bladder, colorectum, lung, and breast (Arts, 2008; Bouzari et al., 2009; Coyle et al., 2008; Sukhthankar et al., 2008; Velho et al., 2008; Wu et al., 2008). Polyphenols are a class of antioxidants that include tannins and flavonoids (Tangney & Rosenson, 2010) and are found in many plants. New medical research focuses on polyphenol extract from various types of tea. Tea is made from the tea plant (*Camellia sinensis*), and many tea varieties, including green tea and black tea, are derived from this plant (Sivasubramaniam et al., 2009). Teas and their beneficial properties differ in terms of fermentation, processing, and added ingredients. Thus, herbal teas contain different properties because they are derived from herbs, fruits, and flowers but not from the tea plant; they may contain plant polyphenols depending on what herbs are used (Sivasubramaniam et al., 2009).

The multitudes of studies that have been undertaken because the potential for cancer prevention using antioxidants have shown much promise. The current body of evidence to support the recommendation of the use of polyphenols in the field of oncology, specifically primary cutaneous melanoma, is so far insufficient, but the growing incidence of cancer and the need for improved prevention and treatment modalities add to the importance of conducting more research in this field.

Although prevention and polyphenols are keys to working with an integrative approach to skin cancer, many other approaches exist. Although it is hard to test the role of nutrients in preventing various forms of skin cancer, several studies have looked at antioxidants (including vitamin C, vitamin E, beta-carotene, zinc, and vitamin A), folic acid, fats and proteins, and a variety of whole foods. Antioxidants may offer some protection from skin cancer (Asgari et al., 2009a, 2009b; Baglia & Katiyar, 2006). Foods such as fish, beans, carrots, chard, pumpkin, cabbage, broccoli, and vegetables containing beta-carotene and vitamin C may also help protect skin (Birt et al. 1996). Studies on animals suggest that lignans, substances found in foods such as soy and flaxseed, may help fight cancer in general, including the spread of melanoma from one part of the body to another (Bain et al., 1993).

Substances found in plants that may help protect the skin from sun-related damage include apigenin, a flavonoid found in vegetables and fruits, including broccoli, celery, onions, tomatoes, apples, cherries, and grapes, and in tea and wine, curcumin, found in the spice turmeric, resveratrol, found in grape skins, red wine, and peanuts, and quercetin, a flavonoid found in apples and onions.

REFERENCES

Arts, I. C. (2008). A review of the epidemiological evidence on tea, flavonoids, and lung cancer. *Journal of Nutrition, 138,* 1561S–1566S.

Asgari, M. M., Maruti, S. S., Kushi, L. H., et al. (2009a). A cohort study of vitamin D intake and melanoma risk. *Journal of Investigative Dermatology, 129*(7), 1675–1680.

Asgari, M. M., Maruti, S. S., Kushi, L. H., et al. (2009b). Antioxidant supplementation and risk of incident melanomas: results of a large prospective cohort study. *Archives of Dermatology, 145*(8), 879–882.

Baglia, M. S., & Katiyar, S. K. (2006). Chemoprevention of photocarcinogenesis by selected dietary botanicals. *Photochemical & Photobiological Science, 5*(2), 243–253.

Bain, C., Green, A., Siskind, V., et al. (1993). Diet and melanoma: an exploratory case-control study. *Annals of Epidemiology, 3,* 235–238.

Birt, D. F., Pelling, J. C., Nair, S., et al. (1996). Diet intervention for modifying cancer risk. *Progress in Clinical & Biological Research, 395*, 223–234.

Bouzari, N., Romagosa, Y., & Kirsner, R. S. (2009). Green tea prevents skin cancer by two mechanisms. *Journal of Investigative Dermatology, 129*, 1054. doi:10.1038/jid.2009.64

Coyle, C. H., Philips, B. J., Morrisroe, S. N., Chancellor, M. B., & Yoshimura, N. (2008). Antioxidant effects of green tea and its polyphenols on bladder cells. *Life Sciences, 83*, 12–18. doi:10.1016/j.lfs.2008.04.010

Marieb, E. N., & Hoehn, K. (2009). *Human anatomy & physiology* (8th ed.). San Francisco, CA: Pearson Benjamin Cummings.

National Cancer Institute. (n.d.). Melanoma. Retrieved from http://www.cancer.gov

Sivasubramaniam, S., Parrott-Sheffer, C., Singh, S., & the editors of Encyclopaedia Britannica. (2009). Tea. In Encyclopaedia Britannica. Retrieved from http://www.britannica.com/EBchecked/topic/585115/tea

Snowden, R. V. (2010). Annual report: US cancer death rates still declining. Retrieved from http://www.cancer.org/Cancer/news/annual-report-us-cancer-death-rates-still-declining

Sukhthankar, M., Yamaguchi, K., Lee, S., et al. (2008). A green tea component suppresses posttranslational expression of basic fibroblast growth factor in colorectal cancer. *Gastroenterology, 134*, 1972–1980. doi:10.1053/j.gastro.2008.02.095

Tangney, C. C., & Rosenson, R. S. (2010). Lipid lowering with diet or dietary supplements. UpToDate. Retrieved from http://www.uptodate.com.ezproxylocal.library.nova.edu/online/content/topic.do?topicKey=lipiddis/6831&selectedTitle=1~150&source=search_result#H12

Velho, A. V., Hartmann, A. A., & Kruel, C. D. (2008). Effect of black tea in diethylnitrosamine-induced esophageal carcinogenesis in mice. *Acta Cirurgica Brasileira, 23*(4), 329–336.

Wu, A. H., Ursin, G., Koh, W., et al. (2008). Green tea, soy, and mammographic density in Singapore Chinese women. *Cancer Epidemiology, Biomarkers, & Prevention, 17*(12), 3358–3365. doi:10.1158/1055-9965.EPI-08-0132

26

Integrative Management of Stasis Dermatitis

ROBERT A. NORMAN AND PATRICK BRENNAN

Key Concepts

♣ Stasis dermatitis, also known as gravitational eczema, originates from chronic venous insufficiency.

♣ Approximately 7% of older adults, often the obese, experience the disease.

♣ Chronic edema and venous incompetence set the stage for the development of stasis dermatitis.

♣ Doppler ultrasound, sonography, and venography are used as adjunctive diagnostic measures.

♣ Leg elevation, compression stockings, topical steroids and emollients, and aspirin or pentoxifylline may be helpful.

♣ Integrative therapies include horse chestnut tree, calendula, aloe vera, and Unna boots.

♣ Lifestyle changes, including diet, exercise, yoga, and massage, have been found quite useful in the overall plan of improvement.

Introduction

Stasis dermatitis stems from chronic venous insufficiency. Chronic edema and venous incompetence set the stage for the development of stasis dermatitis. Patients often exhibit a history of varicose veins and deep venous thrombosis. Other associated factors are pregnancy, increased blood volume, and increased venocaval pressure. Patients will classically first notice stasis dermatitis in the lower extremities over the medial ankles. The initial presenting symptoms here are erythema and pruritus.

During an acute inflammation stasis dermatitis can mimic cellulitis with evidence of exudate and crusting skin. In the chronic state, stasis dermatitis is known for exhibiting dermal fibrosis. The repetitive exudative extravasation of erythrocytes seen in chronic stasis dermatitis leads to progressive pigmentation of the skin from the hemosiderin deposits. Complications of stasis dermatitis often include secondary infection as well as the maturation of venous stasis ulcers (Fauci et al., 2008; Wolf & Johnson, 2009).

Pathogenesis of Stasis Dermatitis

The chronic venous insufficiency that leads to stasis dermatitis exhibits irregular venous flow patterns. Normally, valves of the deep veins in the calves block the retrograde flow of venous blood. Previous deep vein thrombosis can lead to postthrombotic syndrome and incompetent valves of the deep veins of the lower extremities. Communicating veins that unite the superficial calf veins with the deep veins are also damaged in the setting of chronic venous insufficiency. In this case blood will demonstrate retrograde venous flow from the deep calf veins to the superficial venous plexuses. These irregular flow patterns contribute to the pathogenesis of stasis dermatitis.

Fibrin deposited in the face of this vascular damage also contributes to the disease process. Fibrin is laid down in the extravascular space, causing sclerosis. The microvasculature and lymphatic channels become destroyed and nutrition of the epidermis is compromised. Eventually the epidermis breaks down and venous stasis ulcers arise (Fauci et al., 2008; Wolf & Johnson, 2009).

Clinical Presentation

Patients with stasis dermatitis often present with classic clinical signs of chronic venous insufficiency. They will often complain of aches, pains, and heaviness of the legs. These symptoms are provoked by periods of standing still and are relieved by walking. The use of leg musculature helps pump the blood through these compromised vasculature structures. Edema of the legs is also associated with standing and is worst at the end of the day. Patients' shoes fit tightly by the end of the day as a result of the edema, and they often experience night cramps. The edema often resolves or improves to some degree in the morning after the patient has experienced an extended period of time in a horizontal position while sleeping. This position takes the pressure off the veins with nonfunctional valves (Fauci et al., 2008; Wolf & Johnson, 2009).

Crusted and scaly erosions are often seen around the ankles. Inflammatory papules may be present. Dermal sclerosis may also be present and can be painful and limit ankle movement. Varying degrees of pigmentation is also noticeable due to hemosiderin deposits from old and new hemorrhages. Pruritus associated with stasis dermatitis may lead to excoriations from chronic scratching. Irritant dermatitis may also be simultaneously present as a result of secretions from venous stasis ulcers and bacterial colonization (Fauci et al., 2008, Wolf & Johnson, 2009). Allergic contact dermatitis also develops more frequently in stasis dermatitis areas.

Venous stasis ulcers are a frequent complication of chronic venous stasis and stasis dermatitis. These ulcers are frequently found on the calf, most commonly near the medial malleolus. They are described as irregularly shaped with well-defined borders. They are usually shallow but can be quite large and may involve the entire circumference of the lower leg. Venous stasis ulcers are painful and are usually roofed with necrotic tissue. There is virtually always secondary bacterial colonization, and rarely squamous cell carcinoma can develop from a chronic ulcer (Gyton & Hall, 2006; Wolf & Johnson, 2009).

Laboratory Examinations and Diagnosis

The diagnosis of stasis dermatitis can usually be made with a thorough history and clinical examination. Doppler, color-coded duplex sonography, and venography can also aid in diagnosis.

Venography is a study that uses x-rays to locate thrombi in the venous system. It is performed by injecting dye into the venous system of the examined extremity and then taking x-ray films at timed intervals. Failure of the dye to progress through the venous system indicates an occlusion. In this way, the venous system is visualized for patency. Venography is accurate for diagnosing thrombi below the knee (Pagana & Pagana, 2009).

Doppler ultrasound is useful for detecting the movement of red blood cells within veins. It is able to detect venous occlusion. The characteristic "swish" sound of the patent venous system is absent in the face of venous occlusion. However, the Doppler ultrasound does not provide accurate results for occlusion below the upper calf. A color-coded duplex sonogram allows for a pulsed Doppler probe within the transducer to assess both blood flow velocity and direction. A color is allocated for direction of blood flow within the vessel. The intensity of the color is related to the velocity of the blood traveling in the vessel. Thus, slowing of blood or reversal of its direction can be visualized and venous insufficiency can be detected (Pagana & Pagana, 2006).

Treatment

Stasis dermatitis can be greatly improved by the simple treatment of elevating the leg routinely throughout the course of the day. The use of compression stockings is also beneficial. The stockings should ideally have a minimal gradient of 30 mmHg prescription strength to be effective. However, over-the-counter 20 mmHg stockings are less expensive and are easier to pull on, especially for elderly patients, and are much better than nothing. Mid-potency topical steroids and emollients are also useful. Patients should be instructed to protect the areas from injury and to avoid scratching. The edema may need diuretics for control. When the stasis dermatitis does not respond as readily as expected to treatment, superimposed allergic contact dermatitis should be considered (see Chapter 16 on allergic contact dermatitis).

Venous ulcers can be problematic to treat once they occur. All necrotic tissue that develops over the ulcer should be carefully debrided periodically and covered with a semipermeable compression dressing. Steroids will prolong the healing process of venous ulcers and should not be applied in these areas. Bacteriostatic oral antibiotic therapy should be instituted as all virtually all ulcers will become secondarily infected. Skin grafts may be necessary in the face of chronic ulcers (Fauci et al., 2008; Wolf & Johnson, 2009).

Integrative Approach

Herbal remedies for stasis dermatitis exist. Prepared forms of horse chestnut from the deciduous horse chestnut tree are used by some herbalists to treat venous insufficiency and have been proven to be as effective as compression stockings in double-blind studies in Europe. Proanthocyanidins, tannins, and saponins are the active ingredients that work to constrict veins and improve the venous circulatory problems seen in stasis dermatitis (Wink & Wyk, 2004).

Aloe vera is a plant of African origin that contains leaves full of salve. This gel or liquid contains enzymes that have anti-inflammatory properties that promote wound healing. Topical application of aloe vera salve may help heal the venous ulcers associated with stasis dermatitis and also relieve some of the pruritus associated with the condition (Balch & Balch, 2010).

Calendula is an herb that has a history of usefulness in treating ulcers. It is used topically by herbalists for its anti-inflammatory and wound healing properties and is also available commercially in various cream-based preparations. Calendula is used in stasis dermatitis to reduce the risk of infection and to promote the growth of granulation tissue in ulcers to speed the healing process (Wink & Wyk, 2004).

REFERENCES

Balch, J. F., & Balch, P. A. (2010). *Prescription for nutritional healing* (5th ed.). Philadelphia: Penguin.

Fauci, A. S., et al. (2008). *Harrison's principles of internal medicine* (17th ed., pp. 314–316, 335, 366, 731). New York: McGraw-Hill.

Gyton, A. C., & Hall, J. E. (2006). *Textbook of medical physiology* (11th ed., pp. 459–467). Philadelphia: Elsevier.

Pagana, K. D., & Pagana, T. J. (2006). *Mosby's manual of diagnostic and laboratory tests* (3rd ed., pp. 949–952, 1163–1165). St. Louis, MO: Mosby Elsevier.

Wink, M., & Wyk, B. (2004). *Medicinal plants of the world.* New York: Timber Press.

Wolff, K., & Johnson, R. A. (2009). *Fitzpatrick's color atlas & synopsis of clinical dermatology* (6th ed., pp. 465–477). New York: McGraw-Hill.

27

Integrative Management of Urticaria

ERIN N. WILMER, KACHIU C. LEE, AND PETER A. LIO

Key Concepts

♣ Urticaria can be categorized as acute or chronic, and further subdivided into spontaneous or induced forms.

♣ Chronic spontaneous urticaria is a skin disorder that affects an estimated 0.5% to 1% of the population and is characterized by the sudden appearance of wheals and/or angioedema that present on a regular basis for at least six weeks.

♣ The cause remains unclear in the majority of cases and treatment is consequently aimed at symptom management.

♣ Chronic spontaneous urticaria is the most common, problematic, and long-lasting subtype of the nonacute form of urticaria and therefore the most amenable to complementary and alternative therapies (CAM).

♣ Treatment of chronic spontaneous urticaria with CAM may be effective, specifically when using the modalities of acupuncture, cupping, and dietary changes.

Introduction

Current European Academy of Allergology and Immunology/Global Allergy and Asthma European Network/European Dermatology Forum/World Allergy Organization (EAACI/GA2LEN/EDF/WAO) guidelines categorize urticaria as acute or chronic, and further subdivide acute or chronic urticaria into spontaneous or induced forms (Maurer et al., 2013; Zuberbier et al., 2009).

Chronic spontaneous urticaria is the most common nonacute form of urticaria (Staubach et al., 2011), affecting an estimated 0.5% to 1% of the population (Maurer et al., 2011). The following discussion will focus on chronic spontaneous urticaria because this is the most problematic and long-lasting subtype, and therefore the most amenable to complementary and alternative therapies (CAM). Accordingly, the majority of peer-reviewed research on CAM is on the chronic spontaneous subtype of urticaria.

Chronic spontaneous urticaria is a skin disorder characterized by sudden appearance of wheals and/or angioedema that present on a regular basis for at least six weeks. The cause remains unclear in the majority of cases, and treatment is consequently aimed at symptom management (Zuberbier, 2003).

Antihistamines are first-line conventional therapies used for this condition. However, chronic use of medications is typically required as the underlying etiology is not addressed by antihistamine pharmacotherapy. Fewer than half of patients respond to antihistamines with complete symptom control, while one third to one half of patients are improved but not clear (Maurer et al., 2011). Second-line conventional treatments (e.g., corticosteroids, leukotriene antagonists, cyclosporine, dapsone, and omalizumab) are associated with potentially serious side effects (Zuberbier, 2012). Lack of efficacy and risk of adverse events with medications may encourage patients and practitioners to consider CAM for the treatment of chronic spontaneous urticaria (Ernst, 2000). This chapter reviews various evidence-based CAM for treatment of urticaria.

Acupuncture

Acupuncture is a modality commonly used by practitioners of traditional Chinese medicine (TCM) in the treatment of chronic urticaria. Western scientists hypothesize that acupuncture ameliorates skin disease via both local effects (i.e., change in skin temperature and blood flow) and systemic effects. The systemic effects are thought to result from central nervous system activation and its subsequent influence on the neuroendocrine and immune systems (Iliev, 1998).

Acute urticaria has an estimated 90% cure rate when treated at four specific points: LI11 (*Quchi*), Sp10 (*Xuehai*), Sp6 (*Sanyinjiao*), and S36 (*Zusanli*) (Chen & Yu, 1998). In contrast, chronic urticaria is a more complex and challenging problem. According to TCM theory, the etiology of chronic spontaneous urticaria involves deficiency of *qi* and blood, a combination of pathogenic wind with cold or heat at the skin surface, and a congenital defect that promotes weak *Ying* and *Wei* systems (Tao, 2009; Yang, 2001; Zhao, 2006). Thus, the aim of treatment is to restore *qi*, increase blood circulation, dispel wind, and regulate the *Ying* system (Liu, 2002). Various strategies may be used, including ordinary acupuncture, auricular acupuncture, acupuncture point bleeding, acupuncture point injection, and cupping at an acupuncture point (Chen & Yu, 1998).

Several small studies have examined the therapeutic effects of ordinary acupuncture on chronic spontaneous urticaria. Lai (1993) compared 15 patients treated with acupuncture to 15 patients treated with desensitization therapy and found the short-term cure and "markedly effective" rates were higher in the acupuncture group ($p < 0.05$). Eruption frequency and amount of wheals were also improved in the acupuncture group ($p < 0.01$), although there was no difference in the duration of wheals or severity of pruritus. In another study, Bo's abdominal acupuncture was performed in 31 patients and compared to 30 patients treated with ceterizine. The efficacy rate was 81% in the acupuncture group and 77% in the cetirizine group, showing no statistically significant difference. However, there were no side effects mentioned in the acupuncture cohort, whereas drowsiness, headache, and thirst were reported by the cetirizine cohort (Chen & Guo, 2005).

Tao (2009) treated 31 patients with individualized acupuncture regimens, which included point bleeding and cupping. Complete resolution was achieved in 26% of patients, improvement in 55%, and "failure" (wheals decreased by less than 30% and no significant improvement in pruritus) in 19%. Zhao employed ordinary acupuncture with point injection of diphenhydramine, followed by cupping, in 32 patients and compared the outcomes to those in 32 patients treated with a variety of antihistamines. The outcomes were categorized as "cured," "effective," or "ineffective." The total effective rate (either "cured" or "effective") was 91% for the acupuncture group and 69% for the antihistamine group ($p < 0.05$), with a lower relapse rate in the acupuncture arm ($p < 0.01$) (Zhao, 2006). Another study of 200 patients investigated the efficacy of acupoint injection of autologous blood compared to treatment with topical dexamethasone acetate and oral setastine hydrochloride. The cure rate was 66% in the patients who received acupoint injection and 0% in patients treated with topical and oral medications (Xiu & Wang, 2011). The 0% cure rate is inconsistent with results from other studies examining the efficacy of medications; the control regimen was clearly not optimized. Nevertheless, achievement of cure in two thirds of the experimental patients is notable.

In addition to the reports mentioned above, two recent investigations explored the effect of acupuncture on IgE levels in patients with chronic urticaria. Elevated IgE levels in a subpopulation of patients with chronic urticaria are associated with disease severity and duration (Kessel et al., 2010). In an observational study of 12 patients, Jianli (2006) demonstrated a significant decrease in IgE levels following acupuncture therapy compared to pre-acupuncture baseline levels ($p < 0.05$). In a similar study of 60 subjects with chronic urticaria, 30 experimental subjects received acupuncture therapy, while 30 control-group subjects were treated with an antihistamine (levocetirizine). Symptom scores and serum IgE levels declined in both groups ($p < 0.01$) but were similar between the experimental and control cohorts at zero, two, and six weeks. However, by 12 weeks, patients treated with acupuncture demonstrated significantly decreased symptom scores and IgE levels ($p < 0.05$) (Gao et al., 2009). These studies suggest that the therapeutic mechanism of acupuncture may involve regulation of IgE levels.

These investigations have clinical limitations due to the small number of peer-reviewed studies, small sample sizes, lack of consistent controls, and confounding variables that result from the individually tailored approach to acupuncture. Nonetheless, acupuncture may still be an effective alternative therapy for the treatment of chronic urticaria, with fewer adverse effects than pharmacological agents.

Cupping

Cupping is a non-needle form of treatment used to treat chronic urticaria. The technique involves placing a localized "vacuum" cup against the skin surface. Suction pulls the skin into the cup and causes trauma to the superficial blood vessels, resulting in purpura and ecchymoses (Yoo & Tausk, 2004). In dry cupping, skin is drawn into the cup without bleeding, whereas in wet cupping the skin is lacerated so blood from the cutaneous microcirculation is drawn into the cup (Lee et al., 2011). Yang (2001) reported on seven chronic urticaria patients treated with wet cupping, five of whom were cured and two of whom improved. Yang's theory is that the procedure removes stagnant blood and wind, two causative agents of chronic urticaria. In a larger study of 40 patients, 20 were treated with cupping, while 20 controls received chlorpheniramine and "miraculous pills of Ledebouriella" (防风通圣丸). A cure rate of 55% was achieved in the cupping group, compared to 30% in the control group ($p < 0.01$) (Li & Ding, 2001). Liu (2002) treated 26 patients with a combination of pricking, cupping, and a decoction called *qu feng tiao ying*. Results were compared to 24 patients who received the decoction only (control group I) and to 21 patients who received "Western drugs" including cetirizine, dexamethasone, or clorpheniramine (control group II). The total effectiveness rate (cured or markedly effective) was 85% in the treatment group, 63% in control group I, and 52% in control group II ($p < 0.01$).

Data on the efficacy of cupping in the treatment of chronic urticaria are limited and additional randomized, controlled studies are warranted.

Interestingly, a meta-analysis showed the cure rate of patients with acne who received cupping therapy was significantly superior to treatment with medication. Patients with herpes zoster treated with cupping also had a superior cure rate and superior reduction in postherpetic neuralgia, with no reports of adverse events from cupping (Cao et al., 2012). With additional well-designed studies, similar efficacy of cupping may be observed in patients with chronic urticaria.

Diet

Intolerance to pseudoallergens in the diet is a purported cause of chronic urticaria, particularly in patients who do not respond to antihistamine therapy (Zuberbier, 2001; Zuberbier et al., 1995). Pseudoallergens include salicylates, preservatives, dyes, aromatic compounds, and naturally occurring substances in vegetables, fruits, and spices (Akoglu et al., 2012; Magerl et al., 2010; Zuberbier et al., 2002). Pseudoallergic urticaria likely results from non-IgE-mediated reactions. It is thought that leuokotrienes, kinins, and/or prostaglandins may be involved in the pathogenesis of pseudoallergen-induced urticaria (Pacor et al., 2001).

A low-pseudoallergen diet reduces urticarial activity in a subset of patients, with varying efficacy. Magerl and colleagues (2010) assessed the effects of a pseudoallergen-free diet in 140 patients and reported a strong response in 14%, a partial response in 14%, and a substantial reduction in medication usage in 6%. In a similar study of 104 patients, 17% reported complete remission, 51% partial remission, and 32% no remission after a five-week pseudoallergen-free diet. Furthermore, all responders reported an improved quality-of-life score ($p < 0.001$) (Bunselmeyer et al., 2009). Zuberbier and colleagues (1995) demonstrated complete symptom resolution or significant symptom reduction in 73% of patients administered a pseudoallergen-free diet for two weeks. Six-month follow-up showed complete remission in 46% of patients who remained on the diet and improvement in all but one patient. In a study of 55 patients, 53% responded to a pseudoallergen-free diet, with "response" defined as a lasting response of more than 50% in the skin-symptom score during the diet period (Buhner et al., 2004). Akoglu and colleagues (2012) demonstrated a significant decrease in leukotriene E4 levels in patients who responded to a low-pseudoallergen diet compared to nonresponders ($p < 0.001$), suggesting that leukotriene E4 is involved in the pathogenesis of pseudoallergen-induced chronic urticaria. In the largest study we found (838 patients), 31% experienced symptom improvement on a diet free of food additives (Di Lorenzo et al., 2005).

The range of positive responses to a pseudoallergen-free diet may result from variations in the diet formulation, the duration of diet, patient attributes, and concomitant pharmacotherapy. Importantly, these studies were not placebo-controlled, and urticaria has a significant rate of self-resolution over time, making these findings somewhat less impressive. Regardless, the underlying theory has at least some merit, and these studies suggest that a pseudoallergen-free diet may offer complete resolution in a proportion of patients, with no reports of adverse events.

Psychiatric Comorbidities and Stress Reduction

The role of psychological stress in the pathogenesis of urticaria has been described in the medical literature for decades. In 1957, Rees reported that onset of urticarial symptoms was preceded by stressful life events in 51 of 100 patients (Rees, 1957). Furthermore, up to 81% of patients endorse stress as an aggravating or causative factor of their chronic urticaria (Ozkan et al., 2007). Chung and colleagues (2010) recently examined the relationship between chronic urticaria and posttraumatic stress disorder (PTSD). Patients with chronic urticaria were nearly twice as likely to have a diagnosis of PTSD compared to control patients with allergies, although there was no association between the diagnosis of PTSD and the severity of skin disease. It is hypothesized that the sympathetic nervous system hyperarousal and re-experiencing of traumatic events that occurs with PTSD may manifest as urticaria (Gupta & Gupta, 2012).

Patients with chronic urticaria are also more likely to have comorbid anxiety, depression and psychosomatic disorders (Engin et al., 2008; Hashiro & Okumura, 1994; Pasaoglu et al., 2006; Sperber et al., 1989). In a study of 100 patients with chronic spontaneous urticaria, 48% were found to have one or more mental disorders, and those with a mental disorder showed significantly higher levels of emotional distress compared to those without (Staubach et al., 2011). Other studies examining the prevalence of psychiatric illness in patients with urticaria have identified comorbidity rates ranging from 35% to 70% (Hashiro & Okumura, 1994; Ozkan et al., 2007; Picardi et al., 2000; Uguz et al., 2008). Patients with chronic spontaneous urticaria also have significantly higher levels of life event stress and perceived stress compared to patients with type I allergy (Chung et al., 2009). These studies support the notion of stress as a precipitating and/or exacerbating factor of chronic urticaria, although further investigations are needed to examine the role of stress as a causal agent.

Given the presumed role of stress in chronic spontaneous urticaria, some investigators have examined the effect of hypnosis on disease manifestation. In 15 patients with chronic urticaria of an average duration of nearly eight years, hypnosis with relaxation therapy resulted in complete resolution in six patients and improvement in eight patients, with 80% of the subjects reporting decreased medication requirements (Shertzer & Lookingbill, 1987). To our knowledge, this is the only study that has directly investigated the efficacy of hypnotherapy in treating chronic spontaneous urticaria. Other reports have focused on the ability to alter cutaneous responses to histamine using hypnosis. Zachariae and colleagues (2001) observed smaller flare responses to histamine prick in hypnosis-induced sadness states compared to hypnosis-induced happy or angry states ($p < 0.05$) but no difference in wheal responses. In a separate study by Zachariae and colleagues (1989), hypnotized subjects produced a significant reduction in flare size following a histamine prick test ($p < 0.02$). Similar outcomes were observed in one study by Laidlaw and colleagues (1994): flare size but not wheal size was significantly reduced following hypnotherapy. A later study demonstrated a significant decrease in wheal reaction to histamine following hypnosis ($p < 0.0001$) (Laidlaw et al., 1996).

The effect of hypnotherapy on delayed-type hypersensitivity response has also been investigated with both positive and negative outcomes. In two distinct studies, Locke and colleagues (1987, 1994) observed no change in delayed-type hypersensitivity response following hypnotic suggestion. Conversely, Zachariae and colleagues (1989) reported that hypnotic suggestion increased delayed-type hypersensitivity response on one arm and decreased it on the other arm, resulting in a significant difference in flare size ($p < 0.02$) and induration ($p < 0.01$). These controversial results could be due to differences in patient populations, patient hypnotizability and methods of hypnosis, wheal and flare induction, and outcome measurement.

Clinicians have successfully used hypnosis for the treatment of a wide spectrum of cutaneous diseases, including psoriasis, rosacea, vitiligo, and hyperhidrosis, among others (Shenefelt, 2000). The mechanism by which hypnosis produces symptom improvement in skin disease is unclear. It is thought that the relaxation response induced by hypnosis has an effect on blood flow, autonomic function, and neurohormonal interactions (Shenefelt, 2003; Tausk, 1998). It is important to note that some patients are more hypnotizable than others, and this difference tends to be innate and stable over time (Hoeft et al., 2012). Patient selection, therefore, should be considered prior to engaging in hypnotherapy. The advantages of hypnosis for the treatment of chronic spontaneous urticaria are its safety, absence of toxicity, and ability of the patient to self-treat, providing the patient with a sense of control over his or her illness. Although data on the efficacy of hypnotherapy in treating chronic spontaneous urticaria are limited, it can be considered a safe complementary or alternative approach for patients refractory to traditional therapy.

Homeopathy

Homeopathy is commonly used as a complementary or alternative treatment for skin disease (Simonart et al., 2011). However, studies investigating its safety and efficacy in dermatologic disorders are extremely limited and often of low methodological quality (Simonart et al., 2011; Smolle, 2003). The efficacy of an individualized homeopathic regimen was analyzed in one study with six patients and mean disease duration of 4.6 years. The initial homeopathic medicines used included pulsatilla, sulphus, sepia, bryonia, and apis, although, notably, patients were free to alter their treatment. Efficacy was measured using both patient and physician assessment. One patient was cured, four patients achieved moderate improvement, and one patient achieved mild improvement (Itamura 2007). The results of this single, small, no-randomized study are not suitable for generalization. However, the basic tenet of homeopathy, treating a patient as a whole being (Stibbe, 1999), may be a beneficial approach, particularly in addressing the psychosocial aspects of chronic spontaneous urticaria. Based on the lack of peer-reviewed studies examining the effects of homeopathy on urticaria, no recommendation on its use can be made without further study.

Herbal Remedies

Herbal therapies have been used for thousands of years in the treatment of skin disorders. As is the case with homeopathy, scientific evidence is primarily limited to anecdotal results, although a few randomized, controlled trials have shown a positive response to herbal remedies (Bedi & Shenefelt, 2002). We identified only two studies reporting treatment of chronic spontaneous urticaria with herbal medicine. Zhong and colleagues (2011) evaluated the efficacy of *Tripterygium hypoglaucum Hutch* (THH) in a randomized, double-blind, placebo-controlled trial. THH is a traditional Chinese medicinal herb with anti-inflammatory, anti-allergic, and immunosuppressive properties. Sixty-nine patients with a poor response to antihistamine therapy were divided into a treatment group (n = 37) and a control group (n = 32); all patients received cetirizine therapy. After four weeks, there was a 63% improvement in the experimental group compared to a 24% improvement in the control group ($p < 0.001$). THH also significantly reduced the mean pruritus scores each study week ($p < 0.005$). Importantly, THH may not be a totally benign treatment: its main chemical components are alkaloids, terpenes, and pigments, and it has been shown to have a strong ability to induce chromosomal nondisjunction, chromosomal aberrations, and aneuploidy in mice and to show clear cytotoxicity and genotoxicity in human cell lines (Liu et al., 2003).

Kato and colleagues (2010) reported five cases of chronic urticaria successfully treated with the Japanese medicinal herb *yokukansan*, in addition to antihistamines. Disease activity was scored according to EAACI/GA2LEN/EDF guidelines; complete resolution was reported in two cases, marked improvement in one case, and mild improvement in three cases. *Yokukansan* has traditionally been used as an anxiolytic and recent reports suggest it is effective in treating psychiatric illness (Miyaoka et al., 2009; Monji et al., 2009). The beneficial effect of *yokukansan* in the treatment of chronic urticaria may be related to its modulation of psychiatric symptoms.

Conclusion

Urticaria can present as both an acute and chronic disease. Treatment of chronic spontaneous urticaria with CAM may be effective, specifically when using the modalities of acupuncture, cupping, and dietary changes. Hypnotherapy has limited data, but both clinical and experimental responses are supportive. Homeopathy cannot be recommended, as there is a lack of evidence on its effectiveness in the treatment of urticaria. Herbal remedies may be effective, although the different herbal preparations used in each study pose a significant limitation to evidence-based reviews, and possible toxicity warrants caution in this domain.

REFERENCES

Akoglu, G., Atakan, N., et al. (2012). Effects of low pseudoallergen diet on urticarial activity and leukotriene levels in chronic urticaria. *Archives of Dermatology Research, 304*(4), 257–262.

Bedi, M. K., & Shenefelt, P. D. (2002). Herbal therapy in dermatology. *Archives of Dermatology, 138*(2), 232–242.

Buhner, S., Reese, I., et al. (2004). Pseudoallergic reactions in chronic urticaria are associated with altered gastroduodenal permeability. *Allergy, 59*(10), 1118–1123.

Bunselmeyer, B., Laubach, H. J., et al. (2009). Incremental build-up food challenge—a new diagnostic approach to evaluate pseudoallergic reactions in chronic urticaria: a pilot study: stepwise food challenge in chronic urticaria. *Clinical & Experimental Allergy, 39*(1), 116–126.

Cao, H., Li, X., et al. (2012). An updated review of the efficacy of cupping therapy. *PLoS One, 7*(2), e31793.

Chen, C. J., & Yu, H. S. (1998). Acupuncture treatment of urticaria. *Archives of Dermatology, 134*(11), 1397–1399.

Chen, L. Y., & Guo, Y. G. (2005). [Observation on short-term therapeutic effect of Bo's abdominal acupuncture on chronic urticaria]. *Zhongguo Zhen Jiu, 25*(11), 768–770.

Chung, M. C., Symons, C., et al. (2009). Stress, psychiatric co-morbidity and coping in patients with chronic idiopathic urticaria. *Psychology & Health, 25*(4), 477–490.

Chung, M. C., Symons, C., et al. (2010). The relationship between posttraumatic stress disorder, psychiatric comorbidity, and personality traits among patients with chronic idiopathic urticaria. *Comprehensive Psychiatry, 51*(1), 55–63.

Di Lorenzo, G., Pacor, M. L., et al. (2005). Food-additive-induced urticaria: a survey of 838 patients with recurrent chronic idiopathic urticaria. *International Archives of Allergy & Immunology, 138*(3), 235–242.

Engin, B., Uguz, F., et al. (2008). The levels of depression, anxiety and quality of life in patients with chronic idiopathic urticaria. *Journal of the European Academy of Dermatology & Venereology, 22*(1), 36–40.

Ernst, E. (2000). The usage of complementary therapies by dermatological patients: a systematic review. *British Journal of Dermatology, 142*(5), 857–861.

Gao, H., Li, X. Z., et al. (2009). [Influence of penetrative needling of Shendao (GV 11) on the symptom score and serum IgE content in chronic urticaria patients]. *Zhen Ci Yan Jiu, 34*(4), 272–275.

Gupta, M. A., & Gupta, A. K. (2012). Chronic idiopathic urticaria and post-traumatic stress disorder (PTSD), an under-recognized comorbidity. *Clinics in Dermatology, 30*(3), 351–354.

Hashiro, M., & Okumura, M. (1994). Anxiety, depression, psychosomatic symptoms and autonomic nervous function in patients with chronic urticaria. *Journal of Dermatology Science, 8*(2), 129–135.

Hoeft, F., Gabrieli, J. D., et al. (2012). Functional brain basis of hypnotizability. *Archives of General Psychiatry, 69*(10), 1064–1072.

Iliev, E. (1998). Acupuncture in dermatology. *Clinics in Dermatology, 16*(6), 659–688.

Itamura, R. (2007). Effect of homeopathic treatment of 60 Japanese patients with chronic skin disease. *Complementary Therapy in Medicine, 15*(2), 115–120.

Jianli, C. (2006). The effect of acupuncture on serum IgE level in patients with chronic urticaria. *Journal of Traditional Chinese Medicine, 26*(3), 189–190.

Kato, S., Kato, T. A., et al. (2010). Successful treatment of chronic urticaria with a Japanese herbal medicine, yokukansan. *Journal of Dermatology, 37*(12), 1066–1067.

Kessel, A., Helou, W., et al. (2010). Elevated serum total IgE—a potential marker for severe chronic urticaria. *International Archives of Allergy & Immunology, 153*(3), 288–293.

Lai, X. (1993). Observation on the curative effect of acupuncture on type I allergic diseases. *Journal of Traditional Chinese Medicine, 13*(4), 243–248.

Laidlaw, T. M., Richardson, D. H., et al. (1994). Immediate-type hypersensitivity reactions and hypnosis: problems in methodology. *Journal of Psychosomatic Research, 38*(6), 569–580.

Laidlaw, T. M., Booth, R. J., et al. (1996). Reduction in skin reactions to histamine after a hypnotic procedure. *Psychosomatic Medicine, 58*(3), 242–248.

Lee, M. S., Kim, J. I., et al. (2011). Is cupping an effective treatment? An overview of systematic reviews. *Journal of Acupuncture & Meridian Studies, 4*(1), 1–4.

Li, L., & Ding, J. (2001). Treatment of urticaria with cupping at back-shu points—a report of 40 cases. *Journal of Traditional Chinese Medicine, 21*(1), 37–38.

Liu, D. (2002). Pricking, cupping and qu feng tiao ying decoction for treatment of chronic urticaria. *Journal of Traditional Chinese Medicine, 22*(4), 269–271.

Liu, S. X., Cao, J., et al. (2003). Molecular analysis of *Tripterygium hypoglaucum* (level) Hutch-induced mutations at the HPRT locus in human promyelocytic leukemia cells by multiplex polymerase chain reaction. *Mutagenesis, 18*(1), 77–80.

Locke, S. E., Ransil, B. J., et al. (1987). Failure of hypnotic suggestion to alter immune response to delayed-type hypersensitivity antigens. *Annal of the New York Academy of Science, 496*, 745–749.

Locke, S. E., Ransil, B. J., et al. (1994). Effect of hypnotic suggestion on the delayed-type hypersensitivity response. *Journal of the American Medical Association, 272*(1), 47–52.

Magerl, M., Pisarevskaja, D., et al. (2010). Effects of a pseudoallergen-free diet on chronic spontaneous urticaria: a prospective trial. *Allergy, 65*(1), 78–83.

Maurer, M., Bindslev-Jensen, C., et al. (2013). Chronic idiopathic urticaria (CIU) is no longer idiopathic: time for an update! *British Journal of Dermatology, 168*(2), 455–456.

Maurer, M., Weller, K., et al. (2011). Unmet clinical needs in chronic spontaneous urticaria. A GA(2)LEN task force report. *Allergy, 66*(3), 317–330.

Miyaoka, T., Furuya, M., et al. (2009). Yi-gan san as adjunctive therapy for treatment-resistant schizophrenia: an open-label study. *Clinical Neuropharmacol, 32*(1), 6–9.

Monji, A., Takita, M., et al. (2009). Effect of yokukansan on the behavioral and psychological symptoms of dementia in elderly patients with Alzheimer's disease. *Progress in Neuropsychopharmacology & Biological Psychiatry, 33*(2), 308–311.

Ozkan, M., Oflaz, S. B., et al. (2007). Psychiatric morbidity and quality of life in patients with chronic idiopathic urticaria. *Annals of Allergy, Asthma, & Immunology, 99*(1), 29–33.

Pacor, M. L., Di Lorenzo, G., et al. (2001). Efficacy of leukotriene receptor antagonist in chronic urticaria. A double-blind, placebo-controlled comparison of treatment with montelukast and cetirizine in patients with chronic urticaria with intolerance to food additive and/or acetylsalicylic acid. *Clinical & Experimental Allergy, 31*(10), 1607–1614.

Pasaoglu, G., Bavbek, S., et al. (2006). Psychological status of patients with chronic urticaria. *Journal of Dermatology, 33*(11), 765–771.

Picardi, A., Abeni, D., et al. (2000). Psychiatric morbidity in dermatological outpatients: an issue to be recognized. *British Journal of Dermatology, 143*(5), 983–991.

Rees, L. (1957). An aetiological study of chronic urticaria and angioneurotic oedema. *Journal of Psychosomatic Research, 2*(3), 172–189.

Shenefelt, P. D. (2000). Hypnosis in dermatology. *Archives of Dermatology, 136*(3), 393–399.

Shenefelt, P. D. (2003). Biofeedback, cognitive-behavioral methods, and hypnosis in dermatology: is it all in your mind? *Dermatologic Therapy, 16*(2), 114–122.

Shertzer, C. L., & Lookingbill, D. P. (1987). Effects of relaxation therapy and hypnotizability in chronic urticaria. *Archives of Dermatology, 123*(7), 913–916.

Simonart, T., Kabagabo, C., et al. (2011). Homoeopathic remedies in dermatology: a systematic review of controlled clinical trials. *British Journal of Dermatology, 165*(4), 897–905.

Smolle, J. (2003). Homeopathy in dermatology. *Dermatologic Therapy, 16*(2), 93–97.

Sperber, J., Shaw, J., et al. (1989). Psychological components and the role of adjunct interventions in chronic idiopathic urticaria. *Psychotherapy & Psychosomatic, 51*(3), 135–141.

Staubach, P., Dechene, M., et al. (2011). High prevalence of mental disorders and emotional distress in patients with chronic spontaneous urticaria. *Acta Dermato-Venereologica, 91*(5), 557–561.

Stibbe, J. R. (1999). Homeopathy in dermatology. *Clinics in Dermatology, 17*(1), 65–68.

Tao, S. (2009). Acupuncture treatment for 35 cases of urticaria. *Journal of Traditional Chinese Medicine, 29*(2), 97–100.

Tausk, F. A. (1998). Alternative medicine. Is it all in your mind? *Archives of Dermatology, 134*(11), 1422–1425.

Uguz, F., Engin, B., et al. (2008). Axis I and Axis II diagnoses in patients with chronic idiopathic urticaria. *Journal of Psychosomatic Research, 64*(2), 225–229.

Xiu, M. G., & Wang, D. F. (2011). [Observation on therapeutic effect of acupoint injection desensitization with autoblood on chronic urticaria]. *Zhongguo Zhen Jiu, 31*(7), 610–612.

Yang, R. (2001). Treatment of obstinate diseases by acupuncture and cupping. *Journal of Traditional Chinese Medicine, 21*(2), 118–121.

Yoo, S. S., & Tausk, F. (2004). Cupping: East meets West. *International Journal of Dermatology, 43*(9), 664–665.

Zachariae, R., Bjerring, P., et al. (1989). Modulation of type I immediate and type IV delayed immunoreactivity using direct suggestion and guided imagery during hypnosis. *Allergy, 44*(8), 537–542.

Zachariae, R., Jorgensen, M. M., et al. (2001). Skin reactions to histamine of healthy subjects after hypnotically induced emotions of sadness, anger, and happiness. *Allergy, 56*(8), 734–740.

Zhao, Y. (2006). Acupuncture plus point-injection for 32 cases of obstinate urticaria. *Journal of Traditional Chinese Medicine, 26*(1), 22–23.

Zhong, J., Xian, D., et al. (2011). Efficacy of *Tripterygium hypoglaucum Hutch* in adults with chronic urticaria. *Journal of Alternative & Complementary Medicine, 17*(5), 459–464.

Zuberbier, T. (2001). The role of allergens and pseudoallergens in urticaria. *Journal of Investigative Dermatology Symposium Proceedings, 6*(2), 132–134.

Zuberbier, T. (2003). Urticaria. *Allergy, 58*(12), 1224–1234.

Zuberbier, T. (2012). Chronic urticaria. *Currenty Allergy & Asthma Reports, 12*(4), 267–272.

Zuberbier, T., Asero, R., et al. (2009). EAACI/GA(2)LEN/EDF/WAO guideline: definition, classification and diagnosis of urticaria. *Allergy, 64*(10), 1417–1426.

Zuberbier, T., Chantraine-Hess, S., et al. (1995). Pseudoallergen-free diet in the treatment of chronic urticaria. A prospective study. *Acta Dermato-Venereologica, 75*(6), 484–487.

Zuberbier, T., Pfrommer, C., et al. (2002). Aromatic components of food as novel eliciting factors of pseudoallergic reactions in chronic urticaria. *Journal of Allergy & Clinical Immunology, 109*(2), 343–348.

28

Integrative Management of Verrucae (Warts)

PHILIP D. SHENEFELT

Key Concepts

♣ Treatment of warts often requires patience. Warn patients that multiple treatments may be required before their cell-mediated immune response against the wart virus becomes sufficient to obtain resolution.

♣ For nongenital warts, salicylic acid topical treatment is moderately effective, with about the same effectiveness as cryosurgery. Both can cause pain, irritation, pigmentary changes, or scarring. Other methods, including alternative and complementary methods, are of lower proven efficacy.

♣ Genital warts involving certain viral strains are associated with cervical cancer. Women who have had genital warts should have regular Pap smears as recommended by their primary care physician or gynecologist.

♣ Genital warts and the risk of subsequent cervical cancer can be reduced substantially by vaccination of early teen girls and boys with wart vaccine. No vaccine is currently available for nongenital warts.

♣ Perform surgical removal of warts with caution because of the increased likelihood of scarring without an increased rate of wart resolution compared with topical treatments or cryosurgery.

♣ For a wart that is extremely large and resistant to therapy, consider an incisional biopsy to rule out a diagnosis of verrucous carcinoma.

Introduction

Verrucae or warts are benign tumors of skin and mucosa caused by the human papilloma virus (HPV). HPV is a double-stranded DNA virus. More than 120 types of HPV have been identified, of which more than 40 types can infect the genital area. Although certain HPV types tend to occur mainly at specific anatomic sites, warts associated with any HPV type may occur at any site. Frequent clinical manifestations of HPV infection include common warts, genital warts, flat warts, and deep, painful palmoplantar warts (myrmecia).

Genital warts or condylomata acuminata are the most common sexually transmitted disease, with an estimated exposure of up to 75% of sexually active adults. Malignant transformation associated with certain HPV types can lead to cervical cancer and other anogenital and oral cancers. Pap smears can often detect early cervical transformation toward malignancy. Over 90% of cervical cancers are associated with HPV and half of those are associated with types 16 and 18 (Nebesio et al., 2001).

Less common manifestations of HPV infection include focal epithelial hyperplasia (Heck's disease) (Cohen et al., 1993), epidermodysplasia verruciformis, and plantar cysts. The wart viruses are transmitted by direct or indirect contact. Disruption to the normal epithelial barrier predisposes to infection. Common warts are usually asymptomatic but may occasionally cause tenderness or cosmetic disfigurement. Plantar warts on weight-bearing surfaces of the foot can be painful with ambulation.

Malignant transformation in nongenital warts is rare but does occur and is known as verrucous carcinoma (Guadara et al., 1992; Kolker et al., 1998; Noel et al., 1994). Verrucous carcinoma is a slow-growing, locally invasive, well-differentiated squamous cell carcinoma that most commonly occurs on the plantar sole of the foot. It may be easily mistaken for a large common wart. It can occur anywhere on the skin. Although verrucous carcinoma rarely metastasizes, it can be locally destructive and should be excised. A deep incisional biopsy of any wart that is extensive, persistent, and not responsive to treatment is indicated to rule out carcinoma.

In some cases, treatment of warts can be difficult, with frequent failures and recurrences. Immunosuppressed individuals have more difficulty in ridding themselves of warts. Most warts, however, resolve spontaneously within a few years as delayed cellular immunity to the wart virus becomes activated and destroys them.

Epidemiology

Warts are endemic worldwide and are estimated to affect approximately 7% to 12% of the population (Kilkenny & Marks, 1996). Nongenital warts are more frequent in school-aged children, with a prevalence of 10% to 20% (Schachner et al., 1983). Warts also occur with increased frequency among immunosuppressed patients and meat handlers. HPV is spread by direct skin-to-skin contact or indirect contact through fomites. Any break in the skin, whether a cut, scratch, abrasion, or blister, facilitates entry of the wart virus. The HPV is quite hardy and can survive desiccation, freezing, and prolonged storage outside of host cells. When host immune response is low, autoinoculation may occur. The incubation period for HPV commonly ranges from one to six months, but latency periods of up to three years or more may occur. Common warts appear approximately twice as frequently in whites as in blacks or Asians (Mallory et al., 1991). Focal epithelial hyperplasia (Heck's disease) is more prevalent among American Indians and Inuit (Cohen et al., 1993). The male-to-female ratio approaches 1:1. Warts can occur at any age. They are unusual in infancy and early childhood; the incidence increases among school-aged children and peaks at age 12 to 16 years for nongenital warts (Silverberg, 2004). The incidence of nongenital warts then generally declines slowly with age. Genital warts in children should raise suspicion of possible sexual abuse. Sexual transmission of genital warts is most common in teenagers and those in their early twenties but can happen at any age. Most individuals are exposed to genital warts at some point.

Cause and Prevention

Warts are caused by infection on the skin or mucous membranes with HPV, a double-stranded, circular, supercoiled DNA virus enclosed in an icosahedral capsid with 72 capsomers that belongs to the Papovaviridae. Warts can infect any area, with the infection confined to the epithelium and with no systemic dissemination of the virus. Viral replication occurs in differentiated epithelial cells in the upper level of the epidermis, although viral particles can be found in the basal layer. More than 120 types of HPV have been identified. They are numbered in the order of their discovery based on genotype, with at least a 10% difference required in the nucleotide sequences compared with other types (Tyring, 2000). Those that cause common warts are most commonly HPV types 2 and 4, followed by types 1, 3, 27, 29, and 57. Deep palmoplantar warts (myrmecia) are most commonly associated with HPV type 1, followed by types 2, 3, 4, 27, 29, and 57. Flat warts are caused by HPV types 3, 10, and 28. Butcher's warts are associated with HPV type 7. Focal epithelial hyperplasia (Heck's disease) is caused by HPV types 13 and 32. Cystic warts are associated with HPV type 60. Genital warts most commonly are HPV type 6, 11, 16, and 18, although other HPV types can also infect the anogenital tract. A few HPV types are associated with the development of malignancies, including types 6, 11, 16, 18, 31, and 35. Types 16 and 18 are the HPV types most frequently associated with squamous cell carcinoma of the cervix, genitalia, anus, and oropharynx. Malignant transformation is seen most commonly in patients with genital warts and in immunocompromised patients. Vaccination at puberty against the oncogenic strains of HPV with Gardasil™ or Cervarix™ offers a preventive measure against these HPV-induced genital/anal/oral malignancies. Vaccination with Gardasil™ is for HPV types 6, 11, 16, and 18 while Cervarix™ is for HPV types 16 and 18. In patients with epidermodysplasia verruciformis, HPV types 5, 8, 20, and 47 have oncogenic potential. So far no vaccine has been developed and approved for the prevention of nongenital warts.

Diagnosis

Verruca vulgaris or common warts appear as hyperkeratotic papules with a rough, irregular surface. They range in size from smaller than 1 mm to larger than 1 cm and are seen most commonly on the hands and knees at sites of prior minor trauma. They can occur on any part of the body. The diagnosis of warts is made primarily on the basis of clinical findings (Melton & Rasmussen 1991; Young et al., 1998). Careful paring of the wart surface may reveal minute black dots, which represent thrombosed capillaries. If the diagnosis is in doubt, obtain a biopsy. Immunohistochemical detection of HPV structural proteins may confirm the presence of virus in a lesion, but this has low sensitivity. Polymerase chain reaction may be used to amplify viral DNA for testing and allows identification of the specific HPV type viral DNA using Southern blot. HPV may usually be detected in younger lesions but may not be detectable in older lesions. Filiform warts are slender threadlike upward growths, usually seen on the face around the lips, eyelids, or nares. Myrmecia or deep palmoplantar warts (Holland et al., 1992) begin as small shiny papules and enlarge to become deep endophytic, sharply defined, round lesions with a rough keratotic surface, surrounded by a smooth collar of callus. Those that occur on the plantar surface on weight-bearing areas, such as the metatarsal head and heel, can be painful. Palmoplantar warts on the hand tend to be subungual or periungual. Verruca plana or flat warts are flat or slightly elevated flesh-colored papules that may be smooth or slightly hyperkeratotic. Their size ranges from 1 to 5 mm or more; there may be a few to hundreds of lesions that may become grouped or confluent. Flat warts are most common on the face, hands, and shins but may occur anywhere. They may have a linear distribution as a result of scratching or trauma (Koebner phenomenon). They may be spread by shaving. Butcher's warts are seen most commonly on the hands of raw-meat handlers, often with hyperproliferative cauliflower-like lesions. A mosaic wart is a plaque of closely grouped warts. When the skin surface of a mosaic wart is carefully pared, the angular outlines of tightly compressed individual warts can be seen. Mosaic warts usually occur on the palms and soles. Focal epithelial hyperplasia (Heck's disease) (Cohen et al., 1993) is an HPV infection occurring in the oral cavity, often on the lower labial mucosa or on the buccal or gingival mucosa and rarely on the tongue, appearing as multiple flat-topped or dome-shaped pink-white papules, usually 1 to 5 mm, with some lesions coalescing into plaques. A cystic wart (plantar epidermoid cyst) appears as a smooth nodule with visible rete ridges on the weight-bearing surface of the sole. When the nodule is incised, keratinous material may be expressed. The etiology of these lesions is uncertain. One theory holds that a cyst forms, originating from the eccrine duct, and secondary HPV infection occurs; another theory maintains that epidermis infected with HPV becomes implanted into the dermis, forming an epidermal inclusion cyst (Matsukura et al., 1992; Yanagihara et al., 1989). Differential diagnoses for warts include acquired digital fibrokeratoma, actinic keratosis, arsenical keratosis, cutaneous horn, lichen niditus, hypertrophic lichen planus, molluscum contagiosum, prurigo nodularis, seborrheic keratosis, and squamous cell carcinoma.

Conventional Treatment Options

While many types of treatments are available for warts, none is effective for every patient (Bellew et al., 2004; Benton, 1997; Brodell & Johnson, 2003; Drake et al., 1995; Gibbs & Harvey, 2006; Goldfarb et al., 1991; Jablonska et al., 1997; Rivera & Tyring, 2004, Stone et al., 1990). Beginning with the least painful, least expensive, and least time-consuming methods is recommended, reserving the more expensive and invasive procedures for resistant extensive warts. In general, a single nonspreading wart probably reflects that the patient has a better cell-mediated immune (CMI) response to the wart virus, while multiple spreading warts reflect less CMI response (Bouwes Bavinck & Berkhout, 1997). Offering no treatment is certainly safe and cost-effective, since 65% of warts may regress spontaneously within two years. However, warts may enlarge or spread to other areas. Treatment is recommended for patients with extensive, spreading, or symptomatic warts or warts that have been present for more than two years. When warts resolve without treatment, no scarring is seen. Scarring can result when treatment methods cause dermal injury, such as with strong acids, electrocautery, excision, and laser, and less commonly with cryosurgery. Treatment failures and wart recurrences are common, especially among immunocompromised patients. Normal-appearing perilesional skin

Table 28.1. Recommended Treatments for Warts

Wart Type	First Line	Second Line	Third Line
Genital	Liquid nitrogen	Imiquimod	Sinecatechins Hypnosis
Common	Salicylic acid Liquid nitrogen	Imiquimod* or 5-fluorouracil with occlusion	Contact sensitizers** Hypnosis
Flat	Imiquimod*	Topical retinoid*	Liquid nitrogen
Plantar	Salicylic acid Liquid nitrogen	Intralesional immunotherapy*	Bleomycin* Hypnosis

*Off-label
**Considered experimental

may harbor HPV, which helps explain recurrences. Table 28.1 gives an overview of recommended first-, second-, and third-line treatments for warts. For the most recent information on prescription medicines and their indications, interactions, and adverse effects see the current *Physicians' Desk Reference* (PDR Staff, 2011) or similar source.

Psychological Treatment of Warts

Suggestion and its associated placebo effect have a long history of enhancing wart resolution both in folklore and in the medical literature. Belief can change brain electrochemistry, leading to modification of CMI through psycho-neuro-endocrine effects on the immune system. The case series literature supports suggestion (Meineke et al., 2002), and the effectiveness of placebo has been supported by case series but not by a small randomized control trial (RCT) (Spanos et al., 1990). There are no contraindications or adverse effects for appropriate suggestion. Combining suggestion with other treatment modalities may be synergistic. The small RCT by Spanos and colleagues (1990) is one of several RCTs that demonstrated the efficacy of hypnosis in inducing wart resolution; in this trial it was significantly superior to salicylic acid and placebo and control. Hypnosis has been used to treat warts resistant to other treatments (Ewin, 1992). Resolution rates have been reported from 27% to 55%, with prepubertal children more likely to respond than adults. For warts not responsive to hypnosis, a case series with resolution in 33 of 41 cases demonstrated the efficacy of psychosomatic hypnoanalysis (Ewin, 1992; Ewin & Eimer, 2006). For genital warts in women, hypnosis has been shown to be equally effective to medical treatments at reducing wart sizes and numbers and more effective than medical treatments for complete clearance at 12 weeks

(Barabasz et al., 2009). Hypnosis and psychosomatic hypnoanalysis should be used only by those suitably trained and should be used with great caution in patients with psychosis. Hypnosis has minimal adverse effects such as occasional posthypnotic mild headache.

Nonprescription Patient-Applied Topical Agents

Keratolytic agents are the most commonly used nonprescription wart treatments. Salicylic acid is a first-line therapy used to treat warts. It is available without a prescription and can be applied by the patient at home. The local inflammatory reaction created by the treatment attracts various inflammatory cells that may in turn help to develop the CMI response. Cure rates in RCTs from 70% to 80% are reported, compared with about 30% to 50% in controls. Multiple RCTs support its effectiveness (Gibbs & Harvey, 2006). Salicylic acid (Compound W and similar) is available in 5% to 40% concentration in creams, paints, gels, karaya gum, impregnated plasters, collodion, or sodium carboxycellulose tape. Lactic acid is a second keratolytic ingredient in some wart varnishes. By dissolving the intercellular cement substance, salicylic acid desquamates the outer horny layer of skin. The therapeutic effect may be enhanced by mechanical removal of some of the surface keratin by filing or carefully paring prior to application. Treatment for adults and children is topically to the wart daily for several weeks. No drug interactions are reported. Contraindications include documented hypersensitivity and prolonged use in diabetics or those with impaired circulation. Do not use on moles, nevi, or birthmarks. Do not use strong acids on the genital area, face, or mucous membranes. Do not use on irritated skin or infected skin. It is Pregnancy Category C (fetal risk was revealed in studies in animals but not established or not studied in humans). It may be used if the benefits outweigh the risk to the fetus. Also avoid contact with normal skin surrounding warts. If contact with eyes or mucous membranes occur, immediately flush with water for 15 minutes. Avoid inhaling vapors of the solvents. Side effects may include irritation and maceration of surrounding normal skin or contact dermatitis to the colophony in collodion bases.

Adhesiotherapy consists of applying duct tape to cover the wart daily overnight. This method is painless and inexpensive and has published reports of good success (Focht et al., 2002; Wenner et al., 2007). The topical occlusion of warts overnight causes the cornified epithelium to swell, soften, and macerate. Removal of the tape causes the tape to gently strip off the macerated epidermis. Mild irritation from the tape adhesive may attract inflammatory cells that help to induce CMI against the wart virus. Two RCTs found no significant difference between duct tape and placebo occlusion (de Haen et al., 2006; Wenner et al., 2007).

Herbal home remedies such as raw minced garlic or banana inner peel, lemon slice, vinegar, lime juice, raw potato slice, tea tree oil, aloe, castor oil, dandelion stem milk, milkweed stem milk, crushed chickweed, or strong calendula tea applied topically to the wart with or without duct tape or adhesive tape occlusion have so far not been tested by RCTs to determine if they surpass the placebo effect. Raw garlic cloves have been shown to have antiviral activity and can be rubbed onto the wart nightly, followed by occlusion (Silverberg, 2002). Topical tea tree oil has also been reported as successful in some cases (Millar & Moore, 2008).

Hyperthermia treatment involves immersing the involved skin in hot water (113 degrees F [45 degrees C]) for 30 to 45 minutes, two or three times per week, and has been reported effective in some cases in inducing wart resolution.

Prescription Patient-Applied Topical Agents

Immunomodulators are agents that stimulate the release of key factors that regulate aspects of the immune system (Rivera & Tyring, 2004). Imiquimod (Aldara) 5% cream is an immunomodulator that is approved by the U.S. Food and Drug Administration for treating genital and perianal warts in patients 12 years or older. It induces skin cells to secrete interferon alpha and other cytokines. While it has not received FDA approval for treatment of nongenital warts, off-label use has resulted in successful treatment of nongenital warts in some cases (Perrett et al., 2004). It is applied topically at bedtime three times a week with or without duct tape or adhesive tape occlusion. Irritation may be increased with more frequent use. There are no reported interactions with other drugs. Contraindications are documented hypersensitivity. It is Pregnancy Category C and may be used if the benefits outweigh the risk to the fetus. Local irritation may occur at application sites, including redness, itching, and burning. In many cases treatment may have to continue for up to six months to achieve clearing of warts.

5-Fluorouracil (Efudex) is a topical antineoplastic chemotherapeutic agent that inhibits cell growth and proliferation. It has been reported to be effective as an off-label use in treating genital and common warts and was recently developed as a non-FDA-approved combination topical prescription agent with salicylic acid (Wart-Off™), available at certain specialty pharmacies. For nongenital warts it may be effective when used under occlusion and has been more successful in treating flat warts than plantar and common nongenital warts. Adult application of the 5% solution or cream is daily for up to one month. It may be used under occlusion, but the risk of irritation increases. Successful pediatric usage has also been reported. There have been no reported drug interactions when used topically. Contraindications include documented hypersensitivity and breastfeeding. It is Pregnancy Category X, contraindicated, and benefit does not outweigh risk. Moderate to severe skin irritation may occur locally.

Podophyllotoxin (Podofilox) is a purified ingredient of podophyllin and is less irritating than podophyllum resin (see under "Provider-Applied Topical Agents"). Podophyllotoxin is a cytotoxic compound that tends to work better on mucosal surfaces and is used more commonly in the treatment of genital warts (Tyring et al., 1998). It may be applied topically twice daily for three consecutive days per week and repeated weekly, not to exceed four weeks. Little information is available regarding its use to treat nongenital warts. There are no reported drug interactions. Contraindications are documented hypersensitivity, prolonged use in diabetics and those with impaired circulation; do not use on nevi or birthmarks or on irritated or infected skin. It is Pregnancy Category X, contraindicated, and benefit does not outweigh risk.

Sinecatechins (Veregen) 15% ointment is a water extract of green tea leaves from *Camellia sinensis*. The polyphenolic sinecatechins have been shown to inhibit enzymes related to viral replication and inflammatory mediators (Tyring, 2012). It is approved for anogenital warts and has a clearance rate of 55% and a low recurrence rate of 5% (Tatti et al., 2008).

Tretinoin (Retin-A) is a topical retinoic acid that has been successful in off-label use in treating flat warts. It is applied topically daily. Contraindications include documented hypersensitivity and breastfeeding. It is Pregnancy Category X, contraindicated, and benefit does not outweigh risk. Mild to moderate skin irritation may occur locally.

Cidofovir (Vistide), an antiviral agent, is a nucleotide analogue that inhibits viral DNA polymerase and induces apoptosis. Currently it is only available for intravenous administration to HIV-positive patients for treatment of cytomegalovirus infection. A topical gel has been evaluated in clinical trials for use in treatment of HPV infection. In two patients with recurrent persistent nongenital warts that did not respond to multiple standard therapies, the warts resolved with the use of topical cidofovir gel applied once or twice per day (Zabawski et al., 2006). It remains an investigational drug for warts (Roark & Pandya, 1998). Dosages in adults and children are not established. Interactions and contraindications other than documented hypersensitivity with topical use have not been established. It is Pregnancy Category C. Other precautions for topical use have not been determined. Intralesional injection use to treat warts has also been proposed.

Provider-Applied Topical Agents

Trichloroacetic acid (Tri-Chlor) is a caustic compound that causes immediate superficial tissue necrosis. It is available as an 80% solution that is painted onto lesions in the office after excess keratotic debris is carefully pared. Repeat therapy is performed weekly as needed until the wart resolves. Pediatric use is not established. There are no reported drug interactions. Contraindications include documented hypersensitivity and prolonged use in diabetic persons and those with impaired circulation. Do not use on nevi or birthmarks, face, or mucous membranes. Do not use on irritated skin or infected skin. It is Pregnancy Category C. Application may cause pain, burning, and ulceration. If not applied carefully, destruction with resultant scarring of normal surrounding skin may occur.

Podophyllum resin (Podocon-25) is a resin extract derived from *Podophyllum peltatum,* the may apple plant, that contains several cytotoxic compounds. It works better on mucosal surfaces than keratinized surfaces and is therefore more commonly used for treatment of genital warts. Trained personnel must apply it topically in adults and children because of adverse effects and oral toxicity. It may be left on the skin for one to six hours before being washed off. There are no reported drug interactions. Contraindications are documented hypersensitivity and prolonged use in diabetics and those with impaired circulation. Do not use on nevi or birthmarks or on irritated skin or infected skin. It is Pregnancy Category X, contraindicated, and benefit does not outweigh risk. Other precautions include that podophyllum resin may cause significant irritation, local erosion, ulceration, and scarring. Systemic side effects of excessive absorption may include fever, nausea, vomiting, confusion, coma, ileus, renal failure, paresthesias, polyneuritis, and leukopenia. Avoid extensive application because of the risk of systemic absorption.

Cantharidin (Canthacur) is a dried extract of blister beetle (Spanish fly) 0.7% solution in flexible collodion. It is applied sparingly with the wooden end of a cotton-tipped applicator in the provider's office, after which the area is allowed to completely dry. Tape occlusion after application can enhance penetration in large or plantar warts but should be used with caution. Cantharidin causes epidermal necrosis and blistering. Repeat applications at three- to four-week intervals may be required. There are no reported drug interactions. Contraindications include documented hypersensitivity. It should not be used near the eyes. It is Pregnancy Category C. It is a strong blistering agent and should be used with caution in intertriginous areas due to possible smearing or occlusion. Adverse effects include blistering, epidermal necrosis at sites of application, and possible "ring wart phenomenon," in which the virus is spread circumferentially in adjacent tissue damaged by the treatment process.

Aminolevulinic acid (Levulan Kerastick) is a photosensitizer that has been successfully used topically off-label in combination with blue light to treat flat warts (Mizuki et al., 2003). Several RCTs on other nongenital warts have produced conflicting results (Gibbs & Harvey, 2006). The main adverse events have been burning pain during and mild discomfort following the treatments. There are no reported drug interactions. It is Pregnancy Category C. Photosensitivity occurs after application and before blue light treatment.

Allergic contact sensitizers may induce wart resolution by inducing allergic contact dermatitis, causing a localized inflammation and immune response. Dibutyl squaric acid, also known as squaric acid dibutyl ester (SADBE), and diphencyclopropenone (DCP) are contact sensitizers that are not mutagenic nor carcinogenic. Dinitrochlorobenzene (DNCB) is a contact sensitizer that is mutagenic according to the Ames test and possibly carcinogenic and should be avoided when dealing with a potential oncogenic type of wart virus. Older RCTs with DNCB showed that it was more than twice as effective as placebo (Gibbs & Harvey, 2006). None of these contact sensitizers is FDA approved for medical use; they are considered experimental. To achieve initial sensitization, apply topical solution under occlusion on the inner upper arm, then apply to warts every one to two weeks as needed until the wart resolves. For SADBE typically a 4% solution is used for sensitization and a 4% or 1% solution is applied topically to the wart. There are no reported drug interactions. It is Pregnancy Category C. Erythema and pruritus occur at treated sites, and occasionally allergic contact dermatitis may be severe (blistering) or rarely may become disseminated. Recall dermatitis may occur commonly at the initial sensitization site. Regional lymphadenopathy may occur.

Intralesional Injections

Interferons alfa-2a and alfa-2b (Roferon and Intron A) are naturally occurring cytokines with antiviral, antibacterial, antitumor, and immunomodulatory actions. Intralesional administration is more effective than systemic administration and is associated only with mild flulike symptoms. Treatments may be required for several weeks to months before beneficial results are seen. Consider this treatment as third line, and reserve it for warts resistant to standard treatments. Cure rates of 36% to 63% have been reported. In adults it is injected directly into warts up to three times a week for three to six weeks. Pediatric dosing is not established. Interactions are minimal with the small amounts injected. Contraindications include documented hypersensitivity. It is to be used with caution in patients with brain metastases, severe hepatic or renal insufficiencies, seizure disorders, multiple sclerosis, or a compromised central nervous system. It is Pregnancy Category C and may be used if the benefits outweigh the risk to the fetus. Transient flulike symptoms may occur after initial injections, although tolerance usually develops. Pain at injection sites may occur.

Intralesional immunotherapy off-label using injections of *Candida,* mumps, or *Trichophyton* skin test antigens has been shown to be effective in the treatment of warts, with reports of success in up to 74% of patients (Horn et al., 2005). The initial intradermal injection of the skin test antigen can establish the patient's reactivity to it. A small amount of the antigen is injected intralesionally at the base of the wart every two to four weeks until resolution. It is variably effective.

Bleomycin (Blenoxane) is an antineoplastic cytotoxic polypeptide chemotherapeutic agent that inhibits DNA synthesis in cells and viruses. It has an affinity for HPV-infected tissue and induces vascular changes that result in epidermal necrosis. Bleomycin has been beneficial in treating resistant nongenital warts, especially plantar warts. It is recommended to be held in reserve as a third-line treatment when standard therapies have failed. Wart resolution rates have ranged from 33% to 92% (James et al., 1993; Munn et al., 1996). In adults the treatment involves injecting 0.5 to 1 mg/mL of the solution directly into the wart, not to exceed 1.5 mg per treatment. This treatment is usually painful. Less painful administration involves placing a 1 mg/mL drop onto the wart and pricking it into the wart with a needle. Pediatric usage is not established. Interactions are unlikely when small amounts are injected intralesionally. Contraindications include documented hypersensitivity and breastfeeding. It is Pregnancy Category D, with fetal risk shown in humans; not recommended in pregnancy. It may cause pain with injection, local urticaria, and vaso-occlusive phenomenon (Raynaud phenomenon) with possible distal necrosis of the digit. Permanent damage to the nail matrix may occur when used periungually. It may cause mutagenesis and pulmonary toxicity (10%). Idiosyncratic reactions similar to anaphylaxis (1%) may occur, so it is important to monitor for adverse effects during and after treatment.

Systemic Agents

Cimetidine is a type 2 histamine receptor antagonist commonly used to treat peptic ulcer disease. Because of its immunomodulatory effects at higher doses, cimetidine was considered a possible treatment for warts, but study results have varied. Double-blind placebo-controlled studies have shown no benefit (Yilmaz et al., 1996). Dosing in adults and children is 20 to 40 mg/kg orally per day in divided doses every six hours, not to exceed 2,400 mg/day in adults.

It can increase blood levels of theophylline, warfarin, tricyclic antidepressants, triamterene, phenytoin, quinidine, propranolol, metronidazole, procainamide, and lidocaine. Multiple potential drug interactions exist (see full prescribing information for more details). Contraindication is documented hypersensitivity. It is Pregnancy Category B with fetal risk not confirmed in studies in humans but shown in some studies in animals. Serious reactions may include neutropenia, thrombocytopenia, agranulocytosis, and anemia. Common reactions include headache, nausea, vomiting, diarrhea, and rash. Older patients may experience confusional states. It may cause impotence and gynecomastia in young males. It may increase levels of many drugs. The dose should be adjusted or discontinued if changes in renal function occur.

Two reports have described off-label intravenous cidofovir used for the treatment of extensive, disfiguring, and refractory warts in immunocompromised patients. It should be used with caution because of the risk of nephrotoxicity (Kottke & Parker, 2006; Zabawski et al., 1997). Contraindications include hypersensitivity and elevated creatinine levels. Warnings include nephrotoxicity as well as neutropenia. It is Pregnancy Category C; it should be used during pregnancy only if the potential benefit justifies the potential risk to the fetus. It may cause decreased ocular pressure, anterior uveitis/iritis, or metabolic acidosis.

Isotretinoin (Accutane) may help off-label with extensive disabling hyperkeratotic warts in immunocompromised patients. It may help alleviate the pain related to the hyperkeratosis and facilitate the use of other treatments. Retinoids also have helped reduce the number of wart lesions in immunosuppressed renal transplant patients. The limiting side effects include liver function abnormalities, increased serum lipid levels, and teratogenicity. An FDA-mandated registry called iPLEDGE is now in place for all individuals prescribing, dispensing, or taking isotretinoin. This registry aims to further decrease the risk of pregnancy and other unwanted and potentially dangerous adverse effects during a course of isotretinoin therapy. Dosage for adults is 0.5 to 2 mg/kg/day orally divided into two doses and taken with food. Drug interactions include toxicity that may occur with vitamin A or acitretin coadministration. Pseudotumor cerebri or papilledema may occur when coadministered with tetracyclines. Reduced plasma levels of carbamazepine may occur. Contraindications include documented hypersensitivity, pregnancy, breastfeeding, paraben sensitivity, or a history of psychiatric disturbance such as depression. It is Pregnancy Category X, contraindicated, and benefit does not outweigh risk. Common reactions include dry skin, cheilitis, photosensitivity, hypertriglyceridemia, hair loss, and decreased night vision. Inflammatory bowel disease may be unmasked. It may be associated with development of hepatitis. Diabetics may experience problems in controlling blood glucose levels while on therapy. It is to be discontinued if rectal bleeding, abdominal pain, or severe diarrhea occurs. Use with caution if there is a history of depression or other psychiatric disorder. It is associated with severe birth defects, so females must use two forms of birth control throughout therapy, and pregnancy tests must be checked monthly.

Surgical Options

Cryosurgery with liquid nitrogen (–196 degrees C) is the most effective method of cryosurgery (Bourke et al., 1995). Less cold cryo substances generally do not achieve sufficient freezing of tissue. Liquid nitrogen is applied using a cotton-bud applicator or cryospray device with freezing including a 1- to 2-mm rim of normal skin tissue around the wart. Repeat every one to four weeks for approximately three months, as needed. Warn patients about pain and possible blistering after treatment. Use with caution on the sides of fingers, since it can injure underlying structures and nerves. Other side effects may include scarring, ulceration, or hypopigmentation. Wart resolution rates of 50% to 80% have been reported. Paring the wart, in addition to two freeze–thaw cycles, has been a valuable adjunct to cryosurgery for plantar warts (Berth-Jones & Hutchinson, 1992).

Electrodesiccation and curettage may be more effective than cryosurgery, but it is painful and more likely to scar, and HPV can be isolated from the plume. Retreatment may be necessary.

Surgical excision should be avoided in most circumstances because of the risks of scarring and the high rate of recurrence. Exceptions include debulking of giant condylomata acuminata.

Lasers are an expensive treatment method and are reserved for large or resistant warts. Multiple treatments may be required. Local or general anesthesia may be necessary. A potential risk of airborne wart infection exists for healthcare workers and patients, since HPV can be isolated in the smoke plume and can be inhaled (Gloster & Roenigk, 1995). Carbon dioxide lasers have successfully treated resistant warts, but the procedure can be painful and leave scarring. One retrospective study revealed a cure rate of 64% at 12 months with carbon dioxide lasers (Sloan et al., 1998). The flashlamp-pumped pulse dye laser has shown mixed results in treating warts, with a decreased risk of scarring and transmission of HPV in the smoke plume (Hughes & Hughes, 1998). The Nd:YAG laser may be used for deeper, larger warts.

Conclusion

Prevention of infection with common strains of oncogenic genital wart virus by vaccination of both males and females at puberty is desirable.

Treatment of warts can be difficult. Multiple treatments often may be required. The patient must build a CMI response against the wart virus to obtain resolution. Salicylic acid topical treatment of nongenital warts is moderately efficacious. Treatments may result in pain, irritation, blistering, ulceration, and even scarring. Cryosurgery can also be efficacious, but with associated pain and a risk of scarring or hypopigmentation. Other methods are of lower proven efficacy. Integrating conventional and alternative treatments sometimes has a synergistic effect.

Perform surgical removal of warts with caution, since an increased risk of scarring exists, without an increased rate of wart resolution.

If a wart is extremely large and resistant to conventional therapies, consider an incisional biopsy to rule out the diagnosis of verrucous carcinoma.

REFERENCES

Barabasz, A., Higley, L., Christensen C., et al. (2009). Efficacy of hypnosis in the treatment of human papillomavirus (HPV) in women: rural and urban samples. *International Journal of Clinical & Experimental Hypnosis, 58*(1), 102–121.

Bellew, S. G., Quartarolo, N., & Janniger, C. K. (2004). Childhood warts: an update. *Cutis, 73*(6), 379–384.

Benton, E. C. (20). Therapy of cutaneous warts. *Clinics in Dermatology, 15*(3), 449–455.

Berth-Jones, J., & Hutchinson, P. E. (1992). Modern treatment of warts: cure rates at 3 and 6 months. *British Journal of Dermatology, 127*(3), 262–265.

Bourke, J. F., Berth-Jones, J., & Hutchinson, P. E. (1995). Cryotherapy of common viral warts at intervals of 1, 2 and 3 weeks. *British Journal of Dermatology, 132*(3), 433–436.

Bouwes Bavinck, J. N., & Berkhout, R. J. (1997). HPV infections and immunosuppression. *Clinics in Dermatology, 15*(3), 427–437.

Brodell, R. T., & Johnson, S. M. (Eds.) (2003). *Warts: diagnosis and management: an evidence-based approach.* London: Martin Dunitz; 2003.

Cohen, P. R., Hebert, A. A., & Adler-Storthz, K. (1993). Focal epithelial hyperplasia: Heck disease. *Pediatric Dermatology, 10*(3), 245–251.

de Haen, M., Spigt, M., van Uden, C., et al. (2006). Efficacy of duct tape vs placebo in the treatment of verruca vulgaris (warts) in primary school children. *Archives of Pediatric & Adolescent Medicine, 160*(11), 1121–1125.

Drake, L. A., Ceilley, R. I., Cornelison, R. L., et al. (1995). Guidelines of care for warts: human papillomavirus. Committee on Guidelines of Care. *Journal of the American Academy of Dermatology, 32*(1), 98–103.

Edwards, I., Ferenczy, A., Eron, L., et al. (1998). Self-administered topical 5% imiquimod cream for external anogenital warts. HPV study group. Human Papilloma Virus. *Archives of Dermatology, 134,* 25–30.

Ewin, D. M. (1992). Hypnotherapy for warts (verruca vulgaris), 41 consecutive cases with 33 cures. *American Journal of Clinical Hypnosis, 35*(1), 1–10.

Ewin, D. M., & Eimer, B. N. (2006). *Ideomotor signals for rapid hypnoanalysis: a how-to manual.* Springfield, IL: Charles C. Thomas Publishers.

Focht, D. R. 3rd, Spicer, C., & Fairchok, M. P. (2002). The efficacy of duct tape vs cryotherapy in the treatment of verruca vulgaris (the common wart). *Archives of Pediatric & Adolescent Medicine, 156*(10), 971–974.

Gibbs, S., & Harvey, I. (2006). Topical treatments for cutaneous warts. *Cochrane Database of Systematic Reviews.* Issue 3. Art. No.: CD001781. DOI: 10.1002/14651858. CD001781.pub2 http://cochrane.org/reviews (accessed Dec. 7, 2009).

Gloster, H. M. Jr., & Roenigk, R. K. (1995). Risk of acquiring human papillomavirus from the plume produced by the carbon dioxide laser in the treatment of warts. *Journal of the American Academy of Dermatology, 32*(3), 436–441.

Goldfarb, M. T., Gupta, A. K., Gupta, M. A., et al. (1991). Office therapy for human papillomavirus infection in nongenital sites. *Dermatology Clinics, 9*(2), 287–296.

Guadara, J., Sergi, A., Labruna, V., et al. (20). Transformation of plantar verruca into squamous cell carcinoma. *Journal of Foot Surgery, 31*(6), 611–614.

Holland, T. T., Weber, C. B., & James, W. D. (1992). Tender periungual nodules. Myrmecia (deep palmoplantar warts). *Archives of Dermatology, 128*(1), 105–106, 108–109.

Horn, T. D., Johnson, S. M., Helm, R. M., et al. (20). Intralesional immunotherapy of warts with mumps, Candida, and Trichophyton skin test antigens: a single-blinded, randomized, and controlled trial. *Archives of Dermatology, 141*(5), 589–594.

Hughes, P. S., & Hughes, A. P. (1998). Absence of human papillomavirus DNA in the plume of erbium:YAG laser-treated warts. *Journal of the American Academy of Dermatology,* Mar 1998; 38(3), 426–428.

Jablonska, S., Majewski, S., Obalek, S., et al. (1997). Cutaneous warts. *Clinics in Dermatology, 15*(3), 309–319.

James, M. P., Collier, P. M., Aherne, W., et al. (1993). Histologic, pharmacologic, and immunocytochemical effects of injection of bleomycin into viral warts. *Journal of the American Academy of Dermatology, 28*(6), 933–937.

Kilkenny, M., & Marks, R. (1996). The descriptive epidemiology of warts in the community. *Australasian Journal of Dermatology, 37*(2), 80–86.

Kolker, A. R., Wolfort, F. G., Upton, J., et al. (20). Plantar verrucous carcinoma following transmetatarsal amputation and renal transplantation. *Annals of Plastic Surgery, 40*(5), 515–519.

Kottke, M. D., & Parker, S. R. (2006). Intravenous cidofovir-induced resolution of disfiguring cutaneous human papillomavirus infection. *Journal of the American Academy of Dermatology, 55*(3), 533–536.

Mallory, S. B., Baugh, L. S., & Parker, R. K. (1991). Warts in blacks versus whites. *Pediatric Dermatology, 8*(1), 91.

Matsukura, T., Iwasaki, T., & Kawashima, M. (1992). Molecular cloning of a novel human papillomavirus (type 60) from a plantar cyst with characteristic pathological changes. *Virology, 190*(1), 561–564.

Meineke, V., Reichrath, J., Reinhold, U., et al. (20). Verruca vulgares in children: successful simulated X-ray treatment (a suggestion-based therapy). *Dermatology, 204*(4), 287–289.

Melton, J. L., & Rasmussen, J. E. (1991). Clinical manifestations of human papillomavirus infection in nongenital sites. *Dermatology Clinics, 9*(2), 219–233.

Millar, B. C., & Moore, J. E. (2008). Successful topical treatment of hand warts in a paediatric patient with tea tree oil (*Melaleuca alternifolia*). *Complement Therapy in Clinical Practice, 14*(4), 225–227.

Mizuki, D., Kaneko, T., & Hanada, K. (2003). Successful treatment of topical photodynamic therapy using 5-aminolevulinic acid for plane warts. *British Journal of Dermatology, 149*(5), 1087–1088.

Munn, S. E., Higgins, E., Marshall, M., et al. (1996). A new method of intralesional bleomycin therapy in the treatment of recalcitrant warts. *British Journal of Dermatology, 135*(6), 969–971.

Nebesio, C. L., Mirowski, G. W., & Chuang, T. Y. (2001). Human papillomavirus: clinical significance and malignant potential. *International Journal of Dermatology, 40,* 373–379.

Noel, J. C., Detremmerie, O., Peny, M. O., et al. (1994). Transformation of common warts into squamous cell carcinoma on sun-exposed areas in an immunosuppressed patient. *Dermatology, 189*(3), 308–311.

PDR Staff. (2011). *2012 Physician's Desk Reference* (66th ed.). Montvale, NJ: Thompson.

Perrett, C. M., Harwood, C., & Brown, V. (2004). Topical 5% imiquimod treatment for refractory cutaneous warts. *Journal of the American Academy of Dermatology, 50*(3), P41.

Rivera, A., & Tyring, S. K. (2004). Therapy of cutaneous human Papillomavirus infections. *Dermatologic Therapy, 17*(6), 441–448.

Roark, T. R., & Pandya, A. G. (1998). Combination therapy of resistant warts in a patient with AIDS. *Dermatologic Surgery, 24*(12), 1387–1389.

Schachner, L., Ling, N. S., & Press, S. (1983). A statistical analysis of a pediatric dermatology clinic. *Pediatric Dermatology, 1*(2), 157–164.

Silverberg, N. B. (2002). Garlic cloves for verruca vulgaris. *Pediatric Dermatology, 19*(2), 183.

Silverberg, N. B. (2004). Human papillomavirus infections in children. *Current Opinion Pediatrics, 16*(4), 402–409.

Sloan, K., Haberman, H., & Lynde, C. W. (1998). Carbon dioxide laser-treatment of resistant verrucae vulgaris: retrospective analysis. *Journal of Cutaneous Medicine & Surgery, 2*(3), 142–145.

Spanos, N., Williams, V., & Gwynn, M. I. (1990). Effects of hypnotic, placebo, and salicylic acid treatments on wart regression. *Psychosomatic Medicine, 52.* 109–114.

Stone, K. M., Becker, T. M., Hadgu, A., et al. (1990). Treatment of external genital warts: a randomized clinical trial comparing podophyllin, cryotherapy, and electrodessication. *Genitourinary Medicine, 66,* 16–19.

Tatti, S., Swineheart, J. M., Thielert, C., et al. (2008). Sinecatechins, a defined green tea extract, in the treatment of external anogenital warts: a randomized controlled trial. *Obstetrics & Gynecology, 111,* 1371–1379.

Tyring, S., Edwards, L., Cherry, K., et al. (1998). Safety and efficacy of 0.5% podofilox gel in the treatment of anogenital warts. *Archives of Dermatology, 134,* 33–38.

Tyring, S. K. (2000). Human papillomavirus infections: epidemiology, pathogenesis, and host immune response. *Journal of the American Academy of Dermatology, 43,* S18–S26.

Tyring, S. K. (2012). Sinecatechins: effects on HPV-induced enzymes involved in inflammatory mediator generation. *Journal of Clinical & Aesthetic Dermatology, 5*(1), 19–26.

Wenner, R., Askari, S. K., Cham, P. M., et al. (2007). Duct tape for the treatment of common warts in adults: a double-blind randomized controlled trial. *Archives of Dermatology, 143*(3), 309–313.

Yanagihara, M., Sumi, A., & Mori, S. (1989). Papillomavirus antigen in the epidermoid cyst of the sole. Immunohistochemical and ultrastructural study. *Journal of Cutaneous Pathology, 16*(6), 375–381.

Yilmaz, E., Alpsoy, E., & Basaran, E. (1996). Cimetidine therapy for warts: a placebo-controlled, double-blind study. *Journal of the American Academy of Dermatology, 34*(6), 1005–1007.

Young, R., Jolley, D., & Marks, R. (1998). Comparison of the use of standardized diagnostic criteria and intuitive clinical diagnosis in the diagnosis of common viral warts (verrucae vulgaris). *Archives of Dermatology, 134*(12), 1586–1589.

Zabawski, E. J. Jr., Sands, B., Goetz, D., et al. (20). Treatment of verruca vulgaris with topical cidofovir [letter]. *Journal of the American Medical Association, 278*(15), 1236.

29

Integrative Management of Vitiligo

RAMAN MADAN AND FALGUNI ASRANI

Key Concepts

♣ Vitiligo is a condition that has been referenced for centuries and is the most common pigmentary disorder worldwide. There is a strong psychosocial stigma associated with it. Different treatments have been attempted, although most have been inadequate.

♣ Vitiligo is caused by an absence of functional melanocytes in the lesional skin. Several pathogenic mechanisms are hypothesized; they include autoimmune mechanisms, oxidant–antioxidant mechanisms, transepidermal melanocytorrhagy, neural mechanisms, and intrinsic defects of melanocytes.

♣ Topical steroids, phototherapy, and oral immunosuppressants are the most common treatments currently used for vitiligo. Surgical therapies and total depigmentation are available but less commonly used.

♣ *Ginkgo biloba* has been used to treat vitiligo because of its anti-inflammatory, immunomodulatory, antioxidant, and anxiolytic effects.

♣ Ayurvedic therapy centering on establishing equilibrium among the three energy components of *vayu* (wind), *pitta* (bile), and *kapha* (phlegm) has also been used to treat vitiligo. This involves herbal medication, detoxification, and external application of herbal powders and oils.

♣ Dead Sea climatotherapy has been a popular treatment for vitiligo. This is likely due to the solar radiation and the high salt concentration. While effective, the treatment is not considered practical for many.

♣ Different herbs have been combined, and several products are currently available to treat vitiligo. Such products include Anti-vitiligo®, Kalawalla®, and Melagenina®.

Introduction

The term *vitiligo* was first used by the Roman physician Celsus in the Latin medical classic *De Medicina* in the first century C.E. The origin may be from the word *vituli* or *vitelius*, both of which refer to the white patches in the fur of calves (Kopera, 1997). For centuries, there has been mention of vitiligo. The first description of "white patches" dates back to 2200 B.C.E., when it was described in *Tarikh-e-Tibb-Iran*, the prescribed book of medicine at the time (Seghal & Srivastava, 2007). The Ebers Papyrus from Egypt, dating back to 1500 B.C.E., provides detailed reports of two types of patchy skin diseases that had color change. One condition was described as being untreatable and was likely referring to leprosy, a disease commonly confused with vitiligo in the past. The other condition was described as having light patches and considered treatable, which was likely vitiligo. Numerous other references to vitiligo can be found from India in 1300 B.C.E., the Far East in 1200 B.C.E., Greek literature from 450 B.C.E., the Bible, and various Chinese literatures (Kopera, 1997).

By the end of the 19th century, more was understood about vitiligo and it was defined as a pigmentary dystrophy. Louis Brocq expanded on this term as a lack of pigmentation, or achromy, accompanied with an increase in pigmentation, or dyschromy (Kopera, 1997). Eventually, the histological features of vitiligo were described by Moritz Kaposi, who stated that "the only anatomic change in vitiliginous skin is the lack of pigment granules in deep rete cells" (Kaposi, 1899).

Different treatments for vitiligo have been attempted throughout history, although most have been inadequate. Phototherapy was used in ancient times but did not come into use in the Western world until the development of PUVA and UVB therapy in the latter half of the 20th century (Millington, 2007). Extract from the fruit of the plant *Ammi majus* was used in the 13th century in Egypt as an attempt to treat vitiligo. Mixtures of bromides, iodides, mercury, croton oil, sublimate, and naphthol were also used in the past without great results (Kopera, 1997). Homeopathic medicine and natural remedies still play a large role in treatment.

While reference to vitiligo dates back centuries, there is still much to be learned about the pathophysiology, pathogenesis, and treatment of this very common skin condition. Vitiligo is a chronic disorder characterized by a complete absence of melanocytes in the epidermis. It presents initially with white macules that can enlarge and eventually affect the entire skin (Wolff et al., 2009). While the disease can start at any time, vitiligo most commonly begins in childhood or young adulthood, with peak ages of onset between 10 and 30 years (Wolff et al., 2007). The disease is rare in infancy and in the elderly (Tonsi,

2004). Given the cosmetic concerns, this disease can cause severe psychological distress, especially in those with dark skin (Halder & Taliaferro, 2008).

With an incidence rate between 0.1% and 2%, vitiligo is the most common pigmentary disorder worldwide. Men and women are both equally afflicted with vitiligo. Females have been presumed to be more often affected, but this is likely due to the fact they are more likely to seek treatment for cosmetic reasons (Halder & Taliaferro, 2008). In the United States, the incidence of vitiligo is estimated at 1% (Wolff et al., 2009). Although all races are affected, the incidence is higher in racially pigmented skin and has been reported to be as high as 4% in some South Asian and Mexican populations. The highest worldwide prevalence is considered to be in Gujarat, India, with a prevalence of approximately 8.8% (Alikhan et al., 2011; Yaghoobi et al., 2011). This increased prevalence may be secondary to the increased number of diagnoses in these populations, due to contrast between white vitiligo macules and dark skin (Wolff et al., 2009).

Pathophysiology

Vitiligo is a multifactorial polygenic disorder with both genetic and nongenetic factors. Familial clustering is observed in vitiligo but inheritance occurs in a non-Mendelian pattern (Passeron & Ortonne, 2005; Zhang et al., 2005). Approximately 20% of patients with vitiligo have at least one first-degree relative with vitiligo (Wolff et al., 2009). An autosomal dominant gene of variable penetrance has also been reported, as well as cases of vitiligo in monozygotic twins (Yaghoobi et al., 2011). Multiple other potential gene associations have been reported, but there is still much left to study.

There is general agreement that vitiligo is caused by an absence of functional melanocytes in the lesional skin, which is evidenced by a loss of histochemically recognizable melanocytes. There are several leading pathogenic hypotheses for vitiligo, such as autoimmune mechanisms, oxidant–antioxidant mechanisms, transepidermal melanocytorrhagy, neural mechanisms, and intrinsic defects of melanocytes. Other theories include dysregulation of melanocyte apoptosis, lipid membrane alterations in melanocytes, deficiencies of melanocytic growth factors, and destruction of melanocytes by viral infection (possibly cytomegalovirus). A few of the main theories are highlighted below; however, the data to date favor a combination of several different pathogenic mechanisms "converging" to cause the vitiligo skin lesions (Kopera, 1997).

AUTOIMMUNE DESTRUCTION OF MELANOCYTES

The autoimmune theory proposes an alteration in humoral or cellular immunity, which results in melanocyte destruction. Dysfunction in the humoral pathway is supported by the association of vitiligo with other autoimmune conditions such as hypo/hyperthyroidism and, less often, pernicious anemia, Addison's disease, diabetes mellitus, alopecia areata, and autoimmune polyglandular syndrome (Kemp et al., 2001; Ongenae et al., 2003). Additionally, autoantibodies directed against several different melanocyte antigens have been found in the sera of patients with vitiligo (Ongenae et al., 2003).

There is also strong evidence suggesting abnormal cellular immunity in the pathogenesis of vitiligo. T cells have been found to infiltrate perilesional skin, with activated CD8+T cells representing the predominant cell type (Lang et al., 2001; Ogg et al., 1998; van den Boorn et al., 2009). In addition, skin-homing melanocyte-specific cytotoxic T cells can be detected in the peripheral blood of patients with autoimmune vitiligo (Antelo et al., 2011).

DEFECTIVE OXIDANT–ANTIOXIDANT SYSTEM IN VITILIGO

The role of oxidative damage to melanocytes in lesional skin was first considered because vitiligo exhibits a characteristic yellow/green or bluish fluorescence under Wood's lamp illumination. This Wood's lamp finding led to the discovery that skin fluorescence is secondary to the accumulation of two oxidized pteridines—6-biopterin (blue) and 7-biopterin (yellow/green) (Schallreuter et al., 1994a, 1994b). The overproduction of these tetrahydrobiopterins suggests a metabolic defect in tetrahydrobiopterin homeostasis in patients with vitiligo. This defect can result in overproduction of hydrogen peroxide (H_2O_2), which can be toxic to melanocytes, potentially leading to their destruction. Several studies in this area have shown high levels of oxidative stress in vitiligo (Hasse et al., 2004; Spencer et al., 2007; Sravani et al., 2009).

TRANSEPIDERMAL MELANOCYTORRHAGY

Recent studies have found a chronic detachment and transepidermal loss of epidermal melanocytes in patients with generalized vitiligo. It is thought that mechanical stress or friction induces detachment of melanocytes and then the damaged melanocytes are eliminated from the area via transepidermal migration, leading to patches of vitiligo (Cario-André et al., 2007; Gauthier et al., 2003).

NEURAL MECHANISM

There is evidence that peripheral nerve endings may secrete a substance that is cytotoxic to melanocytes, which leads to their destruction. This theory is supported by the segmental variety of vitiligo, which occurs in specific dermatomes, indicating the nerves in that dermatome may lead to the skin lesions.

Nerve endings in depigmented areas have been shown to produce abnormal neuropeptides and nerve growth factors and displayed axonal degeneration. It is proposed that these abnormal chemicals may be toxic to melanocytes. Additionally, depigmented areas showed some abnormal autonomic function, such as increased adrenergic tone, increased norepinephrine, and an increased concentration of catecholamines. These data suggest that neurotransmitter release could have an effect on melanocyte destruction and therefore depigmentation (Taieb, 2000).

INTRINSIC DEFECT OF MELANOCYTES

This theory suggests that melanocytes in vitiligo have an intrinsic defect leading to melanocyte death. Vitiligo melanocytes have shown various abnormalities such as dilation of the rough endoplasmic reticulum, which may play a role in vitiligo (van den Wiingaard et al., 2000). Studies have also shown abnormal expression of tyrosinase-related protein 1 (TYRP1) in vitiligo melanocytes as well as increased sensitivity to oxidative stress (UVB), resulting in early cell death (Jimbow et al., 2001). Based on these findings, it has been proposed that melanocytes disappear secondary to abnormal synthesis and processing of TYRP1 and its abnormal interaction with the melanogenesis within the rough endoplasmic reticulum.

Clinical Findings

There are multiple forms of vitiligo; the most common form is described as discrete amelanotic milky-white macules ranging from 5 mm to 5 cm or greater surrounded by normal skin. Trichrome vitiligo is a variant that has three colors (white, light brown, dark brown) representing the stages of evolution of vitiligo. Inflammatory vitiligo is a variant with an elevated erythematous potentially pruritic margin. Vitiligo ponctué is characterized by multiple small confetti-like discrete amelanotic macules occurring on normal or hyperpigmented skin. Isomorphic Koebner phenomenon (development of lesions at the site of trauma) is a notable manifestation of vitiligo (Gauthier, 1995). Patients often attribute the onset of vitiligo to a specific event such as physical injury, sunburn, emotional trauma, illness, or pregnancy (Yaghoobi et al., 2011), but aside from the Koebner phenomenon, none of these factors has been proven to precipitate vitiligo. This disease progresses by growth of current lesions or by development of new lesions. Patients are considered to have stable disease when they have trichrome or inflammatory lesions and no growing or new lesions for six months to one year (Bolognia et al., 2008).

DISTRIBUTION

There are three main patterns of depigmentation in vitiligo: focal, segmental, and generalized. The focal type is characterized by one to several macules present at a single site. The segmental type is characterized by one or several macules present in a bandlike distribution on one side of the body. The most common form is generalized vitiligo, which is characterized by widespread distribution of depigmented macules, often symmetrical, with a predilection around the eyes and mouth and on digits, elbows, knees, lower back, and genitalia. The "lip-tip" pattern involves the skin around the mouth and the distal fingers and toes; lips, nipples, and genitalia can also be involved. Vitiligo universalis is the term used when lesional skin becomes confluent, leaving only a few areas of normally pigmented skin (Bolognia et al., 2008; Wolff et al., 2005).

The Wood's lamp examination can be helpful in making the diagnosis, particularly in fair-skinned individuals. The normal function of melanin is to block and absorb the light; however, there is less or no epidermal melanin in the vitiligo-affected patches. The vitiligo-affected skin appears blue white with sharp margins. Wood's light can also be helpful to detect vitiligo at a very early stage for preemptive treatment. It can similarly be used for an early assessment of the success of treatment. In certain cases skin biopsy may be required. However, the findings are not diagnostic; they simply support the clinical diagnosis. Histopathological examination will show normal skin with an absence of melanocytes. Electron microscopy will show an absence of melanocytes and an absence of melanosomes in the keratinocytes (Bolognia et al., 2008).

Although most patients with vitiligo are otherwise healthy, associated autoimmune endocrinopathies can occur in some individuals. The patients should be educated on signs and symptoms to look out for. The strongest association is thyroid disease; therefore, a screening with review of systems and possible TSH assessment is indicated. There are also studies showing an association of vitiligo with diabetes mellitus and cases of vitiligo associated with Addison's disease, gonadal failure, and pernicious anemia (Bolognia et al., 2008; James et al., 2011).

Differential Diagnosis

Complete depigmentation of the skin can occur in other conditions. Chemical leukoderma, or occupational vitiligo, is caused by exposure to agents such as phenolic germicides, thiols, catecholsmercatoamines, and several quinines. Typically, depigmented patches will occur only in areas where the skin has had contact with chemical agents. Clinically, it may be very difficult to differentiate chemical leukoderma from vitiligo; therefore, a detailed history is needed.

Leukodermas associated with melanoma or scleroderma can also mimic vitiligo. Piebaldism has a similar clinical presentation, but it is congenital and typically present at birth. Early lesions of vitiligo, where there is only partial loss of pigment, may resemble postinflammatory hypopigmentation, tinea versicolor, leprosy, nevus depigmentosus, hypopigmented mycosis fungoides, and pityriasis alba. Vitiligo ponctué may resemble the confetti macules seen in tuberous sclerosis (Bolognia et al., 2008; James et al., 2011).

Treatment

Vitiligo is a chronic disease with a highly variable course. Overall it can be a challenging condition to treat. Spontaneous repigmentation can occur in 15% to 25% of cases. The major concern for patients is cosmetic; therefore, multiple cosmetic cover-up options have been developed to temporarily camouflage skin lesions. Topical dyes resistant to being washed off are often used, and self-tanning creams containing dihydroxyacetone are useful for patients with lighter to olive skin tones.

The main goals of vitiligo treatment are repigmentation and stabilization of disease progression. Although there is currently no cure for vitiligo, there are multiple treatment options. We will briefly visit the "conventional" medical treatment options and then focus on the myriad of "alternative" medicine treatment and remedies for vitiligo.

Topical steroids are mainstay treatments for focal/limited disease. A two-month trial of mid- to super-high-potency steroids should be implemented. Typically lesions on the face respond better than those on the extremities or trunk. The use of topical calcipotreinene daily may increase the efficacy of topical steroids. Tacrolimus 0.1% ointment, which is an immunomodulating agent, is an effective treatment in especially cosmetically sensitive areas such as the face because it avoids the side effects, such as atrophy and acne, that can be induced by prolonged steroid use.

PUVA, also called photochemotherapy or phototherapy, is an effective radiation treatment for vitiligo. It involves exposure of the skin to UVA under medical supervision. The effective agent in PUVA treatment is psoralen, a light-sensitizing medication that is taken orally or applied topically. Worldwide, PUVA treatment is the one of the most popular treatments for vitiligo; the concept for this treatment dates back thousands of years, when the plants *Psoralea coryifolia* Linn. and *Ammi majus* Linn. were eaten or used topically in Egypt and India to treat vitiligo. Today, isolates of the plants are used topically or orally in conjunction with a synthetic compound to chemically increase sensitivity to light. The patient is then exposed to a measured amount of natural sunlight (PUVASOL) or PUVA to induce repigmentation. Topical application of 8-methoxypsoralen to the affected areas followed by UVA exposure has also been effective for focal or limited disease. For widespread disease, systemic PUVA, where the patient takes methoxsalen capsules two hours before the appointment for treatment, is a more practical treatment choice. One main drawback for these therapies is burns and blistering, which commonly occur during treatment. Additionally, patients will have tanned skin from the treatment, which often lasts for several months. In many ethnicities tanned skin is seen as less "beautiful," so this may be a considerable drawback for some patients. PUVA treatments may increase the risk of premature skin aging and skin cancer.

Narrow-band UVB (311 nm), also a phototherapy, is beginning to replace PUVA/PUVASOL therapy in many countries because of its safety profile and convenience. Narrow-band UVB therapy twice weekly is an effective therapy. Repigmentation may begin after 15 to 25 treatments, but significant improvement can take up to 200 treatments (Scherschun et al., 2001; Westerhof & Nieuweboer-Krobotova, 1997). The Excimer laser (308 nm), which can deliver high doses of light to single lesions, can be used for localized disease. Lesions are treated twice weekly for an average of 24 to 48 sessions. This treatment can help eliminate the side effects also.

Surgical therapies are used in specific cases where patients have failed to respond to other treatments and have limited and stable disease. Stable disease is defined as no new lesions and no growing lesions for at least six months to one year (Gupta et al., 2002). In minigrafting, the simplest method, small punch grafts (1 to 2 mm) are taken from nonlesional skin and implanted into lesional skin. Each graft is placed about 5 to 8 mm apart, creating a cobblestone effect. Donor sites should be chosen carefully as there will be scarring and possible pigment alteration (Falabella et al., 1995). Suction blister epidermal grafting is another technique; it is effective and avoids scarring at the donor site. Grafting of cultures of autologous melanocytes is yet another technique that can be used, but it is expensive and requires highly skilled laboratory expertise (Gauthier & Surleve-Bazeille, 1992; Guerra et al., 2000).

Total depigmentation is a favorable treatment option for patients with greater than 50% body surface involvement. The most commonly used agent is 20% monobenzyl ether of hydroquinone (MBEH) applied twice daily to the affected areas for 9 to 12 months. MBEH is a potent irritant and/or allergen, so an open use test should be done before starting therapy. Patients must understand that this therapy requires strict lifelong photoprotection (Bolognia et al., 2001; Mosher et al., 1977).

Although these traditional medical practices have been able to help treat this disease, no cure has been discovered. Vitiligo is a disease that dates back many centuries, and even before the era of modern medicine various treatments and remedies were tried worldwide.

One of the most popular and most studied "natural" treatments for vitiligo is *Ginkgo biloba*. Its therapeutic effects are related to its unique polyphenol compounds, including terpenoids (ginkgolides and bilobalides), flavonoids, and flavonol extracts. Studies have shown that gingko extracts can have an antioxidant effect by decreasing oxidative stress in macrophages and endothelial cells. Ginkgolides specifically have this antioxidant effect because of their superoxide scavenging effect. Biflavones has been shown to protect from UVB-induced cytotoxicity (Szczurko et al., 2011). While the exact reason *G. biloba* is useful in the treatment of vitiligo is unknown, but several theories have been proposed. Its anti-inflammatory, immunomodulatory, antioxidant, and anxiolytic effects all are suggested mechanisms contributing to its effectiveness (Szczurko et al., 2011). In one study, *G. biloba* 40 mg given three times a day orally was found to significantly affect repigmentation and arrest of the disease (Parsad et al., 2003). In another study *G. biloba* 60 mg twice daily for 12 weeks stopped the progression of disease in all participants and produced an average repigmentation in 15% of vitiligo lesions. The treatment is inexpensive and has relatively few side effects, making it an appealing treatment option.

Gingko's anxiolytic effect has also been suspected to contribute to its efficacy in treatment for vitiligo. Some believe one of the proposed mechanisms for the pathogenesis of vitiligo is related to stress and anxiety (Szczurko et al., 2011). *G. biloba* has been found to decrease the effects of learned helplessness as well as the negative effects of increased plasma concentrations of epinephrine, norepinephrine, and corticosterone (Jezova et al., 2002).

One study showed that vitamin E can be effective in treating vitiligo. Patients were given PUVA and 900 IU/day vitamin E while control patients were given PUVA three times a week for six months. The results showed that PUVA and vitamin E produced good improvement in 60% of the treatment group versus 40% of the control group (Akyol et al., 2002).

Vitamin E is often noted for its antioxidant properties. A study was done giving patients antioxidant- and mitochondrial-stimulating cream, oral antioxidants, and phenylalanine. The oral antioxidants included vitamin A 20,000 IU, vitamin C 1,000 mg, vitamin E 400 IU, zinc 15 mg, selenium 50 µg, magnesium 2 mg, CoQ10 75 mcg, and pycnogenol 1 mg. The results showed that the use of the antioxidant and mitochondrial cream and oral antioxidants and phenylalanine provided the best results (Rojas et al., 2007).

Vitamin B12, vitamin C, and folic acid have also been used for their antioxidant effects in the treatment of vitiligo (Whitton et al., 2010).

Ayurvedic therapy has been used for centuries in India for many different diseases. It involves exploring the patient's background and trying to establish equilibrium among the three energy components: *vayu* (wind), *pitta* (bile), and *kapha* (phlegm). When these energies exist in equal quantities, the body will remain healthy. It is believed that a healthy metabolic system, good digestion, proper excretion, and a focus on exercise, yoga, and meditation all help achieve this vitality (Carrier, 2011). Ayurvedic treatments generally involve plant-based or herbal medicines, although animal products such as milk may be used (Dhanik et al., 2011). There are three major therapies for vitiligo in the Ayurvedic texts. The first involves using herbal medication and minerals as pacification therapy. The second involves detoxification therapies such as purgation and bloodletting. The third involves external applications of herbal powder and oil (Narahari et al., 2011).

Many different oral herbal combinations have been recommended for vitiligo. The oral herbal therapies are thought to be effective by stimulating melanoblastic cells. Liquid extract of *Acacia catechu* bark is one treatment that has been shown to be effective. Other herbs that have been used include *Psoralea corylifolia* leaves with psoralens, Usheer tea prepared from *Vetivexia zizaniodis*, and Brahmi tablets containing *Eclipta alba*. Despite their effectiveness, some of these herbs may be associated with side effects such as hepatotoxicity (Teschke & Bahre, 2009).

The activity of vitiligo is described in Ayurvedic texts by the number of coalescing lesions and reduced digestive ability (Szczurko & Boon, 2008). Ayurveda *panchakarma* involves detoxification therapies for the treatment of vitiligo. One method involves therapeutic vomiting to cleanse the gastrointestinal tract by clearing toxins from the liver and gallbladder. Enemas, nasal drops, and bloodletting are all recommended as well to cleanse the body. Drinking water kept overnight in a copper vessel was also often practiced (Narahari et al., 2011).

Several external applications for vitiligo are also recommended by Ayurvedic medicine. One such preparation consists of dried ginger, black pepper, pippali, and leadwort root fermented in cow's urine (Donata et al., 1990). *P. corylifolia*, a combination of turmeric powder and mustard powder, sweet basil leaves with juice, and radish seeds with vinegar are some of the many applications that are recommended to be applied to the white patches of skin (Narahari et al., 2011).

Bathing in the Dead Sea (Dead Sea climatotherapy) is another treatment that has been used for years. For best results, patients should go for several weeks between late February and mid-November. The high salt concentration, high $MgCl_2$ concentration of water, and solar radiation have all been proposed as mechanisms for the efficacy of treatment. The high salt concentration (346 g/L) has been proposed to release pro-inflammatory and chemotactic mediators. $MgCl_2$ modifies the activity of antigen-presenting Langerhans cells. The solar radiation at the Dead Sea is considered beneficial because the UVB spectrum at the basin of the Dead Sea becomes scattered in a manner that is inversely proportional to the wavelength; therefore, the erythemal spectral range becomes attenuated more than the rest of the UVB spectral range (Czarnowicki et al., 2011). Pseudocatalase cream can be added to Dead Sea climatotherapy. The proposed mechanism involves removing high levels of H_2O_2 from patients, which leads to the initiation of repigmentation (Schallreuter et al., 2002). Dead Sea climatotherapy is relatively safe and has no long-term side effects, but it may be impractical for patients due to its high cost, long distance, and time required for travel (Czarnowicki et al., 2011).

In China, several different remedies have been used in the treatment of vitiligo. A mixture of Xiaobai, 160 mL, taken orally daily has been found to be effective. It contains 30 g walnut, 10 g red flower, 30 g black sesame, 30 g black beans, 10 g zhibeifu ping, 10 g lulu tong, and 5 plums. Chinese herbal mixtures and corticosteroids have been shown to improve vitiligo as well (Szczurko & Boon, 2008). The practice of Chinese cupping, which involves providing suction over the skin, can be used to induce blisters on the thigh, whose roofs are subsequently used for epithelial grafts in the treatment of vitiligo (Awad, 2008).

Herbal products have been used for the treatment of vitiligo for centuries. Anti-vitiligo®, a treatment that has been available since November 2003, is effective in treating both recent-onset and longstanding cases. The main ingredients—coconut oil, *P. corylifolia*, black cumin, and barberry root—all contribute to its efficacy (Tahir et al., 2010). Coconut oil is easily dissolved by the skin and is rich in vitamin E and therefore has a strong antioxidant activity. *P. corylifolia* is a natural psoralen that can be used topically or orally. It is another source of antioxidant activity. In addition, it can sensitize human skin to the tanning effect of UV and sunlight. The efficacy of black cumin or the seeds of *Nigella sativa* is due to its immunomodulatory effect. It has been known to mediate T-cell and natural killer cell immune responses. Lastly, barberry root, or the root of *Berberis vulgaris,* is an herb that in addition to its antioxidant and cytoprotective properties is effective because of the chemicals and other bioactive compounds it contains. Alkaloids such as berbamine, berberine, and oxycacanthine can be found in barberry root. Tannins, chelifonic acid, resins, thiamine, lutein, vitamin C, beta-carotene, zeacanthin, zinc, chromium, and cobalt can all be found as well (Tahir et al., 2010).

Bavachi (*P. carylifolia*), a psoralen derivative, is a popular ingredient in commercially available products for vitiligo. This ingredient helps induce pigmentation in hypopigmented skin. It is believed that the hyperemia caused by psoralens increases the melanin-producing activity in skin.

Vitilo© lotion and Bonzastrong© lotion are two commercially available lotions that have been used with success. Vitilo© lotion is composed of 4%

Bavachi (*P. carylifolia*), 1% Karanja (*Pongamia glabra*), 2% Neem (*Azadirachta indica*), 2% Manjistha (*Rubia cordifolia*), 1% Haldi (*Curcuma longa*), 1% AmbaHaldi (*Curcuma amada*), 2% Raktachandan (*Pterocarpus santalinum*), 1% Vacha (*Acorus calamus*), and 4% processed JasadBhasma (ZnO). The ingredients in Bonzastrong© lotion are similar.

The patient should apply a thin layer of lotion two or three times to the affected area of skin. After waiting roughly 30 minutes, or until the lotion dries, the patient should then expose the area to sunlight for five to 20 minutes. Aside from itching, which should be treated with coconut oil, no serious side effects have been reported. Patients should not apply the product to mucous membranes.

Polypodium leucotomos is a fern native to the tropical and subtropical regions of the Americas. It has a long history of use as a folk remedy in Honduras. In one study, patients were given PUVA and *P. leucotomos*, with controls being given PUVA for 12 weeks. The percentage of patients with skin repigmentation greater than 50% was significantly higher with PUVA and *Polypodium* (Reyes et al., 2006).

Kalawalla®, another herbal product used in vitiligo, contains *P. leucotomos* and works as a natural immunomodulator. It works by increasing lymphocyte levels and regulating the CD4/CD8 levels to a normal ratio. This product, taken orally, contains 120 mg *P. leucotomos* extract and 280 mg *P. leucotomos* rhizome. Pruritus has been reported as a side effect (Tahir et al., 2010).

Piperine, the major alkaloid of black pepper (*Piper nigrum* L.; Piperaceae), stimulates melanocyte proliferation and dendrite formation in vitro. This property renders it a potential treatment for vitiligo. When combined with ultraviolet radiation treatment, piperine has been shown to promote pigmentation of the skin by stimulating melanocyte replication. The analogues tetrahydropiperine (THP) and reduced cyclohexylpiperdine (rCHP) were particularly effective (Faas et al., 2008).

The amino acid L-phenylalanine is also used to treat vitiligo. It is known that phenylalanine is a precursor for melanin via L-tyrosine, and it is suggested there is a problem with L-phenylalanine metabolism in vitiligo. A combination of topical application and oral ingestion of phenylalanine with natural sunlight exposure has been shown to aid in repigmentation with relatively few side effects (Siddigui et al., 1994). It was also noticed that with this therapy there were decreased Langerhans cells present in lesional skin. L-phenylalanine can have a role in the treatment of vitiligo in any patient with access to natural or UVA light (Felsten et al., 2011).

Melagenina® (now Melagenina Plus®) was developed in Cuba about 20 years ago. It was initially extracted from human placenta tissue, and now other animal placental tissues are also used (Nordlund & Halder, 1990). It is applied topically and is thought to work by stimulating the proliferation and differentiation of immature melanocytes and melanoblasts (Zhao et al., 2008). There are claims of high success rates, but these cannot be verified. The product instructions indicate that the cream should be applied and then the affected skin should be exposed to 15 minutes of natural sunlight.

Conclusion

Alternative and complementary medicine has been used for centuries for vitiligo. Although there have not been many strong formal studies, the therapeutic benefit of many of these treatments must not be overlooked. These historical and cultural treatments need not replace our conventional medical therapies, but they can certainly expand our armamentarium of treatment options for this chronic and difficult-to-treat disease.

REFERENCES

Akyol, M., Celik, V. K., Ozcelik, S., et al. (2002). The effects of vitamin E on the skin lipid peroxidation and the clinical improvement in vitiligo patients treated with PUVA. *European Journal of Dermatology, 12*, 24–26.

Alikhan, A., et al. (2011). Vitiligo: A comprehensive overview. *Journal of the American Academy of Dermatology, 65*(3), 473–514.

Antelo, D. P.,Filgueira, A. L., & Cunha, J. M. (2011). Reduction of skin-homing cytotoxic T cells (CD8+ -CLA+) in patients with vitiligo. *Photodermatology, Photoimmunology, & Photomedicine, 27*(1), 40–44.

Awad, S. S. (2008). Chinese cupping: a simple method to obtain epithelial grafts for the management of resistant localized vitiligo. *Dermatologic Surgery, 34*(9), 1186–1192.

Bolognia, J. L., LaPia, K., & Somma, S. (2001). Depigmentation therapy. *Dermatologic Therapy, 14*, 29–34.

Bolognia, J., Jorizzo, J. L., & Rapini, R. P. (2008). *Dermatology* (2nd ed., pp. 913–920). St. Louis, MO: Mosby/Elsevier.

Cario-André, M., et al. (2007). The melanocytorrhagic hypothesis of vitiligo tested on pigmented, stressed, reconstructed epidermis. *Pigment Cell Research, 20*(5), 385–393.

Carrier, M. (2011). Ayurvedic medicine. *Skeptic, 16*(2), 17.

Czarnowicki, T., et al. (2011). Dead Sea climatotherapy for vitiligo: a retrospective study of 436 patients. *Journal of the European Academy of Dermatology & Venereology, 25*(8), 959–963.

Dhanik, A., Sujatha, N., & Rai, N. P. (2011). Clinical evaluation of the efficacy of *Shvitrahara kashaya* and *lepa* in vitiligo. *Ayu, 32*(1), 66–69.

Donata et al. (1990). Clinical trial of certain ayurvedic medicines indicated in vitiligo. *Ancient Science of Life, 9*(4), 202–206.

Faas, L., et al. (2008). In vivo evaluation of piperine and synthetic analogues as potential treatments for vitiligo using a sparsely pigmented mouse model. *Br J Dermatol. 2008;158*(5), 941–950.

Falabella, R., et al. (1995). The minigrafting test for vitiligo: detection of stable lesions for melanocyte transplantation. *Journal of the American Academy of Dermatology, 32*(2 Pt 1), 228–232.

Felsten, M. L., Alikhan, A., & Petronic-Rosic, V. (2011). Vitiligo: A comprehensive overview- Part II: Treatment options and approach to treatment. *Journal of the American Academy of Dermatology, 65*(3), 493–514.

Gauthier, Y. (1995). The importance of Koebner's phenomenon in induction of vitiligo vulgaris lesions. *European Journal of Dermatology, 5*, 704–708.

Gauthier, Y., & Surleve-Bazeille, J. E. (1992). Autologous grafting with noncultured melanocytes: a simplified method for treatment of depigmented lesions. *Journal of the American Academy of Dermatology, 26*(2 Pt 1), 191–194.

Gauthier, Y., et al. (2003). Melanocyte detachment after skin friction in nonlesional skin of patients with generalized vitiligo. *British Journal of Dermatology, 148*(1), 95–101.

Guerra, L., et al. (2000). Treatment of "stable" vitiligo by timed surgery and transplantation of cultured epidermal autografts. *Archives of Dermatology, 136*(11), 1380–1389.

Gupta, S., Honda, S., & Kumar, B. (2002). A novel scoring system for evaluation of results of autologous transplantation methods in vitiligo. *Indian Journal of Dermatology, Venereology, Leprology, 68*(1), 33–37.

Halder, R. M., & Taliaferro, S. J. (2008) Chapter 72: Vitiligo. In K. Wolff et al. (Eds.), *Fitzpatrick's dermatology in general medicine* (7th ed.). New York: McGraw-Hill.

Hasse, S., et al. (2004). Perturbed 6-tetrahydrobiopterin recycling via decreased dihydropteridine reductase in vitiligo: more evidence for H2O2 stress. *Journal of Investigative Dermatology, 122*(2), 307–313.

James, W. D., et al. (2011). *Andrews' diseases of the skin: clinical dermatology*. London: Saunders.

Jezova, D., et al. (2002). Reduction of the rise in blood pressure and cortisol release during stress by *Ginkgo biloba* extract (EGb 761) in healthy volunteers. *Journal of Physiology & Pharmacology, 53*(3), 337–348.

Jimbow, K., et al. (2001). Increased sensitivity of melanocytes to oxidative stress and abnormal expression of tyrosinase-related protein in vitiligo. *British Journal of Dermatology, 144*(1), 55–65.

Kaposi, M. (1899). *Pathologie und Therapie der hautkrankheiten.* (pp. 703–707). Berlin/Wien: Urban and Schwarzcnberg.

Kemp, E. H. Waterman, E. A., & Weetman, A. P. (2001). Autoimmune aspects of vitiligo. *Autoimmunity, 34*(1), 65–77.

Kopera, D. (1997). Historical aspects and definition of vitiligo. *Clinics in Dermatology, 15*(6), 841–843.

Lang, K. S., et al. (2001). HLA-A2 restricted, melanocyte-specific CD8(+) T lymphocytes detected in vitiligo patients are related to disease activity and are predominantly directed against MelanA/MART1. *Journal of Investigative Dermatology, 116*(6), 891–897.

Millington, G. (2007). Vitiligo: the historical curse of depigmentation. *International Journal of Dermatology, 46*(9), 990–995.

Mosher, D. B., Parrish, J. A., & Fitzpatrick, T. B. (1977). Monobenzylether of hydroquinone. A retrospective study of treatment of 18 vitiligo patients and a review of the literature. *British Journal of Dermatology, 97*(6), 669–679.

Narahari, S. R., et al. (2011). Integrating modern dermatology and Ayurveda in the treatment of vitiligo and lymphedema in India. *International Journal of Dermatology, 50*(3), 310–334.

Nordlund, J. J., & Halder, R. (1990). Melagenina. An analysis of published and other available data. *Dermatologica, 181*(1), 1–4.

Ogg, G. S., et al. (1998). High frequency of skin-homing melanocyte-specific cytotoxic T lymphocytes in autoimmune vitiligo. *Journal of Experimental Medicine, 188*(6), 1203–1208.

Ongenae, K., Van Geel, N., & Naeyaert, J. (2003). Evidence for an autoimmune pathogenesis of vitiligo. *Pigment Cell Research 16*(2), 90–100.

Parsad, D., Pandhi, R., & Juneja, A. (2003). Effectiveness of oral *Ginkgo biloba* in treating limited, slowly spreading vitiligo. *Clinical & Experimental Dermatology, 28*(3), 285–287.

Passeron, T., & Ortonne, J. (2005). Physiopathology and genetics of vitiligo. *Journal of Autoimmunity, 25*(Suppl), 63–68.

Reyes, E., Jaén, P., de las Heras, E., et al. (2006). Systemic immunomodulatory effects of *Polypodium leucotomos* as an adjuvant to PUVA therapy in generalized vitiligo: a pilot study. *Journal of Dermatological Science, 41*, 213–216.

Rojas-Urdaneta, J. E., & Poleo-Romero, A. G. (2007). Evaluation of an antioxidant and mitochondria-stimulating cream formula on the skin of patients with stable common vitiligo [in Spanish]. *Investigacion Clinica, 48*, 21–31.

Schallreuter, K. U., et al. (1994a). Defective tetrahydrobiopterin and catecholamine biosynthesis in the depigmentation disorder vitiligo. *Biochimica et Biophysica Acta, 1226*(2), 181–192.

Schallreuter, K. U., et al. (2002). Rapid initiation of repigmentation in vitiligo with Dead Sea climatotherapy in combination with pseudocatalase (PC-KUS). *International Journal of Dermatology, 41*(8), 482–487.

Schallreuter, K. U., et al. (1994b). Regulation of melanin biosynthesis in the human epidermis by tetrahydrobiopterin. *Science, 263*(5152), 1444–1446.

Scherschun, L., Kim, J. J., & Lim, H. W. (2001). Narrow-band ultraviolet B is a useful and well-tolerated treatment for vitiligo. *Journal of the American Academy of Dermatology, 44*(6), 999–1003.

Seghal, V., & Srivastava, G. (2007). Vitiligo: compendium of clinico-epidemiological features. *Indian Journal of Dermatology, Venereology, Leprology, 73*(3), 149–156.

Siddigui, A. H., et al. (1994). L-phenylalanine and UVA irradiation in the treatment of vitiligo. *Dermatology, 188*(3), 215–218.

Spencer, J. D., et al. (2007). Oxidative stress via hydrogen peroxide affects proopiomelanocortin peptides directly in the epidermis of patients with vitiligo. *Journal of Investigative Dermatology, 127*(2), 411–420.

Sravani, P. V., et al. (2009). Determination of oxidative stress in vitiligo by measuring superoxide dismutase and catalase levels in vitiliginous and non-vitiliginous skin. *Indian Journal of Dermatology, Venereology, Leprology, 75*(3), 268–271.

Szczurko, O., & Boon, H. S. (2008). A systematic review of natural health product treatment for vitiligo. *BMC Dermatology, 8,* 2.

Szczurko, O., et al. (2011). *Ginkgo biloba* for the treatment of vitiligo vulgaris: an open label pilot clinical trial. *BMC Complementary & Alternative Medicine, 11,* 21.

Tahir, M. A., et al. (20). Current remedies for vitiligo. *Autoimmunity Review, 9*(7), 516–520.

Taieb, A. (2000). Intrinsic and extrinsic pathomechanisms in vitiligo. *Pigment Cell Research, 13*(Suppl 8), 41–47.

Teschke, R., & Bahre, R. (2009). Severe hepatotoxicity by Indian Ayurvedic herbal products: a structured causality assessment. *Annals of Hepatology, 8*(3), 258–266.

Tonsi, A. (2004). Vitiligo and its management update: a review. *Pakistan Journal of Medical Science, 20,* 242–247.

van den Boorn, J. G., et al. (2009). Autoimmune destruction of skin melanocytes by perilesional T cells from vitiligo patients. *Journal of Investigative Dermatology, 129*(9), 2220–2232.

van den Wiingaard, R. M., et al. (2000). Expression and modulation of apoptosis regulatory molecules in human melanocytes: significance in vitiligo. *British Journal of Dermatology, 143*(3), 573–581.

Westerhof, W., & Nieuweboer-Krobotova, L. (1997). Treatment of vitiligo with UV-B radiation vs topical psoralen plus UV-A. *Archives of Dermatology, 133*(12), 1525–1528.

Whitton, M. E., et al. (2010). Interventions for vitiligo. *Cochrane Database of Systematic Reviews,* 1.

Wolff, K., et al. (2007). *Fitzpatrick's dermatology in general medicine* (7th ed., pp. 616–621). New York: McGraw Hill.

Wolff, K., Johnson, R. A., & Suurmond, D. (2009). Section 13: Pigmentary disorders: Vitiligo. In K. Wolff et al., *Fitzpatrick's color atlas & synopsis of clinical dermatology* (6th ed.). New York: McGraw-Hill.

Wolff, K., et al. (2005). *Fitzpatrick's color atlas and synopsis of clinical dermatology.* New York: McGraw-Hill Medical Pub. Division.

Yaghoobi, R., Omidian, M., & Bagherani, N. (2011). Vitiligo: A review of published work. *Journal of Dermatology, 38,* 419–431.

Zhang, Z-J., Chen, J-J., & Lui, J-B. (2005). The genetic concept of vitiligo. *Journal of Dermatologic Science, 39,* 137–146.

Zhao, D., et al. (2008). Melagenine modulates proliferation and differentiation of melanoblasts. *International Journal of Molecular Medicine, 22*(2), 193–197.

30

The History, Research, Education, and Future of Integrative Dermatology

ALAN M. DATTNER

Key Concepts

- ♣ Integrative dermatology looks beyond Western diagnoses, using other healing perspectives, to seek the etiology and specific treatment for a patient's skin condition.
- ♣ Sensitization by food, microbial, and environmental antigens may direct cross-reactive attack against highly specific skin targets, causing inflammation there. Using this perspective in taking a history of the events preceding an outbreak, one can obtain valuable clues to the cause of an individual's skin inflammation.
- ♣ A number of resources within and outside the dermatology world already exist that are good entry points for this evolving field.
- ♣ The future of integrative dermatology rests on both the scientific breakthroughs in areas such as gut flora, immune recognition, and control of skin physiology and observations on how to find the most relevant healing system and treatment for a given individual and how to combine that with other therapies.

Introduction

Integrative dermatology is a recent term. It emerged from the term "integrative medicine," which is currently the most medically acceptable perspective and nomenclature for the incorporation of nonallopathic healing methods into current Western standard of care. Its origins go back not only to dermatology before the advent of "miracle drugs," but also to the very earliest use of plants and incantations for healing the skin. Before the acceleration of the development of modern medical therapeutics via science, herbs were one of the main forms of treatment (Dattner, 2003). Specific indications for choice of which herbs to use were championed by groups like the "eclectics" in the early 1900s (Winston & Dattner, 1999). This chapter will focus on more recent forms of integrative skin care since the advent of the specialty of dermatology.

Definition

Integrative dermatology is as much a philosophy as it is a method; it looks to reverse causal factors rather than just stop symptoms. The truest nature of integrative dermatology is to approach the patient with an all-encompassing and more diverse worldview than is available or offered in modern Western practice. Grappling with the central generative principle behind a chronic skin disorder could yield better results than treating according to the diagnosis, or worse, merely endeavoring to suppress or control the presenting symptoms. Many healing philosophies, including Western herbalism, consider the skin to be an organ of elimination and, as such, view skin disorders as the result of improper accumulation of toxins from food or environment, in concert with faulty function of eliminative organs such as the kidneys and liver. Some healing systems would consider acne to be a symptom of an underlying condition rather than as a primary "diagnosis."

Just as a different operating system on our phones or computers may simplify a previously complex operation into a one-step process, a modified and holistic philosophical approach to healing could greatly simplify the understanding of how to alleviate a patient's skin disease. Although much of this chapter focuses on the use of various remedies that are not central to current practice, it is important to consider and incorporate different perspectives from various healing systems just as we might consult with different specialists according to the organ system involved.

Evolution of Modern Medicine and Dermatology

The development of vaccination, followed by sulfonamides and then antibiotics in the mid-1900s, dramatically changed our ability to control infectious diseases of the skin such as staph and smallpox. Soon it was discovered that antibiotics could control acne without the need for painful and difficult dietary restrictions. Inflammatory disorders, no matter what their cause, were calmed by corticosteroids, while a succession of more potent anti-inflammatories with higher specificity have enabled control of diseases that previously defied treatment. Application of statistics, controlled methodology and double-blind studies, coupled with basic research to validate underlying mechanisms of a therapy, became the gold standard for evaluation of not only these but any form of treatment.

A deeper understanding of the pathophysiology of various diseases advanced the concept of a disease to that of an actual entity. The public as well as physicians and insurance companies began thinking of diseases as specific entities with exact treatments that at least controlled the symptoms, and sometimes induced remission. This perspective differs from that of other healing systems such as Chinese medicine, Ayurveda, and homeopathy, which view patients as reaching the phenotypic presentation we call a disease by very individualized paths.

History of Integrative Dermatology

Integrative medicine was initially known as holistic medicine, alternative or complementary medicine, and then complementary and alternative medicine (CAM). Dermatology followed the same path as unproven remedies from other healing systems were found to help control skin disorders. In the United States, dietary restrictions and supplementation, along with "cleansing" and vitamins, were the first approaches used in this new dermatology practice. The evolution of diet and specific nutritional biochemical supplementation to augment organ function that was inadequate but did not present with anatomical or biochemical abnormalities, such as insufficient hepatic ability to biotransform and eliminate specific drugs (i.e., griseofulvin toxicity), was termed "functional medicine" by Jeffry Bland, PhD, one of the founders of this approach (Jones & Bland, 2010).

Integrative dermatology/medicine is a more useful and acceptable term because it encompasses the coordination and inclusion of other methodologies with traditional or conventional dermatology/medicine. Although specific distinctions apply, integrative dermatology emerged from alternative, complementary, herbal, nutritional, holistic, and psychological dermatology.

Many aspects of integrative medicine reflect cyclical trends in both science and dermatology. The use of herbs came, went, and returned. Eliminating dairy to treat acne was a key component of acne treatment regimens for a significant fraction of the older dermatologists who taught during the 1970s. The use of bioflavonoids for their protective effects on the skin was championed by the Nobel Prize-winning Albert Szent-Gyorgyi at a New York Academy of Science meeting and in a compendium published in 1955 (Szent-Gyorgyi, 1955). Naturopaths and herbalists used these plant-derived substances as food and supplements long before the recent upsurge in interest in free radical binding anti-aging compounds.

Silymarin, a bioflavonoid from milk thistle, had been available for treating liver toxicity for mushroom poisoning. Dr. Haines Ely discussed its use for liver damage associated with skin disease at "What's New" at an American Academy of Dermatology (AAD) meeting. By the 1990s, there were 500 articles describing its use on PubMed before dermatologists began discussing it on RxDerm, an Internet forum hosted by Art Huntly.

HISTORICAL CONTRIBUTION OF MOLECULAR RESEARCH TO AN INTEGRATIVE UNDERSTANDING

Research on the specificity of immune recognition has given an understanding of the unique HLA-associated specificity of lymphocytic cellular immune attack (Shaw et al., 1978). This primed sensitization in one part of the body could lead to attack against a specific disease-associated biochemical site on the skin (or anywhere else) and accounts for the reason a food, chemical, or microbe might provoke inflammation in one individual and not in another with the same disease. The antigenic hapten stimulating a response is recognized in conjunction with the HLA antigens of the presenting leukocytes, creating a unique spectrum of specificity (Dattner et al., 1979). Thus, there is a unique but limited biochemical spectrum of specific targets on the skin that could be attacked in a cross-reactive manner (molecular mimicry). The possibility that chemicals, microbial products, or food-derived molecules could escape intact and act as either stimulators or targets for specific immune attack, as well as differ among individuals, becomes much more plausible (Walker & Isselbacher, 1974).

Along with understanding how molecular mimicry provides a way to search a patient's history for exposures precipitating skin disease, a number of other discoveries over the past decades have expanded therapeutic understanding and tools to heal the skin. Prostaglandin activity's effect on increasing or calming inflammation and the role of gamma linoleic (omega-6) (Senapati et al., 2008) and omega-3 unsaturated fatty acids from dietary oils provided nutritional tools to assuage some conditions. Antioxidants, primarily from plants, have been shown to slow some aging processes and are being incorporated into numerous cosmeceutical products. Improved understanding of yeasts like *Malasezzia* and the role of probiotics (Kalliomaki et al., 2001) is bringing dermatology closer to recognizing the relationship between the "yeast syndrome" and skin disease. Cross-reaction between *Malasezzia* in the skin and *Candida* (Huang et al., 1995) and dietary yeast byproducts in the gut may be one of the reasons why administration of probiotics and reduction of yeast exposure calms many forms of inflammation in the skin.

Our current models of inflammatory disease development take into account genetic variation of antigen-presenting transplantation antigens and enzyme variations such those used in chemical biotransformation. Combined with the responses and epigenetic changes induced by food, chemical, and microbial exposure and environmental shifts in cellular and organ function at every level, the possibility emerges that individuals have very different paths to developing a given skin disorder. Integrative dermatology explores different perspectives on an individual's path to a specific skin condition and attempts to clear it by reversing the conditions that led to it. Treatment intended only to suppress symptoms is used far less than in conventional dermatology.

Education

If dermatologists are to integrate other treatment modalities, training in these methods and/or developing a trustworthy network of alternative providers for referrals is critical. Acupuncture, for example, has come to be accepted as a "black box" of diagnostic modalities and treatments that clearly help some people after other methods fail. With techniques such as pulse diagnosis, in addition to skill, knowledge, sensitivity, and experience, there is a kind of intuitive summation leading to diagnostic information. Becoming comfortable with these techniques, and knowing whom/when/where to refer, may take years of practice and trial and error.

Dermatologists and residents interested in integrative dermatology would benefit first from developing a broad understanding of integrative medicine, and then proficiency in at least one other healing discipline.

Dermatology Committees and Conference Presentations

In 1997, the AAD created a task force on nutrition and the evaluation of alternative medicine. The main objective was to develop presentations for the AAD meeting in 1998 on nutrition and alternative medicine in dermatology. This task force was ultimately dissolved, but in 2013 a new AAD work group on CAM was established to explore integrative modalities in both medical and cosmetic dermatology.

Over the past 14 years there have been a number of other forums and short presentations on herbs, antioxidants, cosmeceuticals, *Pityrosporum*, nutrition, Chinese medicine, and emotional factors in skin disease at the AAD. All of these, given the right perspective, are components of a model of integrative dermatology. Dr. Bill Danby spoke about the relationship between milk and acne and the hormonal mechanisms thought to be involved. Dr. Ely was an early pioneer in using both herbs and drugs in novel ways based on scientific understanding of the underlying mechanisms in skin disease. He presented his observations at the AAD and the Massachusetts Academy of Dermatology, and wrote about them in the publication *Dermatologic Therapy* (Ely, 1989). Other presentations relevant to integrative dermatology have included Jan Faegermann on *Pityrosporum* yeasts and Stephen Wright on evening primrose oil.

Other Boards and Integrative Training Opportunities

Various groups and conferences around the country hold meetings that often include topics related to integrative dermatology. Examples of recent events include:

- The American Board of Holistic Medicine was founded in 1996; it officially changed its name to the American Board of Integrative Holistic Medicine in 2008.
- The Institute for Functional Medicine (http://www.functional-medicine.org/) offers a program of weekend and weeklong modules throughout the year on a variety of topics bridging the naturopathic and integrative approaches in shifting organ and cellular function to calm disease. They continuously mine the scientific literature for studies regarding biochemical and nutritional supplementation of the digestive, immune, and eliminative systems.
- Various supplement companies hold seminars and speakers who discuss the use of their supplement formulations as well as a functional overview of various disorders or systems. These forums may be good opportunities for learning and networking with other practitioners with similar perspectives.
- The American College for Advancement in Medicine (ACAM) holds biannual meetings focused on various topics. Their November 2009 meeting "Autoimmune Diseases: 21st-Century Approaches" provided a clinically useful and fairly well-documented understanding of the

reasons for and the methods for diagnosing and treating the pathology underlying the rising tide of allergic and autoimmune disorders.

- The University of Arizona in Tucson offers a two-year distance learning fellowship in Integrative Medicine for physicians in practice that is open to generalists as well as specialists. There is a licensing board exam under development as well.
- Working with a skilled practitioner in another healing discipline, and experiencing irrefutable improvements in yourself or a patient that are confirmed by laboratory data, is another way to become more receptive to healing methods that are generally regarded as quackery by mainstream medical professionals.

Historical Meetings

At the 2013 AAD meeting in Miami, there was a forum on integrative dermatology that gave a broad overview of the topic and defined key terminology.

In September of 2012, **Advances in Integrative Dermatology** was presented at the 100th Anniversary of the Brazilian Dermatology Society Rio de Janeiro, Brazil (Norman, 2012).

On December 5, 2011, the First International Congress on Integrative and Holistic Dermatology was held at Manipal University in India. Also in December 2011, the 5th National Symposium on Evidence-Based and Integrative Medicine for Lymphatic Filariasis and Chronic Dermatoses occurred at the Institute for Applied Dermatology, Kasaragod, India (Dattner, 2011).

The World Congress of Dermatology in Buenos Aires in 2007 held a session on alternative (nonconventional) therapy in dermatology (Dattner, 2006). There was a session on antioxidants and one on probiotics and skin.

The International Academy of Cosmetic Dermatology in Paris in 2005 had a session on nutrition and the skin (Dattner, 2005).

In 2000, the University of New Mexico sponsored "Integrative Medicine and the Skin 2000" in Santa Fe (Dattner, 2000). It was the first and only such conference in the United States to this author's knowledge.

Selected Published Resources

The chapter in *Fitzpatrick's Dermatology in General Medicine* on "Complementary and Alternative Medicine in Dermatology" offers an introduction to the field and a discussion of the treatment of common and uncommon dermatoses (Dattner, 2012).

Rakel's *Integrative Medicine* (3rd ed.) contains several chapters devoted to dermatologic disorders (Dattner, 1997). A complete issue on alternative medicine and dermatology was published in the *Archives of Dermatology* in November 1998.

Evidence-based medicine emerged as a way of legitimatizing observations of treatments that did not seem to make sense in terms of the science of the time. Homeopathy, with dilutions beyond Avogadro's number, makes little sense in terms of Newtonian physics but begins to sound valid with higher physics (Shapiro & Shear, 2002). We ultimately have to apply the lens of scientific thinking to our studies, but not necessarily at first evaluation.

Numerous studies support the use of plants and their constituents in correcting digestive, eliminative, physiological, and immunological abnormalities leading to skin disorders. Much less is written, and far less is proven, regarding philosophical issues of integrative medicine such as vitalism and the force of nature as it pertains to healing. A look at the medical research literature will reveal that savvy scientists are applying insights from a wide variety of alternative disciplines to both the clinical and mechanistic understanding of pathophysiology related to the skin.

A functional medicine approach to integrative dermatology includes fostering elimination of potentially toxic and reactive compounds out of the body. These compounds can bind to skin molecules or interfere with enzymatic and other processes in the skin and elsewhere. That removal is a major role of the liver, which via the p450 enzymes (Ivanov et al., 2009) makes these compounds more soluble or more reactive to bind to a carrier molecule such as a glucuronide or glutathione in phase II liver detoxification. If this process is slow, or if there are not enough of the required carriers, the toxic molecule, being now even more reactive than before, can bind elsewhere in the skin or body and cause havoc, interfering with enzymatic and physiological processes or modifying self to create neoantigens. Silymarin, the active ingredient in *Silybum marianum* (milk thistle), actually slows p450 3A4, preventing generation of more active molecules. Further, a number of studies from India show that traditional foods such as chutneys also enhance phase II liver detoxification. This is just one example of what may be considered integrative dermatology research.

The Future

Approach is key to the concept of integrative medicine. Which patient receives which treatment and how that treatment is administered are as important as the treatment itself. Herbs, antioxidants, diet, supplements and the like are appearing more and more in the literature and marketplace.

Integrative dermatology promises to enrich the diagnosis and treatment of skin diseases by vastly expanding the models we use to explore and interpret the factors creating and perpetuating a skin disorder. Diet, long neglected as a constant in dermatologic studies, is emerging as an important contributor to skin disease. P450 hepatic degradation enzymes are regulated by foods like grapefruit. Viruses, bacteria, and yeast affect the permeability of the intestinal barrier to food and microbial antigens. Food affects bacterial species' growth selection, which in turn regulates the degree of autoreactivity (Ivanov et al., 2009). Sugar influences AGE (advanced glycosylation end product) formation, insulin sensitivity, microbial populations, and IGF-1 levels. Toxic chemicals and minerals in the diet accumulate and poison various enzyme systems, altering immune response or depleting the ability of those enzymes to perform eliminative and other functions. The supply of cofactors such as vitamins, minerals, or specific biochemicals in the form of food or concentrates offers the possibility of enhancing impaired enzyme function and restoring normal cellular and organ function to correct underlying causes of skin disease.

Asking clinical research questions with the additional perspective of both functional medicine and basic immunology allows much greater depth and improves the odds of getting to the cause of inflammatory skin disorders. For example, early studies showed that breastfeeding, as reflected in the recommendations of many European countries, has protective effects against atopy in infants. Later, larger studies showed that it does not protect, except in the more severe cases (Flohr et al., 2011). The possibility exists that there has actually been a shift in this protective effect, but some experts prefer to deny previous common public impressions and early studies regarding such protection.

From an integrative dermatology perspective, the more relevant question is this: How can breastfeeding protect against childhood atopy? We know that the infant gut is more permeable to food antigens and becomes less so with age. What is less obvious is that there has been a shift toward increased permeability of the maternal intestinal wall with time, possibly paralleling the increase of sugar in the diet as well as antibiotic, steroid, and birth-control pill use. A series of papers from Isolauri's group (Rautava et al., 2012) showed a host of ways in which probiotics fed to mother or infant reduced the incidence of atopy in the infants. Less clear is the implied hypothesis that overgrowth of yeast inflames and disrupts the intestinal barrier.

Potential study design here is complicated by other factors: the infant gut is also hyperpermeable to food antigen, and this permeability is improving with time and worsening with inflammation. The development of sensitivity and tolerance to food antigens in the infant gut is also likely to be dependent on timing, dose, and informational factors such as cytokines from the maternal gut. From classical immunology, one would expect that the dose of antigen inducing tolerance would be a U-shaped curve, with both very low and very high doses inducing a degree of tolerance, and increased sensitization occurring in the middle. The way to explore the potential pertinent variables is to observe mothers whose infants' gastrointestinal distress and atopic symptoms vary according to what the breastfeeding mother eats. Future research regarding breastfeeding in atopy will have to ask immunological and functional medicine questions about the timing and dosage of food, immune signals, and antigen leakage through both the maternal and infant gut. Along with an understanding of the immunology and the role of the gut microbiome, more complete and actionable information will emerge.

The integrative approach begs to include and also surpass the reductionist tendency to search for the single factor or mechanism involved in the increased prevalence of disorders such as atopic dermatitis. A wider context might include immunophysiological confusion and self-reactivity due to system overload of the affected individual. This is likely from distress, the 80,000 legal chemicals in our environment, electromagnetic pollution, and excesses and deficiencies in our so-called "normal" diet. When molecular and cellular immunology is applied to questions from this wider view, we will have a better understanding of causes and how to address or eliminate them.

With 60 to 1,000 different species in the roughly 100 trillion organisms in the human gut, it is folly to believe that we will ever have the kind of scientific proof we imagined possible with the double-blind studies of old, while controlling *all* of the relevant variables. Diet can affect flora (Turnbaugh et al., 2009), and certain flora, like segmented filamentous bacteria, can favor TH17 cells and the development of autoimmune diseases (Ivanov et al., 2009). Molecular cross-reactivity between gut-derived antigens and targets in the skin is a likely cause of skin inflammation. Digestive function adequacy and intestinal barrier integrity determine which food and microbe molecules leak out of the gut into the blood and Peyer's patches. Variations in histocompatibility antigens, which present these molecules for recognition, make each individual's skin sensitivity unique. That accounts for why it has been impossible to assign specific food aggravators to specific skin diseases.

Just as the dermatologist learns science and practices the art of medicine, integrative dermatology can lend a much wider perspective to the art of understanding the etiology of skin disorders, as well as evaluating and treating them.

It is clear that the future is now, and there is a steady commercialization and incorporation of effective remedies into dermatologic practice. Integration of natural substances and other methods that are not quite ready for prime time is inevitable in dermatology. The development by cosmetic companies and nutrition companies of a whole range of skin products that are biologically active but not tested or approved by the U.S. Food and Drug Administration ("cosmeceuticals" and "nutraceuticals") over the past two decades is ample proof that people want and will use these to attempt to improve their skin beyond what their dermatologist suggests. The bigger question is whether a wider group of dermatologists will use these techniques and products, and which additional health philosophy they will employ to most effectively choose how and when to use them in a given patient.

Integrative dermatology considers the multiple constituents of herb formulations, and that is often lost in the pharmaceutical philosophy that emphasizes a single active constituent for a specific symptom or disease. Often the characteristics of the whole extract are referred to as the "energetics" of the herb—how they warm or cool, moisten or dry different organs, and thus how they might best work for or aggravate according to the corresponding state of the organs of that individual.

Another trend in integrative dermatology is to seek safer ingredients and delivery system components in topical formulations. Incorporation of protective herbal products such as green tea and bioflavonoids, and of ceramides to replace those not produced by eczematous skin, is already an ongoing trend. Removal of potentially allergenic or toxic preservatives is part of the design of new lines of natural and organic cosmetics and topical formulations.

Medical centers with both conventional and integrative medicine departments in communication with one another and with basic scientists will have the best chance of forging new integrative treatments for skin disease. The dermatology department in Manipal communicates with the Ayurvedic department and the yoga department, but this mutual respect is only beginning in India. We have looked to the universities to conduct research and companies to produce products. Ultimately, we need to equip astute clinicians with the ability to collaborate with basic scientists in laboratories to elucidate the likely interactive relationships they are observing and experiencing.

Integrative dermatology includes flexible use of nutritional biochemicals, vitamins, cofactors, as well as other substances that influence enzymatic reactions in the body. It enables the correction of some enzymatic defects due to SNPs, infections, or drugs in an individual-specific manner. For example, 13-cis retinoic acid is known to affect over 200 different enzyme systems in the body. For those adversely affected by this drug, we need a much broader therapeutic tool kit than that available in the pharmacy. Integrative dermatology brings a broad access to relevant cofactors and substrates for the enzymatic processes involved.

Contact dermatitis has always been an area in which dermatologists practice environmental medicine. Understanding occupational, consumer, and industrial chemistry is important for identifying the sources of contact allergy. Environmental medicine is crucial to the integrative medicine world for finding the cause of various sensitivities, chronic toxicity, and autoimmune disorders. There has been a trend of not only incorporating more chemicals into foods and toiletries, but also, in many cases, a trend to make it harder to identify these ingredients on the label. Bucking this trend of more chemicals and less government oversight has been a push by major personal care product companies to hire integrative-minded dermatologists to advise them on various issues. An integrative approach to skin disease at the highest level means identifying broad social trends that lead to more skin disease, and speaking out to warn consumers, legislators, and manufacturers and to help industry to produce safer products.

Integrative dermatologists of the future will need to list their clinical, alternative, and basic science skills so that they are accessible and can be easily found by both other physicians and people in need of their help. For pharmaceutical companies, integrative dermatologists will lead the development of methods to help spot those people who are potentially at risk with specific drugs, help combine natural products to prevent side effects, and help rescue those patients who have side effects from one or a series of drugs. These actions could avoid untold morbidity, reduce support costs for those returned to productive lives, reduce lawsuit damages, and even prevent certain drugs from being removed from the market if the rare but onerous side effects can be predicted, avoided, prevented, or remedied. Some financial saving is available to insurance companies who can avoid paying for expensive medications. The savings to the economy could justify allowing adequate compensation for integrative dermatologists who need to spend vastly larger amounts of time with patients with chronic skin diseases, eliciting information, investigating basic science and integrative approaches, and treating, reeducating, and coaxing patients to make lifestyle changes to control their skin and underlying issues.

The AAD has made it a point to participate in public health programs for the greater good. Sun protection, skin cancer warnings and screenings, legislation against tanning for minors, and camps for those with serious skin disease are just some of the public health efforts it has taken on. As there is a direct correlation between harmful chemicals in our environment and what enters our skin and bodies, there is room for dermatologists, as the world experts on the skin, to collectively take a stand on reducing harmful chemicals in our environment that accumulate in and/or otherwise harm the skin. With much of the world represented at AAD meetings, integrative dermatology has the opportunity to explore a systems approach to aiding industry in shifting to less toxic products and processes for the benefit of the skin of our species.

A century ago, pharmaceutical companies packaged herbs for patient use. Over time this morphed into the targeting of disease mechanisms with increasingly specific inhibitors of the disease process. In dermatology, this has often meant inhibiting the last phase of symptomatic inflammatory processes with everything from corticosteroids to biologics. While this approach has given dermatologists tools to provide great relief from suffering and saving lives, it also has come with many unintended adverse effects. In an integrative dermatology model, forward-thinking pharmaceutical companies could also apply their vast resources to help dermatologists unearth the network of underlying factors contributing to an individual patient's inflammatory skin disorders. This would create a team approach to controlling chronic inflammatory skin disorders with additional systemic benefits rather than side effects, and return patients from the purely alternative treatment arena to a more effective integrative dermatology treatment model.

Integrative dermatologists versed in at least one additional healing modality, with a background in functional medicine and an understanding of other methods, will make observations to populate the information space between conventional dermatology practice and their modality of choice. If they also have a basic science background, it will be easier to answer questions about the fundamental changes that are occurring. Together with allies in the nutritional, supplement, and forward-thinking pharmaceutical industry and with the perspective of other healing systems, new paradigms will emerge for understanding and reversing the causes of skin disorders that have challenged dermatologists and their patients.

REFERENCES

Dattner, A. M. (1997). Immunologic studies support homeopathic medicine. *Archives of Dermatology, 133*(2), 244–245.

Dattner, A. M. (2000). How I integrate nutrition and alternative medicine into my practice: 21 years of "holistic" dermatology. *Integrative Medicine and the Skin,* Santa Fe, NM.

Dattner, A. M. (2002). Seborrheic dermatitis. In D. Rakel (Ed.), *Integrative medicine* (p. 491). Philadelphia: Saunders.

Dattner, A. M. (2003). From medical herbalism to phytotherapy in dermatology: Back to the future. *Dermatologic Therapy, 16,* 106.

Dattner, A. M. (2005). Nutritional anti-inflammatory strategies for anti-aging of the skin. Presented at Nutrition and Anti-aging. IV World Congress of the International Academy of Cosmetic Dermatology, July 2 to 5, 2005, Paris, France.

Dattner, A. M. (2006). The IVth International Academy of Cosmetic Dermatology Congress—a holistic perspective. *Journal of Cosmetic Dermatology, 5*(2), 178–180.

Dattner, A. M. (2011). A holistic model for integrating nutritional and energy treatments into the care of inflammatory skin disorders. Presented at 5th National Symposium on Evidence-Based and Integrative Medicine for Lymphatic Filariasis and Chronic Dermatoses, Institute for Applied Dermatology, Kasaragod, India, Dec. 3, 2011.

Dattner, A. M. (2012). Complementary and alternative medicine in dermatology. In L. A. Goldsmith, S. I. Katz, B. A. Gilchrest, et al. (Eds), *Fitzpatrick's dermatology in general medicine* (8th ed., pp. 2899–2904). New York: McGraw Hill.

Dattner, A. M., Mann, D. L., & Levis, W. R. (1979). Studies on the contact sensitization of man with simple chemicals: V. Clonal priming allows direct in vitro assessment of autologous HLA-associated factors required for immune response to dinitro-chlorobenzene. *Journal of Investigative Dermatology, 73*(3), 246–249.

Ely, H. (1989). Therapies you've probably never heard of. *Dermatologic Clinics, 7*(1), 19–35.

Flohr, C., Nagel, G., Weinmayr, G., et al. (2011). Lack of evidence for a protective effect of prolonged breastfeeding on childhood eczema: lessons from the International Study of Asthma and Allergies in Childhood. *Journal of Dermatology, 165*(6), 1280–1289.

Huang, X., et al. (1995). Allergen cross-reactivity between *Pityrosporum orbiculare* and *Candida albicans*. *Allergy, 50,* 50:648.

Ivanov, I. I., Atarashi, K., Littman, D. R., et al. (2009). Induction of intestinal Th17 cells by segmented filamentous bacteria cell. *Cell, 139*(3), 485–498.

Jones, D. S., & Bland, J. S. (2010). What is functional medicine? In S. M. Baker, P. Bennett, & J. S. Bland (Eds.), *Textbook of functional medicine.* Institute for Functional Medicine.

Kalliomaki, M., et al. (2001). Probiotics in primary prevention of atopic disease: A randomized placebo-controlled trial. *Lancet, 357,* 1076.

Rautava, S., Kainonen, E., Salminen, S., et al. (2012). Maternal probiotic supplementation during pregnancy and breast-feeding reduces the risk of eczema in the infant. *Journal of Allergy & Clinical Immunology* [E-pub before print, Oct. 16].

Senapati, S., Banerjee, S., & Gangopadhyay, D. N. (2008). Evening primrose oil is effective in atopic dermatitis: a randomized placebo-controlled trial. *Indian Journal of Dermatology, Venereology, Leprology, 74*(5), 447–452.

Shapiro, L. E., & Shear, N. H. (2002). Drug interactions: Proteins, pumps, and P-450s. *Journal of the American Academy of Dermatology, 47*(4): 467–484.

Shaw, S., Levis, W. R., Dattner, A. M., et al. (1978). Specificity of human cytotoxic responses to chemically modified autologous cells. *Transplant Proceedings, 10*(4), 937–941.

Szent-Györgyi, A. (1955). Perspectives for the bioflavanoids. In: *Annals of the New York Academy of Sciences. Bioflavonoids and the Capillary, 61,* 732–735.

Turnbaugh, P. J., Ridaura, V. K., Faith, J. J., et al. (2009). The effect of diet on the human gut microbiome: a metagenomic analysis in humanized gnotobiotic mice. *Science Translational Medicine, 1*(6), 6–14.

Walker, W. A., & Isselbacher, K. J. (1974). Uptake and transport of macromolecules by the intestine. Possible role in clinical disorders. *Gastroenterology, 67*(3), 531–550.

Winston, D., & Dattner A. M. (1999). The American system of medicine. *Clinics in Dermatology, 17,* 53.

INDEX

Wholistic Hybrid, 215
wild milky oats, for pruritus, 368
willow bark
    for postherpetic neuralgia (PHN),
        360–361
    salicylate in, 149
Wilson, J.W., 298*t*
wintergreen, salicylate in, 149
witch hazel
    for acne, 127
    for CVI, 132
    for dermatitis, 136
    for neuropathic and psychogenic
        neurodermatitis, 351
    for pruritus, 368
    for rosacea, 404
Wolf, J., 195
wolf's bane. *See* arnica *(Arnica montana)*
woodruff, coumadin in, 149
Wood's lamp examination, 475
World Congress of Dermatology, 492
wounds and burns
    aloe vera for, 67, 147–148
    chamomile for, 81
    Chinese rhubarb for, 149
    goldenrod for, 149
    herbal medicines for, 147–149
    honey for, 148
    Labrador tea for, 149
    lavender *(Lavendula spp.)* for, 149
    magnesium lactate for, 148
    marigold for, 148–149
    mullein for, 149
    oak bark for, 149
    psychoneuroimmunology for, 96–98
    rhatany for, 149
    St. John's wort for, 149
    tannins for, 149

yellow dock for, 149
Wright, S., 491

Xiaobai, for vitiligo, 480
Xu, X.J., 137
Xuehai, 114
xylocaine patches, for postherpetic neu-
    ralgia (PHN), 357

Yang, R., 442
yellow dock
    for dermatitis, 136
    for wounds and burns, 149
Yeong, Y.S., 215–216
yin and yang, 111
Ying system, 441
yoga, 185, 335
yohimbe, as hypertension inducer, 150
Yokota, T., 78
Yoon, S., 68

Zachariae, R., 445
Zawahry, M.E., 418
zeaxanthin, 25
Zemophyte, 113–114, 135, 265, 265*b*
Zhao, Y., 441
Zhong, J., 446
Zimmerman, J., 218
zinc
    about, 20, 30–31
    for acne, 227
    for psoriasis, 377
Zostavax, 356, 362
Zostrix, for postherpetic neuralgia
    (PHN), 357
Zovirax (acyclovir), for postherpetic neu-
    ralgia (PHN), 361–362
Zuberbier, T., 443

DATE DUE

210018	
	PRINTED IN U.S.A.